Ototoxicity: Basic Science and Clinical Applications

Ototoxicity: Basic Science and Clinical Applications

Edited by Niklaus Richards

STATES
ACADEMIC PRESS
www.statesacademicpress.com

States Academic Press,
109 South 5th Street,
Brooklyn, NY 11249, USA

Visit us on the World Wide Web at:
www.statesacademicpress.com

ISBN: 978-1-63989-401-7

Cataloging-in-Publication Data

Ototoxicity : basic science and clinical applications / edited by Niklaus Richards.
p. cm.
Includes bibliographical references and index.
ISBN 978-1-63989-401-7
1. Ototoxic agents. 2. Ear--Effect of drugs on. 3. Drugs--Side effects.
4. Ear--Diseases--Chemotherapy. I. Richards, Niklaus.
RF285.O83 O86 2022
617.806 1--dc23

Table of Contents

Preface

Over the recent decade, advancements and applications have progressed exponentially. This has led to the increased interest in this field and projects are being conducted to enhance knowledge. The main objective of this book is to present some of the critical challenges and provide insights into possible solutions. This book will answer the varied questions that arise in the field and also provide an increased scope for furthering studies.

The property of being toxic to the ear, especially, to the auditory nerve or cochlea and the vestibular system, is termed as ototoxicity. The effects of toxicity can be permanent and irreversible or temporary and reversible. There are many drugs used in clinical situations that are ototoxic and are prescribed for very serious health conditions despite the risk of hearing disorders. A few of these drugs are antibiotics such as tobramycin, streptomycin, gentamicin, platinum-based chemotherapy agents such as carboplatin and cisplatin and loop diuretics such as furosemide. Several nonsteroidal anti-inflammatory drugs have also been found to be ototoxic. This may result in dysequilibrium, sensorineural hearing loss, or both. This book traces the progress of this field and highlights some of its key concepts. It will also provide interesting topics for research which interested readers can take up. This book will prove to be immensely beneficial to students and researchers in this field.

I hope that this book, with its visionary approach, will be a valuable addition and will promote interest among readers. Each of the authors has provided their extraordinary competence in their specific fields by providing different perspectives as they come from diverse nations and regions. I thank them for their contributions.

Editor

1

Inhibition of Mitochondrial Division Attenuates Cisplatin-Induced Toxicity in the Neuromast Hair Cells

Jonathon W. Vargo[1]*, Steven N. Walker*[1]*, Suhasini R. Gopal*[1]*, Aditi R. Deshmukh*[1]*, Brian M. McDermott Jr.*[1,2,3,4]*, Kumar N. Alagramam*[1,3,4] *and Ruben Stepanyan*[1,3]*

[1]Department of Otolaryngology—Head and Neck Surgery, University Hospitals Cleveland Medical Center, Cleveland, OH, United States, [2]Department of Biology, Case Western Reserve University, Cleveland, OH, United States, [3]Department of Neurosciences, Case Western Reserve University, Cleveland, OH, United States, [4]Department of Genetics and Genome Sciences, Case Western Reserve University, Cleveland, OH, United States

Edited by:
Lisa Cunningham,
National Institutes of Health (NIH),
United States

Reviewed by:
Leonard Rybak,
Southern Illinois University School of Medicine, United States
Jing Wang,
INSERM Délégation Languedoc-Roussillon, France

***Correspondence:**
Ruben Stepanyan
rxs690@case.edu

Cisplatin and other related platinum antineoplastic drugs are commonly used in the treatment of a variety of cancers in both adults and children but are often associated with severe side effects, including hearing loss. Cisplatin's ototoxic effects are multifaceted, culminating in irreversible damage to the mechanosensory hair cells in the inner ear. Platinum drugs act on cancerous cells by forming nuclear DNA adducts, which may initiate signaling leading to cell cycle arrest or apoptosis. Moreover, it was reported that cisplatin may induce mitochondrial DNA damage in non-cancerous cells. Therefore, protecting mitochondria may alleviate cisplatin-induced insult to non-proliferating cells. Thus, it is important to identify agents that shield the mitochondria from cisplatin-induced insult without compromising the anti-tumor actions of the platinum-based drugs. In this study we tested the protective properties of mitochondrial division inhibitor, mdivi-1, a derivative of quinazolinone and a regulator of mitochondrial fission. Interestingly, it has been reported that mdivi-1 increases the apoptosis of cells that are resistant to cisplatin. The ability of mdivi-1 to protect hair cells against cisplatin-induced toxicity was evaluated in a fish model. Wild-type (Tübingen strain), *cdh23* mutant, and transgenic *pvalb3b*::GFP zebrafish stably expressing GFP in the hair cells were used in this study. Larvae at 5–6 days post fertilization were placed in varying concentrations of cisplatin (50–200 μM) and/or mdivi-1 (1–10 μM) for 16 h. To evaluate hair cell's viability the number of hair bundles per neuromast were counted. To assess hair cell function, we used the FM1-43 uptake assay and recordings of neuromast microphonic potentials. The results showed that mdivi-1 protected hair cells of lateral line neuromasts when they were challenged by 50 μM of cisplatin: viability of hair cells increased almost twice from 19% ± 1.8% to 36% ± 2.0% ($p < 0.001$). No protection was observed when higher concentrations of cisplatin were used. In addition, our data were in accord with previously reported results that functional mechanotransduction strongly potentiates cisplatin-induced hair cell toxicity. Together, our results suggest that mitochondrial protection may prevent cisplatin-induced damage to hair cells.

Keywords: cisplatin, mdivi-1, hair cells, zebrafish, mechanotransduction, mitochondria

INTRODUCTION

Cisplatin and other related platinum drugs are common antineoplastic agents that are used in the treatment of a variety of cancers in both adults and children (for a review see Jamieson and Lippard, 1999). However, these drugs are associated with various side effects including nephrotoxicity and ototoxicity (for review see Rybak et al., 2009; Schacht et al., 2012; Karasawa and Steyger, 2015; Francis and Cunningham, 2017). Although nephrotoxicity can be managed to some extent (Cornelison and Reed, 1993; Wong and Giandomenico, 1999), mitigating ototoxicity in patients treated with cisplatin remains an unmet medical need (Brock et al., 2012; Schacht et al., 2012; Karasawa and Steyger, 2015). The platinum drugs act on cancerous cells mainly by forming adducts within the DNA (Huang et al., 1995; Jamieson and Lippard, 1999) and, possibly, by increasing reactive oxygen species (ROS) levels (Kopke et al., 1997; Rybak et al., 1999; Devarajan et al., 2002). In addition, cisplatin leads to cytotoxicity in normal cells that are not actively proliferating, inducing mitochondrial DNA damage and ROS elevation (Marullo et al., 2013; Wisnovsky et al., 2013).

Platinum-based antineoplastics irreversibly damage the cochlear hair cells starting in the basal turn—the outer hair cells appear to be more susceptible to this class of drug than other cell types in the cochlear duct, including the inner hair cells (Hinojosa et al., 1995; Li et al., 2004; Rybak et al., 2007). However, cisplatin-induced insult could extend beyond the hair cells and damage cells of the *stria vascularis*, a critical organ within the cochlea that is essential for maintaining the endocochlear potential and function of the cochlea (Laurell and Engstrom, 1989; Laurell et al., 2007). Although, damage to mostly outer hair cells is observed when low doses of cisplatin are used in rodents (Laurell and Engstrom, 1989; Cardinaal et al., 2000; Laurell et al., 2000; Park et al., 2002).

Routes of cisplatin entry into the hair cell could include the organic cation transporter Oct2 or the influx copper transporter Ctrl (Riedemann et al., 2007; Ciarimboli et al., 2010; More et al., 2010; Xu et al., 2012). In addition, it was reported that in the absence of hair cell mechanotransduction (MET) cisplatin-induced hair cell death is reduced in zebrafish neuromast (Thomas et al., 2013; Stawicki et al., 2014). Gentamicin, which is bigger in size and weight than cisplatin, is known to permeate MET channels (Marcotti et al., 2005; Alharazneh et al., 2011; Vu et al., 2013); similarly, it is possible that cisplatin can permeate hair cell MET channels, although other routes could exist (Thomas et al., 2013). Using the zebrafish lateral line system, we test whether cisplatin affects hair cell MET currents, which might implicate its interaction with MET channels.

Attempts to find and develop otoprotective strategies for platinum-based drugs have been ongoing. One area of interest is antioxidant molecules. These include N-acetyl-cysteine (Feghali et al., 2001), alpha-lipoic acid (Kim et al., 2014), D-methionine (Lorito et al., 2011) and sodium thiosulfate (Muldoon et al., 2000). The most important consideration is to find a protection method or a drug that does not compromise the anti-tumor actions of the platinum-based drugs. For that reason, using mdivi-1, an inhibitor of the mitochondrial fission protein Drp1, could be a promising strategy to mitigate cisplatin-induced ototoxicity (Qian et al., 2015). One interesting aspect of mdivi-1 is that it has been reported to increase the apoptosis of tumor cells that are resistant to cisplatin (Qian et al., 2014). In general, mitochondrial dynamics were found to modulate antineoplastic activity of cisplatin (Qian et al., 2015; Han et al., 2017). Interestingly, cisplatin-induced tubular cell apoptosis and acute kidney injury were reduced by mdivi-1 (Brooks et al., 2009). Some recent work has shown promise for mdivi-1 in ameliorating the adverse effects of ototoxic aminoglycosides on hair cells of the inner ear (Nuttall et al., 2015). Here we test whether mdivi-1 could protect hair cells against cisplatin toxicity using the zebrafish lateral line system.

MATERIALS AND METHODS

Animals

Experiments were conducted using the Tübingen strain of zebrafish of either sex provided by the McDermott zebrafish core facility. Transgenic zebrafish stably expressing GFP in the hair cell body (*pvalb3b*::GFP) were previously generated (McDermott et al., 2010), and *cdh23*^{tj264a} mutant (Söllner et al., 2004) was a kind gift from Dr. Teresa Nicolson (Oregon Health and Science University). Fish were maintained and bred at 28°C according to standard procedures (Nüsslein-Volhard and Dahm, 2002). This study was carried out in accordance with the recommendations in the Guide for the Care and Use of Laboratory Animals of the National Institutes of Health and animal welfare guidelines of the Committee of Case Western Reserve University (CWRU), USA. The protocol was approved by the Institutional Animal Care and Use Committee at CWRU (Protocol Number: 2012-0187).

Cisplatin Treatment

Zebrafish larvae at days post fertilization (dpf) 5–6, were placed in varying concentrations of cisplatin (50–200 μM,

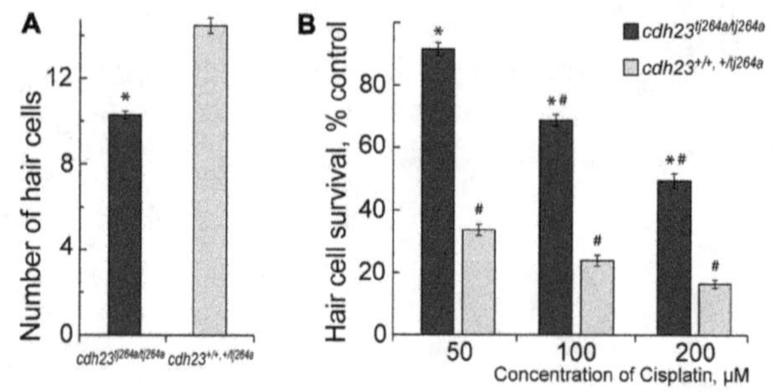

FIGURE 1 | Mechanotransduction (MET) potentiates cisplatin-induced hair cell death. **(A)** Untreated *cdh23*$^{tj264a/tj264a}$ have fewer hair cells per neuromast when compared to wild-type and heterozygous fish. **(B)** When treated with increasing concentrations of cisplatin, *cdh23* mutants, which do not have functional MET, have significantly greater hair cell survival in comparison to wild-type or heterozygous animals, which have normal MET. Data are mean, error bars indicate SEM. $^{*}p < 0.001$, in comparison to wild-type and normal heterozygous larvae within the same treatment concentration. $^{\#}p < 0.001$, in comparison to untreated controls within larvae of the same genotype (see Supplementary Table S1).

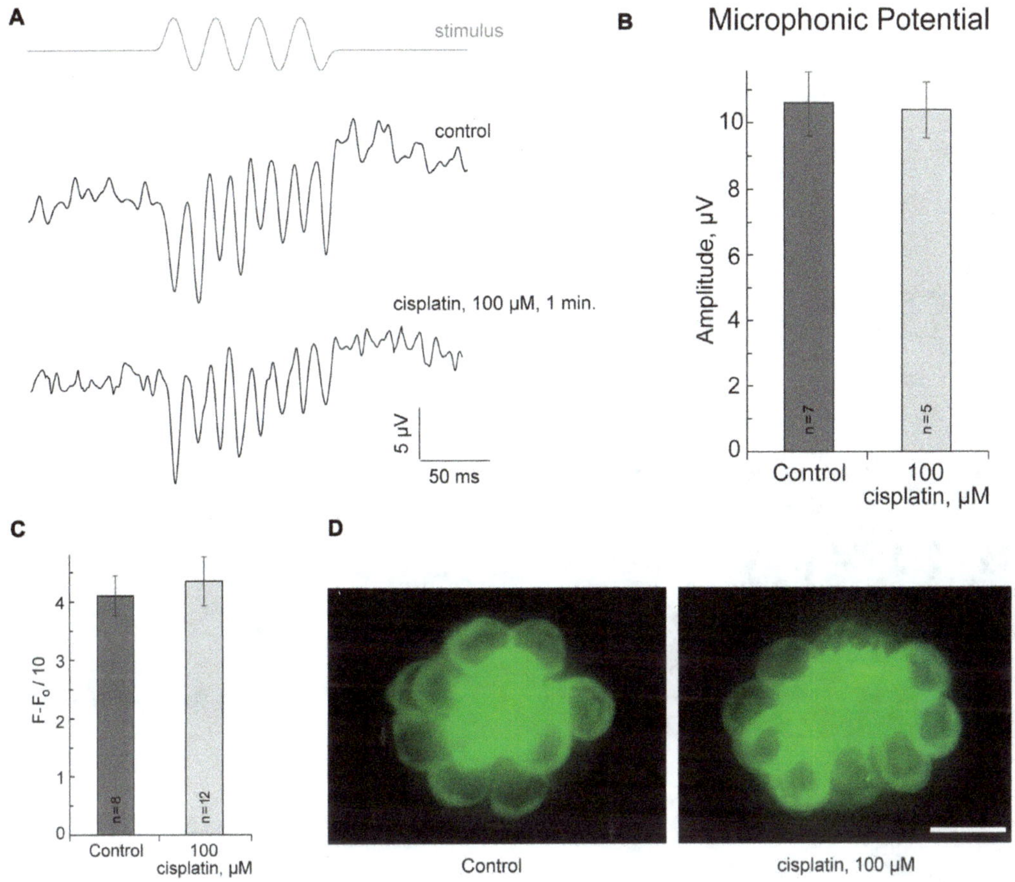

FIGURE 2 | Cisplatin does not affect MET in neuromast hair cells. **(A)** Neuromast microphonic potentials are not affected after 100-μM-cisplatin application. The top trace shows pressure applied to the stimulating puff pipette. **(B)** Summary of microphonic potential peak-to-peak amplitudes at twice the stimulus frequency obtained from lateral line neuromasts (controls and after 100-μM-cisplatin application). **(C)** Summary of fluorescent signal of FM1-43FX in live lateral line neuromasts of control and after 100-μM-cisplatin application. **(D)** Representative maximum-intensity projection images of FM1-43FX-treated live neuromasts: control and after 100-μM-cisplatin. Data are mean, error bars indicate SEM. *n* = 5–12 larvae (noted on bar graphs, from three to six clutches) per data point. Scale bar: 10 μm.

ThermoFisher Scientific, Waltham, MA, USA) and/or mdivi-1 (1–10 μM, Enzo Life Sciences, Farmingdale, NY, USA) overnight for 16 h. The next day, the larvae were transferred to another dish, anesthetized with MS-222 (Sigma-Aldrich, St. Louis, MO, USA), and secured in a recording chamber using strands of dental floss tie downs (Ricci and Fettiplace, 1997) and placed under the microscope, an upright Olympus BX51WI microscope equipped with 100× 1NA objective for observation. To assess viability, blood flow and heart rate were visually monitored. Images were observed with a Grasshopper3 CMOS camera (Point Grey, Richmond, BC, Canada) and captured with manufacturer provided software. Starting with the eye neuromasts and moving caudal, the number of hair bundles were counted in approximately 10 neuromasts per fish.

FM1-43 Labeling and Image Analyses

After overnight treatment with cisplatin and/or Mdivi-1, fish were placed into wells containing FM1-43 (ThermoFisher Scientific, Waltham, MA, USA) in fish water. After 30 s, fish were transferred to fish solution containing MS-222 and BSA. The larvae were then secured in a recording chamber and placed under the microscope for imaging as described above. Approximately 3–4 neuromasts were imaged, and maximal projection images were generated using ImageJ (NIH, Bethesda, MD, USA). For lateral line neuromasts, raw images were gathered using an Olympus BX51WI microscope and a Grasshopper3 CMOS camera as described above. Fluorescence measurements were obtained using ImageJ. A region of interest was used to obtain measurements from the cells in each neuromast (I_{cell}) and an area without cells ($I_{background}$) in the same image. Fluorescence intensity of FM1-43FX (I_{load}) for each neuromast was normalized ($I_{load} = I_{cell} - I_{background}$).

Recordings of Neuromast Microphonic Potential in Zebrafish

We anesthetized zebrafish larvae (5–7 dpf) using MS-222 dissolved in a standard bath solution containing (in mM): NaCl (120), KCl (2), HEPES (10), $CaCl_2$ (2), NaH_2PO_4 (0.7), adjusted to pH ~7.2. The larvae were secured in a recording

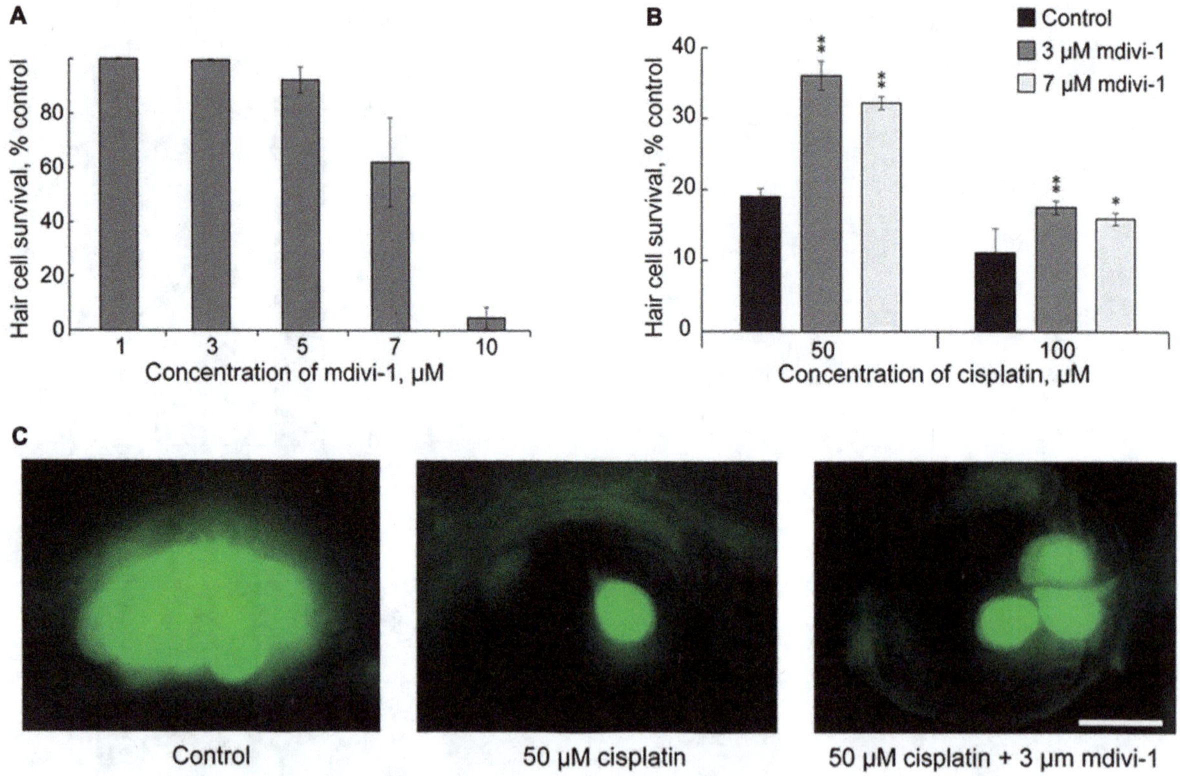

FIGURE 3 | Mdivi-1 protects against cisplatin-induced hair cell death. **(A)** Concentrations of mitochondrial division inhibitor mdivi-1 between 1–5 μM are well tolerated by zebrafish; whereas 10 μM of mdivi-1 is toxic to hair cells (n = 5 larvae per data point, from three clutches). **(B)** Application of 3 or 7 μM of mdivi-1 allowed significantly more hair cells to survive treatment with 50 and 100 μM of cisplatin. **(C)** Representative maximum-intensity projection images of *pvalb3b*::GFP neuromast hair cells treated with 50-μM-cisplatin and/or 50-μM-mdivi-1 (middle and right images). Data are mean, error bars indicate SEM. $^{**}p < 0.001$ and $^{*}p < 0.05$, in comparison to no mdivi-1 treatment within the same cisplatin concentration (see Supplementary Table S1). Scale bar: 10 μm.

chamber and placed under the microscope for observation as described above. Viability, blood flow and heart rate of larvae were visually monitored. Images were observed with a Grasshopper3 CMOS camera and captured with manufacturer provided software. We recorded from posterior neuromasts; kinocilia tufts were deflected with a fluid jet (Nicolson et al., 1998; Trapani and Nicolson, 2010) delivered via a glass pipette with a diameter of approximately 5–7 μm and controlled by HSPC-1 (ALA Scientific Instruments, Farmingdale, NY, USA). Fluid jet pipette was placed approximately 75 μm near the neuromast and used to deliver sinusoidal stimuli of 50 Hz frequency. The microphonic potentials were recorded at room temperature (22°C). We used borosilicate glass electrodes with a resistance of 3–6 MΩ, which were filled with standard bath solution and placed near the apical edges of the lateral line neuromasts. We recorded microphonic potentials using a PC-505B amplifier (Warner Instruments, Hamden, CT, USA) and a PCI-6221 digitizer (National Instruments, Austin, TX, USA). Microphonic potentials were amplified by 20 (SIM983, Stanford Research, Sunnyvale, CA, USA), measured by a jClamp (Scisoft, Yale University, New Haven, CT, USA) in a current-clamp mode, and low-pass filtered at 100 Hz. All records represent an average of at least 500 trials.

Statistics

All statistical analyses were performed using GraphPad Prism 7. Data are reported as mean ± SEM. Comparisons between groups were analyzed by ANOVA with Tukey *post hoc* testing.

RESULTS AND DISCUSSION

Mechanotransduction Potentiates Cisplatin-Induced Hair Cell Death

Our data show that functional MET potentiate cisplatin-induced hair cell toxicity in lateral line neuromasts in a zebrafish (**Figure 1**), in accordance with published reports (Thomas et al., 2013; Stawicki et al., 2014). $cdh23^{tj264a/tj264a}$ mutant zebrafish do not have functional MET in hair cells, because Cdh23 is an integral part of mechanosensitive stereocilia bundles in hair cells (Siemens et al., 2004; Söllner et al., 2004; Kazmierczak et al., 2007; Indzhykulian et al., 2013). Notably, *cdh23* mutants have smaller numbers of hair cells per neuromast in comparison to wild-type or heterozygous fish (**Figure 1**). Despite the fact that treatment with 50 μM of cisplatin did not significantly change the number of hair cells in neuromasts of $cdh23^{tj264a/tj264a}$ zebrafish, whereas in wild-type fish this dose of cisplatin considerably reduced the number of hair cells (**Figure 1A**). This result indicates that

MET channels may be involved in cisplatin entry into the hair cell. Alternatively, cisplatin entry into the hair cell is largely independent of the MET channel, but the ion flow carried out by functional MET potentiates cisplatin-induced damage.

Cisplatin and Mechanotransduction in Neuromast Hair Cells

If cisplatin enters hair cells via MET channels, it could interact with the channel directly and attenuate ion flow through the channel. To test this hypothesis, the microphonic potentials of neuromast hair cells (**Figures 2A,B**) were measured with and without application of 50 μM or 100 μM of cisplatin. The microphonic potential is an evoked electrical potential elicited by hair bundle deflections. The microphonic potential results from modulation of the cationic current flowing into stimulated hair cells via functional MET channels. Our results show that microphonic potentials were not affected by cisplatin application (**Figures 2A,B**). An alternate approach using FM1-43FX was also employed to test the hypothesis. FM1–43FX is a derivative of FM1-43, an amphipathic styryl dye that is known to rapidly accumulate in sensory hair cells via the MET channels that are partially open at rest in non-stimulated hair bundles (Gale et al., 2001; Meyers et al., 2003). Loading of FM1-43FX in live hair cells of lateral line neuromasts of controls and after 100-μM-cisplatin was not significantly different (**Figures 2C,D**). Our results did not reveal any evidence that cisplatin enters hair cells via MET channels. It is known that aminoglycosides enter hair cells via MET channels and are permeant blockers of these channels. Our results, however, do not rule out the possibility cisplatin may enter hair cells via the MET channel but this amount may not be sufficient to affect measured microphonic potentials.

When MET is functional, substantial amounts of calcium can enter hair cells through MET channels. Intracellular calcium balance is critical for hair cell function; it was found that calcium homeostasis is rapidly disrupted following ototoxic aminoglycoside exposure (Esterberg et al., 2014). It is possible that hair cell mitochondria continuously buffer calcium entering cell via functional MET channels, causing hair cells to become more vulnerable to toxic insult. Drugs that could reduce mitochondrial stress and/or protect mitochondria in other ways, may potentially increase hair cell viability when faced with ototoxic drugs.

Mitochondrial Division Inhibitor 1 Protects against Cisplatin-Induced Hair Cell Death

Here we tested whether mdivi-1 can protect hair cells against cisplatin induced toxicity in neuromast hair cells. Mdivi-1 is an inhibitor of mitochondrial division that selectively attenuates dynamin-related protein 1 activity, a fission protein that involved in the constriction and cleavage of mitochondria (Cassidy-Stone et al., 2008). First, we tested different doses of mdivi-1 for neuromast hair cell toxicity. High doses of mdivi-1, more than 10 μM, were toxic to the 5–6 dpf larvae (**Figure 3A**); therefore, we used lower doses of mdivi-1, 3 and 7 μM. Our data show that these doses of mdivi-1 protected hair cells of lateral line neuromast against toxicity of 50 μM of cisplatin (**Figures 3B,C**). These data demonstrated that modulating mitochondria dynamics may increase viability of hair cells against cisplatin toxicity in a zebrafish model. This finding is interesting also because it is known that mdivi-1 assists the abilities of cisplatin to trigger apoptosis in certain platinum-resistant tumor cells (Qian et al., 2014). Future studies, incorporating mammalian models, will be of further value in corroborating our results and revealing the mechanism of mdivi-1-mediated protection.

CONCLUSION

MET potentiates cisplatin-induced damage of neuromast hair cells. However, cisplatin, in contrast to aminoglycosides, does not affect MET of neuromast hair cells. Our data suggests that mitochondrial protection may prevent cisplatin-induced damage to hair cells.

AUTHOR CONTRIBUTIONS

JWV and RS: conceived and designed the experiments and wrote the article. JWV, RS and SNW: performed the experiments and analyzed the data. JWV, SNW, SRG, ARD, BMM, KNA and RS: discussion and contributed reagents, materials, animal work.

ACKNOWLEDGMENTS

The authors thank Carol Fernando and members of Brian McDermott Laboratory for their help with zebrafish core facility. We thank Joseph Santos-Sacchi, Yale University, for providing us with the license to run jClamp. This research was supported by NIH grants DC015016 (RS) and DC009437 (BMM).

REFERENCES

Alharazneh, A., Luk, L., Huth, M., Monfared, A., Steyger, P. S., Cheng, A. G., et al. (2011). Functional hair cell mechanotransducer channels are required for aminoglycoside ototoxicity. *PLoS One* 6:e22347. doi: 10.1371/journal.pone.0022347

Brock, P. R., Knight, K. R., Freyer, D. R., Campbell, K. C., Steyger, P. S., Blakley, B. W., et al. (2012). Platinum-induced ototoxicity in children: a consensus review on mechanisms, predisposition, and protection, including a new International Society of Pediatric Oncology Boston ototoxicity scale. *J. Clin. Oncol.* 30, 2408–2417. doi: 10.1200/JCO.2011.39.1110

Brooks, C., Wei, Q., Cho, S. G., and Dong, Z. (2009). Regulation of mitochondrial dynamics in acute kidney injury in cell culture and rodent models. *J. Clin. Invest.* 119, 1275–1285. doi: 10.1172/JCI37829

Cardinaal, R. M., de Groot, J. C., Huizing, E. H., Veldman, J. E., and Smoorenburg, G. F. (2000). Histological effects of co-administration of an ACTH$_{(4-9)}$ analogue, ORG 2766, on cisplatin ototoxicity in the albino guinea pig. *Hear. Res.* 144, 157–167. doi: 10.1016/s0378-5955(00)00061-7

Cassidy-Stone, A., Chipuk, J. E., Ingerman, E., Song, C., Yoo, C., Kuwana, T., et al. (2008). Chemical inhibition of the mitochondrial division dynamin reveals its role in Bax/Bak-dependent mitochondrial outer membrane permeabilization. *Dev. Cell* 14, 193–204. doi: 10.1016/j.devcel.2007.11.019

Ciarimboli, G., Deuster, D., Knief, A., Sperling, M., Holtkamp, M., Edemir, B., et al. (2010). Organic cation transporter 2 mediates cisplatin-induced oto- and nephrotoxicity and is a target for protective interventions. *Am. J. Pathol.* 176, 1169–1180. doi: 10.2353/ajpath.2010.090610

Cornelison, T. L., and Reed, E. (1993). Nephrotoxicity and hydration management for cisplatin, carboplatin and ormaplatin. *Gynecol. Oncol.* 50, 147–158. doi: 10.1006/gyno.1993.1184

Devarajan, P., Savoca, M., Castaneda, M. P., Park, M. S., Esteban-Cruciani, N., Kalinec, G., et al. (2002). Cisplatin-induced apoptosis in auditory cells: role of death receptor and mitochondrial pathways. *Hear. Res.* 174, 45–54. doi: 10.1016/s0378-5955(02)00634-2

Esterberg, R., Hailey, D. W., Rubel, E. W., and Raible, D. W. (2014). ER-mitochondrial calcium flow underlies vulnerability of mechanosensory hair cells to damage. *J. Neurosci.* 34, 9703–9719. doi: 10.1523/JNEUROSCI.0281-14.2014

Feghali, J. G., Liu, W., and Van De Water, T. R. (2001). L-N-acetyl-cysteine protection against cisplatin-induced auditory neuronal and hair cell toxicity. *Laryngoscope* 111, 1147–1155. doi: 10.1097/00005537-200107000-00005

Francis, S. P., and Cunningham, L. L. (2017). Non-autonomous cellular responses to ototoxic drug-induced stress and death. *Front. Cell. Neurosci.* 11:252. doi: 10.3389/fncel.2017.00252

Gale, J. E., Marcotti, W., Kennedy, H. J., Kros, C. J., and Richardson, G. P. (2001). FM1-43 dye behaves as a permeant blocker of the hair-cell mechanotransducer channel. *J. Neurosci.* 21, 7013–7025.

Han, X. J., Shi, S. L., Wei, Y. F., Jiang, L. P., Guo, M. Y., Wu, H. L., et al. (2017). Involvement of mitochondrial dynamics in the antineoplastic activity of cisplatin in murine leukemia L1210 cells. *Oncol. Rep.* 38, 985–992. doi: 10.3892/or.2017.5765

Hinojosa, R., Riggs, L. C., Strauss, M., and Matz, G. J. (1995). Temporal bone histopathology of cisplatin ototoxicity. *Am. J. Otol.* 16, 731–740.

Huang, H., Zhu, L., Reid, B. R., Drobny, G. P., and Hopkins, P. B. (1995). Solution structure of a cisplatin-induced DNA interstrand cross-link. *Science* 270, 1842–1845. doi: 10.1126/science.270.5243.1842

Indzhykulian, A. A., Stepanyan, R., Nelina, A., Spinelli, K. J., Ahmed, Z. M., Belyantseva, I. A., et al. (2013). Molecular remodeling of tip links underlies mechanosensory regeneration in auditory hair cells. *PLoS Biol.* 11:e1001583. doi: 10.1371/journal.pbio.1001583

Jamieson, E. R., and Lippard, S. J. (1999). Structure, recognition, and processing of cisplatin-DNA adducts. *Chem. Rev.* 99, 2467–2498.

Karasawa, T., and Steyger, P. S. (2015). An integrated view of cisplatin-induced nephrotoxicity and ototoxicity. *Toxicol. Lett.* 237, 219–227. doi: 10.1016/j.toxlet.2015.06.012

Kazmierczak, P., Sakaguchi, H., Tokita, J., Wilson-Kubalek, E. M., Milligan, R. A., Muller, U., et al. (2007). Cadherin 23 and protocadherin 15 interact to form tip-link filaments in sensory hair cells. *Nature* 449, 87–91. doi: 10.1038/nature06091

Kim, J., Cho, H.-J., Sagong, B., Kim, S.-J., Lee, J.-T., So, H.-S., et al. (2014). α-lipoic acid protects against cisplatin-induced ototoxicity via the regulation of MAPKs and proinflammatory cytokines. *Biochem. Biophys. Res. Commun.* 449, 183–189. doi: 10.1016/j.bbrc.2014.04.118

Kopke, R. D., Liu, W., Gabaizadeh, R., Jacono, A., Feghali, J., Spray, D., et al. (1997). Use of organotypic cultures of Corti's organ to study the protective effects of antioxidant molecules on cisplatin-induced damage of auditory hair cells. *Am. J. Otol.* 18, 559–571.

Laurell, G., Ekborn, A., Viberg, A., and Canlon, B. (2007). Effects of a single high dose of cisplatin on the melanocytes of the stria vascularis in the guinea pig. *Audiol. Neurootol.* 12, 170–178. doi: 10.1159/000099020

Laurell, G., and Engstrom, B. (1989). The combined effect of cisplatin and furosemide on hearing function in guinea pigs. *Hear. Res.* 38, 19–26. doi: 10.1016/0378-5955(89)90124-x

Laurell, G., Viberg, A., Teixeira, M., Sterkers, O., and Ferrary, E. (2000). Blood-perilymph barrier and ototoxicity: an *in vivo* study in the rat. *Acta Otolaryngol.* 120, 796–803. doi: 10.1080/000164800750061624

Li, Y., Womer, R. B., and Silber, J. H. (2004). Predicting cisplatin ototoxicity in children: the influence of age and the cumulative dose. *Eur. J. Cancer* 40, 2445–2451. doi: 10.1016/j.ejca.2003.08.009

Lorito, G., Hatzopoulos, S., Laurell, G., Campbell, K. C. M., Petruccelli, J., Giordano, P., et al. (2011). Dose-dependent protection on cisplatin-induced ototoxicity—an electrophysiological study on the effect of three antioxidants in the Sprague-Dawley rat animal model. *Med. Sci. Monit.* 17, BR179–BR186. doi: 10.12659/msm.881894

Marcotti, W., van Netten, S. M., and Kros, C. J. (2005). The aminoglycoside antibiotic dihydrostreptomycin rapidly enters mouse outer hair cells through the mechano-electrical transducer channels. *J. Physiol.* 567, 505–521. doi: 10.1113/jphysiol.2005.085951

Marullo, R., Werner, E., Degtyareva, N., Moore, B., Altavilla, G., Ramalingam, S. S., et al. (2013). Cisplatin induces a mitochondrial-ROS response that contributes to cytotoxicity depending on mitochondrial redox status and bioenergetic functions. *PLoS One* 8:e81162. doi: 10.1371/journal.pone.0081162

McDermott, B. M. Jr., Asai, Y., Baucom, J. M., Jani, S. D., Castellanos, Y., Gomez, G., et al. (2010). Transgenic labeling of hair cells in the zebrafish acousticolateralis system. *Gene Expr. Patterns* 10, 113–118. doi: 10.1016/j.gep.2010.01.001

Meyers, J. R., MacDonald, R. B., Duggan, A., Lenzi, D., Standaert, D. G., Corwin, J. T., et al. (2003). Lighting up the senses: FM1-43 loading of sensory cells through nonselective ion channels. *J. Neurosci.* 23, 4054–4065.

More, S. S., Akil, O., Ianculescu, A. G., Geier, E. G., Lustig, L. R., and Giacomini, K. M. (2010). Role of the copper transporter, CTR1, in platinum-induced ototoxicity. *J. Neurosci.* 30, 9500–9509. doi: 10.1523/JNEUROSCI.1544-10.2010

Muldoon, L. L., Pagel, M. A., Kroll, R. A., Brummett, R. E., Doolittle, N. D., Zuhowski, E. G., et al. (2000). Delayed administration of sodium thiosulfate in animal models reduces platinum ototoxicity without reduction of antitumor activity. *Clin. Cancer Res.* 6, 309–315.

Nicolson, T., Rüsch, A., Friedrich, R. W., Granato, M., Ruppersberg, J. P., and Nüsslein-Volhard, C. (1998). Genetic analysis of vertebrate sensory hair cell mechanosensation: the zebrafish circler mutants. *Neuron* 20, 271–283. doi: 10.1016/s0896-6273(00)80455-9

Nüsslein-Volhard, C., and Dahm, R. (2002). *Zebrafish: A Practical Approach.* New York, NY: Oxford University Press.

Nuttall, A., Foster, S., Zhang, Y., and Wilson, T. (2015). "Points, strands and donuts: the mitochondria dynamics of cochlear cells," in *Association for Research in Otolaryngology 38th MedWinter Meeting* (Barltimore, MD).

Park, M. S., De Leon, M., and Devarajan, P. (2002). Cisplatin induces apoptosis in LLC-PK1 cells via activation of mitochondrial pathways. *J. Am. Soc. Nephrol.* 13, 858–865.

Qian, W., Salamoun, J., Wang, J., Roginskaya, V., Van Houten, B., and Wipf, P. (2015). The combination of thioxodihydroquinazolinones and platinum drugs reverses platinum resistance in tumor cells by inducing mitochondrial apoptosis independent of Bax and Bak. *Bioorg. Med. Chem. Lett.* 25, 856–863. doi: 10.1016/j.bmcl.2014.12.072

Qian, W., Wang, J., Roginskaya, V., McDermott, L. A., Edwards, R. P., Stolz, D. B., et al. (2014). Novel combination of mitochondrial division inhibitor 1 (mdivi-1) and platinum agents produces synergistic pro-apoptotic effect in drug resistant tumor cells. *Oncotarget* 5, 4180–4194. doi: 10.18632/oncotarget.1944

Ricci, A. J., and Fettiplace, R. (1997). The effects of calcium buffering and cyclic AMP on mechano-electrical transduction in turtle auditory hair cells. *J. Physiol.* 501, 111–124. doi: 10.1111/j.1469-7793.1997.111bo.x

Riedemann, L., Lanvers, C., Deuster, D., Peters, U., Boos, J., Jürgens, H., et al. (2007). Megalin genetic polymorphisms and individual sensitivity to the ototoxic effect of cisplatin. *Pharmacogenomics J.* 8, 23–28. doi: 10.1038/sj.tpj.6500455

Rybak, L. P., Mukherjea, D., Jajoo, S., and Ramkumar, V. (2009). Cisplatin ototoxicity and protection: clinical and experimental studies. *Tohoku J. Exp. Med.* 219, 177–186. doi: 10.1620/tjem.219.177

Rybak, L. P., Whitworth, C. A., Mukherjea, D., and Ramkumar, V. (2007). Mechanisms of cisplatin-induced ototoxicity and prevention. *Hear. Res.* 226, 157–167. doi: 10.1016/j.heares.2006.09.015

Rybak, L. P., Whitworth, C., and Somani, S. (1999). Application of antioxidants and other agents to prevent cisplatin ototoxicity. *Laryngoscope* 109, 1740–1744. doi: 10.1097/00005537-199911000-00003

Schacht, J., Talaska, A. E., and Rybak, L. P. (2012). Cisplatin and aminoglycoside antibiotics: hearing loss and its prevention. *Anat. Rec.* 295, 1837–1850. doi: 10.1002/ar.22578

Siemens, J., Lillo, C., Dumont, R. A., Reynolds, A., Williams, D. S., Gillespie, P. G., et al. (2004). Cadherin 23 is a component of the tip link in hair-cell stereocilia. *Nature* 428, 950–955. doi: 10.1038/nature02483

Söllner, C., Rauch, G. J., Siemens, J., Geisler, R., Schuster, S. C., Müller, U., et al. (2004). Mutations in cadherin 23 affect tip links in zebrafish sensory hair cells. *Nature* 428, 955–959. doi: 10.1038/nature02484

Stawicki, T. M., Owens, K. N., Linbo, T., Reinhart, K. E., Rubel, E. W., and Raible, D. W. (2014). The zebrafish merovingian mutant reveals a role for pH regulation in hair cell toxicity and function. *Dis. Model. Mech.* 7, 847–856. doi: 10.1242/dmm.016576

Thomas, A. J., Hailey, D. W., Stawicki, T. M., Wu, P., Coffin, A. B., Rubel, E. W., et al. (2013). Functional mechanotransduction is required for cisplatin-induced hair cell death in the zebrafish lateral line. *J. Neurosci.* 33, 4405–4414. doi: 10.1523/JNEUROSCI.3940-12.2013

Trapani, J. G., and Nicolson, T. (2010). Physiological recordings from zebrafish lateral-line hair cells and afferent neurons. *Methods Cell Biol.* 100, 219–231. doi: 10.1016/B978-0-12-384892-5.00008-6

Vu, A. A., Nadaraja, G. S., Huth, M. E., Luk, L., Kim, J., Chai, R., et al. (2013). Integrity and regeneration of mechanotransduction machinery regulate aminoglycoside entry and sensory cell death. *PLoS One* 8:e54794. doi: 10.1371/journal.pone.0054794

Wisnovsky, S. P., Wilson, J. J., Radford, R. J., Pereira, M. P., Chan, M. R., Laposa, R. R., et al. (2013). Targeting mitochondrial DNA with a platinum-based anticancer agent. *Chem. Biol.* 20, 1323–1328. doi: 10.1016/j.chembiol.2013.08.010

Wong, E., and Giandomenico, C. M. (1999). Current status of platinum-based antitumor drugs. *Chem. Rev.* 99, 2451–2466. doi: 10.1021/cr980420v

Xu, X., Ren, H., Zhou, B., Zhao, Y., Yuan, R., Ma, R., et al. (2012). Prediction of copper transport protein 1 (CTR1) genotype on severe cisplatin induced toxicity in non-small cell lung cancer (NSCLC) patients. *Lung Cancer* 77, 438–442. doi: 10.1016/j.lungcan.2012.03.023

2

PI3K and Inhibitor of Apoptosis Proteins Modulate Gentamicin-Induced Hair Cell Death in the Zebrafish Lateral Line

Heather Wiedenhoft[1†], Lauren Hayashi[2] and Allison B. Coffin[1,3*]

[1] College of Arts and Sciences, Washington State University, Vancouver, WA, United States, [2] Knight Cancer Institute, Oregon Health & Science University, Portland, OR, United States, [3] Department of Integrative Physiology and Neuroscience, Washington State University, Vancouver, WA, United States

Edited by:
Lisa Cunningham,
National Institutes of Health (NIH),
United States

Reviewed by:
Su-Hua Sha,
Medical University of South Carolina,
United States
Rafael Linden,
Federal University of Rio de Janeiro,
Brazil

***Correspondence:**
Allison B. Coffin
allison.coffin@wsu.edu

Inner ear hair cell death leads to sensorineural hearing loss and can be a direct consequence of aminoglycoside antibiotic treatment. Aminoglycosides such as gentamicin are effective therapy for serious Gram-negative bacterial infections such as some forms of meningitis, pneumonia, and sepsis. Aminoglycosides enter hair cells through mechanotransduction channels at the apical end of hair bundles and initiate intrinsic cell death cascades, but the precise cell signaling that leads to hair cell death is incompletely understood. Here, we examine the cell death pathways involved in aminoglycoside damage using the zebrafish (*Danio rerio*). The zebrafish lateral line contains hair cell-bearing organs called neuromasts that are homologous to hair cells of the mammalian inner ear and represents an excellent model to study ototoxicity. Based on previous research demonstrating a role for p53, Bcl2 signaling, autophagy, and proteasomal degradation in aminoglycoside-damaged hair cells, we used the Cytoscape GeneMANIA Database to identify additional proteins that might play a role in neomycin or gentamicin ototoxicity. Our bioinformatics analysis identified the pro-survival proteins phosphoinositide-dependent kinase-1 (PDK1) and X-linked inhibitor of apoptosis protein (Xiap) as potential mediators of gentamicin-induced hair cell damage. Pharmacological inhibition of PDK1 or its downstream mediator protein kinase C facilitated gentamicin toxicity, as did *Xiap* mutation, suggesting that both PI3K and endogenous Xiap confer protection. Surprisingly, aminoglycoside-induced hair cell death was highly attenuated in wild type Tupfel long-fin (TL fish; the background strain for the *Xiap* mutant line) compared to wild type *AB zebrafish. Pharmacologic manipulation of p53 suggested that the strain difference might result from decreased p53 in TL hair cells, allowing for increased hair cell survival. Overall, our studies identified additional steps in the cell death cascade triggered by aminoglycoside damage, suggesting possible drug targets to combat hearing loss resulting from aminoglycoside exposure.

Keywords: zebrafish, hair cell protection, hearing loss, aminoglycosides, lateral line, ototoxicity, programmed cell death, strain difference

INTRODUCTION

Aminoglycosides antibiotics, including neomycin and gentamicin, cause hearing loss and vestibular dysfunction in 20–30% of patients who take these drugs (Rizzi and Hirose, 2007; Xie et al., 2011; Schacht et al., 2012). However, these antibiotics are still frequently used world-wide because of their relatively low cost and high efficacy in fighting devastating infectious diseases such as tuberculosis, sepsis, and other severe Gram-negative bacterial infections (Maurin and Raoult, 2001; Rizzi and Hirose, 2007). Aminoglycosides cause hearing loss by killing sensory hair cells in the inner ear, which eliminates the first neural step in transforming acoustic energy into neural impulses (Schacht et al., 2012). Damage to mammalian hair cells is permanent, as they do not regenerate. It is therefore critical that we understand how aminoglycosides cause hair cell death so that we may develop targeted therapies to intervene in the damage process and preserve hearing.

Cell death signaling is traditionally broken into two domains: apoptosis and necrosis. Apoptosis is classified morphologically by nuclear condensation and biochemically by caspase activation, while necrosis is distinct, with nuclear and plasma membrane swelling (Zimmermann et al., 2001; Danial and Korsmeyer, 2004). However, this binary classification fails to fully encompass the complexity of cell death signaling that occurs in many tissues, including the ear (Forge and Schacht, 2000; Matsui et al., 2002; Jiang et al., 2006a; Coffin et al., 2013b). Studies in the past decade demonstrate that aminoglycosides activate a complex set of signaling cascades in damaged hair cells, and that not all hair cells respond to aminoglycosides in the same biochemical manner (Jiang et al., 2006a; Taylor et al., 2008; Coffin et al., 2013b). For example, *in vitro* and *in vivo* studies in chickens and rodents suggest that classical apoptosis plays a dominant role in aminoglycoside damage, primarily activating the mitochondrial cell death pathway driven by caspase-9 and caspase-3 (e.g., Forge and Li, 2000; Cunningham et al., 2002; Matsui et al., 2002, 2004; Cheng et al., 2003). However, other research in mammals and zebrafish demonstrates caspase-independent cell death *in vivo*, albeit with involvement of mitochondrial proteins (Jiang et al., 2006a; Owens et al., 2007; Tabuchi et al., 2007; Coffin et al., 2013a,b). These contradictory data likely result from differences in species and experimental conditions, including *in vitro* vs. *in vivo* differences and differences in drug treatment paradigms. Reactive oxygen species formation is a hallmark feature in many aminoglycoside ototoxicity studies, and antioxidants confer some level of protection (Hirose et al., 1999; McFadden et al., 2003; Choung et al., 2009; Poirrier et al., 2010; Esterberg et al., 2016). Other studies suggest involvement of numerous cell death and survival cascades, including c-Jun N-terminal kinase (JNK) and p53 signaling (Wang et al., 2003; Sugahara et al., 2006; Coffin et al., 2013a; Anttonen et al., 2016). Despite these studies, we still have an incomplete picture of the signaling events that occur in aminoglycoside-damaged hair cells. A better understanding of cell death and survival signaling due to aminoglycoside exposure will provide more targets for therapeutic intervention.

The present study uses the larval zebrafish lateral line to better understand cell death processes after aminoglycoside exposure. The lateral line is used by zebrafish to detect near field vibrations in the water caused by abiotic or biotic sources such as prey, predators, or water current (Montgomery et al., 1997; Coombs et al., 2014). The lateral line system contains clusters of neuromasts—sensory hair and supporting cells encapsulated in a jelly-like cupula—that are arranged along the head and trunk of the fish. Lateral line hair cells are structurally and functionally similar to the hair cells of the mammalian inner ear and show similar responses to aminoglycosides and other hair cell toxins (Harris et al., 2003; Ou et al., 2007; Coffin et al., 2010). In the lateral line, neomycin and gentamicin activate distinct, yet somewhat overlapping, responses in damaged hair cells, suggesting that not all cell death responses are common across aminoglycosides and that a greater understanding of these differences is necessary to develop appropriate therapeutics (Coffin et al., 2009, 2013a,b; Owens et al., 2009; Hailey et al., 2017). Neomycin induces changes in calcium mobilization, mitochondrial membrane potential, and reactive oxygen species generation, and damage is dependent on the mitochondrial protein Bax (Owens et al., 2007; Coffin et al., 2013a; Esterberg et al., 2013, 2014, 2016). Although gentamicin toxicity in the lateral line is less well-studied, prior research shows that gentamicin-induced damage is independent of Bax and substantially dependent on p53 signaling (Coffin et al., 2013a).

In a previous study, we screened a cell death inhibitor library to identify novel regulators of aminoglycoside-induced hair cell death in the lateral line (Coffin et al., 2013b). This study identified several compounds that modulate aminoglycoside-induced hair cell death in the lateral line, including a Bax channel blocker, the p53 inhibitor pifithrin-α (PFTα), the Omi/HtrA2 inhibitor Ucf-101, and the autophagy inhibitor 3-MA (Coffin et al., 2013a,b). Here, we used this cell death inhibitor dataset as the input for pathway analysis using Cytoscape GeneMANIA to identify additional protein targets that may modulate aminoglycoside ototoxicity. We generated a list of molecular targets for each pharmacological reagent from the inhibitor dataset, basing our target selection on the literature demonstrating specific targets for each inhibitor. Our list contains 36 genes that our previous work suggests may modulate aminoglycoside ototoxicity, with some gene products implicated in neomycin toxicity, some in gentamicin toxicity, and some in response to either aminoglycoside. Pathway analysis yielded a complex network of potentially interacting signaling molecules in response to neomycin or gentamicin application.

We then used pharmacological or genetic manipulation to examine how these protein targets influence aminoglycoside-induced hair cell death. We selected two candidate classes of molecules: phosphoinositide-dependent kinase-1 (PDK1) and inhibitor of apoptosis proteins (IAPs), for further analysis, based on the potentially central role of these molecules, the paucity of information about these molecules in the auditory periphery, and the availability of pharmacological and genetic reagents for experimental use. We elected to focus on modulators of gentamicin damage because there is relatively little information on gentamicin ototoxicity in the lateral line, while neomycin damage is more understood (e.g., Harris et al., 2003; Esterberg et al., 2013, 2014, 2016). We found that PDK1 plays a protective role in gentamicin-damaged hair cells, as does X-linked inhibitor of apoptosis protein (Xiap). The *Xiap* mutant fish were created on a Tupfel long-fin (TL) background, and through comparisons with other wild type fish lines we discovered that hair cells in TL fish are less sensitive to aminoglycoside damage than hair cells in *AB fish, likely owing to differences in p53.

MATERIALS AND METHODS

Pathway Analysis

Based on our previous work (Coffin et al., 2013a,b), we generated a list of 36 genes that may modulate neomycin or gentamicin toxicity in the lateral line. Accession numbers and nucleotides for each gene were collected from the NCBI database (Brown et al., 2015). We used this gene list as input for pathway analysis of hair cell responses to neomycin or gentamicin damage. Supplementary Table 1 contains the list of input genes. Functional annotation of genes was performed using The Database for Annotation, visualization and Integrated Discovery (DAVID) Gene-Enrichment and Functional Annotation Analysis (Dennis et al., 2003; Huang et al., 2007; Wilhelm et al., 2012). The default EASE threshold of 0.1.0 was used. Global co-expression networks were then constructed using the Cytoscape app GeneMANIA (Campanaro et al., 2007; Montojo et al., 2010; Vied et al., 2014; Hausen et al., 2017). The desired organism used was human, with the options to display up to 50 related genes, 20 related attributes, and automatic weighting. Interactions were designated as genetic interactions, shared protein domains, pathway, co-expression, physical interactions, and predicted interactions. These different interactions are represented by different colored lines in the final output. From this analysis, we selected candidate proteins for pharmacological or genetic manipulation during aminoglycoside exposure in larval zebrafish.

Animals

Experiments were conducted on *AB wild type fish unless specifically noted. The *Xiap*^{sa2739} mutant fish, which have a premature stop codon in the *Xiap* gene, were created by the Sanger Institute on a TL background (zfin.org). *Xiap* mutants were purchased through the Zebrafish International Resource Center (ZIRC) and bred as a homozygous line. Wild type TL fish were also purchased through ZIRC. All fish were reared in the zebrafish facility at Washington State University, Vancouver. Larvae were produced through group matings and raised at 28°C in Petri dishes containing fish water. All experiments were performed in E2 embryo medium (EM: 1 mM $MgSO_4$, 0.15 mM KH_2PO_4, 1 mM $CaCl_2$, 0.5 mM KCl, 15 mM NaCl, 0.05 mM Na_2HPO, and 0.7 mM $NaHCO_3$ in dH_2O, pH 7.2; Westerfield, 2000). Animals were used at 5–6 days post-fertilization (dpf) because at this age their hair cells exhibit mature sensitivity to known hair cell toxins (Murakami et al., 2003; Santos et al., 2006; Ou et al., 2007). This study was carried out in accordance with the recommendations of the American Veterinary Medical Association and the Institutional Animal Care and Use Committee at Washington State University. The protocol was approved by the Institutional Animal Care and Use Committee at Washington State University.

Drug Exposure

Stock solutions of the aminoglycosides gentamicin and neomycin (Sigma-Aldrich, St. Louis, MO, United States) were diluted in EM to final concentrations of 25–400 μM. The ototoxic chemotherapy agent cisplatin was also used for one set of experiments. Cisplatin (MWI Animal Health, Boise, ID, United States) was diluted in EM to final concentrations of 250–1000 μM. For all experiments, fish were divided into treatment groups of 6–20 fish per group and placed in custom transfer baskets in a six-well plate. In order to understand the differences between neomycin- and gentamicin-induced hair cell death, we used either an acute treatment paradigm (30 min drug exposure, 60 min recovery in EM), or a continuous treatment paradigm (6 h drug exposure), as previous research demonstrates that these treatments activate distinct sets of cell death events (Coffin et al., 2009, 2013a,b; Owens et al., 2009). The acute exposure paradigm was used for neomycin treatment, while the continuous exposure paradigm was used for gentamicin.

In order to examine cell death, we used the following cell signaling modulators: PHT-427, which is a dual inhibitor of Akt and PDK1 proteins (Selleck Chemicals, Houston, TX, United States), LCL-161, a Smac/Diablo mimetic that acts as an antagonist of IAPs (Selleck Chemicals), an Akt inhibitor (Akt Inhibitor VIII, EMD Millipore, Billerica, MA, United States), the PDK1 inhibitor BX795 (UBPBio, Aurora, CO, United States), the protein kinase C (PKC) inhibitor Calphostin C (EMD Millipore), the p53 inhibitor PFTα, or the Mdm2 inhibitor nutlin-3a, which stabilizes p53. PFTα and nutlin-3a were purchased from Sigma. Cell death modulators were added 1 h prior to drug treatment and remained present during aminoglycoside exposure. Cell death modulators were reconstituted in DMSO. Control fish were given a corresponding amount of DMSO, ranging from 0.001 to 1% total volume to match the DMSO concentrations in the inhibitor treatment.

Hair Cell Assessment

To quantify hair cell survival, fish were treated with the vital dye 2-(4-(dimethylamino)styryl)-*N*-ethylpyridinium iodide (DASPEI, Life Technologies, Grand Island, NY, United States). Fish were incubated in 0.005% DASPEI for 15 min, then rinsed twice in fresh EM and anesthetized with 0.001% buffered 3-aminobenzoic acid ethyl ester methanesulfonate (MS-222, Argent Labs, Redmond, WA, United States) prior to imaging with a Leica M165FC fluorescent stereomicroscope (Leica Microsystems, Buffalo Grove, IL, United States). Ten pre-determined anterior neuromasts (IO1, IO2, IO3, M2, IO4, O2, MI1, MI2, SO1, and SO2; Raible and Kruse, 2000) per fish were then assigned a score from 0 to 2 based on brightness of DASPEI labeling, with 0 being no visible neuromast, 1 indicating visible but faint labeling, and 2 indicating bright labeling (Harris et al., 2003; Coffin et al., 2009; Owens et al., 2009). Aggregate scores were given per fish as a sum of its 10 neuromast scores (score of 0–20 per fish), and data were normalized to the control group for each experiment.

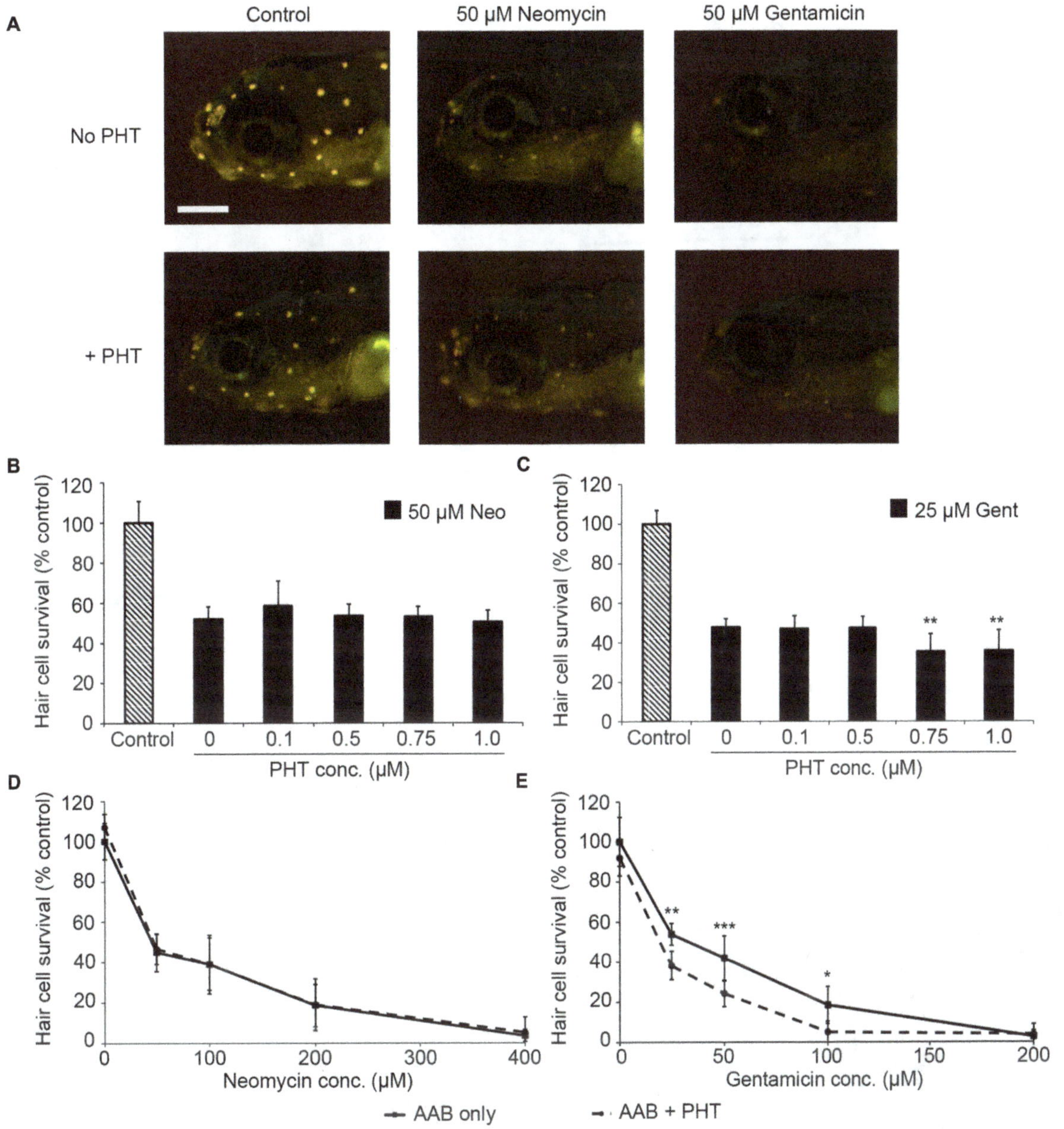

FIGURE 1 | The PDK1/Akt inhibitor PHT-427 sensitizes hair cells to gentamicin damage but not to neomycin. **(A)** Representative images showing DASPEI-labeled fish from the indicated groups. Scale bar = 200 μm and applies to all panels. **(B)** PHT dose–response function with 50 μM neomycin. PHT does not alter neomycin sensitivity (one-way ANOVA, $F_{4,50} = 1.68$, $p = 0.17$). **(C)** PHT increases sensitivity to gentamicin toxicity (one-way ANOVA, $F_{4,43} = 6.94$, $p < 0.001$). Bonferroni-corrected *post hoc* analysis demonstrates significant sensitization at 0.75 or 1 μM PHT. **(D)** 0.75 μM PHT does not alter the neomycin dose–response function (two-way ANOVA, $F_{1,86} = 1.04$, $p = 31$). **(E)** 0.75 μM PHT significantly sensitizes hair cells to gentamicin (two-way ANOVA with inhibitor presence as the factor, $F_{1,67} = 31.95$, $p < 0.001$). In panels **(D,E)**, solid lines are aminoglycoside (AAB) only, dashed lines are aminoglycoside with 0.75 μM PHT. Bonferroni-corrected *post hoc* analysis shows significant differences at 25, 50, and 100 μM gentamicin. $^{*}p < 0.05$, $^{**}p < 0.01$, $^{***}p < 0.001$. $N = 6$–12 fish/treatment.

For a sub-set of experiments, direct hair cells counts were used to validate DASPEI scores (Coffin et al., 2009, 2013a). Fish were euthanized with 0.002% buffered MS-222 and fixed in 4% paraformaldehyde overnight at 4°C. Fish were then rinsed in phosphate-buffered saline (PBS, Life Technologies) and blocked in PBS supplemented with 5% normal goat serum and 0.1% Triton-X (both from Sigma-Aldrich). Fish were then incubated overnight at 4°C in anti-parvalbumin, a specific hair cell label, in PBS with 0.1% Triton-X and 1% goat serum (1:500 antibody dilution, EMD Millipore). Fish were rinsed in fresh PBS + Triton-X, incubated in secondary antibody (Alexa Fluor goat anti-mouse 488 or 568, Life Technologies) for 4 h at room temperature, rinsed again, and stored at 4°C in a 1:1 solution of PBS:glycerol. The fish were then mounted on

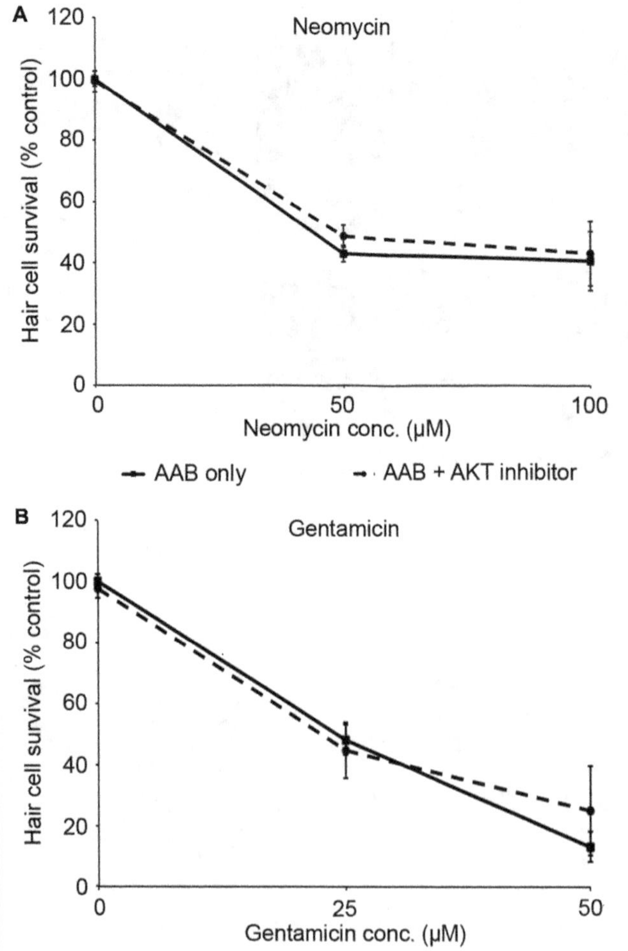

FIGURE 2 | Akt inhibition does not modulate aminoglycoside-induced hair cell death. Fish were treated with 1 μM Akt inhibitor and variable concentrations of neomycin **(A)** or gentamicin **(B)**. Solid lines are aminoglycoside (AAB) only, dashed lines are aminoglycoside with Akt inhibitor. Data were analyzed by two-way ANOVA with inhibitor presence as the factor. $F_{1,55} = 2.31$, $p = 0.13$ (neomycin), $F_{1,59} = 0.89$, $p = 0.35$ (gentamicin). $N = 10$–12 fish/treatment.

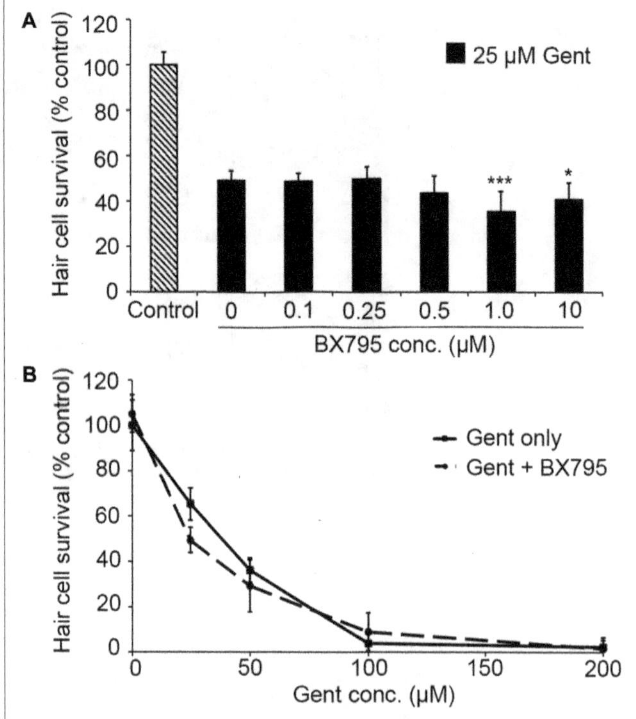

FIGURE 3 | The PDK1 inhibitor BX795 sensitizes hair cells to gentamicin damage. **(A)** BX795 exhibits dose-dependent sensitization (one-way ANOVA, $F_{5,60} = 8.807$, $p < 0.001$). Significant sensitization is seen with 1 or 10 μM BX795 against 25 μM gentamicin (***$p < 0.001$ and *$p < 0.05$, respectively). **(B)** A trend toward BX795 sensitization is seen across the gentamicin dose–response function, although this effect is not significant (two-way ANOVA with inhibitor presence as the factor, $F_{1,101} = 3.501$, $p = 0.06$). Solid lines are gentamicin only, dashed lines are gentamicin with BX795. $N = 8$–13 fish/treatment.

bridged coverslips and viewed using a Leica DMRB compound fluorescent microscope at 40× magnification, or with a Leica SP8 scanning confocal microscope. Hair cells from the same five neuromasts situated under the eye (IO1, IO2, IO3, M2, and OP1; Raible and Kruse, 2000) were counted and summed to arrive at one value per fish.

UV-Induced Cell Death

In order to examine cell death in other cells, we used UV light exposure, which causes DNA damage and cell death in a variety of cell types (Zeng et al., 2009; Yabu et al., 2015; Mao et al., 2017). Three dpf larvae (*AB or TL) were exposed to UV light for 90 s, then allowed to recover in either EM or PFTα for 3 h. Fish were then labeled with 5 μg/ml acridine orange (AO) for 45 min (Life Technologies; Kong et al., 2016), rinsed twice in fresh EM, anesthetized with MS-222, and imaged on a Leica SP8 confocal microscope. Identical laser, gain, and offset setting were used for all images. AO-labeled cells were quantified from a 10,000 μm^2 region of the ventral surface of the head, where the gill arches meet.

Data Analysis

Data were analyzed by one- or two-way ANOVA (as appropriate) using GraphPad Prism version 7. All data are presented as mean ± 1 SD. With power analysis using 10 animals per group, our standard sample size, we can detect a difference of 12% with 95% power, with type I and type II errors of 0.05. For experiments with $N = 6$, this allows us to detect a 15% difference.

RESULTS

PI3K or IAP Inhibition Modulates Hair Cell Death

Pathway analysis yielded a complex network of potentially interacting signaling molecules in response to neomycin or gentamicin application (Supplementary Figure 1 and Data Sheets 1, 2). Here, we focus on PDK1 and IAP as potential

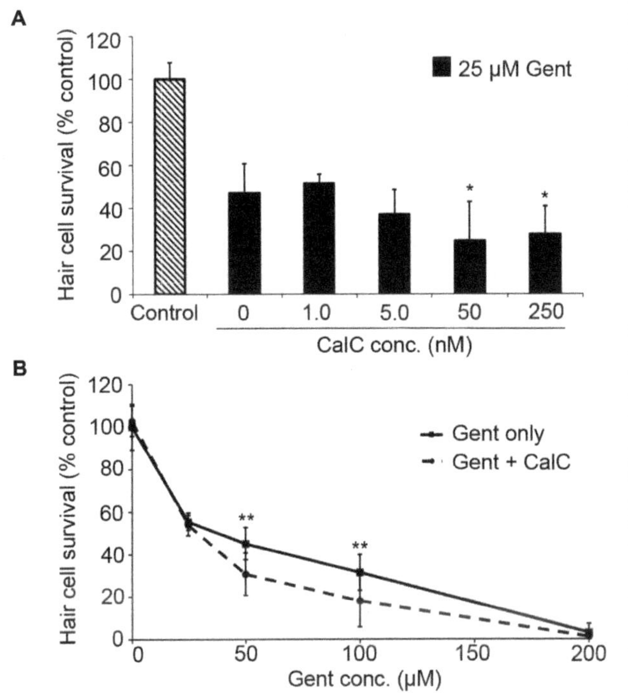

FIGURE 4 | The PKC inhibitor Calphostin C (CalC) facilitates gentamicin-induced hair cell death. **(A)** CalC significantly sensitizes hair cells to damage from 25 μM gentamicin (one-way ANOVA, $F_{4,31} = 6.16$, $p = 0.0009$). Either 50 or 250 nM CalC facilitates damage (*$p < 0.05$ in each case). $N = 5$–8 fish/treatment. **(B)** 250 nM CalC sensitizes hair cells to varying concentrations of gentamicin (two-way ANOVA with inhibitor presence as the factor, $F_{1,81} = 12.48$, $p = 0.0007$). Significant sensitization is seen at 50 or 100 μM gentamicin (**$p < 0.01$). $N = 8$–10 fish/treatment.

modulators of hair cell death, as both molecules appeared on one or both pathway diagrams (for neomycin and gentamicin).

PHT-427, a dual inhibitor of PDK1 and Akt, sensitized hair cells to gentamicin damage, with 750 nM PHT conferring significant sensitization (**Figure 1**; one-way ANOVA, $p < 0.001$). 750 nM PHT increased gentamicin-induced hair cell damage by 13–17%, depending on the gentamicin concentration (**Figure 1E**). There was no sensitization observed with 200 μM gentamicin, as this concentration damaged all hair cells without PHT, meaning that a further reduction in hair cell survival could not be detected. PHT did not sensitize hair cells to neomycin toxicity (**Figure 1**; one-way ANOVA, $p = 0.17$). PHT was not ototoxic on its own ("zero AAB" data points in **Figures 1D,E** and data not shown). These data suggest that either PDK1 or Akt normally protect hair cells specifically from gentamicin toxicity. Using 1 μM Akt inhibitor, which has been previously used in the zebrafish lateral line, we found that Akt-specific inhibition did not modulate aminoglycoside-induced hair cell death (Uribe et al., 2015, and **Figure 2**; two-way ANOVA, $p = 0.13$ and $p = 0.35$ for neomycin and gentamicin, respectively). By contrast, the PDK1 inhibitor BX795 significantly sensitized hair cells to 25 μM gentamicin, with a 13.7% decreased in hair cell survival in the presence of 1 μM BX795 (**Figure 3A**; one-way ANOVA, $p < 0.001$). However, this sensitization was not evident at higher gentamicin concentrations (**Figure 3B**; two-way ANOVA, $p = 0.06$). Collectively, our data suggest PDK1 as the endogenously protective component of this pathway.

PDK1 can activate both Akt and PKC. As our data in **Figure 3** suggest that gentamicin damage does not rely on Akt, we next assessed the role of PKC using the specific inhibitor Calphostin C (Schmidt et al., 2004). Calphostin C significantly facilitated gentamicin toxicity (**Figure 4A**; one-way ANOVA, $p = 0.0009$), with approximately a 20% reduction in hair cell survival with 50 or 250 nM Calphostin C, respectively. 250 nM Calphostin C sensitized hair cells to variable concentrations of gentamicin (two-way ANOVA, $p = 0.0007$; **Figure 4B**), with a 14.5% reduction in hair cell survival seen at 50 μM gentamicin and a 13.6% reduction observed with 100 μM gentamicin. These data suggest that PDK1 may protect hair cells by activation of PKC.

We then examined the role of IAPs in aminoglycoside toxicity. The Smac mimetic LCL-161, which targets cIAP1 and cIAP2 for degradation and leads to caspase activation, modestly sensitized hair cells to gentamicin damage (**Figure 5**; one-way ANOVA, $p = 0.28$), with 10 μM LCL reducing hair cell survival by 18.4% over gentamicin only. 10 μM LCL appeared to protect hair cells from neomycin damage, at least at 100 μM neomycin, with 14.8% more hair cells surviving when LCL was present (**Figure 5C**; two-way ANOVA, $p = 0.041$). Higher concentrations of LCL were ototoxic on their own (data not shown). More substantial results were observed in *Xiap* loss of function mutant fish. Hair cells in *Xiap* mutants were significantly more sensitive to gentamicin than were hair cells in wild type TL fish, the background strain on which the *Xiap* mutant line was created (**Figure 6**; two-way ANOVA, $p < 0.0001$). There was a modest effect of genotype on neomycin sensitivity (two-way ANOVA, $p = 0.002$). However, this effect resulted from a difference in neomycin susceptibility between *AB and TL fish, while *Xiap* mutant and TL hair cells did not differ in neomycin sensitivity (two-way ANOVA, $p = 0.12$). These data suggest that endogenous *Xiap* expression may protect hair cells from gentamicin, but not from neomycin damage. We also found that TL hair cells were resistant to gentamicin when compared to wild type *AB fish, demonstrating strain-specific differences in aminoglycoside susceptibility (**Figure 6**; see figure legend for pairwise statistical comparisons).

Strain Differences in p53 Signaling

We went on to explore the differences between *AB and TL strains in more detail, focusing on the more robust differences observed in gentamicin-exposed fish. Previous studies demonstrate that p53 modulates gentamicin-induced hair cell death in zebrafish (Coffin et al., 2013a,b). There was a significant effect of fish strain on the response to p53 manipulation (**Figure 7**; two-way ANOVA, $p < 0.001$). Inhibiting p53 with PFTα significantly protected *AB hair cells from gentamicin damage (**Figure 7A**; $p < 0.0001$), with PFT-treated *AB fish having 19.7% more hair cells than *ABs treated with gentamicin only. By contrast, there was no increase in hair cell survival in TL fish ($p = 0.14$). Similarly, stabilizing p53 with nutlin-3a greatly sensitized *AB hair cells to gentamicin damage, with a 23.9% reduction in hair cells in nutlin-3a-treated fish (**Figure 7**;

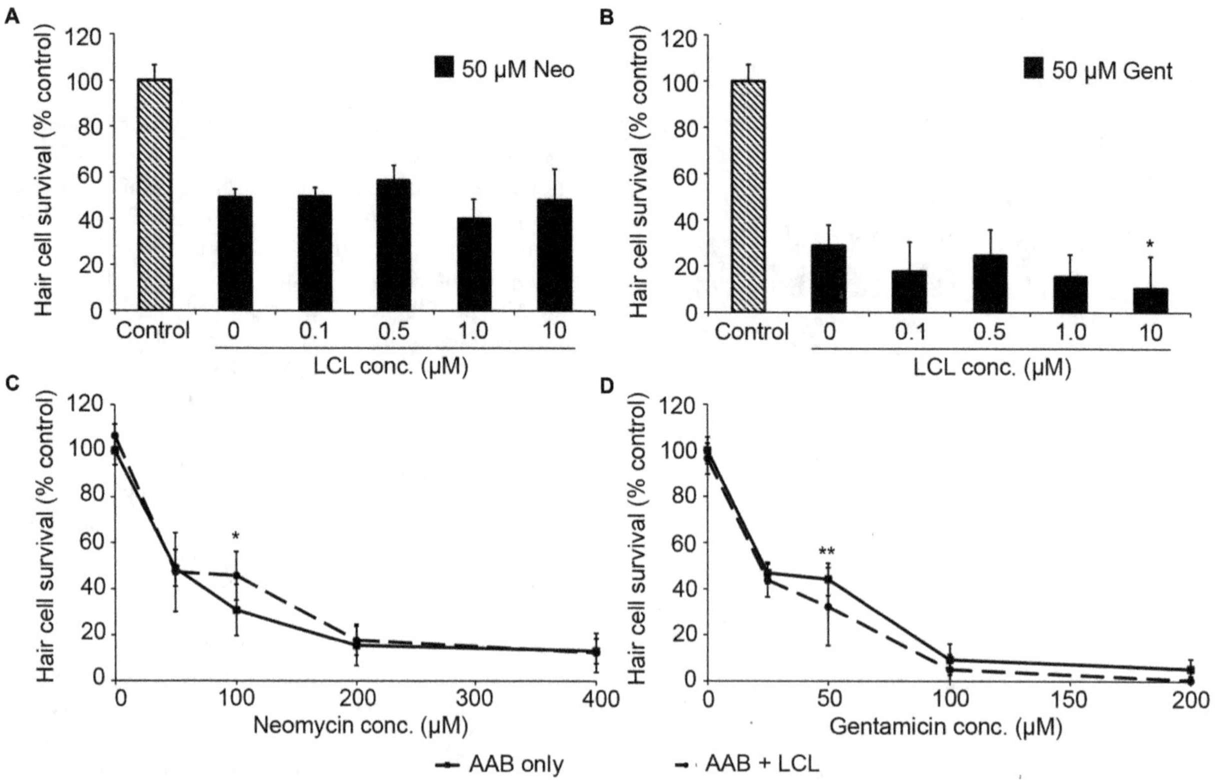

FIGURE 5 | The Smac mimetic LCL-161, which inhibits cIAP1, modestly sensitizes hair cells to gentamicin damage. **(A)** Variable LCL-161 concentrations do not affect toxicity to 50 μM neomycin (one-way ANOVA, $F_{4,69} = 1.54$, $p = 0.199$). **(B)** Variable LCL has a modest but significant effect on gentamicin toxicity (one-way ANOVA, $F_{4,31} = 3.14$, $p = 0.028$), with 10 μM LCL conveying significant sensitization (*$p < 0.05$). **(C)** 10 μM LCL appears to modestly protect hair cells from 100 μM neomycin (two-way ANOVA, $F_{1,74} = 4.34$, $p = 0.041$, *post hoc* analysis *$p < 0.05$). **(D)** 10 μM LCL increases susceptibility to gentamicin (two-way ANOVA with inhibitor presence as the factor, $F_{1,88} = 12.93$, $p < 0.001$). Sensitization is only apparent at 50 μM gentamicin (**$p < 0.01$). Solid lines are aminoglycoside (AAB) only, dashed lines are aminoglycoside with LCL. $N = 6$–12 fish/treatment.

$p < 0.0001$). Nutlin-3a did not affect gentamicin damage in TL hair cells ($p = 0.99$). These experiments suggest that p53 signaling may be altered in TL hair cells, or that gentamicin-induced hair cell death is independent of p53 in this line.

We next asked if TL hair cells are resistant to cisplatin damage. Cisplatin is an ototoxic chemotherapy drug that, in the lateral line, kills hair cells in a p53-independent manner (Ou et al., 2007; Coffin et al., 2013a). As shown in **Figure 8**, there was no difference in cisplatin-induced hair cell death between TL and *AB fish (two-way ANOVA, $p = 0.084$), suggesting that the relative resistance of TL hair cells to damage is specific for aminoglycosides and may be related to differences in p53.

Finally, we asked if cell death in response to UV light exposure was altered in TL fish. UV light kills multiple cell types through p53-dependent signaling cascades (Zeng et al., 2009; Gong et al., 2015). There was a significant effect of treatment for either fish strain (**Figure 9**; one-way ANOVA, $p < 0.001$ for each strain). UV light caused a threefold increase in the number of AO-labeled cells in the ventral head region of *AB fish ($p < 0.0001$), and this increase was attenuated by treatment with PFTα, with no significant difference observed between control fish and fish exposed to UV but treated with PFTα (**Figure 9B**, $p = 0.87$). In TL fish, UV exposure also led to a significant fourfold increase in AO labeling ($p < 0.0001$), but PFTα did not significantly reduce the magnitude of cell death (**Figure 9C**; $p = 0.99$). In neither case did PFTα itself alter the number of AO-labeled cells. Collectively, these data point to strain-specific differences in p53-dependent cell death signaling.

DISCUSSION

Cell Death and Survival in Aminoglycoside-Damaged Hair Cells

The goal of this study was to identity new candidate molecules involved in aminoglycoside-damaged hair cells of the zebrafish lateral line, and to experimentally manipulate them to determine their effect on hair cell death. We used DAVID and GeneMANIA to construct hypothetical genetic interaction pathways for neomycin and gentamicin damage, using known hair cell death molecules from the Bcl2 family and pharmacological modulators of aminoglycoside ototoxicity in the lateral line as the basis for selecting input genes (Coffin et al., 2013a,b). Our pathway analysis yielded several signaling proteins known to modulate aminoglycoside ototoxicity in mammalian systems, such as JNK and heat shock proteins (e.g., Wang et al., 2003; Cunningham

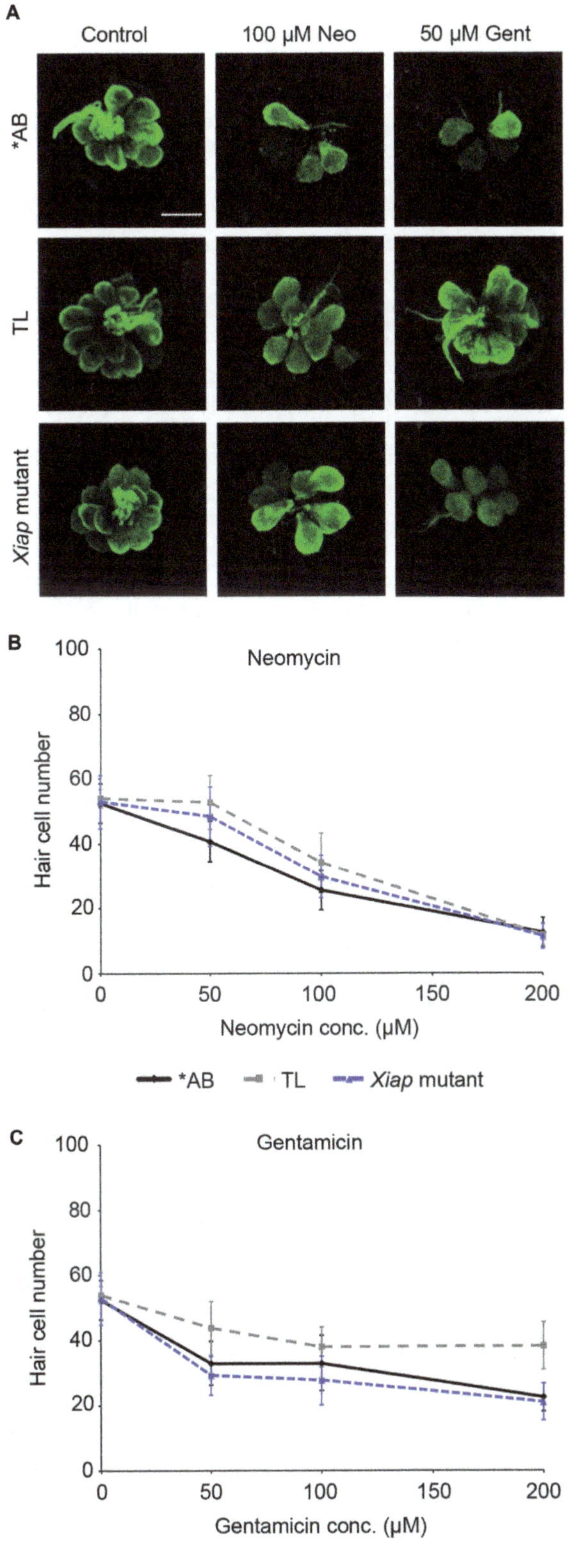

FIGURE 6 | Ototoxin sensitivity differs by genotype. *AB, TL, or *Xiap* mutant fish (created on a TL background) were treated acutely with neomycin or continuously with gentamicin. Hair cells were assessed by direct counts of anti-parvalbumin-labeled cells.

(Continued)

FIGURE 6 | Continued

(A) Representative confocal images of anti-parvalbumin-labeled hair cells from *AB, TL, and *Xiap* mutant fish. The scale bar = 10 μm and applies to all panels. **(B)** Genotype significantly effects hair cell sensitivity to neomycin (two-way ANOVA, $F_{2,102} = 6.363$, $p = 0.002$). Significant pairwise comparisons: 50 μM neo: AB vs TL $p < 0.001$, AB vs. *Xiap* $p < 0.05$; 100 μM neo: AB vs. TL $p < 0.05$. **(C)** There is a significant difference of genotype on gentamicin sensitivity (two-way ANOVA with genotype as the factor, $F_{3,96} = 24.15$, $p < 0.0001$). There is also a significant interaction between genotype and gentamicin concentration ($F_{6,96} = 3.028$, $p = 0.009$). Significant pairwise comparisons: 50 μM gent: AB vs. TL $p < 0.01$, TL vs. *Xiap* $p < 0.001$; 100 μM gent: TL vs. *Xiap* $p < 0.01$; 200 μM gent: AB vs. TL $p < 0.001$, TL vs. *Xiap* $p < 0.001$. In panels **(B,C)**, black solid lines are *AB fish, gray dashed lines are TL fish, and blue dashed lines are *Xiap* mutant fish. $N = 7–11$ fish/treatment.

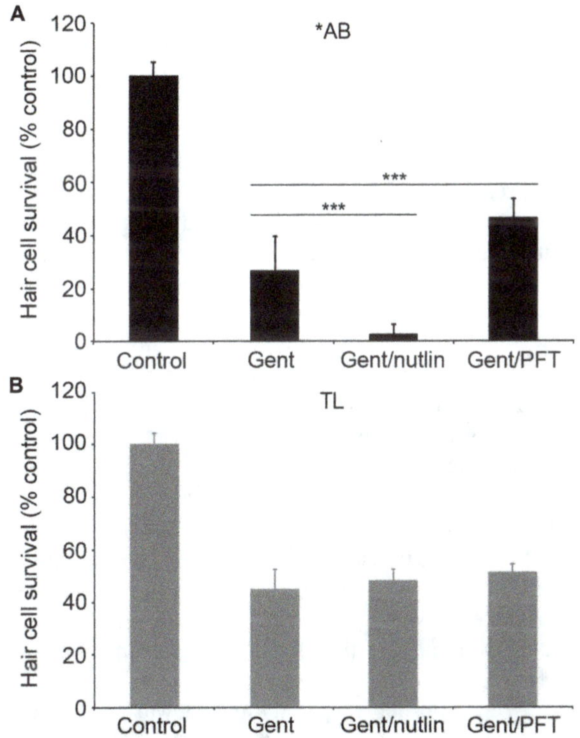

FIGURE 7 | p53 modulation does not affect gentamicin-induced hair cell death in TL fish. Fish were treated with 25 μM gentamicin either alone, with **(A)** 50 μM nutlin-3a, or with **(B)** 25 μM PFTα. Data are normalized to untreated *AB fish. There is a significant effect of treatment, genotype, and the interaction between the two ($F_{3,112} = 705.1$, $F_{1,112} = 149.7$, $F_{3,112} = 47.07$ for treatment, genotype, and the interaction term, respectively, $p < 0.001$ in all cases). Asterisks denote significant differences from gentamicin-only treatment, not including controls. ***$p < 0.001$. $N = 10–20$ fish/group.

and Brandon, 2006; Sugahara et al., 2006; Taleb et al., 2008). However, our analysis also yielded other candidate genes for future exploration. Collectively, the pathway analysis provides new molecular targets for ototoxicity research.

The pathway analysis diagrams in Supplementary Figure 1 differ for gentamicin and neomycin, because our previous research demonstrates that in the lateral line, these

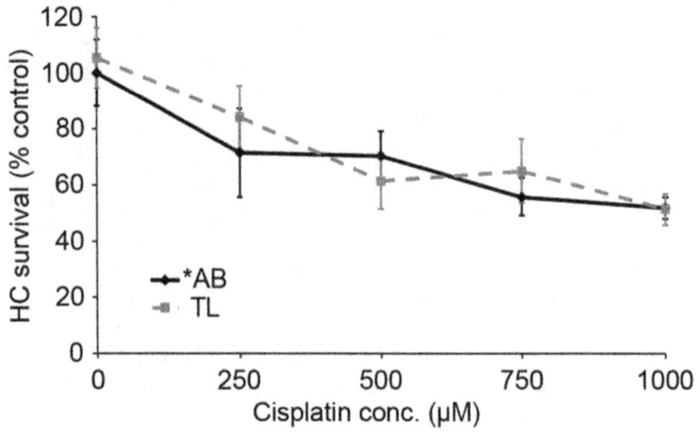

FIGURE 8 | There is no strain difference in cisplatin ototoxicity. Six hours continuous exposure to cisplatin results in dose-dependent hair cell death, with no significant difference between *AB and TL fish (two-way ANOVA with genotype as a factor, $F_{1,92} = 3.049$, $p = 0.084$). $N = 9$–13 fish/treatment.

aminoglycosides activate only partially overlapping suites of cell death regulators (Coffin et al., 2009, 2013a,b; Owens et al., 2009). For the present study, we focused on proteins from the gentamicin analysis, as gentamicin ototoxicity is relatively understudied in the lateral line, and gentamicin is in widespread clinical use. We selected three candidates for manipulation: the PI3K signaling protein PDK1, the inhibitor of apoptosis protein Xiap, and the mitochondrial protein Smac. We found that PDK1 inhibition sensitized hair cells to gentamicin damage but not neomycin toxicity, suggesting that endogenous PDK1 may protect hair cells from gentamicin exposure. In rodent models, aminoglycoside exposure can alter expression of PI3K signaling components and PI3K inhibition sensitizes cochlear explants to gentamicin damage (Chung et al., 2006; Jiang et al., 2006b; Jadali and Kwan, 2016). Our data suggest that PDK1, which activates downstream members of the PI3K pathway, may be responsible for the PI3K-dependent modulation of aminoglycoside ototoxicity.

PDK1 can phosphorylate multiple downstream targets, including Akt and PKC (Mora et al., 2004). Akt inhibition does not alter aminoglycoside susceptibility in the lateral line (**Figure 3**; Uribe et al., 2015), suggesting that PKC or other downstream PDK1 targets are responsible for the modulatory effect we observed. In mammals, multiple studies have implicated Akt in aminoglycoside ototoxicity, although the evidence for a protective role comes primarily from neonatal cochlear cultures, which may not accurately represent the mature *in vivo* condition (Chung et al., 2006; Brand et al., 2011, 2015; Heinrich et al., 2015). Our data suggest that endogenous Akt does not attenuate aminoglycoside ototoxicity *in vivo*, and that the effect of PDK1 manipulation is dependent on PKC, consistent with *in vitro* data from Chung et al. (2006). PDK1-dependent PKC signaling mediates mechanical hypersensitivity in a neuropathic pain model, demonstrating a role for this signaling cascade in nervous system injury (Ko et al., 2016). PDK1 activation of PKC also contributes to increased cell survival in some tumor types, likely by interacting with Bcl2-family proteins (Desai et al., 2011; Zabiewicz et al., 2014). Our previous data demonstrate that over-expression of Bcl2 protects hair cells from gentamicin toxicity (Coffin et al., 2013a), and the current research suggests that PKC signaling may play a role in this protective effect.

Our data do not allow us to determine the cell type(s) specifically responsible for PI3K-dependent protection. The effect could be cell-autonomous and confined to hair cells, but previous studies demonstrate that supporting cells are critical for hair cell survival in the undamaged ear and play an important role in hair cell responses to ototoxic damage (Haddon et al., 1998; May et al., 2013; Jadali et al., 2017). PI3K signaling is dependent on an extracellular ligand binding to a membrane-bound receptor to initiate the intracellular cascade (reviewed in Gamper and Powerll, 2012; Cunningham and Ruggero, 2013). Therefore, PDK1 modulation of hair cell survival depends on an upstream signal that could originate in neighboring supporting cells, or in a potentially distant cell population. A similarly cooperative mechanism was proposed by Jadali and Kwan (2016), who suggested that IGF-1 or another excreted ligand may be necessary for PI3K-dependent hair cell protection. Future experiments are necessary to further examine PI3K signaling in ototoxicity and to determine the source of the ligand and the cell types involved.

The IAPs play roles in cell proliferation, differentiation, and survival. The Smac mimetic LCL-161, which targets cIAP1 and cIAP2 for degradation (Vince et al., 2007; West et al., 2016), modestly altered hair cell responses to aminoglycosides, with differing responses for neomycin and gentamicin. It is unclear if these modest but opposing differences are biologically relevant, and future experiments are needed to further probe the role of these IAPs in ototoxicity. However, *Xiap* loss-of-function significantly sensitized hair cells to gentamicin damage, but not to neomycin toxicity, suggesting a protective role for endogenous *Xiap* during gentamicin exposure. Xiap can modulate cell death via both caspase-dependent and caspase-independent pathways, and plays diverse roles in cellular responses to stresses such as toxin exposure (Dubrez-Daloz et al., 2008). *Xiap* over-expression protects hair cells from cisplatin damage, and modestly reduces neomycin ototoxicity in P8-P14 mice (Cooper et al., 2006; Sun et al., 2014). It is possible that *Xiap* over-expression in zebrafish would prevent neomycin-induced hair cell loss, as increasing pro-survival factors can confer protection even if endogenous levels appear insufficient to modulate hair cell damage (Uribe et al., 2015). However, our results provide further evidence for differences in cell signaling responses to neomycin vs. gentamicin in zebrafish hair cells.

Xiap can function as an ubiquitin ligase, consistent with our previous data demonstrating a role for proteasomal degradation in aminoglycoside toxicity (Galbán and Duckett, 2010; Coffin et al., 2013b). Xiap ubiquitinates multiple targets, including apoptosis-inducing factor (AIF), leading to AIF activation and caspase-independent programmed cell death (Lewis et al., 2011). In the lateral line, aminoglycoside-induced hair cell death is independent of caspase activation, implicating this caspase-independent role of Xiap in gentamicin damage (Coffin et al., 2013b). AIF translocates from the mitochondria to the nucleus in damaged cells, and AIF translocation is reported in hair cells in response to amikacin administration *in vivo* or to gentamicin

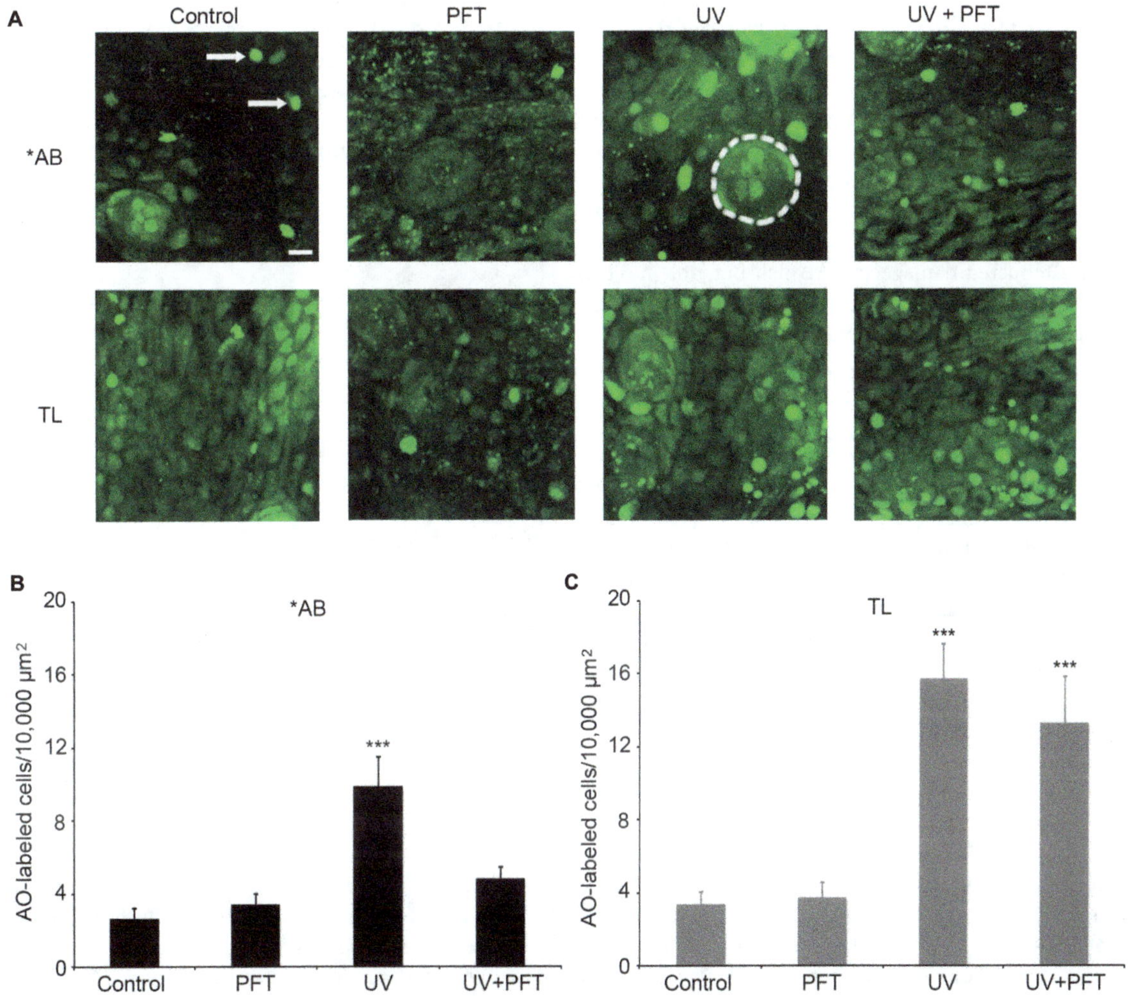

FIGURE 9 | p53 differentially modulates UV-induced cell death between AB and TL fish. **(A)** Representative confocal images of the ventral head region, showing the differences in AO labeling between groups. Each box is 100 × 100 μm; the actual size of the regions used to collect the quantitative data in panels **(B,C)**. Arrows in the upper left panel point to examples of AO-labeled cells. Dashed line in the upper middle panel (AB/UV group) outlines a neuromast for reference. Scale bar in the upper left panel = 10 μm and applies to all panels. **(B)** UV exposure in *AB fish significantly kills cells, and PFTα treatment returns cell death to baseline levels. One-way ANOVA, $F_{3,25} = 11.27$, $p < 0.001$. **(C)** UV exposure also increase the number of AO-labeled cells in TL fish, and PFTα does not prevent cell death. One-way ANOVA, $F_{3,26} = 13.96$, $p < 0.001$. For both panels, asterisks "***" indicate different from controls of the same strain, $p < 0.001$. $N = 6$–8 fish/group.

in vitro, suggesting that AIF may mediate hair cell damage (Lecain et al., 2007; Zhang et al., 2012). However, an *in vivo* study in mice did not find AIF translocation after kanamycin ototoxicity, but did note a decrease in cochlear AIF expression (Jiang et al., 2006a). It is unclear if these differences are due to species differences or to the aminoglycoside used. Future research is necessary to determine if an Xiap–AIF interaction plays a role in aminoglycoside ototoxicity in the lateral line.

GeneMANIA predicts interactions between genes, yielding potential candidates for experimental follow-up. Our bioinformatics analysis of the different cell signaling genes associated with aminoglycoside damage helped identify potential molecular targets for modulation of hair cell responses to neomycin or gentamicin. Both *PDK1* and *Xiap* appeared on the gentamicin signaling diagram but not the neomycin diagram, and modulation of PDK1 or Xiap influenced hair cell death in response to gentamicin but not neomycin. These data further highlight the toxin-specific nature of hair cell damage, and the utility of the bioinformatics approach to identify potential candidate molecules for experimental validation.

Strain-Specific Responses to Aminoglycoside Damage

During our cell signaling investigation, we found strain-specific differences in aminoglycoside sensitivity, with TL fish being modestly resistant to neomycin-induced hair cell death, and substantially resistant to gentamicin damage. Our previous work demonstrated that p53 inhibition conferred modest protection from neomycin and substantial protection from gentamicin in *AB fish (Coffin et al., 2013a). We therefore investigated p53 modulation in *AB vs. TL fish here and found that p53 modulation did not alter hair cell responses to gentamicin in TL fish, in contrast to the marked effect on hair cell death in *AB animals. Our p53 manipulation experiments suggest that ~40% of gentamicin-induced hair cell death in the lateral line is independent of p53, since in *AB fish p53 inhibition partially rescues gentamicin damage, leading to hair cell loss on par with gentamicin-treated TL hair cells that did not receive p53 inhibitor. Cell death due to UV exposure is also p53-dependent, and UV exposure induced cell death in both *AB and TL larvae. p53 inhibition attenuated damage in *AB fish but not in TLs, further evidence for strain-specific differences in p53 signaling, leading to strain-specific responses to damaging agents.

Strain-specific differences in aminoglycoside sensitivity were previously noted in rodents (Sullivan et al., 1987; Wu et al., 2001). For example, Fisher-344 rats are more susceptible to gentamicin ototoxicity and nephrotoxicity than are Sprague-Dawley rats, and BALB/c mice are more susceptible to kanamycin damage than C57BL/6 mice (Sullivan et al., 1987; Wu et al., 2001). Human genetic differences in ototoxic sensitivity are well-known, particularly mitochondrial mutations that convey increased susceptibility to aminoglycoside-induced hearing loss (Fischel-Ghodsian, 1998). To our knowledge, this is the first report of a strain difference in aminoglycoside susceptibility in zebrafish. Monroe et al. (2016) demonstrated that different strains of adult zebrafish differ in hearing sensitivity, with TL fish having greater sensitivity than age-matched *ABs. However, the cause of these differences is unknown.

Zebrafish exhibit strain-specific responses to several behavioral tasks, such as inhibitory avoidance learning or startle response habituation (Gorissen et al., 2015; van den Bos et al., 2017). TL fish have reduced resting cortisol levels and decreased expression of stress-related genes when compared to AB fish, and our unpublished results suggest that cortisol may increase aminoglycoside susceptibility in lateral line hair cells (Gorissen et al., 2015; van den Bos et al., 2017; Hayward and Young, unpublished data). Therefore, in addition to differences in p53 signaling, increased cortisol levels in *AB animals may further sensitize their hair cells to aminoglycoside damage. Future experiments are needed to dissect the relative contributions of stress-related factors and strain-specific aminoglycoside sensitivity.

CONCLUSION

Our pathway analysis suggests several novel candidates for modulation of aminoglycoside ototoxicity, and our pharmacological and genetic manipulations demonstrate likely roles for the PI3K proteins PDK1 and PKC, and the IAPs Xiap, as endogenous regulators of gentamicin toxicity. We further demonstrate that strain-specific differences in p53 signaling likely underlie differential susceptibility to gentamicin damage. These studies increase understanding of cell signaling in ototoxic damage and suggest molecular targets for possible therapeutic intervention.

AUTHOR CONTRIBUTIONS

HW, LH, and AC all participated in the research design, conducted experiments, performed data analysis, and wrote or contributed to the writing of this manuscript.

ACKNOWLEDGMENTS

We thank A. Young, E. Cooper, and M. Sokolova for fish husbandry assistance, B. Villalpando for technical assistance, and A. Groves for early discussion on the pathway analysis. We also thank two reviewers for their feedback, which helped to improve this manuscript.

REFERENCES

Anttonen, T., Herranen, A., Virkkala, J., Kirjavainen, A., Elomaa, P., Laos, M., et al. (2016). c-Jun N-terminal phosphorylation: biomarker for cellular stress rather than cell death in the injured cochlea. *eNeuro* 3:ENEURO.0047-16.2016. doi: 10.1523/ENEURO.0047-16.2016

Brand, Y., Levano, S., Radojevic, V., Naldi, A. M., Setz, C., Ryan, A. F., et al. (2015). All Akt isoforms (Akt1, Akt2, Akt3) are involved in normal hearing, but only Akt2 and Akt3 are involved in auditory hair cell survival in the mammalian inner ear. *PLOS ONE* 10:e0121599. doi: 10.1371/journal.pone.0121599

Brand, Y., Setz, C., Levano, S., Listyo, A., Chavez, E., Pak, K., et al. (2011). Simvastatin protects auditory hair cells from gentamicin-induced toxicity and activates Akt signaling *in vitro*. *BMC Neurosci.* 12:114. doi: 10.1186/1471-2202-12-114

Brown, G. R., Hem, V., Katz, K. S., Ovetsky, M., Wallin, C., Ermolaeva, O., et al. (2015). Gene: a gene-centered information resource at NCBI. *Nucleic Acids Res.* 43, D36–D42. doi: 10.1093/nar/gku1055

Campanaro, S., Picelli, S., Torregrossa, R., Colluto, L., Ceol, M., Del Prete, D., et al. (2007). Genes involved in TGF beta1-driven epithelial-mesenchymal transition of renal epithelial cells are topologically related in the human interactome map. *BMC Genomics* 8:383. doi: 10.1186/1471-2164-8-383

Cheng, A. G., Cunningham, L. L., and Rubel, E. W. (2003). Hair cell death in the avian basilar papilla: characterization of the *in vitro* model and caspase activation. *J. Assoc. Res. Otolaryngol.* 4, 97–105. doi: 10.1007/s10162-002-3016-8

Choung, Y. H., Taura, A., Pak, K., Choi, S. J., Masuda, M., and Ryan, A. F. (2009). Generation of highly-reactive oxygen species is closely related to hair cell damage in rat organ of Corti treated with gentamicin. *Neuroscience* 161, 214–226. doi: 10.1016/j.neuroscience.2009.02.085

Chung, W.-H., Pak, K., Lin, B., Webster, N., and Ryan, A. F. (2006). A PI3K pathway mediates hair cell survival and opposes gentamicin toxicity in neonatal rat organ of Corti. *J. Assoc. Res. Otolaryngol.* 7, 373–382. doi: 10.1007/s10162-006-0050-y

Coffin, A. B., Ou, H., Owens, K. N., Santos, F., Simon, J. A., Rubel, E. W., et al. (2010). Chemical screening for hair cell loss and protection in the zebrafish lateral line. *Zebrafish* 7, 3–11. doi: 10.1089/zeb.2009.0639

Coffin, A. B., Reinhart, K. E., Owens, K. N., Raible, D. W., and Rubel, E. W. (2009). Extracellular divalent cations modulate aminoglycoside-induced hair cell death in the zebrafish lateral line. *Hear. Res.* 253, 42–51. doi: 10.1016/j.heares.2009.03.004

Coffin, A. B., Rubel, E. W., and Raible, D. W. (2013a). Bax, Bcl2, and p53 differentially regulate neomycin- and gentamicin-induced hair cell death in the zebrafish lateral line. *J. Assoc. Res. Otolaryngol.* 14, 645–659. doi: 10.1007/s10162-013-0404-1

Coffin, A. B., Williamson, K. L., Mamiya, A., Raible, D. W., and Rubel, E. W. (2013b). Profiling drug-induced cell death pathways in the zebrafish lateral line. *Apoptosis* 18, 393–408. doi: 10.1007/s10495-013-0816-8

Coombs, S., Bleckmann, H., Fay, R. R., and Popper, A. N. (2014). *The Lateral Line System*. New York, NY: Springer. doi: 10.1007/978-1-4614-8851-4

Cooper, L. B., Chan, D. K., Roediger, F. C., Shaffer, B. R., Fraser, J. F., Musatov, S., et al. (2006). AAV-mediated delivery of the caspase inhibitor XIAP protects against cisplatin ototoxicity. *Otol. Neurotol.* 27, 484–490.

Cunningham, J. T., and Ruggero, D. (2013). New connections between old pathways: PDK1 signaling promotes cellular transformation through PLK1-dependent MYC stabilization. *Cancer Discov.* 3, 1099–1102. doi: 10.1158/2159-8290.CD-13-0581

Cunningham, L. L., and Brandon, C. S. (2006). Heat shock inhibits both aminoglycoside- and cisplatin-induced sensory hair cell death. *J. Assoc. Res. Otolaryngol.* 7, 299–307. doi: 10.1007/s10162-006-0043-x

Cunningham, L. L., Cheng, A. G., and Rubel, E. W. (2002). Caspase activation in hair cells of the mouse utricle exposed to neomycin. *J. Neurosci.* 22, 8532–8540.

Danial, N. N., and Korsmeyer, S. J. (2004). Cell death: critical control points. *Cell* 116, 205–219. doi: 10.1016/S0092-8674(04)00046-7

Dennis, G. Jr., Sherman, B. T., Hosack, D. A., Yang, J., Gao, W., Lane, H. C., et al. (2003). DAVID: database for annotation, visualization, and integrated discovery. *Genome Biol.* 4:R60. doi: 10.1186/gb-2003-4-9-r60

Desai, S., Pillai, P., Win-Piazza, H., and Acevedo-Duncan, M. (2011). PKC-I promotes glioblastoma cell survival by phosphorylating and inhibiting BAD through a phosphatidylinositol 3-kinase pathway. *Biochem. Biophys. Acta* 1813, 1190–1197. doi: 10.1016/j.bbamcr.2011.03.007

Dubrez-Daloz, L., Dupoux, A., and Cartier, J. (2008). IAPs: more than just inhibitors of apoptosis proteins. *Cell Cycle* 7, 1036–1046. doi: 10.4161/cc.7.8.5783

Esterberg, R., Hailey, D. W., Coffin, A. B., Rubel, E. W., and Raible, D. W. (2013). Disruption of intracellular calcium regulation is integral to aminoglycoside-induced hair cell death. *J. Neurosci.* 33, 7513–7525. doi: 10.1523/JNEUROSCI.4559-12.2013

Esterberg, R., Hailey, D. W., Rubel, E. W., and Raible, D. W. (2014). ER-mitochondrial calcium flow underlies vulnerability of mechanosensory hair cells to damage. *J. Neurosci.* 34, 9703–9719. doi: 10.1523/JNEUROSCI.0281-14.2014

Esterberg, R., Linbo, T., Pickett, S. B., Wu, P., Ou, H. C., Rubel, E. W., et al. (2016). Mitochondrial calcium uptake underlies ROS generation during aminoglycoside-induced hair cell death. *J. Clin. Invest.* 126, 3556–3566. doi: 10.1172/JCI84939

Fischel-Ghodsian, N. (1998). Mitochondrial mutations and hearing loss: paradigm for mitochondrial genetics. *Am. J. Hum. Genet.* 62, 15–19. doi: 10.1086/301695

Forge, A., and Li, L. (2000). Apoptotic death of hair cells in mammalian vestibular sensory epithelia. *Hear. Res.* 139, 97–115. doi: 10.1016/S0378-5955(99)00177-X

Forge, A., and Schacht, J. (2000). Aminoglycoside antibiotics. *Audiol. Neurootol.* 5, 3–22. doi: 10.1159/000013861

Galbán, S., and Duckett, C. S. (2010). XIAP as a ubiquitin ligase in cellular signaling. *Cell Death Differ.* 17, 54–60. doi: 10.1038/cdd.2009.81

Gamper, C. J., and Powerll, J. D. (2012). All PI3Kinase signaling is not mTOR: dissecting mTOR-dependent and independent signaling pathways in T cells. *Front. Immunol.* 3:312. doi: 10.3389/fimmu.2012.00312

Gong, L., Gong, H., Pan, X., Chang, C., Ou, Z., Ye, S., et al. (2015). p53 isoform Δ113p53/Δ133p53 promotes DNA double-strand break repair to protect cell from death and senescence in response to DNA damage. *Cell Res.* 25, 351–369. doi: 10.1038/cr.2015.22

Gorissen, M., Manuel, R., Pelgrim, T. N. M., Mes, W., de Wolf, M. J. S., Zethof, J., et al. (2015). Differences in inhibitory avoidance, cortisol, and brain gene expression in TL and AB zebrafish. *Genes Brain Behav.* 14, 428–438. doi: 10.1111/gbb.12220

Haddon, C., Jiang, Y.-J., Smithers, L., and Lewis, J. (1998). Delta-Notch signalling and the pattering of sensory cell differentiation in the zebrafish ear: evidence from the *mind bomb* mutant. *Development* 125, 4637–4644.

Hailey, D. W., Esterberg, R., Linbo, T., Rubel, E. W., and Raible, D. W. (2017). Fluorescent aminoglycosides reveal intracellular trafficking routes in mechanosensory hair cells. *J. Clin. Invest.* 127, 472–486. doi: 10.1172/JCI85052

Harris, J. A., Cheng, A. G., Cunningham, L. L., MacDonald, G., Raible, D. W., and Rubel, E. W. (2003). Neomycin-induced hair cell death and rapid regeneration in the lateral line of zebrafish (*Danio rerio*). *J. Assoc. Res. Otolaryngol.* 4, 219–234. doi: 10.1007/s10162-002-3022-x

Hausen, J., Otte, J. C., Legradi, J., Yang, L., Strahle, U., Fenske, M., et al. (2017). Fishing for contaminants: identification of three mechanism specific transcriptome signatures using *Danio rerio* embryos. *Environ. Sci. Pollut. Res. Int.* doi: 10.1007/s11356-017-8977-6 [Epub ahead of print].

Heinrich, U.-R., Strieth, S., Schmidtmann, I., Li, H., and Helling, K. (2015). Gentamicin alters Akt-expression and its activation in the guinea pig cochlea. *Neuroscience* 311, 490–498. doi: 10.1016/j.neuroscience.2015.10.050

Hirose, K., Westerum, L. E., Stone, J. S., Zirpel, L., and Rubel, E. W. (1999). Dynamic studies of ototoxicity in mature avian auditory epithelium. *Ann. N. Y. Acad. Sci.* 884, 389–409. doi: 10.1111/j.1749-6632.1999.tb08657.x

Huang, D. W., Sherman, B. T., Tan, Q., Kir, J., Liu, D., Bryant, D., et al. (2007). DAVID bioinformatics resources: expanded annotation database and novel algorithms to better extract biology from large gene lists. *Nucleic Acids Res.* 35, W169–W175. doi: 10.1093/nar/gkm415

Jadali, A., and Kwan, K. Y. (2016). Activation of PI3K signaling prevents aminoglycoside-induced hair cell death in the murine cochlea. *Biol. Open* 5, 698–708. doi: 10.1242/bio.016758

Jadali, A., Ying, Y.-L. M., and Kwan, K. Y. (2017). Activation of CHK1 in supporting cells indirectly promotes hair cell survival. *Front. Cell. Neurosci.* 11:137. doi: 10.3389/fncel.2017.00137

Jiang, H., Sha, S.-H., Forge, A., and Schacht, J. (2006a). Caspase-independent pathways of hair cell death induced by kanamycin *in vivo*. *Cell Death Differ.* 13, 20–30.

Jiang, H., Sha, S.-H., and Schacht, J. (2006b). Kanamycin alters cytoplasmic and nuclear phosphoinositide signaling in the organ of Corti *in vivo*. *J. Neurochem.* 99, 269–276.

Ko, M., Yang, M. L., Youn, S. C., Lan, C. T., and Tseng, T. J. (2016). Intact subepidermal nerve fibers mediated mechanical hypersensitivity via the activation of protein kinase C gamma in spare nerve injury. *Mol. Pain* 12:1744806916656189. doi: 10.1177/1744806916656189

Kong, E. Y., Yeung, W. K., Chan, T. K. Y., Cheng, S. H., and Yu, K. N. (2016). Exogenous nitric oxide suppresses *in vivo* x-ray-induced targeted and non-targeted effects in zebrafish embryos. *Int. J. Mol. Sci.* 17:1321. doi: 10.3390/ijms17081321

Lecain, E., Omri, B., Behar-Cohen, F., Tran Ba Huy, P., and Crisanti, P. (2007). The role of PKCζ in amikacin-induced apoptosis in the cochlea: prevention by aspirin. *Apoptosis* 12, 333–342. doi: 10.1007/s10495-006-0580-0

Lewis, E. M., Wilkinson, A. S., Davis, N. Y., Horita, D. A., and Wilkinson, J. C. (2011). Nondegradative ubiquitination of apoptosis inducing factor (AIF) by X-linked inhibitor of apoptosis at a residue critical for AIF-mediated chromatin degradation. *Biochemistry* 50, 11084–11096. doi: 10.1021/bi201483g

Mao, P., Wyrick, J. J., Roberts, S. A., and Smerdon, M. J. (2017). UV-induced DNA damage and mutagenesis in chromatin. *Photochem. Photobiol.* 93, 216–228. doi: 10.1111/php.12646

Matsui, J. I., Gale, J. E., and Warchol, M. E. (2004). Critical signaling events during the aminoglycoside-induced death of sensory hair cells *in vitro*. *J. Neurobiol.* 61, 250–266. doi: 10.1002/neu.20054

Matsui, J. I., Ogilvie, J. M., and Warchol, M. E. (2002). Inhibition of caspases prevents ototoxic and ongoing hair cell death. *J. Neurosci.* 22, 1218–1227.

Maurin, M., and Raoult, D. (2001). Use of aminoglycosides in treatment of infections due to intracellular bacteria. *Antimicrob. Agents Chemother.* 45, 2977–2986. doi: 10.1128/AAC.45.11.2977-2986.2001

May, L. A., Kramarenko, I. I., Brandon, C. S., Voelkel-Johnson, C., Roy, S., Truong, K., et al. (2013). Inner ear supporting cells protect hair cells by secreting HSP70. *J. Clin. Invest.* 123, 3577–3587. doi: 10.1172/JCI68480

McFadden, S. L., Ding, D., Salvemini, D., and Salvi, R. J. (2003). M40403, a superoxide dismutase mimetic, protects cochlear hair cells from gentamicin, but not cisplatin toxicity. *Toxicol. Appl. Pharmacol.* 186, 46–54. doi: 10.1016/S0041-008X(02)00017-0

Monroe, J. D., Manning, D. P., Uribe, P. M., Bhandiwad, A., Sisneros, J. A., Smith, M. E., et al. (2016). Hearing sensitivity differs between zebrafish lines used in auditory research. *Hear. Res.* 341, 220–231. doi: 10.1016/j.heares.2016.09.004

Montgomery, J. C., Baker, C. F., and Carton, A. G. (1997). The lateral line can mediate rheotaxis in fish. *Nature* 389, 960–963. doi: 10.1038/40135

Montojo, J., Zuberi, K., Rodriguez, H., Kazi, F., Wright, G., Donaldson, S. L., et al. (2010). GeneMANIA Cytoscape plugin: fast gene function predictions on the desktop. *Bioinformatics* 26, 2927–2928. doi: 10.1093/bioinformatics/btq562

Mora, A., Komander, D., van Aalten, D. M., and Alessi, D. R. (2004). PDK1, the master regulator of AGC kinase signal transduction. *Semin. Cell Dev. Biol.* 15, 161–170. doi: 10.1016/j.semcdb.2003.12.022

Murakami, S. L., Cunningham, L. L., Werner, L. A., Bauer, E., Pujol, R., Raible, D. W., et al. (2003). Developmental differences in susceptibility to neomycin-induced hair cell death in the lateral line neuromasts of zebrafish (*Danio rerio*). *Hear. Res.* 186, 47–56. doi: 10.1016/S0378-5955(03)00259-4

Ou, H. C., Raible, D. W., and Rubel, E. W. (2007). Cisplatin-induced hair cell loss in zebrafish (*Danio rerio*) lateral line. *Hear. Res.* 233, 46–53. doi: 10.1016/j.heares.2007.07.003

Owens, K. N., Coffin, A. B., Hong, L. S., O'Connell Bennett, K., Rubel, E. W., and Raible, D. W. (2009). Response of mechanosensory hair cells of the zebrafish lateral line to aminoglycosides reveals distinct cell death pathways. *Hear. Res.* 253, 32–41. doi: 10.1016/j.heares.2009.03.001

Owens, K. N., Cunningham, D. E., MacDonald, G., Rubel, E. W., Raible, D. W., and Pujol, R. (2007). Ultrastructural analysis of aminoglycoside- induced hair cell death in the zebrafish lateral line reveals an early mitochondrial response. *J. Comp. Neurol.* 502, 522–543. doi: 10.1002/cne.21345

Poirrier, A. L., Pincemail, J., Van Den Ackerveken, P., Lefebvre, P. P., and Malgrange, B. (2010). Oxidative stress in the cochlear: an update. *Curr. Med. Chem.* 17, 3591–3604. doi: 10.2174/092986710792927895

Raible, D. W., and Kruse, G. J. (2000). Organization of the lateral line system in embryonic zebrafish. *J. Comp. Neurol.* 421, 189–198. doi: 10.1002/(SICI)1096-9861(20000529)421:2<189::AID-CNE5>3.0.CO;2-K

Rizzi, M. D., and Hirose, K. (2007). Aminoglycoside ototoxicity. *Curr. Opin. Otolaryngol. Head Neck Surg.* 15, 352–357. doi: 10.1097/MOO.0b013e3282ef772d

Santos, F., MacDonald, G., Rubel, E. W., and Raible, D. W. (2006). Lateral line hair cell maturation is a determinant of aminoglycoside susceptibility in zebrafish (*Danio rerio*). *Hear. Res.* 213, 25–33. doi: 10.1016/j.heares.2005.12.009

Schacht, J., Talaska, A., and Rybak, L. (2012). Cisplatin and aminoglycoside antibiotics: hearing loss and its prevention. *Anat. Rec.* 295, 1837–1850. doi: 10.1002/ar.22578

Schmidt, J. T., Fleming, M. R., and Leu, B. (2004). Presynaptic protein kinase C controls maturation and branch dynamics of developing retinotectal arbors: possible role in activity-driven sharpening. *J. Neurobiol.* 58, 328–340. doi: 10.1002/neu.10286

Sugahara, K., Rubel, E. W., and Cunningham, L. L. (2006). JNK signaling in neomycin-induced vestibular hair cell death. *Hear. Res.* 221, 128–135. doi: 10.1016/j.heares.2006.08.009

Sullivan, M. J., Rarey, K. E., and Conolly, R. B. (1987). Comparative ototoxicity of gentamicin in the guinea pig and two strains of rats. *Hear. Res.* 31, 161–167. doi: 10.1016/0378-5955(87)90122-5

Sun, S., Sun, M., Zhang, Y., Cheng, C., Waqas, M., Yu, H., et al. (2014). *In vivo* overexpression of X-linked inhibitor of apoptosis protein protects against neomycin-induced hair ell loss in the apical turn of the cochlea during the ototoxic-sensitive period. *Front. Cell. Neurosci.* 8:248. doi: 10.3389/fncel.2014.00248

Tabuchi, K., Pak, K., Chavez, E., and Ryan, A. F. (2007). Role of inhibitor of apoptosis protein in gentamicin-induced cochlear hair cell damage. *Neuroscience* 149, 213–222. doi: 10.1016/j.neuroscience.2007.06.061

Taleb, M., Brandon, C. S., Lee, F. S., Lomax, M. I., Dillmann, W. H., and Cunningham, L. L. (2008). Hsp70 inhibits aminoglycoside-induced hair cell death and is necessary for the protective effect of heat shock. *J. Assoc. Res. Otolaryngol.* 9, 277–289. doi: 10.1007/s10162-008-0122-2

Taylor, R. R., Nevill, G., and Forge, A. (2008). Rapid hair cell loss: a mouse model for cochlear lesions. *J. Assoc. Res. Otolaryngol.* 9, 44–64. doi: 10.1007/s10162-007-0105-8

Uribe, P., Kawas, L., Harding, J., and Coffin, A. B. (2015). Hepatocyte growth factor mimetic protects lateral line hair cells from aminoglycoside exposure. *Front. Cell. Neurosci.* 9:3. doi: 10.3389/fncel.2015.00003

van den Bos, R., Mes, W., Galligani, P., Heil, A., Zethof, J., Flik, G., et al. (2017). Further characterization of differences between TL and AB zebrafish (*Danio rerio*): gene expression, physiology and behavior at day 5 of the larval stage. *PLOS ONE* 12:e0175420. doi: 10.1371/journal.pone.0175420

Vied, C. M., Freudenberg, F., Wang, Y., Raposo, A. A., Feng, D., and Nowakowski, R. S. (2014). A multi-resource data integration approach: identification of candidate genes regulating cell proliferation during neocortical development. *Front. Neurosci.* 8:257. doi: 10.3389/fnins.2014.00257

Vince, J. E., Wong, W. W.-L., Khan, N., Feltham, R., Chau, D., Ahmad, A. U., et al. (2007). IAP antagonists target cIAP1 to induced TNFα-dependent apoptosis. *Cell* 131, 682–693. doi: 10.1016/j.cell.2007.10.037

Wang, J., Van de Water, T. R., Bonny, C., de Ribaupierre, F., Puel, J. L., and Zine, A. (2003). A peptide inhibitor of c-Jun N-terminal kinase protects against both aminoglycoside and acoustic trauma-induced auditory hair cell death and hearing loss. *J. Neurosci.* 23, 8596–8607.

West, A. C., Martin, B. P., Andrews, D. A., Hogg, S. J., Banerjee, A., Grigoriadis, G., et al. (2016). The SMAC mimetic, LCL-161, reduces survival in aggressive MYC-driven lymphoma while promoting susceptibility to endotoxic shock. *Oncogenesis* 5, e216. doi: 10.1038/oncsis.2016.26

Westerfield, M. (2000). *The Zebrafish Book: A Guide for Laboratory Use of Zebrafish (Danio rerio)*, 4th Edn. Eugene, OR: University of Oregon Press.

Wilhelm, C. J., Choi, D., Huckans, M., Manthe, L., and Loftis, J. M. (2012). Adipocytokine signaling is altered in Flinders sensitive line rats, and adiponectin correlates in humans with some symptoms of depression. *Pharmacol. Biochem. Behav.* 103, 643–651. doi: 10.1016/j.pbb.2012.11.001

Wu, W.-J., Sha, S.-H., McLaren, J. D., Kawamoto, K., Raphael, Y., and Schacht, J. (2001). Aminoglycoside ototoxicity in adult CBA, C57BL and BALB mice and the Sprague-Dawley rat. *Hear. Res.* 158, 165–178. doi: 10.1016/S0378-5955(01)00303-3

Xie, J., Talaska, A. E., and Schacht, J. (2011). New developments in aminoglycoside therapy and ototoxicity. *Hear. Res.* 281, 28–37. doi: 10.1016/j.heares.2011.05.008

Yabu, T., Shiba, H., Shibasaki, Y., Nakanishi, T., Imamura, S., Touhata, K., et al. (2015). Stress-induced ceramide generation and apoptosis via the phosphorylation and activation of sSMase1 by JNK signaling. *Cell Death Differ.* 22, 258–273. doi: 10.1038/cdd.2014.128

Zabiewicz, J., Pearn, L., Hills, R. K., Morgan, R. G., Tonks, A., Burnett, A. K., et al. (2014). The PDK1 master kinase is over-expressed in acute myeloid leukemia and promotes PKC-mediated survival of leukemic blasts. *Haematologica* 99, 858–864. doi: 10.3324/haematol.2013.096487

Zeng, Z., Richardson, J., Verduzco, D., Mitchell, D. L., and Patton, E. E. (2009). Zebrafish have a competent p53-dependent nucleotide excision repair pathway to resolve ultraviolet B-induced DNA damage in the skin. *Zebrafish* 6, 405–415. doi: 10.1089/zeb.2009.0611

Zhang, D., Fan, Z., Han, Y., Bai, X., Liu, W., Lu, S., et al. (2012). Apoptosis-inducing factor is involved in gentamicin-induced vestibular hair cell death. *ORL J. Otorhinolaryngol. Relat. Spec.* 74, 1–5. doi: 10.1159/000333251

Zimmermann, K. C., Bonzon, C., and Green, D. R. (2001). The machinery of programmed cell death. *Pharmacol. Ther.* 92, 57–70. doi: 10.1016/S0163-7258(01)00159-0

3

Hydrogen Inhalation Protects against Ototoxicity Induced by Intravenous Cisplatin in the Guinea Pig

Anette E. Fransson[1], Marta Kisiel[1], Kristian Pirttilä[2], Curt Pettersson[2], Pernilla Videhult Pierre[3†] and Göran F. E. Laurell[1†]*

[1] Department of Surgical Science, Uppsala University, Uppsala, Sweden, [2] Division of Analytical Pharmaceutical Chemistry, Department of Medical Chemistry, Uppsala University, Uppsala, Sweden, [3] Division of Audiology, Department of Clinical Science, Intervention and Technology, Karolinska Institutet, Stockholm, Sweden

Edited by:
Lisa Cunningham,
National Institutes of Health (NIH),
United States

Reviewed by:
Leonard Rybak,
Southern Illinois University School of Medicine, United States
Shikha Tarang,
Creighton University, United States

***Correspondence:**
Anette E. Fransson
anette.fransson@surgsci.uu.se

†Shared senior authorship.

Introduction: Permanent hearing loss and tinnitus as side-effects from treatment with the anticancer drug cisplatin is a clinical problem. Ototoxicity may be reduced by co-administration of an otoprotective agent, but the results in humans have so far been modest.

Aim: The present preclinical *in vivo* study aimed to explore the protective efficacy of hydrogen (H_2) inhalation on ototoxicity induced by intravenous cisplatin.

Materials and Methods: Albino guinea pigs were divided into four groups. The Cispt ($n = 11$) and Cispt+H_2 ($n = 11$) groups were given intravenous cisplatin (8 mg/kg b.w., injection rate 0.2 ml/min). Immediately after, the Cispt+H_2 group also received gaseous H_2 (2% in air, 60 min). The H_2 group ($n = 5$) received only H_2 and the Control group ($n = 7$) received neither cisplatin nor H_2. Ototoxicity was assessed by measuring frequency specific ABR thresholds before and 96 h after treatment, loss of inner (IHCs) and outer (OHCs) hair cells, and by performing densitometry-based immunohistochemistry analysis of cochlear synaptophysin, organic transporter 2 (OCT2), and copper transporter 1 (CTR1) at 12 and 7 mm from the round window. By utilizing metabolomics analysis of perilymph the change of metabolites in the perilymph was assessed.

Results: Cisplatin induced electrophysiological threshold shifts, hair cell loss, and reduced synaptophysin immunoreactivity in the synapse area around the IHCs and OHCs. H_2 inhalation mitigated all these effects. Cisplatin also reduced the OCT2 intensity in the inner and outer pillar cells and in the stria vascularis as well as the CTR1 intensity in the synapse area around the IHCs, the Deiters' cells, and the stria vascularis. H_2 prevented the majority of these effects.

Conclusion: H_2 inhalation can reduce cisplatin-induced ototoxicity on functional, cellular, and subcellular levels. It is proposed that synaptopathy may serve as a marker for cisplatin ototoxicity. The effect of H_2 on the antineoplastic activity of cisplatin needs to be further explored.

Keywords: ABR, inner hair cells, outer hair cells, synaptophysin, organic cation transporter 2, copper transporter 1, perilymph metabolomics, *in vivo*

INTRODUCTION

Hearing disabilities can be the result of exogenous factors such as exposure to noise and treatment with drugs that have ototoxic side effects. Oncologic treatment using cisplatin-based therapy, is a common cause of drug-induced hearing loss, especially when high doses are given. Cisplatin is among the first generation of platinum-based anticancer agents and is widely used to treat different tumors in both children and adults. Cisplatin can enter the cochlea (Laurell et al., 1995; Hellberg et al., 2013), likely via passive membrane diffusion and active uptake to vulnerable cells. The details of this transport are still not fully elucidated, but organic cation transporter 2 (OCT2) (Ciarimboli et al., 2010) and copper transporter 1 (CTR1) (More et al., 2010) have been implicated in cisplatin uptake to the inner ear.

Inside the cochlea, cisplatin can damage the organ of Corti, spiral ganglion, stria vascularis, and spiral ligament (van Ruijven et al., 2005; Rybak, 2007). At the cellular level, cisplatin-induced ototoxicity typically manifests as loss of outer hair cells (OHCs), mainly in the basal turn of the cochlea, resulting in high-frequency hearing loss (Rybak, 2007). Effects on subcellular compartments are less understood. Recent data suggest that cochlear synaptopathy is a key to acquired hearing loss (Liberman and Kujawa, 2017); however, its role in cisplatin-induced ototoxicity is unknown.

Preclinical experiments suggest that underlying mechanisms of cisplatin-induced ototoxicity include the formation of platinum-DNA adducts, inflammation, and oxidative stress (Rybak, 2007). A number of experimental studies have shown that it is possible to reduce cisplatin ototoxicity by co-administrating an otoprotective drug (Rybak, 2007). However, no otoprotective therapy has clearly attenuated cisplatin ototoxicity in clinical practice.

Pharmacological treatment of the inner ear can involve either systemic or local drug administration, and both have advantages and disadvantages. Systemic administration is a well-established method that can be non-invasive (e.g., oral) or invasive (e.g., intravenous). One challenge is that the cochlea possesses at least two barrier systems, the blood-perilymph and intrastrial fluid-blood barriers (Cohen-Salmon et al., 2007; Shi, 2016), that prevent drugs in systemic circulation from accessing the cochlear compartments. Another challenge is that systemic distribution of a drug may lead to unwanted effects in other systems. Unwanted effects of antioxidant treatment to prevent cisplatin-induced ototoxicity include inhibition of the antineoplastic efficacy of cisplatin (Freyer et al., 2017), stimulation of tumor growth (Sayin et al., 2014), and metastasis (Le Gal et al., 2015). These effects are unacceptable in humans with cancer but difficult to study in experimental models. The literature offers limited information in this area, although there are several experimental studies describing otoprotective (Rybak, 2007) and nephroprotective (dos Santos et al., 2012) effects with concomitant use of drugs with antioxidative effects. An alternative to systemic administration is local drug delivery, which makes it possible to achieve a high drug concentration in the target organ, thereby reducing the risk of unwanted effects in other parts of the body. Some pharmacological agents that have been applied systemically have also been tested for intratympanic administration. Local treatment of the inner ear can only be performed with invasive techniques, and its clinical use is currently limited to steroid treatment for sudden sensorineural hearing loss after failure of systemic steroid treatment (Li et al., 2015) and destructive treatment of vertigo with gentamicin in Ménière's disease (Pullens and van Benthem, 2011).

Multiple candidate substances, mostly antioxidants, have been tested to prevent cisplatin-induced ototoxicity, but little is known about the importance of different physicochemical properties for otoprotective efficacy. One interesting candidate is molecular hydrogen (H_2) as it is expected to easily penetrate the different cochlear barriers and reach the organ of Corti. H_2 can be given as a gas or an aqueous solution, and it has been shown to have antioxidant (Fukuda et al., 2007; Ohsawa et al., 2007; Xie et al., 2010) and anti-inflammatory (Gharib et al., 2001; Xie et al., 2010) properties. Gaseous H_2 is not explosive at a concentration <4% in air or pure oxygen (Huang et al., 2010). Inhaled H_2 reduced organ damage in different animal models of ischemia (Fukuda et al., 2007; Ohsawa et al., 2007; Huang et al., 2011; Hugyecz et al., 2011). Importantly, cisplatin-induced nephrotoxicity was attenuated by aqueous H_2 in rats (Kitamura et al., 2010; Matsushita et al., 2011) and by aqueous and gaseous H_2 in mice (Nakashima-Kamimura et al., 2009), likely by reducing oxidative stress (Nakashima-Kamimura et al., 2009). With regard to effects related to hearing, aqueous H_2 reduced antimycin A-induced production of reactive oxygen species (ROS) and increased the survival of inner hair cells (IHCs) and OHCs in a cochlear explant study (Kikkawa et al., 2009). In a gerbil model of auditory neuropathy, gaseous H_2 reduced ouabain-induced hearing threshold shifts and spiral ganglia damage (Qu et al., 2012a). In guinea pig models of noise-induced hearing loss, aqueous H_2 was shown to reduce hearing threshold shifts (Lin et al., 2011; Zhou et al., 2012; Chen et al., 2014) and hair cell loss (Zhou et al., 2012; Chen et al., 2014), likely by alleviating oxidative stress (Chen et al., 2014, 2017) and/or inflammation (Chen et al., 2017). Gaseous H_2 also reduced noise-induced hearing threshold shifts, OHC loss, and oxidative stress in a guinea pig study (Kurioka et al., 2014). An important advantage of H_2 is that it is considered safe for human use (Huang et al., 2010).

Based on existing findings, we presumed that H_2 therapy exerts different protective effects at subcellular levels in the inner ear when given in conjunction with systemic cisplatin. The present study aimed to study the otoprotective effects of gaseous H_2 in guinea pigs treated with cisplatin by evaluating auditory brainstem response (ABR) threshold shifts, hair cell loss, and immunohistochemical findings in subcellular structures damaged by cisplatin.

MATERIALS AND METHODS

Study Design

Guinea pigs ($n = 34$) were randomly assigned to four treatment groups: Cispt ($n = 11$), Cispt+H_2 ($n = 11$), H_2 ($n = 5$), or Control ($n = 7$). The Cispt and Cispt+H_2 groups received a single intravenous (i.v.) injection of cisplatin. In the Cispt+H_2

group, this injection was immediately followed by 60-min administration of gaseous H_2. The H_2 group only received 60-min administration of H_2, while the Control group received neither cisplatin nor H_2. Auditory function was assessed with frequency-specific ABR measured prior to and approximately 96 h after cisplatin administration. After the final ABR measurement, the Cispt and Cispt+H_2 groups were subjected to perilymph sampling, after which they were euthanized with a high dose of pentobarbital. The H_2 and Control groups were euthanized immediately after the final ABR measurement. Finally, the animals' cochleae were collected for histological analyses. Two of the animals in the Control group were used for ABR recordings, and five animals were processed for immunohistochemistry.

Animals

Guinea pigs (Duncan-Hartley, Lidköpings Kaninfarm, Lidköping, Sweden) of both sexes, 5–8 weeks old and weighing 250–504 g were used. The animals were kept in an enriched environment and housed in small groups with lights on between 7 a.m. and 7 p.m. at a temperature of 21°C and a humidity of 60%. They were given free access to water and standard chow and were allowed to acclimatize for at least 10 days before the experiment started. All procedures were performed under anesthesia and aseptic conditions. The guinea pigs had normal tympanic membranes and hearing as determined by otoscopic examination and ABR assessment. During the experimental procedures, the animals were placed on a homeothermic pad. Body weight was measured daily. The Cispt and Cispt+H_2 groups were hydrated with sterile saline (5 ml, 37°C) subcutaneously (s.c.) each day after cisplatin exposure. All animal procedures were performed in accordance with the ethical guidelines of Uppsala University and consistent with national regulations for animal care and use (ethical permit C 106/13; Uppsala's ethical committee on animal experiments).

Anesthesia

All experiments were performed on anesthetized animals. General anesthesia was achieved with ketamine (40 mg/kg b.w.; Ketalar, 50 mg/ml; Pfizer AB, Sweden) and xylazine (10 mg/kg b.w.; Rompun, 20 mg/ml; Bayer Health Care AG, Denmark) intramuscularly. The depth of anesthesia was determined by measurement of the pedal reflex, and additional doses of ketamine (25 mg/kg b.w.) were given if needed. Bupivacaine (Marcain, s.c., 2.5 mg/ml, AstraZeneca, Sweden) was used as local anesthesia, and buprenorphine, (0.06 mg, Temgesic, 0.3 mg/ml, s.c.; Schering-Plough, NJ, USA) was used as a post-treatment analgesic in animals subjected to cisplatin administration.

Cisplatin Administration

Cisplatin (8 mg/kg b.w.; Platinol 1 mg/ml; Bristol-Myers Squibb AB, Sweden) was administered at an injection rate of 0.2 ml/min through a catheter (PE50, ID = 0.58 mm, OD = 0.965 mm, Intramedic Clay Adams Brand; Becton Dickinson and Company, NJ, USA) inserted into the right jugular vein toward the heart. Immediately after, 1 ml sterile saline was administered through the same catheter. The catheter was then removed, the jugular vein was ligated, and the skin was sutured (Ethilon II polyamide 4-0).

Regulations from the Swedish Work Environment Act (AFS 2005:5) were followed during cisplatin handling and destruction.

H_2 Administration

H_2 was administered over 60 min using a gas mixture of H_2 (2 mol%), oxygen (O_2; 21 mol%), and nitrogen (N_2; 77 mol%; AGA Gas AB, Sweden). The gas was delivered through a facial mask. The flow rate was set at 0.5 l/min using a single-stage pressure regulator (C 200/1 A B 3 BAR DIN 1, Linde AG, Linde Gases Division, Germany).

ABR

Frequency-specific ABR at 3.15, 6.30, 12.5, 20.0, and 30.0 kHz was recorded to monitor auditory function. The animal was anesthetized as previously described and placed in a soundproof box. The stimulus signal was generated through a signal analyzer (Tucker-Davis Technologies, FL, USA) controlled by a personal computer and presented through an electrostatic speaker (EC1; Tucker-Davis Technologies, FL, USA). The speaker was connected to a 10-cm tube positioned in the guinea pig's ear canal. Neural responses were collected using three subdermal electrodes: one placed at the vertex (active), one placed on the mastoid (reference), and a ground electrode placed at the lower back. The ABR threshold was determined as the lowest stimulus intensity that produced a reproducible response for ABR wave II, which was visualized at the same latency after an average of 1,000 recordings.

Metabolomics Analysis of Scala Tympani Perilymph

About 1 h after the last ABR measurement, animals in the Cispt and Cispt+H_2 groups underwent perilymph sampling from the basal turn of the cochlea as previously described (Hellberg et al., 2013). Perilymph (1 μL) was collected from both ears, diluted 1:19 with water, and stored at −80°C until further handling. Some samples were excluded due to contamination or insufficient volume. Samples were thawed in the refrigerator overnight and subjected to protein precipitation by adding cold acetonitrile (4:1 acetonitrile to perilymph, kept on ice) and centrifuged (4°C, 21,000 RCF, 15 min). The supernatant was stored at −80°C pending analysis and analyzed without further treatment. A quality control (QC) sample was prepared as a mixture of aliquots from all samples. Analysis was performed on a UHPLC-Q-ToF-instrument (Waters, Milford, MA, USA). Data were acquired in resolution MS^E-mode with both ESI+ and ESI− acquisition. Chromatography was performed in HILIC mode by gradient elution using a BEH Amide stationary phase (50 × 2.1 mm, 1.7-μm particle size, Waters, Milford, MA, USA). Mobile phase composition was acetonitrile and water with 5 mM ammonium formate and 0.065% formic acid. Data quality was assessed using data acquired from repeated injections at intervals of the QC sample ($n = 15$, corresponding to ~16% of injections) according to previously described methods (Sangster et al., 2006; Engskog et al., 2016). Data preprocessing was performed in the R statistical language (version 3.3.2) using the XCMS package (Smith et al., 2006) followed by normalization to median fold change and filtering of features by retention time and variance in repeated injections. Multivariate data analysis was performed in SIMCA software (ver. 14.1, Umetrics, Umeå, Sweden). Identification of metabolites was achieved by comparing retention time and mass spectral data against in-house and public databases such as the METLIN database (Smith et al., 2005) and Human Metabolome Database (HMDb) (Wishart et al., 2007, 2009, 2013).

Morphological Analysis

After perilymph sampling in the Cispt and Cispt+H_2 groups or after the last ABR measurement in the H_2 and Control groups, the animal was deeply anesthetized with sodium pentobarbital (25 mg/kg, intraperitoneally) and subsequently decapitated. The temporal bones were removed, and the bullae were opened to expose the cochleae. Small fenestrations were made in the apex and round window (RW), and 4% phosphate-buffered formaldehyde was gently flushed through the cochlea. The left and right ears were used for surface preparation and cryosectioning, respectively.

Surface preparation was performed as previously described (Canlon and Fransson, 1995). Briefly, the bone surrounding the organ of Corti, stria vascularis, spiral ligament, and tectorial membrane was removed. The tissue was rinsed in phosphate-buffered saline (PBS) several times before it was placed in a solution of 1% bovine serum albumin (BSA) and 0.3% Triton-X100 for 10 min. It was then rinsed, incubated with fluorescent-labeled phalloidin (TRITC 1:200, Sigma-Aldrich) for 45 min, and subsequently rinsed multiple times. The organ of Corti was dissected in approximately 3-mm-long sections, which were placed on microscope slides in glycerol, covered with a coverslip, and sealed with nail polish. All IHCs and OHCs throughout the cochlea were examined using a Zeiss Axio Observer.Z1 microscope (Carl Zeiss, Germany) equipped with a ×40 objective. A reticule placed in the focus of the microscope eyepiece allowed for 0.25 mm of the coil to be viewed and analyzed at one time. After analyzing all hair cells and scar formations, the percentage of hair cell loss per millimeter was calculated and plotted on a cochleogram.

The right ear was decalcified in 0.1 M EDTA, rinsed, and placed in 15% sucrose for 1 day followed by a gradual infiltration of 15% sucrose and OCT Cryomount (Histolab, Sweden) for 4 days, ending with only OCT overnight before embedding in OCT and sectioning on a cryostat in 12-μm-thick sections throughout the cochlea. The sections were mounted on SuperFrost Plus slides (Menzel-Gläser, Germany).

Immunohistochemistry

To investigate levels of synaptophysin, OCT2, and CTR1, immunohistochemistry labeling was performed in samples from the Cispt, Cispt+H_2, and Control groups. The antibodies used were monoclonal anti-synaptophysin (mouse igG1 isotype, diluted 1:100; Sigma-Aldrich Inc., USA), rabbit anti-rat organic cation transporter OCT-2 (diluted 1:100; Alpha Diagnostic International, USA), and polyclonal rabbit SLC31A1/CTR1 antibody (diluted 1:500; Novus Biologicals, UK).

All staining procedures except rinsing were carried out in a humidified chamber. The slides were incubated at room temperature for 45 min followed by 15 min in 0.1 M PBS. All slides were treated with 0.3% Triton X-100 for 30 min and then rinsed 3 × 5 min in PBS. Thereafter, blocking was performed in 1% BSA with 5% normal goat serum for synaptophysin and in 1% BSA with 5% normal donkey serum for OCT2 and CTR1. The slides were rinsed and then incubated with the primary antibody overnight at 4°C. The following day, the slides were rinsed 3 × 5 min and then incubated with the secondary antibody, which was Alexa 546 (Life Technologies, USA) for synaptophysin, Alexa 488 (Life Technologies, USA) for OCT2, and Dylight 594 (Jackson ImmunoResearch, USA) for CTR1. All secondary antibodies were diluted 1:400 with blocking solution. After the last rinse (3 × 10 min), a cover slip was mounted with Mowiol (Sigma-Aldrich Inc.) mounting medium.

Immunohistochemistry Analysis

Quantification of synaptophysin, OCT2, and CTR1 was performed with densitometry measurement. The cochlea was analyzed at two points on the basilar membrane, 12 mm (middle turn) and 7 mm (basal turn) from the RW (**Figure 1**), which correlate tonotopically to the frequencies 3.15 and 12.5 kHz (von Békésy, 1960). The images were collected and processed using ImageJ software (1.51j8; National Institutes of Health, Bethesda, MD, USA) (Schneider et al., 2012). All sections were stained at the same time, and all images were taken within 5 days of processing staining.

Figure 2A shows a fluorescent image of the organ of Corti from a guinea pig in the Control group stained for synaptophysin and OCT2. Synaptophysin immunoreactivity in the synapses around the IHCs and OHCs are orange, while OCT2 immunoreactivity, which was particularly strong in the inner and outer pillar cells, is green. The software converts the colors to a gray scale (**Figures 2B,C**) and measures pixel intensity ranging from 0 (black) to 255 (white). These counts were used to quantify the fluorescent intensity of the different regions of interest (ROIs), and the values obtained from the densitometry measurements are referred to as intensity.

The outlines of ROIs were manually traced. The ROI for synaptophysin was the synapse area at the IHCs and OHCs. The ROI for the three rows of OHCs was collected together and calculated as one ROI. The ROI for OCT2 included the inner and outer pillar cells and stria vascularis. The ROI for CTR1 was the synapse area at the IHCs, the Deiters' cells, and the stria vascularis.

For each animal, three sections were analyzed using the densitometry method, and the mean was used to calculate the mean intensity of each group.

Statistics

For each guinea pig, the frequency-specific electrophysiological hearing threshold obtained before treatment was subtracted from that obtained after 96 h. A mixed-design analysis of variance (ANOVA) was conducted to measure the influence of treatment group and frequency on threshold shift after verifying that the assumptions of fairly symmetrical data from populations with equal variances were met. Two treatment groups were included in the analysis (Cispt and Cispt+H_2), and frequency consisted of

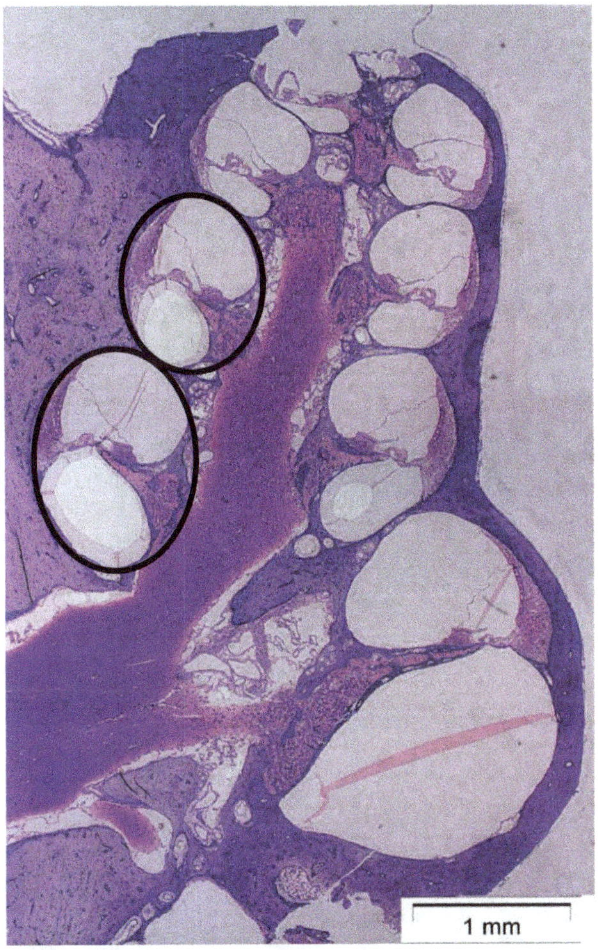

FIGURE 1 | Micrograph showing a mid-modiolar cross-section of a normal guinea pig cochlea. The circles indicate the two points on the basilar membrane, 12 mm (middle turn) and 7 mm (basal turn) from the round window (RW), where the immunoreactivity of synaptophysin, organic cation transporter 2 (OCT2), and copper transporter 1 (CTR1) were analyzed.

five levels: 3.15, 6.30, 12.5, 20.0, and 30.0 kHz. *Post-hoc* analysis was carried out with the Bonferroni test. Statistical analyses were performed using SPSS (v 22, release 22.0.0.1, IBM Corp., USA). To evaluate hair cell loss and immunohistochemistry data, one-way ANOVA was conducted followed by *post-hoc* analysis with the Holm-Sidak method in Sigma (v 13.0, Systat Inc., USA). A two-sided alpha level of 0.05 was used.

RESULTS

The median weight change from the day of cisplatin injection to 96 h after cisplatin injection was −9 g (range: −37–9 g) in the Cispt group and −18 g (−49–10 g) in the Cispt+H_2 group ($p > 0.05$). The values in the H_2 group and two animals in the Control group used for ABR recording were 14 g (2–26 g) and 29 g (26 and 32 g), respectively. Thus, H_2 inhalation did not prevent cisplatin-induced weight loss.

ABR

The differences between the frequency-specific electrophysiological thresholds obtained before and 96 h after cisplatin injection in the Cispt group and the Cispt+H_2 is presented in **Table 1** and the marginal means of threshold shifts are illustrated in **Figure 3**. There was a significant difference across the five frequencies [$F_{(2.01, 40.12)} = 19.34$, $p > 0.001$] and between the Cispt and Cispt+H_2 groups [$F_{(1, 20)} = 6.81$, $p = 0.017$] in threshold shift. There was also a significant interaction between frequency and group [$F_{(2.01, 40.12)} = 6.10$, $p = 0.005$]. *Post-hoc* analysis showed that the threshold shift differed significantly ($p < 0.05$) between different frequencies in the Cispt group but not the Cispt+H_2 group (**Figure 3**). It also showed that the frequency-specific threshold shift was significantly different ($p < 0.05$) between the two groups at 12.5, 20.0, and 30.0 kHz (**Figure 3**). No significant threshold shift was found in the H_2 and Control animals (data not shown).

Metabolomics in Scala Tympani Perilymph

A metabolomics analysis was performed on 14 samples from 10 animals in the Cispt group and 18 samples from 11 animals in the Cispt+H_2 group. Following feature filtering, ~1100 features were used in the multivariate models. Orthogonal Partial Least Squares Discriminant Analysis (OPLS-DA) (Trygg and Wold, 2002) was used to model the difference between the sample groups (R2X 0.219, R2Y 0.375, Q2 0.222 in the predictive component). **Figure 4** shows the sample group separation along the predictive component in the corresponding OPLS-DA scores plot. A total of 50 metabolites were selected by the models as important for class separation using the S-plot for variable selection (Wiklund et al., 2008). Of these, 30 could be putatively identified using database searches. These include choline sulfate, creatinine, methylguanine, methylguanosine, numerous carnitines, proline betaine, methylcytosine, ecgonine, hydroxystachydrine, homostachydrine, creatine, and dimethylarginine.

Morphological Analysis

Quantification of Hair Cell Loss

The morphological changes induced by a single i.v. cisplatin injection were most notable in the basal turn of the cochlea, demonstrating good concordance with the ABR measurements. In the Cispt group, all animals except one showed major OHC loss that was most prominent in the first row. OHC loss started approximately 12 mm from the RW and increased closer to the RW. In this group, five animals showed varying degrees of IHC loss in the basal part of the cochlea. **Figures 5A–C** shows representative cochleograms from animals in the Cispt group.

OHC loss in the Cispt+H_2 group was less pronounced, and no IHC loss was observed. With the exception of one animal, OHC loss was considerably decreased throughout the basilar membrane. The first row of OHC was most affected in this group. In the second and third rows, hair cell loss did not rise above 30% in most animals. The hair cell loss started at 10–12 mm from the RW. **Figures 5D–F** shows representative cochleograms from the Cispt+H_2 group.

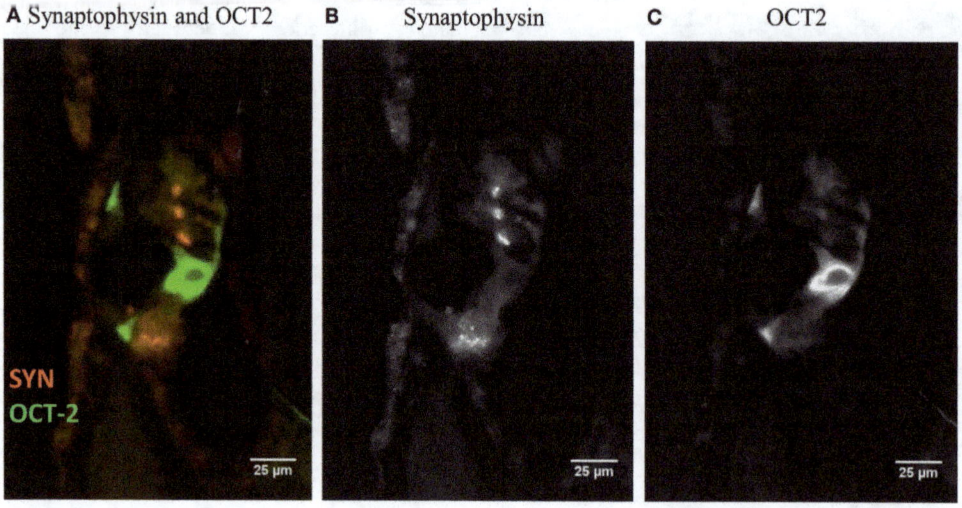

FIGURE 2 | (A) A fluorescent image (40 X) of the organ of Corti from a normal guinea pig. The orange and green labeling indicates immunoreactivity of synaptophysin and OCT2. In order to perform a quantification using densitometry measuring, the software converts the colors to a gray scale, **(B)** synaptophysin and **(C)** OCT2, (CTR1 image not shown). Scale bar: 25 μm.

TABLE 1 | Difference in frequency specific hearing thresholds measured before and 96 h after i.v. injection of cisplatin (8 mg/kg b.w.) to guinea pigs treated with cisplatin only (Cispt group; $n = 11$) or co-treated with hydrogen gas (Cispt+H_2 group; $n = 11$).

	Threshold shift (dB)			
	Cispt		Cispt+H_2	
Frequency (kHz)	Mean	*SD*	Mean	*SD*
3.15	25.9	16.3	15.9	13.2
6.30	29.1	16.3	15.9	16.7
12.5	34.5	14.2	18.2	17.6
20.0	42.3	15.4	20.5	19.0
30.0	44.1	12.8	20.5	17.7

Figure 6 shows the percentages of lost IHCs and OHCs in the first, second, and third rows in the apical, middle, and basal parts of the cochlea. Significantly less loss was noted in the Cispt+H_2 group.

There was a significant difference between the Cispt and Cispt+H_2 groups in total OHC ($p < 0.01$) and IHC ($p < 0.05$) loss, with more intact cells in the Cispt+H_2 group.

Immunoreactivity in the Control group

Three different antibodies were used in this study: synaptophysin, OCT2, and, CTR1. In the Control group, synaptophysin immunoreactivity appeared relatively small and distinct areas under each OHC row (**Figure 7A**). The area of synaptophysin under the IHCs was much larger and lacked distinct borders (**Figure 7A**). OCT2 signal was clearly seen in the inner and outer pillar cells (**Figure 7B**) and was also found in the stria vascularis. CTR1 immunoreactivity was observed in the IHC synapse area, Deiters' cells (**Figure 7C**), and stria vascularis.

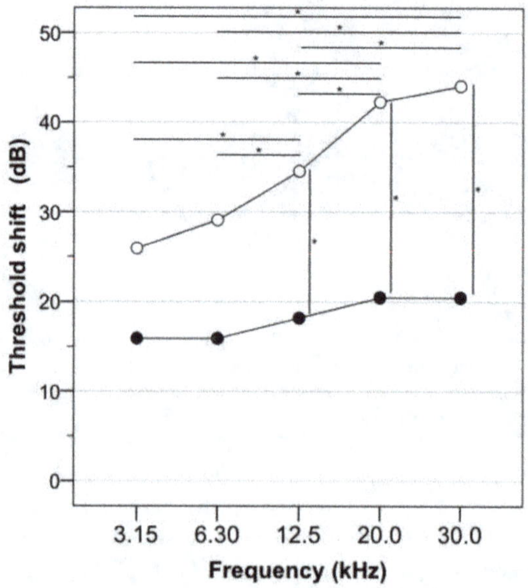

FIGURE 3 | Guinea pigs were subjected to frequency-specific ABR assessment in the left ear before and 96 h after cisplatin injection (8 mg/kg b.w., i.v.). The graph shows the marginal means of the threshold elevations obtained in the Cispt group ($n = 11$; empty circles), which received cisplatin, and in the Cispt+H_2 group ($n = 11$; filled circles), which received cisplatin immediately followed by inhalation of H_2 (2% in air) during 60 min. The horizontal lines with an asterisk indicate a significant difference ($p < 0.05$) between two frequencies, which was obtained only in the Cispt group. The vertical lines with an asterisk indicate a frequency-specific significant difference ($p < 0.05$) between the Cispt group and the Cispt+H_2 group.

Synaptophysin

In the region 12 mm from the RW, there was moderate hair cell loss in the Cispt group and almost no loss in the Cispt+H_2 group. There was a significant difference between these groups in the synapse area of the IHCs ($p < 0.01$, **Figure 8A**) and OHCs ($p < 0.05$, **Figure 8B**). There was also a significant ($p < 0.001$) reduction in the immunoreactivities of both groups compared to Control animals (**Figures 8A,B**).

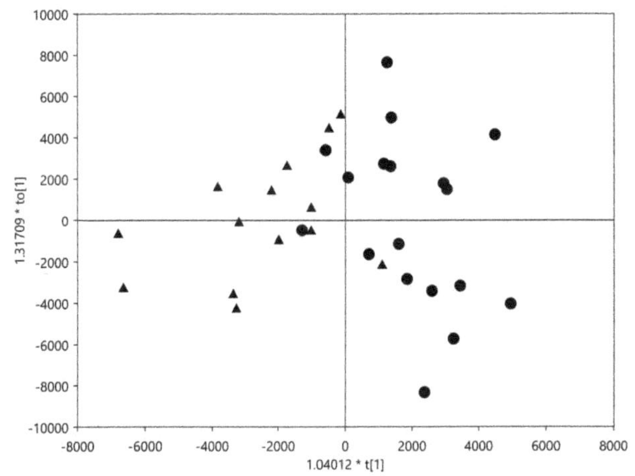

FIGURE 4 | OPLS-DA scores plot (R2X 0.219, R2Y 0.375, Q2 0.222 in the predictive component) of sample Cispt group (triangles) and sample Cispt+H_2 group (circles).

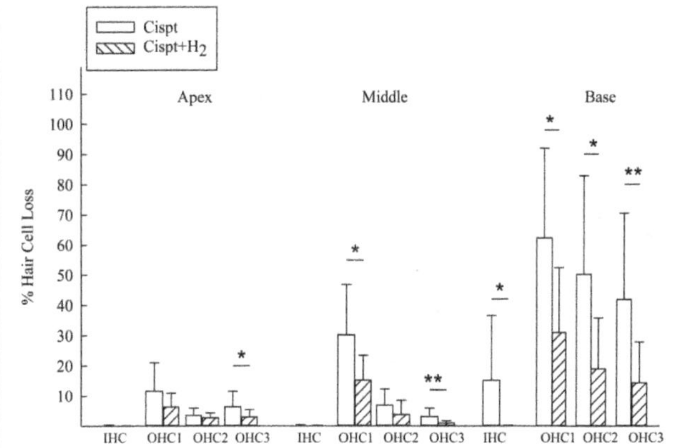

FIGURE 6 | The percentage of lost IHCs and OHCs in the Cispt and Cispt+H_2 groups was summarized in three different regions, Apex (18-14.1 mm from RW), Middle (14-9.1 mm from RW), and Base (9-2.1 mm from RW). *$p < 0.05$ and **$p < 0.01$.

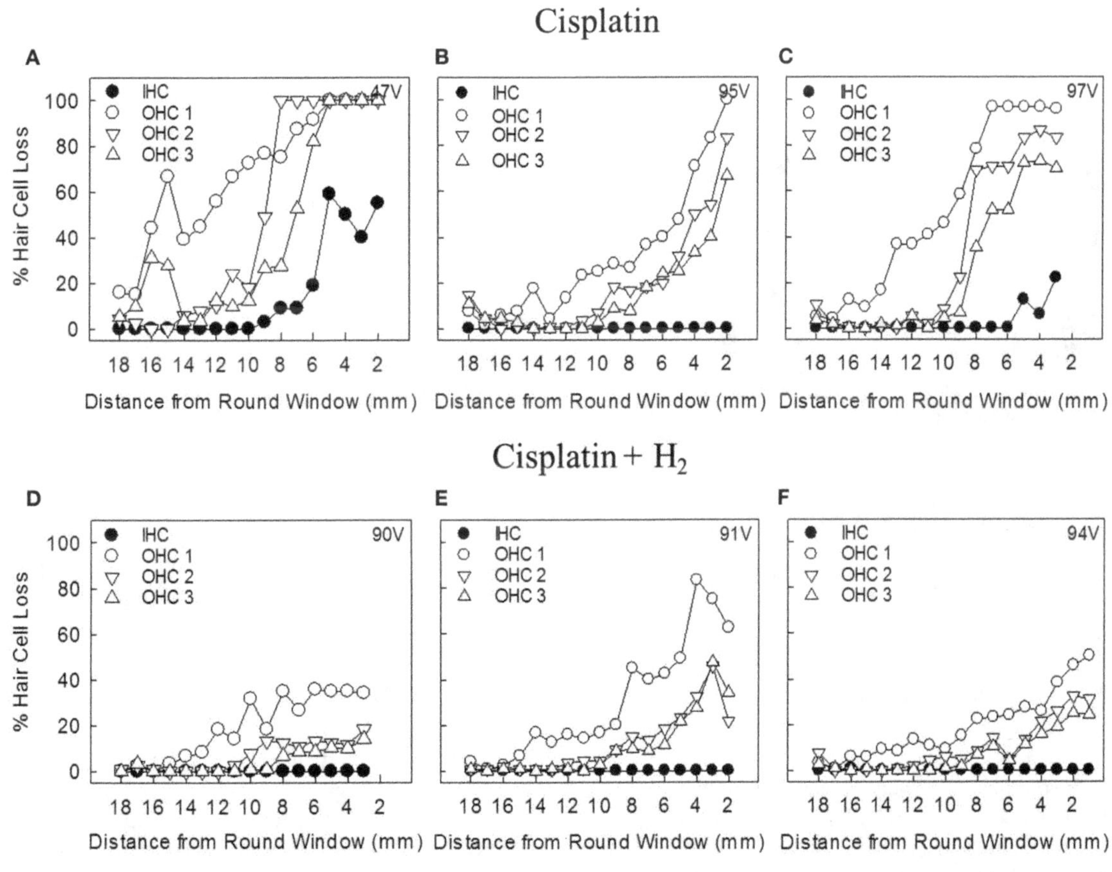

FIGURE 5 | Representative cochleograms from animals in **(A–C)** the Cispt group and **(D–F)** the Cispt+H_2 group. IHC, inner hair cells; OHC 1, outer hair cells of the first row; OHC 2, outer hair cells of the second row; OHC 3, outer hair cells of the third row.

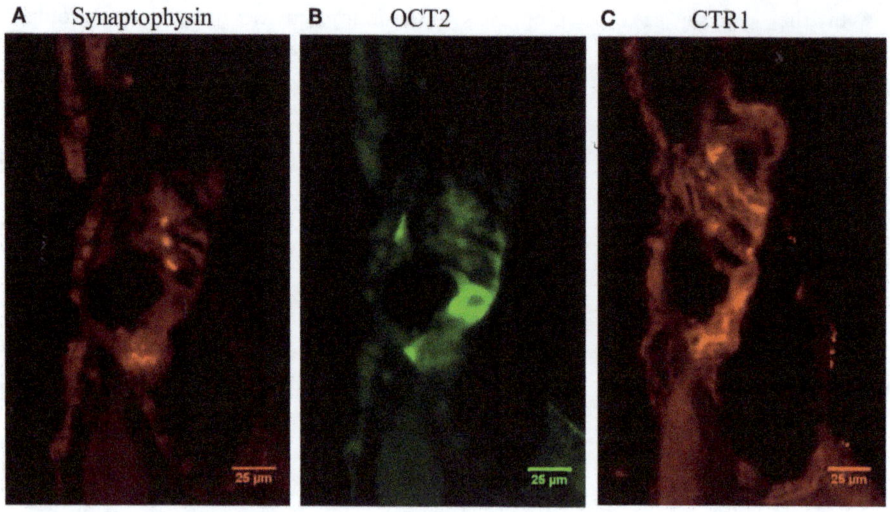

FIGURE 7 | Micrograph (40 X) from a normal guinea pig cochlea (Control group) showing immunoreactivity of **(A)** synaptophysin, **(B)** OCT2, and **(C)** CTR1.

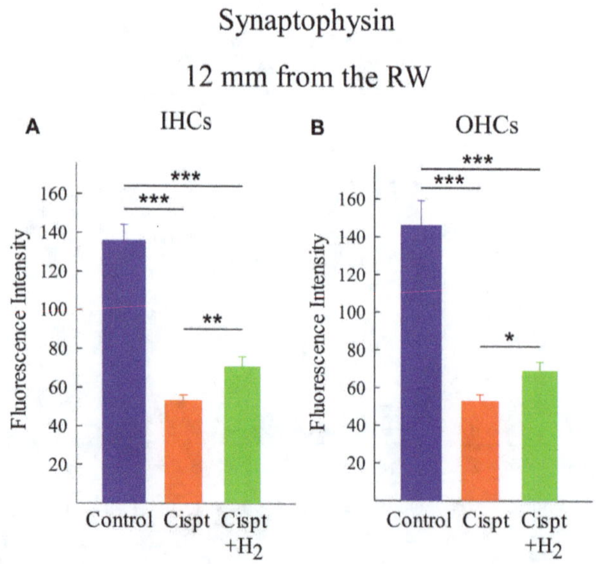

FIGURE 8 | Quantification of the immunoreactivity of synaptophysin, using densitometry, in the synapse area of **(A)** IHCs and **(B)** OHCs at a distance of 12 mm from the RW in the Control group (blue), Cispt group (red), and Cisp+H_2 group (green). The bars illustrate the mean intensity and the error bars represent SD. $^{*}p < 0.05$, $^{**}p < 0.01$, and $^{***}p < 0.001$.

In the region 7 mm from the RW, there was major hair cell loss in the Cispt group, and the organ of Corti had collapsed in some of these animals. Synaptohysin immunoreactivity was seen in most the animals; however, there were too few remaining synapses in the OHC area to perform any statistical comparison with the Cispt+H_2 group. Importantly, immunoreactivity in the Cispt+H_2 was much higher, and synapses were visible around most OHCs. Although the synapse area was reduced, it was still very distinct, but there was a reduction in immunoreactivity compared to the Control group. No statistical difference was found in the IHC synapse areas between the Cispt and Cispt+H_2 groups.

OCT2

In the inner and outer pillar cells 12 mm from the RW, there was a significant difference ($p < 0.05$) between the Control and Cispt groups in OCT2 immunoreactivity, but no difference was found between the Cispt and Cispt+H_2 groups (**Figure 9A**). In the stria vascularis, there was a significant difference between the Control and Cispt groups ($p < 0.001$, **Figure 9B**) and the Control and the Cispt+H_2 groups ($p < 0.01$, **Figure 9B**). In the 7-mm region from the RW, there was a significant decrease ($p < 0.05$) in immunoreactivity of the inner and outer pillar cells in the Cispt group compared to the Control group. In the stria vascularis, there was a significant decrease in both the Cispt and Cispt+H_2 groups compared to Controls (both $p < 0.001$).

CTR1

CTR1 immunoreactivity in the synapse area of IHCs, the Deiters' cells, and the stria vascularis was calculated at 12 and 7 mm from the RW. In the 12-mm region, there was higher immunoreactivity in all areas observed in the Cispt+H_2 group compared to the Cispt group. No significant difference was found in the 7-mm region between the two groups (**Figure 10**).

DISCUSSION

High-dose cisplatin treatment is associated with several toxic insults to the cochlea. Antioxidants were previously shown to protect cochlear structures under experimental conditions. Both systemic and local administration have been employed and demonstrated benefits in experimental animals. Here, we investigated the otoprotective potential of gaseous H_2 given for 60 min starting immediately after albino guinea pigs received

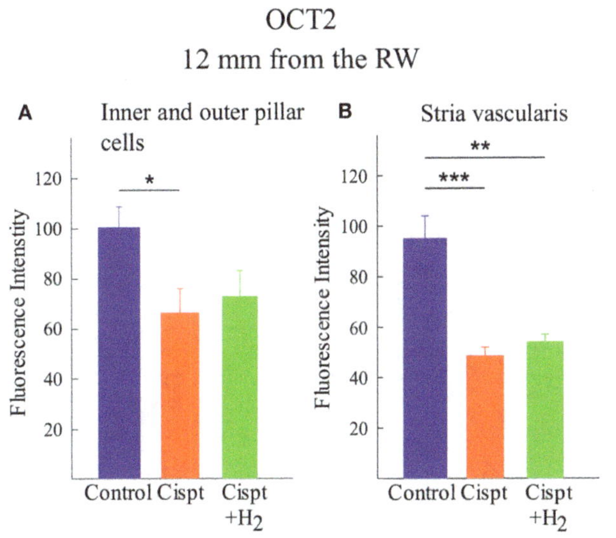

FIGURE 9 | Quantification of the immunoreactivity of OCT2, using densitometry, in **(A)** inner and outer pillar cells and **(B)** stria vascularis at a distance of 12 mm from the RW in the Control (blue), Cispt (red), and Cispt+H_2 (green) groups. The bars illustrate the mean intensity obtained in the three groups and the error bars represent SD. $^{*}p < 0.05$, $^{**}p < 0.01$, and $^{***}p < 0.001$.

a single cisplatin injection. Cisplatin administration caused electrophysiological hearing threshold shifts that were largest at high frequencies. The shifts were partly prevented by H_2 inhalation. The hair cell counts corresponded with the hearing threshold shifts and showed substantial hair cell loss that declined from the base to apex. As previously found (Berglin et al., 2011), OHC loss was greatest in the first row, less in the second row, and least in the third row. There was also some IHC loss in the basal turn of the cochlea, which is less common in cisplatin-treated animals. H_2 inhalation had an important protective effect on OHCs and completely prevented IHC loss. These results agree with those of a previous study, where inhalation of H_2 reduced ABR-assessed threshold shifts and hair cell loss in cisplatin-treated rats (Qu et al., 2012b).

Assessment of threshold shifts and IHC/OHC loss are two rough methods to measure the value of an otoprotective treatment. New, more refined measures are needed to better understand as to the effects of ototoxicologic treatments on cellular and subcellular levels. New insights from animal experiments suggest that synaptopathy plays a key role in hearing damage due to noise, aging, and aminoglycoside treatment, and that it can occur even when hearing thresholds still are normal and hair cells are preserved (Liberman and Kujawa, 2017). These observations indicate that synaptopathy could be an endpoint measure to assess ototoxicological risk and protective treatments. We explored whether synaptopathy may be involved in cisplatin-induced ototoxicity and if it could be prevented by gaseous H_2. We assessed the effect of cisplatin administration without and with concomitant H_2 inhalation on synaptophysin immunoreactivity at the cochlear nerve terminals around the IHCs and OHCs. Measurements were performed 7 and 12 mm from the RW, approximately correlating tonotopically to 12.5 and 3.15 kHz frequencies, respectively (von Békésy, 1960). Although most synapses link IHCs and type I afferent neurons, synapses at the OHCs were also assessed as the OHCs may undergo apoptosis after cisplatin administration. Densitometry analysis was performed to provide a semi-quantitative measure of synaptophysin staining. In many cases, the large destructive effects of cisplatin treatment resulted in collapse of the organ of Corti in the basal turn of the cochlea, which severely hampered the immunohistochemical evaluation at 7 mm. The ROI of synaptophysin was the synapse area of the hair cells. At 12 mm, where threshold changes and OHC loss were less noticeable than at 7 mm and where there was no IHC loss, cisplatin administration still reduced synaptophysin labeling. Notably, this was less pronounced in H_2-treated animals. Evaluation at 7 mm was only possible in the Cispt+H_2 group; there were too few evaluable samples in the Cispt group due to cisplatin cochleotoxicity. Thus, our study shows that synaptopathy might play a role in cisplatin-induced hearing damage. Reduced synaptophysin levels in the inner ear were previously associated with amikacin-induced ototoxicity (Ernfors et al., 1996) and noise trauma (Canlon et al., 1999) in guinea pigs and with aging in mice (Bartolome et al., 2009). Although H_2 inhalation ameliorated the cisplatin-induced change in synaptophysin staining, its protective effect using a post-treatment mode was incomplete. A possible explanation for why partial protection was observed is suboptimal timing. Cisplatin was detected in the scala tympani perilymph just 10 min after i.v. administration in guinea pigs (Laurell et al., 1995; Hellberg et al., 2013). Considering cisplatin's high reactivity, it is possible that a protective agent must already be present in the cochlea to prevent ototoxicity. A second possible explanation is suboptimal dosing. Recognizing the limitations of the methodology and difficulties of knowing the exact pharmacokinetics and pharmacodynamics of H_2 and cisplatin in the inner ear, the results still indicate that H_2 is a promising otoprotective candidate.

Cisplatin is rapidly distributed to the cochlea after systemic administration (Laurell et al., 1995; Hellberg et al., 2013). The details of this transport remain to be elucidated. A study in mice suggested the involvement of the transport protein OCT2 for cochlear uptake of cisplatin (Ciarimboli et al., 2010). Further support for a role of OCT2 was provided by two recent clinical studies that showed an association between a specific gene variant of the OCT2 gene *SLC22A2* and reduced ototoxicity in cisplatin-treated patients (Lanvers-Kaminsky et al., 2015; Spracklen et al., 2016). We therefore wanted to explore the effect of cisplatin administration on OCT2 in the cochlea and whether it was altered by concomitant H_2 inhalation. The ROI of OCT2 included the supporting cells of the organ of Corti (mainly the inner and outer pillar cells) and the stria vascularis. Cisplatin administration reduced OCT2 immunolabeling at 12 mm in both regions, effects that were not prevented by H_2 inhalation. Evaluation at 7 mm was only possible in the Cispt+H_2 group due to extensive cochleotoxicity in the Cispt group. We can only speculate about the causes of reduced OCT2 staining. Possible explanations are that cisplatin alters protein synthesis of OCT2

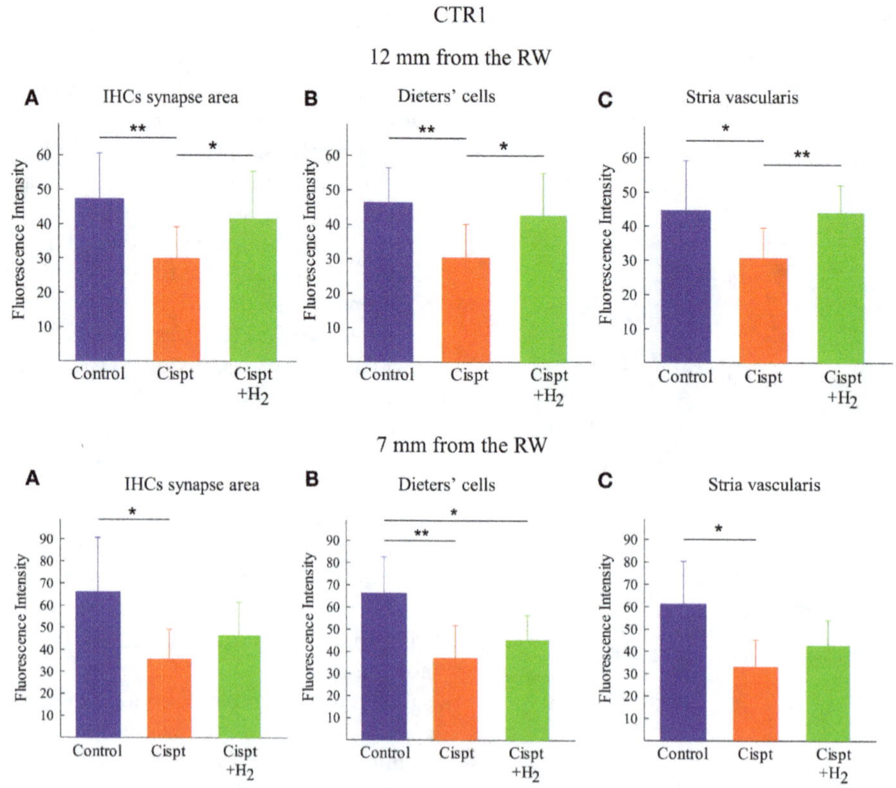

FIGURE 10 | Quantification of immunoreactivity of CTR1, using densitometry. Upper row show the results from the 12 mm region from the RW and the lower row show the results from the 7 mm region from the RW. **(A)** The synapse area of IHCs, **(B)** Dieters' cells, and **(C)** stria vascularis of the cochlea in the control (blue), Cispt (red), and Cispt+H_2 (green) groups. The bars illustrate the mean intensity obtained in the three groups and the error bars represent SD. $^*p < 0.05$ and $^{**}p < 0.01$.

or promotes the apoptosis of OCT2-expressing cells. Another possibility is that cisplatin binds to OCT2 and thereby impairs binding of the OCT2 antibody. The consequences of reduced OCT2 immunolabeling in the cochlea also warrants further investigation. The influence of OCT2 expression on cisplatin-induced nephrotoxicity was first suggested about a decade ago (Yonezawa et al., 2005) and, as recently reviewed, there are many shared feature between cisplatin's ototoxic and nephrotoxic effects (Karasawa and Steyger, 2015). OCT2 is also a determinant of the efficacy of cisplatin-based cancer treatment (Liu et al., 2012). With regard to OCT2 cochlear localization, others have shown that OCT2 can be found in the mouse stria vascularis (Ciarimboli et al., 2010; More et al., 2010) and in IHCs and OHCs (Ciarimboli et al., 2010). Our previous study of guinea pigs revealed OCT2 in the supporting cells of the organ of Corti when using paraffin-sectioning (Hellberg et al., 2015) in contrast to cryosectioning, which was used in the present investigation and in mouse studies (Ciarimboli et al., 2010; More et al., 2010). The tunnel of Corti bordered by the inner and outer pillar cells communicates with the perilymphatic space, and OCT2 expression in these cells indicates that active uptake of cisplatin through this pathway to the endolymphatic space may contribute to OHC toxicity.

Another transporter implicated in cisplatin-induced ototoxicity is CTR1. This protein is abundantly expressed in the mouse cochlea, and pretreatment with the CTR1 substrate copper sulfate decreased cisplatin-induced ototoxicity (More et al., 2010). The ROI of CTR1 was the synapse area of the IHC, Deiters' cells, and the stria vascularis. Cisplatin treatment reduced CTR1 immunolabeling at 12 mm in all these regions, an effect that was prevented by H_2 inhalation. The reduction pattern was similar in the 7-mm region, but the difference between the Cispt and Cispt+H_2 groups did not reach statistical significance. As for the reduction of OCT2 immunolabeling, we can only hypothesize about the causes and consequences of our CTR1 findings. Clinical support for a role of CTR1 in cisplatin-induced ototoxicity remains sparse (Xu et al., 2012), but its importance for cisplatin-induced anticancer efficacy is more established (Liu et al., 2012). There are a number of copper influx and efflux transporters, and several have been shown to be involved in the cellular passage of cisplatin. Future studies that simultaneously investigate both types of copper transporters might increase our understanding in this field. With regard to CTR1 localization within the cochlea, CTR1 was abundantly expressed in the stria vascularis, OHCs, IHCs, and supporting cells in a previous mouse study (More et al., 2010).

As the precise trafficking of cisplatin within the cochlea is not clear, we wanted to further explore the effect of gaseous H_2 on scala tympani perilymph. We aspirated scala tympani perilymph for metabolomics analysis. Although preliminary, the data in the OPLS-DA score plot indicate a clear separation of the Cispt and Cispt+H_2 groups. This finding further supports the possibility that H_2 inhalation can reduce the ototoxic effect of cisplatin within the cochlea before the drug affects the OHCs (i.e., a preventive mechanism before the drug reaches the organ of Corti). This is most likely in line with strategies to prevent cisplatin ototoxicity by intratympanic antioxidant administration. We recently showed that injection of an ototoxic dose of cisplatin to guinea pigs induces a wide range of changes in the blood metabolome (Videhult Pierre et al., 2017).

It is reasonable to speculate that there are important differences between ototoxicity and otoprotection in healthy experimental animals and human beings treated for platinum-sensitive cancer. A major limitation of the study is the focus on the cochlear effects of H_2 administration without an oncologic perspective. We did not evaluate any influence of H_2 on cisplatin cytotoxicity in a tumor target. In cancer research, it is important to assess antitumor activity when introducing a novel co-administrated compound to reduce side effects. Moreover, the hearing situation of patients undergoing cisplatin treatment is more complex, with a number of confounding factors influencing the ototoxic effect. Caution must be taken when interpreting our results obtained in guinea pigs. However, the *in vivo* model reflects a clinically relevant question, although cisplatin administration routes and methods differ from that in clinical practice. For example, we administered a bolus injection of cisplatin, whereas repeated injections are usually given in clinical practice.

The findings in the present investigation raise a number of interesting questions that have to be further studied. Even though our method could be a potentially attractive approach in clinical settings, several issues must be addressed before it can be used as a proof of concept. Antioxidant treatment may have negative effects on cisplatin cytotoxicity in tumors (Freyer et al., 2017) and could even promote tumor growth (Sayin et al., 2014) and metastasis (Le Gal et al., 2015), so more research is needed to develop strategies that circumvent ototoxicity in patients undergoing cisplatin treatment. Substantial effort will be required to assess the effects of H_2 with and without cisplatin on tumor growth and spread. One finding that has not received enough attention is cisplatin's effect on IHC synapses. The observed synaptopathy after a single cisplatin injection could be a target for additional research. In the present study, only H_2 administered after cisplatin was used to prevent ototoxicity. Pre-loading H_2 could be a more effective way to protect hearing. Apart from the discrepancy between the influence of H_2 on OCT2 and CTR1 immunoreactivities, one striking finding in this study was that cisplatin altered immunolabeling of the transport proteins in cochlear tissue. Additional work is needed to clarify the active transport processes involved in cisplatin ototoxicity. Nevertheless, our findings suggest that H_2 administration could prevent cisplatin ototoxicity, but further evaluation is necessary.

CONCLUSION

Although cisplatin is an old drug, it is still frequently used in oncology despite its side effects. There have been no clinical breakthroughs for otoprotection during cisplatin therapy. The present results demonstrate that gaseous H_2 is a promising agent that can protect against cochlear injury. First, H_2 showed an effect on frequency-specific electrophysiological hearing thresholds. Second, surface preparations of the cochlea revealed that OHC loss was attenuated in H_2-treated animals. Third, at the subcellular level, H_2 produced a protective effect on IHC synapses. Hearing loss after cisplatin treatment is multifactorial, and our results implicate synaptopathy as an additional mechanism. Using a guinea pig model for an otoprotective study has some obvious limitations as they cannot be compared with cancer patients. The advantage is the ability to study the inner ear structures in detail after cisplatin treatment, which is not possible in human subjects.

AUTHOR CONTRIBUTIONS

All authors listed, have made substantial, direct and intellectual contribution to the work, and approved it for publication.

ACKNOWLEDGMENTS

The authors wish to thank Mrs. Birgitta Linder for her excellent laboratory work.

REFERENCES

Bartolome, M. V., Zuluaga, P., Carricondo, F., and Gil-Loyzaga, P. (2009). Immunocytochemical detection of synaptophysin in C57BL/6 mice cochlea during aging process. *Brain Res. Rev.* 60, 341–348. doi: 10.1016/j.brainresrev.2009.02.001

Berglin, C. E., Pierre, P. V., Bramer, T., Edsman, K., Ehrsson, H., Eksborg, S., et al. (2011). Prevention of cisplatin-induced hearing loss by administration of a thiosulfate-containing gel to the middle ear in a guinea pig model. *Cancer Chemother. Pharmacol.* 68, 1547–1556. doi: 10.1007/s00280-011-1656-2

Canlon, B., and Fransson, A. (1995). Morphological and functional preservation of the outer hair cells from noise trauma by sound conditioning. *Hear. Res.* 84, 112–124. doi: 10.1016/0378-5955(95)00020-5

Canlon, B., Fransson, A., and Viberg, A. (1999). Medial olivocochlear efferent terminals are protected by sound conditioning. *Brain Res.* 850, 253–260. doi: 10.1016/S0006-8993(99)02091-0

Chen, L., Han, M., Lu, Y., Chen, D., Sun, X., Yang, S., et al. (2017). Molecular mechanisms underlying the protective effects of hydrogen-saturated saline on noise-induced hearing loss. *Acta Otolaryngol.* 137, 1063–1068. doi: 10.1080/00016489.2017.1328743

Chen, J., Yu, N., Lu, Y., Wu, L., Chen, D., Guo, W., et al. (2014). Hydrogen-saturated saline protects intensive narrow band noise-induced hearing loss in guinea pigs through an antioxidant effect. *PLoS ONE* 9:e100774. doi: 10.1371/journal.pone.0100774

Ciarimboli, G., Deuster, D., Knief, A., Sperling, M., Holtkamp, M., Edemir, B., et al. (2010). Organic cation transporter 2 mediates cisplatin-induced oto- and nephrotoxicity and is a target for protective interventions. *Am. J. Pathol.* 176, 1169–1180. doi: 10.2353/ajpath.2010.090610

Cohen-Salmon, M., Regnault, B., Cayet, N., Caille, D., Demuth, K., Hardelin, J. P., et al. (2007). Connexin30 deficiency causes instrastrial fluid-blood barrier disruption within the cochlear stria vascularis. *Proc. Natl. Acad. Sci. U.S.A.* 104, 6229–6234. doi: 10.1073/pnas.0605108104

dos Santos, N. A., Carvalho Rodrigues, M. A., Martins, N. M., and dos Santos, A. C. (2012). Cisplatin-induced nephrotoxicity and targets of nephroprotection: an update. *Arch. Toxicol.* 86, 1233–1250. doi: 10.1007/s00204-012-0821-7

Engskog, M. K. R., Haglöf, J., Arvidsson, T., and Pettersson, C. (2016). LC–MS based global metabolite profiling: the necessity of high quality data. *Metabolomics* 12:114. doi: 10.1007/s11306-016-1058-x

Ernfors, P., Duan, M. L., ElShamy, W. M., and Canlon, B. (1996). Protection of auditory neurons from aminoglycoside toxicity by neurotrophin-3. *Nat. Med.* 2, 463–467. doi: 10.1038/nm0496-463

Freyer, D. R., Chen, L., Krailo, M. D., Knight, K., Villaluna, D., Bliss, B., et al. (2017). Effects of sodium thiosulfate versus observation on development of cisplatin-induced hearing loss in children with cancer (ACCL0431): a multicentre, randomised, controlled, open-label, phase 3 trial. *Lancet Oncol.* 18, 63–74. doi: 10.1016/S1470-2045(16)30625-8

Fukuda, K., Asoh, S., Ishikawa, M., Yamamoto, Y., Ohsawa, I., and Ohta, S. (2007). Inhalation of hydrogen gas suppresses hepatic injury caused by ischemia/reperfusion through reducing oxidative stress. *Biochem. Biophys. Res. Commun.* 361, 670–674. doi: 10.1016/j.bbrc.2007.07.088

Gharib, B., Hanna, S., Abdallahi, O. M., Lepidi, H., Gardette, B., and De Reggi, M. (2001). Anti-inflammatory properties of molecular hydrogen: investigation on parasite-induced liver inflammation. *C. R. Acad. Sci. III* 324, 719–724. doi: 10.1016/S0764-4469(01)01350-6

Hellberg, V., Gahm, C., Liu, W., Ehrsson, H., Rask-Andersen, H., and Laurell, G. (2015). Immunohistochemical localization of OCT2 in the cochlea of various species. *Laryngoscope* 125, E320–E325. doi: 10.1002/lary.25304

Hellberg, V., Wallin, I., Ehrsson, H., and Laurell, G. (2013). Cochlear pharmacokinetics of cisplatin: an *in vivo* study in the guinea pig. *Laryngoscope* 123, 3172–3177. doi: 10.1002/lary.24235

Huang, C. S., Kawamura, T., Toyoda, Y., and Nakao, A. (2010). Recent advances in hydrogen research as a therapeutic medical gas. *Free Radic. Res.* 44, 971–982. doi: 10.3109/10715762.2010.500328

Huang, Y., Xie, K., Li, J., Xu, N., Gong, G., Wang, G., et al. (2011). Beneficial effects of hydrogen gas against spinal cord ischemia-reperfusion injury in rabbits. *Brain Res.* 1378, 125–136. doi: 10.1016/j.brainres.2010.12.071

Hugyecz, M., Mracsko, E., Hertelendy, P., Farkas, E., Domoki, F., and Bari, F. (2011). Hydrogen supplemented air inhalation reduces changes of prooxidant enzyme and gap junction protein levels after transient global cerebral ischemia in the rat hippocampus. *Brain Res.* 1404, 31–38. doi: 10.1016/j.brainres.2011.05.068

Karasawa, T., and Steyger, P. S. (2015). An integrated view of cisplatin-induced nephrotoxicity and ototoxicity. *Toxicol. Lett.* 237, 219–227. doi: 10.1016/j.toxlet.2015.06.012

Kikkawa, Y. S., Nakagawa, T., Horie, R. T., and Ito, J. (2009). Hydrogen protects auditory hair cells from free radicals. *Neuroreport* 20, 689–694. doi: 10.1097/WNR.0b013e32832a5c68

Kitamura, A., Kobayashi, S., Matsushita, T., Fujinawa, H., and Murase, K. (2010). Experimental verification of protective effect of hydrogen-rich water against cisplatin-induced nephrotoxicity in rats using dynamic contrast-enhanced CT. *Br. J. Radiol.* 83, 509–514. doi: 10.1259/bjr/25604811

Kurioka, T., Matsunobu, T., Satoh, Y., Niwa, K., and Shiotani, A. (2014). Inhaled hydrogen gas therapy for prevention of noise-induced hearing loss through reducing reactive oxygen species. *Neurosci. Res.* 89, 69–74. doi: 10.1016/j.neures.2014.08.009

Lanvers-Kaminsky, C., Sprowl, J. A., Malath, I., Deuster, D., Eveslage, M., Schlatter, E., et al. (2015). Human OCT2 variant c.808G>T confers protection effect against cisplatin-induced ototoxicity. *Pharmacogenomics* 16, 323–332. doi: 10.2217/pgs.14.182

Laurell, G., Andersson, A., Engström, B., and Ehrsson, H. (1995). Distribution of cisplatin in perilymph and cerebrospinal fluid after intravenous administration in the guinea pig. *Cancer Chemother. Pharmacol.* 36, 83–86. doi: 10.1007/BF00685738

Le Gal, K., Ibrahim, M. X., Wiel, C., Sayin, V. I., Akula, M. K., Karlsson, C., et al. (2015). Antioxidants can increase melanoma metastasis in mice. *Sci. Transl. Med.* 7:308re8. doi: 10.1126/scitranslmed.aad3740

Li, H., Feng, G., Wang, H., and Feng, Y. (2015). Intratympanic steroid therapy as a salvage treatment for sudden sensorineural hearing loss after failure of conventional therapy: a meta-analysis of randomized, controlled trials. *Clin. Ther.* 37, 178–187. doi: 10.1016/j.clinthera.2014.11.009

Liberman, M. C., and Kujawa, S. G. (2017). Cochlear synaptopathy in acquired sensorineural hearing loss: manifestations and mechanisms. *Hear. Res.* 349, 138–147. doi: 10.1016/j.heares.2017.01.003

Lin, Y., Kashio, A., Sakamoto, T., Suzukawa, K., Kakigi, A., and Yamasoba, T. (2011). Hydrogen in drinking water attenuates noise-induced hearing loss in guinea pigs. *Neurosci. Lett.* 487, 12–16. doi: 10.1016/j.neulet.2010.09.064

Liu, J. J., Lu, J., and McKeage, M. J. (2012). Membrane transporters as determinants of the pharmacology of platinum anticancer drugs. *Curr. Cancer Drug Targets* 12, 962–986. doi: 10.2174/156800912803251199

Matsushita, T., Kusakabe, Y., Kitamura, A., Okada, S., and Murase, K. (2011). Investigation of protective effect of hydrogen-rich water against cisplatin-induced nephrotoxicity in rats using blood oxygenation level-dependent magnetic resonance imaging. *Jpn. J. Radiol.* 29, 503–512. doi: 10.1007/s11604-011-0588-4

More, S. S., Akil, O., Ianculescu, A. G., Geier, E. G., Lustig, L. R., and Giacomini, K. M. (2010). Role of the copper transporter, CTR1, in platinum-induced ototoxicity. *J. Neurosci.* 30, 9500–9509. doi: 10.1523/JNEUROSCI.1544-10.2010

Nakashima-Kamimura, N., Mori, T., Ohsawa, I., Asoh, S., and Ohta, S. (2009). Molecular hydrogen alleviates nephrotoxicity induced by an anti-cancer drug cisplatin without compromising anti-tumor activity in mice. *Cancer Chemother. Pharmacol.* 64, 753–761. doi: 10.1007/s00280-008-0924-2

Ohsawa, I., Ishikawa, M., Takahashi, K., Watanabe, M., Nishimaki, K., Yamagata, K., et al. (2007). Hydrogen acts as a therapeutic antioxidant by selectively reducing cytotoxic oxygen radicals. *Nat. Med.* 13, 688–694. doi: 10.1038/nm1577

Pullens, B., and van Benthem, P. P. (2011). Intratympanic gentamicin for Ménière's disease or syndrome. *Cochrane Database Syst. Rev.* CD008234. doi: 10.1002/14651858.CD008234.pub2

Qu, J., Gan, Y. N., Xie, K. L., Liu, W. B., Wang, Y. F., Hei, R. Y., et al. (2012a). Inhalation of hydrogen gas attenuates ouabain-induced auditory neuropathy in gerbils. *Acta Pharmacol. Sin.* 33, 445–451. doi: 10.1038/aps.2011.190

Qu, J., Li, X., Wang, J., Mi, W., Xie, K., and Qiu, J. (2012b). Inhalation of hydrogen gas attenuates cisplatin-induced ototoxicity via reducing oxidative stress. *Int. J. Pediatr. Otorhinolaryngol.* 76, 111–115. doi: 10.1016/j.ijporl.2011.10.014

Rybak, L. P. (2007). Mechanisms of cisplatin ototoxicity and progress in otoprotection. *Curr. Opin. Otolaryngol. Head Neck Surg.* 15, 364–369. doi: 10.1097/MOO.0b013e3282eee452

Sangster, T., Major, H., Plumb, R., Wilson, A. J., and Wilson, I. D. (2006). A pragmatic and readily implemented quality control strategy for HPLC-MS and GC-MS-based metabonomic analysis. *Analyst* 131, 1075–1078. doi: 10.1039/b604498k

Sayin, V. I., Ibrahim, M. X., Larsson, E., Nilsson, J. A., Lindahl, P., and Bergo, M. O. (2014). Antioxidants accelerate lung cancer progression in mice. *Sci. Transl. Med.* 6:221ra15. doi: 10.1126/scitranslmed.3007653

Schneider, C. A., Rasband, W. S., and Eliceiri, K. W. (2012). NIH image to imagej: 25 years of image analysis. *Nat. Methods* 9, 671–675. doi: 10.1038/nmeth.2089

Shi, X. (2016). Pathophysiology of the cochlear intrastrial fluid-blood barrier (review). *Hear. Res.* 338, 52–63. doi: 10.1016/j.heares.2016.01.010

Smith, C. A., O'Maille, G., Want, E. J., Qin, C., Trauger, S. A., Brandon, T. R., et al. (2005). METLIN: a metabolite mass spectral database. *Ther. Drug Monit.* 27, 747–751. doi: 10.1097/01.ftd.0000179845.53213.39

Smith, C. A., Want, E. J., O'Maille, G., Abagyan, R., and Siuzdak, G. (2006). XCMS: processing mass spectrometry data for metabolite profiling using nonlinear peak alignment, matching, and identification. *Anal. Chem.* 78, 779–787. doi: 10.1021/ac051437y

Spracklen, T. F., Vorster, A. A., Ramma, L., Dalvie, S., and Ramesar, R. S. (2016). Promoter region variation in NFE2L2 influences susceptibility to ototoxicity in patients exposed to high cumulative doses of cisplatin. *Pharmacogenomics J.* doi: 10.1038/tpj.2016.52. [Epub ahead of print].

Trygg, J., and Wold, S. (2002). Orthogonal projections to latent structures (O-PLS). *J. Chemom.* 16, 119–128. doi: 10.1002/cem.695

van Ruijven, M. W., de Groot, J. C., Klis, S. F., and Smoorenburg, G. F. (2005). The cochlear targets of cisplatin: an electrophysiological and morphological time-sequence study. *Hear. Res.* 205, 241–248. doi: 10.1016/j.heares.2005.03.023

Videhult Pierre, P., Haglof, J., Linder, B., Engskog, M. K. R., Arvidsson, T., Pettersson, C., et al. (2017). Cisplatin-induced metabolome changes in serum: an experimental approach to identify markers for ototoxicity. *Acta Otolaryngol.* 137, 1024–1030. doi: 10.1080/00016489.2017

von Békésy, G. (1960). *Experiments in Hearing.* New York, NY: McGraw-Hill.

Wiklund, S., Johansson, E., Sjostrom, L., Mellerowicz, E. J., Edlund, U., Shockcor, J. P., et al. (2008). Visualization of GC/TOF-MS-based metabolomics data for identification of biochemically interesting compounds using OPLS class models. *Anal. Chem.* 80, 115–122. doi: 10.1021/ac0713510

Wishart, D. S., Jewison, T., Guo, A. C., Wilson, M., Knox, C., Liu, Y., et al. (2013). HMDB 3.0–The Human Metabolome Database in 2013. *Nucleic Acids Res.* 41, D801–D807. doi: 10.1093/nar/gks1065

Wishart, D. S., Knox, C., Guo, A. C., Eisner, R., Young, N., Gautam, B., et al. (2009). HMDB: a knowledgebase for the human metabolome. *Nucleic Acids Res.* 37, D603–D610. doi: 10.1093/nar/gkn810

Wishart, D. S., Tzur, D., Knox, C., Eisner, R., Guo, A. C., Young, N., et al. (2007). HMDB: the Human Metabolome Database. *Nucleic Acids Res.* 35, D521–D526. doi: 10.1093/nar/gkl923

Xie, K., Yu, Y., Pei, Y., Hou, L., Chen, S., Xiong, L., et al. (2010). Protective effects of hydrogen gas on murine polymicrobial sepsis via reducing oxidative stress and HMGB1 release. *Shock* 34, 90–97. doi: 10.1097/SHK.0b013e3181cdc4ae

Xu, X., Ren, H., Zhou, B., Zhao, Y., Yuan, R., Ma, R., et al. (2012). Prediction of copper transport protein 1 (CTR1) genotype on severe cisplatin induced toxicity in non-small cell lung cancer (NSCLC) patients. *Lung Cancer* 77, 438–442. doi: 10.1016/j.lungcan.2012.03.023

Yonezawa, A., Masuda, S., Nishihara, K., Yano, I., Katsura, T., and Inui, K. (2005). Association between tubular toxicity of cisplatin and expression of organic cation transporter rOCT2 (Slc22a2) in the rat. *Biochem. Pharmacol.* 70, 1823–1831. doi: 10.1016/j.bcp.2005.09.020

Zhou, Y., Zheng, H., Ruan, F., Chen, X., Zheng, G., Kang, M., et al. (2012). Hydrogen-rich saline alleviates experimental noise-induced hearing loss in guinea pigs. *Neuroscience* 209, 47–53. doi: 10.1016/j.neuroscience.2012.02.028

4

Potential Mechanisms Underlying Inflammation-Enhanced Aminoglycoside-Induced Cochleotoxicity

*Meiyan Jiang[1], Farshid Taghizadeh[1] and Peter S. Steyger[1,2]**

[1] *Oregon Hearing Research Center, Oregon Health & Science University, Portland, OR, United States,* [2] *National Center for Rehabilitative Auditory Research, VA Portland Health Care System, Portland, OR, United States*

Edited by:
Michael E. Smith, Western Kentucky University, United States

Reviewed by:
Karel Allegaert, University Hospitals Leuven, Belgium
Federico Kalinec, University of California, Los Angeles, United States

***Correspondence:**
Peter S. Steyger
steygerp@ohsu.edu

Aminoglycoside antibiotics remain widely used for urgent clinical treatment of life-threatening infections, despite the well-recognized risk of permanent hearing loss, i.e., cochleotoxicity. Recent studies show that aminoglycoside-induced cochleotoxicity is exacerbated by bacteriogenic-induced inflammation. This implies that those with severe bacterial infections (that induce systemic inflammation), and are treated with bactericidal aminoglycosides are at greater risk of drug-induced hearing loss than previously recognized. Incorporating this novel comorbid factor into cochleotoxicity risk prediction models will better predict which individuals are more predisposed to drug-induced hearing loss. Here, we review the cellular and/or signaling mechanisms by which host-mediated inflammatory responses to infection could enhance the trafficking of systemically administered aminoglycosides into the cochlea to enhance the degree of cochleotoxicity over that in healthy preclinical models. Once verified, these mechanisms will be potential targets for novel pharmacotherapeutics that reduce the risk of drug-induced hearing loss (and acute kidney damage) without compromising the life-saving bactericidal efficacy of aminoglycosides.

Keywords: aminoglycosides, gentamicin, ototoxicity, sepsis, infection, bacteriogenic, virogenic, inflammation

INTRODUCTION

In the United States, 12% (~480,000) of ~4 million live births are admitted into the neonatal intensive care unit (NICU) each year (Osterman et al., 2011). NICU patients with confirmed sepsis, or those who develop necrotizing enterocolitis, receive aminoglycosides, typically gentamicin, for 7–10 days or more (Remington, 2011; Blackwood et al., 2017). Yet, clinical use of aminoglycosides carries the risk of permanent hearing loss (cochleotoxicity) that is dose-dependent in preclinical models, and/or acute kidney injury (Forge and Schacht, 2000). The incidence of hearing loss in infants discharged from the NICU ranges between 2 and 15%, compared to 0.3% for full-term babies (Yoon et al., 2003). One factor for this differential prevalence could be cumulative dosing with intravenous administration of aminoglycosides (Garinis et al., 2017c). Another aminoglycoside, tobramycin, induces dose-dependent hearing loss in older pediatric and adult patients with cystic fibrosis that experience repeated severe respiratory infections (Al-Malky et al., 2015; Garinis et al., 2017a). The majority of adults with multi-drug resistant tuberculosis chronically treated with aminoglycosides, typically amikacin or kanamycin over many months, experience permanent hearing loss in a dose-frequency dependent manner (Sagwa et al., 2015).

Only recently have preclinical ototoxicity studies incorporated experimentally induced inflammation (mimicking clinical infections), and found enhanced cochleotoxicity over that in untreated, healthy animals (Oh et al., 2011; Hirose et al., 2014b; Koo et al., 2015). Yet, bacteriogenic induction of experimental systemic sepsis (excluding meningitis and labyrinthitis) has little direct impact on auditory function (Hirose et al., 2014b; Koo et al., 2015). This strongly indicates that systemic inflammatory responses represent a novel co-morbidity that enhances ototoxicity, alongside other better characterized factors such as age, mitochondrial polymorphisms, acoustic trauma, renal dysfunction, and co-therapeutics like loop diuretics or vancomycin (Forge and Schacht, 2000; Garinis et al., 2017b; Jiang et al., 2017). Identifying the factors associated with infection-induced inflammation that increase the risk of aminoglycoside-induced hearing loss will promote new clinical strategies to ameliorate drug-induced ototoxicity. Here, we postulate several mechanisms by which systemic inflammation could exacerbate aminoglycoside-induced cochleotoxicity.

SYSTEMIC INFLAMMATION ENHANCES AMINOGLYCOSIDE-INDUCED COCHLEOTOXICITY

Aminoglycosides are primarily administered systemically to resolve life-threatening bacterial infections that trigger systemic, host-mediated inflammatory responses that rapidly lead to mortality without medical intervention (Mahmoudi et al., 2013). Circulating aminoglycosides readily cross the cochlear blood-labyrinth barrier (BLB) to preferentially load the highly vascularized stria vascularis, and are cleared into endolymph (**Figure 1**). The apical membranes of cochlear hair cells are immersed in endolymph with an electrical potential of +80 mV, while the resting potential of inner and outer hair cells are -45 and -70 mV, respectively (Pickles, 2012). This high potential difference (~135–150 mV) produces a significant electro-repulsive force to drive the cationic aminoglycosides, from endolymph across the apical membranes of hair cells into their electrically negative cytoplasm (Marcotti et al., 2005; Li and Steyger, 2011), with consequent cytotoxic effects (Hiel et al., 1993).

Yet, until recently, most preclinical studies of aminoglycoside-induced cochleotoxicity used healthy preclinical models (Wu et al., 2001; Roy et al., 2013; Duscha et al., 2014). Systemic models of inflammation that mimic infection mediate physiological changes in the blood-brain barrier permeability (Abbott et al., 2006). Bacteriogenic induction of systemic inflammation during chronic aminoglycoside dosing increased the range of frequencies with significant permanent auditory threshold shifts (PTS; **Figure 2**), and extent of outer hair cell death compared to age-matched mice treated with kanamycin alone or saline (Koo et al., 2015). Bacteriogenic induction of systemic inflammation also exacerbated both combinatorial kanamycin/loop diuretic-induced, and also cisplatin-induced, cochleotoxicity (Oh et al., 2011; Hirose et al., 2014b).

A pilot study of NICU subjects (91 subjects) revealed that those with (suspected) sepsis and gentamicin therapy for ≥5 days (18 subjects; 20%) were twice as likely to be referred on a distortion product otoacoustic emission hearing screen compared to all other subjects (Cross et al., 2015). Cystic fibrosis patients with lower lung function scores (indicative of respiratory infection and inflammation) were also more likely to experience cochleotoxicity (Pillarisetti et al., 2011; Al-Malky et al., 2015). The mitochondrial polymorphism most associated with aminoglycoside-induced hearing loss (mt1555A > G) has an incidence between 0.09 and 0.2% (Tang et al., 2002; Bitner-Glindzicz et al., 2009), two orders of magnitude less, and unlikely to statistically influence the number of referred neonates in these studies. Thus, there is an increased risk of drug-induced hearing loss in those receiving aminoglycoside therapy for bacterial infections. Furthermore, 20% of live births with confirmed infection are viral in etiology, yet these infants are empirically treated with aminoglycosides until the causative agent is identified (Remington, 2011). It will be important to determine whether virogenic-induced inflammation enhances cochlear uptake of aminoglycosides and exacerbates cochleotoxicity. To better understand how inflammation could increase cochlear uptake of aminoglycosides, we need to explore inflammatory signaling prior to discussing their potential effect on cochlear uptake mechanisms.

Bacteriogenic and Virogenic Inflammatory Signaling Cascades

Bacterial and viral penetration of blood, tissues and interstitial fluids are typically detected by Toll-like receptors (TLRs) that trigger inflammatory signaling cascades to induce an overwhelming immune response to reduce the risk of pathogenic infection. TLRs are highly conserved pattern-recognition receptors present in diverse cell types, including immune, endothelial, epithelial, and fibrocytes (Atkinson, 2008). There are currently 11 human (and 13 mammalian) TLRs that share common transmembrane domains with leucine-rich repeats that bind to an overlapping array of extracellular (or endosomal) ligands, and a cytosolic signaling domain – the Toll-IL-1 Receptor (TIR) domain (**Figure 3A**). Here, we briefly review the signaling cascades activated by TLR4, the most studied TLR, and also TLR3.

TLR4 (a.k.a CD284, cluster of differentiation 284), was the first to have its specific ligand defined–lipopolysaccharides (LPS) from the cell wall of Gram-negative bacteria (Poltorak et al., 1998). TLR4 is constitutively expressed on the plasma membranes of monocytes, T cells, B cells, and dendritic cells, with induced expression in non-hematopoietic cells (Chakravarty and Herkenham, 2005). Extracellular, soluble LPS-binding protein (LBP) extracts LPS monomers from aggregates released from lyzed bacteria (Schumann et al., 1990). Bound LPS then complexes with CD14 (cluster of differentiation 14), a membrane-anchored glycoprotein, and extracellular lymphocyte antigen 96 (also known as MD2) to activate TLR4 (Shimazu

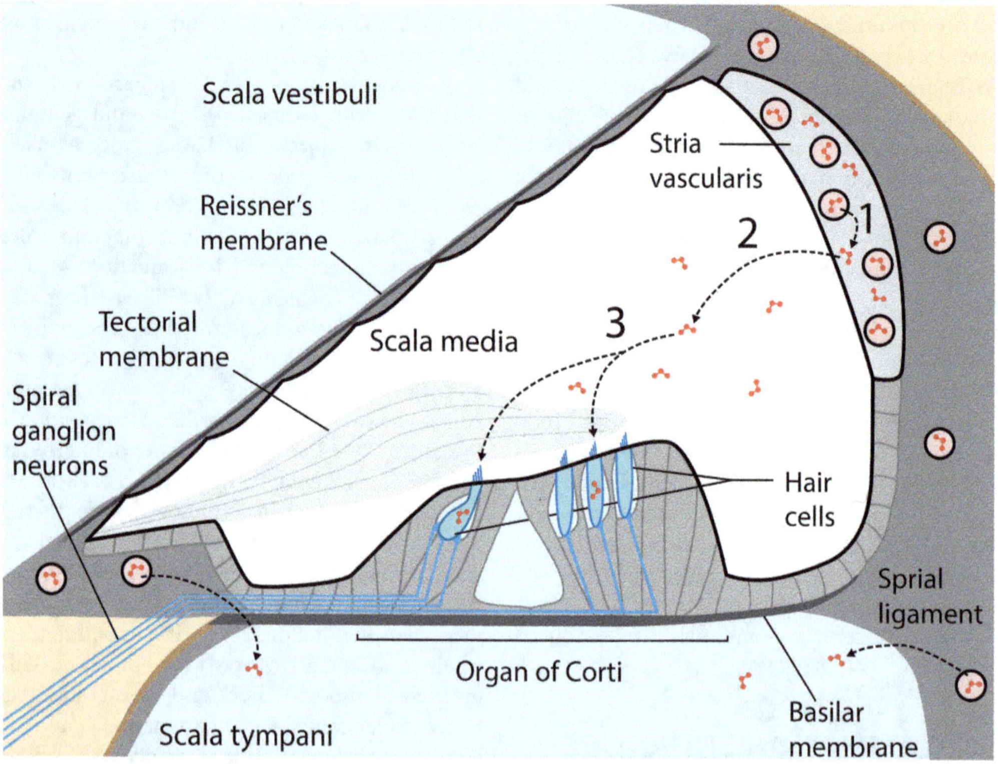

FIGURE 1 | Cross-section of the cochlear duct, with perilymph-filled scala vestibuli and scala tympani (pale blue) separated from the endolymphatic scala media (white) by tight junctions between adjacent cells (thicker black line) in Reissner's membrane, the stria vascularis (light gray) and reticular lamina of the organ of Corti on the basilar membrane. Within the organ of Corti are four longitudinal rows of sensory hair cells (blue), under the tectorial membrane, and innervated by afferent and efferent fibers (blue lines). The highly vascularized stria vascularis has capillaries (pink circles) lined by tight junction-coupled endothelial cells (black lines enclosing pink circles) that form the BLB. Circulating aminoglycosides preferentially cross the BLB into the stria vascularis (1) and are cleared into endolymph (2) prior to entering hair cells across their apical membranes (3). Aminoglycosides also enter perilymph, but this trafficking route is not a major contributor to hair cell uptake in healthy guinea pigs. Diagram not to relative scale, and adapted with permission from Macmillan Publishers Ltd., Li and Steyger (2011).

et al., 1999). The complex facilitates picomolar detection of LPS, otherwise millimolar levels of LPS are required to activate TLR4 directly.

Activated TLR4 triggers one or more TIR domain-containing signaling adaptors: Myeloid Differentiation Primary Response Gene 88 (MyD88), TIR Domain-Containing Adaptor Protein (TIRAP), TIR-domain-containing adaptor inducing interferon-β (TRIF), and TRIF-related Adaptor Molecule (TRAM) that activate individual signaling cascades (Kawai and Akira, 2010; Kim and Sears, 2010; Juskewitch et al., 2012; Hamerman et al., 2016). These cascades are divided into MyD88-*dependent* (MyD88 and TIRAP), and MyD88-*independent* (TRIF and TRAM) signaling cascades (**Figure 3B**). The MyD88-*dependent* pathway signals through IL-1 receptor-associated kinase (IRAK)-4, transforming growth factor-β-activated kinase (TAK) 1, and TAK-binding protein 2 or 3 (TAB2/3) to activate mitogen-activated protein kinase (MAPK) downstream. This in turn leads to the transcription and expression of pro-inflammatory cytokines, such as TNFα, IL-1α, IL-1β, IL-6, or alternatively apoptosis (Takeuchi and Akira, 2009; Guo and Friedman, 2010). The MyD88-*independent* pathway activates IκB kinase (IKK) complex, releasing NF-κB for translocation to the nucleus and transcription of genes for expression of type 1 interferons (O'Neill et al., 2013). Another, complex TIR-domain-containing adaptor protein called Sterile α and HEAT (Armadillo motif; SARM) inhibits the TRIF-mediated (MyD88-*independent*) pathway, and attenuates LPS-mediated signaling to dampen inflammation and abrogate septic shock and multiple organ dysfunction syndrome (Aird, 2003). The time-course of plasma/serum expression profiles for individual acute phase inflammatory (API) cytokines and chemokines changes over hours and days following induction of the inflammatory response (Allan and Rothwell, 2001; Juskewitch et al., 2012).

Viral double-stranded DNA (dsDNA), mRNA, ionizing radiation or hypoxia can activate the ubiquitously expressed TLR3, located on both cell and endosomal membranes, to activate an adaptor protein called TRIF (**Figure 3B**) (Zarember and Godowski, 2002; Kawai and Akira, 2010). TRIF initiates two pathways via IKKα,β and TRAF-3. IKKα,β activates NF-κB subunits that translocate to the nucleus to initiate the transcription of genes for API cytokines and chemokines induced by MyD88 signaling, with differing expression profiles over time (Alexopoulou et al., 2001; Lien and Zipris, 2009; Kawai and Akira, 2010; Kishimoto, 2010). TRAF3 activates TBK1/IKKi to

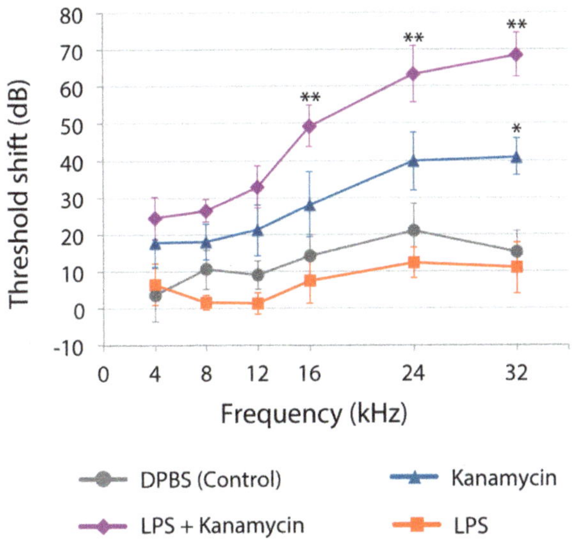

FIGURE 2 | Three weeks after chronic [lipopolysaccharides (LPS) or saline] exposure with or without twice daily kanamycin dosing, ABR threshold shifts for mice treated with LPS-only (red) were not different from saline-treated mice (DPBS, gray). Kanamycin alone (700 mg/kg, twice daily; blue) induced a small but significant PTS at only 32 kHz (*$P < 0.01$) compared to saline-treated mice (gray). that received LPS plus kanamycin (purple) had significant PTS at 16, 24 (**$P < 0.01$), and 32 kHz ($P < 0.05$) compared to mice treated with kanamycin, saline or LPS only (**$P < 0.01$). Mice receiving LPS plus kanamycin also had significant PTS at 12 kHz compared to mice treated with DPBS or LPS only, or LPS-only mice at 8 kHz. Error bars = SD. Figure adapted from Koo et al., 2015, with permission from Science/American Association for the Advancement of Science.

phosphorylate and homodimerize the transcription factors IRF-3 and IRF-7. These dimers then translocate to the nucleus to induce the expression of type I interferon-α (IFN-α [13 subtypes]) and IFN-β. After secretion, these interferons induce the expression of pro-inflammatory cytokines (Assmann et al., 2015). The IFN-α family, and IFN-β, influence a vast spectrum of biological functions, including inhibition of viral replication (Borden et al., 2007), and regulating the homeostatic differentiation of natural killer cells, dendritic cells, B cells, T cells, and osteoclasts (Farrar and Murphy, 2000). Activated IFN-β also phosphorylates the signal transducers and activators of transcription 1 (STAT1) protein (Imaizumi et al., 2016a). IFN-stimulated genes (ISGs) then induce and modulate various biological processes, especially anti-viral activities that target almost all steps in the lifecycle of a virus (Imaizumi et al., 2016a,b).

EXPERIMENTAL MODELS OF SYSTEMIC INFECTION AND COCHLEAR-MEDIATED INFLAMMATORY RESPONSES

Experimental models of infection allow researchers to identify the effect of induced inflammation on normal physiology, a rapidly growing area of research. Classic experimental models of infection use parenteral administration of LPS or polyinosinic:polycytidylic acid (polyI:C) to induce innate immune responses. LPS (a.k.a lipoglycans or endotoxin) is a potent bacteriogenic agonist for TLR4 (Nemzek et al., 2008). PolyI:C is synthetic dsRNA that primarily binds to TLR3, stimulating an innate virogenic immune response (Fortier et al., 2004). The experimental advantages of using LPS and polyI:C as immunogenic stimulants include safety, convenience, control over dose and administration of the immunological challenge, and more importantly reproducibility between individuals within the same group compared to that achieved by inoculation with live bacteria and viruses. The complex interplay between live bacteria or viruses and host immune responses to can lead to wide-ranging experimental outcomes within the same group. LPS-induced inflammation is characterized by time-dependent levels of individual cytokines that are less sustained compared to live bacterial models with polymodal avenues of immunostimulation (Hadjiminas et al., 1994; Nemzek et al., 2008).

The innate immune (inflammatory) response includes secretion of nitric oxide and bacteriotoxic enzymes by immune cells (monocytes, macrophages, neutrophils etc.) that lyze bacteria. Aminoglycosides also lyze bacteria (Martin and Beveridge, 1986; Kadurugamuwa et al., 1993). Lysis of Gram-negative bacteria releases LPS that further stimulates the TLR4-mediated immune response, heightening the systemic host-mediated inflammatory response, analogous to the Jarisch–Herxheimer reaction following penicillin treatment for syphilis (Shenep and Mogan, 1984; Kaplanski et al., 1998; Yang et al., 2010).

Initially, the inner ear was considered an immuno-privileged organ that did not participate in the systemic inflammatory responses (Fujioka et al., 2014). Of 458 articles on cochlear inflammation indexed by PubMed, more than 55% were published in the last 10 years (search conducted June 2017). It is now widely recognized that cochlear inflammation can recruit immune cells into the cochlea (Hirose et al., 2005; Miyao et al., 2008) and, also repair and resolve cochlear damage, as described elsewhere in this Research Topic (Kalinec et al., 2017; Wood and Zuo, 2017).

Experimental models of systemic inflammation were only recently incorporated into preclinical ototoxicity studies (Koo et al., 2011; Quintanilla-Dieck et al., 2013). Crucially, systemic LPS does not significantly modulate the cochlear endolymphatic potential or auditory function (Hirose et al., 2014b; Koo et al., 2015), yet altered BLB physiology that facilitated increased entry of fluorescent markers into perilymph by mechanisms that remain to be directly identified (Hirose et al., 2014a). Systemic administration of also LPS increases cochlear levels of aminoglycosides, particularly in the stria vascularis, without modulating serum levels for these drugs. Furthermore, systemic LPS increased the expression of acute phase inflammatory markers in both serum, and, surprisingly, in cochlear tissues that was not replicated in mice with hypofunctional TLR4 (Koo et al., 2015).

PolyI:C significantly enhances the secretion of thymic stromal lymphopoietin (TSLP), B lymphocyte stimulator (BLyS), IFNγ-inducible protein 10 (IP-10), and macrophage inflammatory protein 1 alpha (MIP-1α) in human inner ear

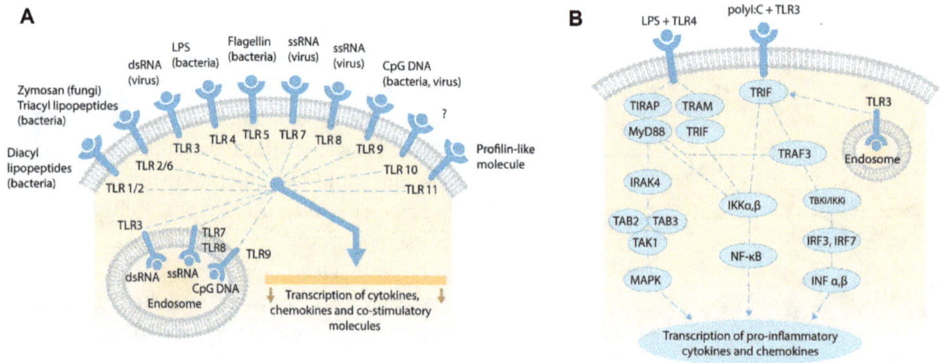

FIGURE 3 | (A) Overview of human TLRs activated by exogenous and endogenous ligands, such as fragmented DNA from necrotic cells; adapted by permission from Macmillan Publishers Ltd, Nature Reviews Gastroenterology and Hepatology, 2006, vol. 3, pp..390–407, Sartor (2006). **(B)** Schematic of TLR4 and TLR3 signaling pathways. LPS binding to membranous TLR4 activates the MyD88-dependent and MyD88-independent signaling pathways via different adaptor proteins. MyD88-dependent pathway activates IRAK-4, transforming TAK1 and TAK-binding protein 2 or 3 (TAB2/3) to stimulate downstream MAPK, and transcription and expression of pro-inflammatory cytokines (e.g., TNFα, IL-1α, IL-1β, IL-2, IL-6, IL-12). The MyD88-independent pathway activates IκB kinase (IKK) complex, releasing NF-κB to translocate to the nucleus and transcribe genes that express type 1 interferons. Viral double-stranded (dsRNA) binds TLR3 on cell or endosomal membranes and recruit the adaptor molecule TRIF. This initiates two pathways via IKKα,β and TRAF-3. IKKα,β activates NF-κB subunits which translocate to the nucleus to trigger transcription of genes encoding pro-inflammatory cytokines. Alternatively, TRIF stimulates TRAF3 to activate TBK1/IKKi and phosphorylate transcription factor IRF-3 and IRF-7. After homodimerization, IRF-3 and-IRF-7 translocate to the nucleus to transcribe type I IFNα,β. Secretion of type 1 IFNα,β leads to further transcription and expression of pro-inflammatory cytokines. Both schematics are not to scale.

endolymphatic sac fibroblasts (Yamada et al., 2017). This suggests that cells in the endolymphatic sac can also produce cytokines and chemokines in response to activated TLR3 (Yamada et al., 2017). Inoculation of cochleae with live or heat-inactivated *Cytomegalovirus* altered BLB permeability, and induced recruitment of inflammatory cells to the spiral ligament, with cochlear inflammation and degeneration present after 5 weeks (Keithley et al., 1989; Fukuda et al., 1992; Keithley and Harris, 1996; Li et al., 2014).

POTENTIAL MECHANISMS UNDERLYING INFLAMMATION-ENHANCED COCHLEOTOXICITY

In the stria vascularis, peri-vascular resident macrophages are thought to modulate the integrity of the strial BLB (and inversely, paracellular flux). The loss of these macrophages decreased the endolymphatic potential, elevated auditory thresholds and increased paracellular flux into the stria vascularis (Zhang et al., 2012). In other tissues, systemic inflammation is associated with decreased expression of tight junctional proteins and increased permeability (Hofer et al., 2008; Singla et al., 2011; Yun et al., 2017). Preclinical models of a disrupted BLB (loss of physical integrity) also results in loss of the endolymphatic potential, elevated auditory thresholds and increased protein expression of genes for ion homeostasis and junctional complexes (Lin and Trune, 1997; Trune, 1997; MacArthur et al., 2006; Cohen-Salmon et al., 2007; MacArthur et al., 2013). However, there is no loss of endolymphatic potential, nor elevated auditory thresholds, during systemic inflammation induced by (lower doses of) LPS that enhanced cochleotoxicity, suggesting that the BLB remained relatively intact (Hirose et al., 2014b; Koo et al., 2015).

For systemically administered aminoglycosides to reach cochlear hair cells, these drugs must first enter endothelial cells forming the BLB, established by tight junctions between adjacent endothelial cells of cochlear blood vessels. The most intense strial uptake of fluorescent gentamicin is within endothelial cells of the strial capillaries, and this uptake can be attenuated by increasing levels of unconjugated aminoglycosides, suggestive of competitive antagonism of saturable cell-regulatable mechanisms (Wang et al., 2010). Aminoglycosides can use one or more cell-regulatable transcellular trafficking routes, including endocytosis and/or permeation through ion channels (e.g., TRPV4) to enter cochlear endothelial cells that form the BLB (Koo et al., 2015).

Aminoglycosides must also be able to exit BLB endothelial cells, and then traffic through the tight junction-coupled marginal cells of the stria vascularis into endolymph (**Figure 4**) prior to entering hair cells across their apical membranes via the aminoglycoside-permeant mechanoelectrical transduction channel. Current flow through most ion channels is passively bi-directional, dependent on the electrophysiological characteristics in which they are situated, e.g., $K_{ir}4.1$ in strial intermediate cells (Ando and Takeuchi, 1999; Marcus et al., 2002), which could facilitate trafficking of aminoglycosides in a similar manner in or out of individual cells within the stria vascularis. Below, we discuss several transmembrane mechanisms that could physiologically modulate the trafficking of the cationic, hydrophilic aminoglycosides.

Endocytosis

Aminoglycosides are readily endocytosed by specific and non-specific mechanisms (Myrdal et al., 2005). Megalin and cubulin are apical membrane receptors that can bind to

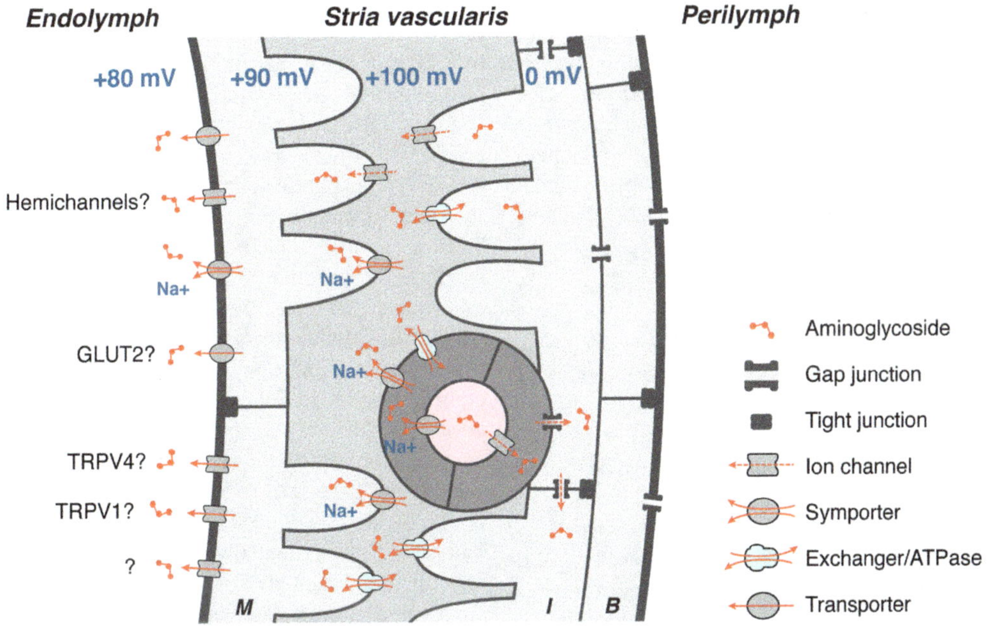

FIGURE 4 | To cross the strial BLB, aminoglycosides must first enter endothelial cells (dark gray), and permeate through gap junctions into intermediate cells (I) and/or basal cells (B). Aminoglycosides could clear endothelial, intermediate and basal cells via transporters, exchangers, and/or cation channels, or by exocytosis of endosomes (not shown), into the intra-strial space. Aminoglycosides are taken up by marginal cells across their basolateral membranes, presumptively by ATPases, exchangers, and transporters (and ion channels?). Once in marginal cells, aminoglycosides clear into endolymph down the electrochemical gradient, presumptively via permeation of hemi-channels, facilitated glucose transporters (GLUT), electrogenic symporters, and at least two TRP channels, TRPV1 and TRPV4. Schematic diagram not to relative scale.

aminoglycosides to induce endocytosis and are expressed in renal and cochlear epithelia, but not in hair cells (Tauris et al., 2009; Nagai and Takano, 2014). Mice lacking megalin show reduced renal uptake of aminoglycosides and attenuated aminoglycoside-induced nephrotoxicity (Nagai et al., 2001; Schmitz et al., 2002), and may represent a partial otoprotective mechanism by sequestering aminoglycosides from endolymph (Tauris et al., 2009). However, blocking endocytosis did not reduce hair cell death *in vitro* (Alharazneh et al., 2011). Blocking trafficking of aminoglycoside-laden endosomes to lysosomes exacerbates hair cell death suggesting that aminoglycoside-induced cytotoxicity proceeds upstream of endosomal and lysosomal activity, which may be partially cytoprotective (Esterberg et al., 2014; Hailey et al., 2017). Although inflammation enhances cochlear uptake of aminoglycosides across the BLB of cochlear endothelial cells, it remains to be determined if inflammation modulates transcytosis of aminoglycosides, especially when LPS exposure can reduce caveolin-mediated endocytosis in lung endothelial cells (Singla et al., 2011).

Endothelial cells and macrophages readily endocytose pathogens and particulates which induce inflammatory responses that further induce endocytotic processes (Majkova et al., 2010; Utech et al., 2010). Binding of the LPS-binding proteins complex to TLR4 induces endocytosis and induction of cytokine expression, as described above. Furthermore, this ligand-receptor binding is also endocytosed with downstream production of cytokines (Tan et al., 2015). In preclinical models, treatment with antibodies to TLR2 and TLR4 attenuate the inflammatory response and promote survival of severe experimental sepsis; however, side-effects include delayed healing from infection (Lima et al., 2015; Gao et al., 2017). Etanercept, an antibody that attenuates the TNFα-mediated inflammation triggered by TLR4, can acutely maintain cochlear blood flow and preserve hearing following acoustic overstimulation that typically induces cochlear inflammation (Arpornchayanon et al., 2013), and also cisplatin-induced cochleotoxicity (Kaur et al., 2011). Investigation of off-target side-effects will be crucial to determine the efficacy and safety of these approaches.

Ion Channels

Any non-selective cation channel on the apical plasma membrane of hair cells (and supporting cells) bathed by endolymph, with a pore diameter larger than the maximum cross-sectional diameter of aminoglycosides (~0.8–0.9 nm), is a candidate ion channel permeant to these drugs. These include the mechanoelectrical transducer (MET) channel of hair cells, and a variety of Transient Receptor Potential (TRP) channels, expressed by hair cells and supporting cells. There are seven subfamilies of TRP channels (TRPC, TRPM, TRPV, TRPA, TRPP, TRPML, and TRPN; all of which are found in mammals except for TRPN). At least four subfamilies are expressed in the cochlea, of which three subfamilies (TRPA, TRPC, TRPV) have a pore diameter larger than the maximum cross-sectional diameter of aminoglycosides, but not the fourth subfamily (TRPML). The very low concentration of calcium ions in endolymph increases the open probability of these non-selective cation channels, enhancing their permeability to aminoglycosides (Marcotti et al., 2005; Myrdal and Steyger, 2005; Karasawa et al., 2008; Banke, 2011). Furthermore, TRP channels can mediate inflammatory responses through multiple mechanisms, including interactions with other TRP channels, immunological receptors (e.g., TLR4) and signaling molecules such as pro-inflammatory cytokines (Numata et al., 2011). These are discussed below.

MET Channels

MET channels are big, multi-subunit complexes, including TMC1 and TMC2 (Kawashima et al., 2011), whose interactions are currently being unraveled, and subject to much debate. Nonetheless, their electrophysiological properties are well-characterized and many accessory components identified (Farris et al., 2006). The MET channels are permeable to a variety of aminoglycosides, including fluorescently tagged aminoglycosides (Marcotti et al., 2005; Coffin et al., 2009; Alharazneh et al., 2011; Vu et al., 2013). Genetic disruptions of essential components of the MET complex, e.g., myosin VIIa, or cadherin-23, reduce aminoglycoside uptake (Richardson et al., 1997; Vu et al., 2013). The conductance of MET channels, and therefore aminoglycoside permeation, can readily be modulated by extracellular cations, and permeant or impermeant MET channel blockers, e.g., tubocurarine, quinine (Farris et al., 2004; Coffin et al., 2009; Alharazneh et al., 2011), and are discussed elsewhere in this Research Topic (Kirkwood et al., 2017; O'Sullivan et al., 2017). The intracellular modulation of the MET channel current by inflammatory signaling (or by any other factors) remains to be determined and, if present, will have wider functional implications besides drug permeation into hair cells.

TRPA1

Transient Receptor Potential Ankyrin 1 (TRPA1) is an inflammatory, irritant, and oxidative stress sensor and has been indirectly localized to the basolateral membrane of outer hair cells (Kwan et al., 2006; Stepanyan et al., 2011). TRPA1 has a pore diameter of 1.1 nm, is dilatable to ~1.4 nm, and is permeable to organic cations under the effect of agonists, see **Tables 1** and **2** (Chen et al., 2009; Karashima et al., 2010; Banke, 2011). TRPA1 channels are required for the release of inflammatory neuropeptides and are activated by inflammatory agents released by damaged or diseased non-neuronal cells (Bautista et al., 2013). TRPA1 channels can be sensitized by inflammatory signals such as protein kinase A (PKA) and phospholipase C (PLC), which can include translocation of TRPA1 from vesicular stores to the plasma membrane (Schmidt et al., 2009). Endogenous TRPA1 agonists, such as methylglyoxal, 4-hydroxynonenal (4-HNE, a product and inducer of oxidative stress), 12-lipoxygenase-derived hepoxilin A3, 5,6-epoxyeicosatrienoic acid and reactive oxygen species (**Table 2**), are generated under various pathophysiological conditions activate TRPA1, contributing to peripheral neurogenic inflammation (Koivisto et al., 2014). *In vitro* experiments show that TRPA1 agonists, cinnamaldehyde, and 4-HNE increase outer hair cell uptake of fluorescent gentamicin (Myrdal and Steyger, 2005; Stepanyan et al., 2011). Thus, insults that induce oxidative stress in outer hair cells could potentially activate basolateral TRPA1 channels to enhance aminoglycoside uptake from the perilymphatic scala tympani, another depository of aminoglycosides *in vivo* (Tran Ba Huy et al., 1986; Ohlemiller et al., 1999). A cochlear expression map for TRPA1 is required to determine its potential involvement in inflammation enhanced cochlear uptake of aminoglycosides.

TRPV1

The Transient Receptor Potential Vanilloid (TRPV) subfamily includes TRPV1, the first TRP channel to be identified as candidate aminoglycoside-permeant channel (Myrdal and Steyger, 2005). TRPV1 has a pore diameter of ~1 nm (Chung et al., 2008; Jara-Oseguera et al., 2008) and can be dilated by agonists (Bautista and Julius, 2008; Moiseenkova-Bell et al., 2008). TRPV1 is activated by high temperatures (>43°C), capsaicin, and protons, see **Table 2** (Caterina et al., 1997; Vellani et al., 2001). Cell lines expressing TRPV1 co-incubated with capsaicin and streptomycin undergo rapid cell death (Caterina et al., 1997), suggestive of TRPV1-facilitation of aminoglycoside-induced cytotoxicity. TRPV1 is expressed in the cuticular plate, stereocilia, and cell bodies of hair cells and selected adjacent supporting cells (Zheng et al., 2003), as well as in marginal cells of

TABLE 1 | Transient Receptor Potential (TRP) channel properties.

	Thermosensitivity	Translocation	Mechanostimulation	Citations
TRPA1	<17°C	Yes	No	Bandell et al., 2004; Rugiero and Wood, 2009; Takahashi and Ohta, 2017
TRPV1	>43°C	Yes	Yes (splice variant)	Caterina et al., 1997; Ji et al., 2002; Sharif Naeini et al., 2006
TRPV4	33°C; >45°C	Yes	Yes	Cohen, 2005; Hartmannsgruber et al., 2007; Sokabe and Tominaga, 2010; Ma et al., 2011
TRPC3/6	None	Yes	Yes	Mio et al., 2007; Goel and Schilling, 2010; Quick et al., 2012; Hanson et al., 2015

the stria vascularis (Jiang et al., 2015). Thus, TRPV1 is expressed at key locations along the strial and endolymphatic trafficking route (**Figure 4**).

Involvement of TRPV1 in inflammation is well documented (Davis et al., 2000). Pro-inflammatory mediators up-regulate TRPV1 expression in chronic inflammatory diseases (Engler et al., 2007; Akbar et al., 2008; Cho and Valtschanoff, 2008). Inflammation can also mobilize the translocation of TRPV1 channels from the vesicular reservoir to the plasma membrane via exocytosis (Planells-Cases et al., 2011). Sensitization and translocation of TRPV1 to plasma membrane can also be induced by pro-inflammatory mediators, nerve growth factor and ATP released from damaged cells following tissue trauma (Julius and Basbaum, 2001; Ji et al., 2002; Zhang et al., 2005). Cytokines such as IL-1β, IL-6, and TNFα increase neuronal excitability via TRPV1 (Schafers and Sorkin, 2008; Miller et al., 2009). After kanamycin challenge, TRPV1 expression is unregulated in cochlear and vestibular sensory cells and neuronal ganglia (Kitahara et al., 2005; Ishibashi et al., 2009), and both native and fluorescently tagged gentamicin can permeate TRPV1 (Jiang et al., 2015).

These data suggest that acoustic overstimulation, or systemic inflammation, that induces cochlear expression of cytokines and chemokines, could sensitize or enhance the expression of TRPV1 at key locations to facilitate trafficking of systemically administered aminoglycosides across the stria vascularis into endolymph, as well as into hair cells independently of the MET channel (Li and Steyger, 2011; Li et al., 2011, 2015). Notably, TRPV1 plays a major role in cellular inflammation during cisplatin-induced ototoxicity, as described elsewhere in this Research Topic (Sheth et al., 2017). Whether an intracellular inflammatory-TRPV1 signaling pathway in hair cells occurs during systemic inflammation and/or aminoglycoside cytotoxicity remains to be determined.

TRPV4

TRPV4 is temperature-sensitive (25–34°C), and mechanically activated by osmotic swelling of cells, as well as by chemically agonists (see **Table 2**), like 4α-phorbol 12,13-didecanoate (Liedtke et al., 2000; Strotmann et al., 2000; Vriens et al., 2004). TRPV4 is expressed by hair cells in the region of the cuticular plate, stereocilia, and cell bodies of hair cells, as well as marginal cells and intermediate cells in the stria vascularis; in addition, TRPV4 is permeable to fluorescently tagged gentamicin (Karasawa et al., 2008). Thus, TRPV4 is expressed at key locations along the strial trafficking route into endolymph and hair cells (**Figure 4**). After kanamycin challenge, the expression of TRPV4 is downregulated in the inner ear sensory cells, neuronal ganglia and stria vascularis (Kitahara et al., 2005; Ishibashi et al., 2009), suggesting that TRPV4 does not enhance cochlear uptake of aminoglycosides during insult, and may represent an otoprotective response. Thus, sepsis-enhanced cochlear uptake of aminoglycosides must overcome any decreased trafficking resulting from inflammatory down-regulated expression of individual aminoglycoside-permeant ion channels.

TRPC Channels

TRPC3 and TRPC6 are canonical TRP channels expressed by hair cells, with a large (~6 nm diameter) inner chamber (Mio et al., 2007; Goel and Schilling, 2010; Quick et al., 2012). Endothelial cells also express TRPC6, and activation by phosphoinositides or products downstream of reactive oxygen species induce translocation from the vesicular reservoir to the plasma membrane via exocytosis (Chaudhuri et al., 2016). This results in endothelial inflammation, increased cellular permeability and disrupted barrier function (Tauseef et al., 2012). Similar translocation and activation has been reported for other members of TRP channels too. For example, TRPC4

TABLE 2 | Regulators of TRP channels, including chemical agents, cytokines, and chemokines.

	Agonists	Antagonists	Citations
TRPA1	Nicotine; mustard oil; cinnamaldehyde (bimodal); cannabinoids; tear gases; zinc; ginger; garlic; 4-HNE; allyl isothiocyanate (AITC); methylglyoxal; 12-lipoxygenase-derived hepoxilin A3; 5,6-epoxyeicosatrienoic acid; reactive oxygen species; bradykinin	HC-030031; AP18; camphor (bimodal)	Bandell et al., 2004; Jordt et al., 2004; McMahon and Wood, 2006; Hu et al., 2009; Talavera et al., 2009; Cao et al., 2012; Sisignano et al., 2012; Alpizar et al., 2013; Koivisto et al., 2014
TRPV1	Anandamide; NADA; capsaicin; piperin; protons; nerve growth factor (sensitization); IL-1β; IL-6; TNFα	Capsazepine; AMG 9810; AMG 517; 5'-iodo-resiniferatoxin	Ahern, 2003; Bonnington and McNaughton, 2003; Reilly et al., 2003; Petho et al., 2004; Gavva et al., 2005; McNamara et al., 2005; Doherty et al., 2007; Schafers and Sorkin, 2008; Hsu et al., 2009; Miller et al., 2009; Lawton et al., 2017
TRPV4	4α-Phorbol 12,13-didecanoate; epoxyeicosatrienoicacids; bisandrographolide; GSK1016790A	Ruthenium Red; Gd^{3+}; La^{3+}; RN-1734	Vriens et al., 2004; Becker et al., 2005; Smith et al., 2006; Thorneloe et al., 2008; Mendoza et al., 2010; Mergler et al., 2011; Zheng et al., 2013
TRPC3/6	Diacylglycerol; GSK1702934A	GSK417651A; GSK2293017A	Hofmann et al., 1999; Mio et al., 2007; Goel and Schilling, 2010; Quick et al., 2012; Tauseef et al., 2012; Chaudhuri et al., 2016

phosphorylation by Src family tyrosine kinases (STKs) following epidermal growth factor receptor stimulation, induces exocytotic insertion of TRPC4 into the plasma membrane (Odell et al., 2005) and TRPV4 translocation happens after shear stress in primary vascular endothelial cells (Baratchi et al., 2016). Thus, the roles of these TRP channels, and their permeability to aminoglycosides and trafficking across the BLB, especially during inflammation remain to be determined.

Vasodilation

Vasodilation is a primary consequence of inflammation in order to facilitate extravasation of plasma (i.e., increased paracellular flux) into the interstitial space of tissues. However, in the tight junction-coupled blood-brain barrier and BLB, vasodilation occurs without major increases in paracellular flux. When inflammation-induced vasodilation in the BLB was abrogated in TLR4-hyporesponsive mice, aminoglycoside-uptake by the cochlea was also attenuated (Koo et al., 2015). Conversely, vasodilators like serotonin and ginkgo biloba enhance cochlear uptake of aminoglycosides and cochleotoxicity (Didier et al., 1996; Miman et al., 2002; Koo et al., 2011). Although, these vasodilators have other confounding cochlear effects, it is intriguing that downstream products of reactive oxygen species (e.g., 4-HNE, peroxidized lipids) also dilated cerebral arterioles via activation of TRPA1 (Sullivan et al., 2015). Thus, it will be important to untangle which feature of these polymodal events directly contributes to the increased strial endothelial uptake of aminoglycosides (Koo et al., 2015).

NEONATE-SPECIFIC FACTORS

Most neonates have a continuing maturation of the BLB up to 27 weeks gestational age (GA). Responses to sounds by the fetus can be first detected to 500 Hz tones at 19 weeks GA and increases in frequency range with continuing gestation to 100 to 3000 Hz by 27 weeks GA (Hepper and Shahidullah, 1994). Extrapolating from preclinical data, this suggests that the BLB is largely functionally mature in order to facilitate onset of hearing with the exquisite three-dimensional organization of cochlear fluids and endolymphatic potentials (Ehret, 1976; Yamasaki et al., 2000; Song et al., 2006). This physiological maturation is supported by the co-expression of cubulin and megalin in the apical membranes of marginal cells in the stria vascularis and Reissner's membrane prior to onset of hearing, as for proximal tubule cells during renal morphogenesis (Christensen and Birn, 2002; Tauris et al., 2009). Neonatal murine pups <2 weeks post-natal age, prior to onset of hearing (Ehret, 1976; Yamasaki et al., 2000; Song et al., 2006), could mimic extremely immature neonates (<27 weeks GA). Neonatal murine pups readily take up fluorescent aminoglycosides compared to adult mice (Dai et al., 2006), however, the effects of this uptake prior to, or during, onset of hearing on mature auditory function remain to be determined.

Substantial evidence demonstrates diminished innate immune responses in neonates to bacterial and viral infections (Levy, 2005), and that individual immune cell types have less capacity to synthesize multiple cytokine responses to immunogenic stimuli. However, empiric data is heterogeneous, with baseline levels and varying immunogenic responses dependent on age, geographical location, race, and TLRs studied (Martino et al., 2012; Georgountzou and Papadopoulos, 2017). The maturing innate immune response during infancy and in specific chronic disease states (e.g., cystic fibrosis) will be an area of immense growth prior to understanding differential effects during developmental maturation of organ systems. Neonates in the NICU may also be exposed to one or more co-therapeutics that can potentiate aminoglycoside-induced hearing loss, including vancomycin, loop diuretics (as an anti-seizure medication), and neuromuscular blocking agents (to facilitate intubation for neonates requiring respiratory assistance), and reviewed by Garinis et al. (2017b). Each of these factors, along with aminoglycoside therapy and inflammation, may contribute to a multiple causative origin of hearing loss proposed for neonates in the NICU (Allegaert et al., 2016).

SUMMARY

In this review, we explored potential mechanisms by which systemic host-mediated inflammatory responses to immunogenic stimuli could exacerbate aminoglycoside trafficking into the cochlea to enhance aminoglycoside-induced cochleotoxicity. Systemic inflammatory signaling cascades induce cochlear expression of cytokines and chemokines that could modulate the rate of endocytosis, and/or, more likely, sensitize/upregulate the expression of selected aminoglycoside-permeant cation channels within the cochlea, particularly TRPV1. The expression of other (candidate) aminoglycoside-permeant cation channels are down-regulated (TRPV4) or remain unknown (e.g., TRPA1, TRPCs) mean that acquisition of further empirical data is needed. The altered expression and physiology of aminoglycoside-permeant channels should modulate the flux of aminoglycosides across the endothelial cells forming the BLB, through the stria vascularis and into endolymph, and thence into hair cells and supporting cells. Once verified, these mechanisms will be potential targets for novel pharmacotherapeutics that reduce the risk of drug-induced cochleotoxicity and acute kidney damage during systemic inflammation without compromising the required bactericidal efficacy of aminoglycosides.

AUTHOR CONTRIBUTIONS

MJ, FT, and PS all conducted the literature review, wrote, revised, edited, and approved submission of the manuscript

ACKNOWLEDGMENTS

The illustrations were designed by Karen Thiebes, Simplified Science Publishing, LLC. The content is solely the responsibility of the authors and do not represent the official views of the NIH, Oregon Health & Science University or the VA Portland Health Care System.

REFERENCES

Abbott, N. J., Ronnback, L., and Hansson, E. (2006). Astrocyte-endothelial interactions at the blood-brain barrier. *Nat. Rev. Neurosci.* 7, 41–53. doi: 10.1038/nrn1824

Ahern, G. P. (2003). Activation of TRPV1 by the satiety factor oleoylethanolamide. *J. Biol. Chem.* 278, 30429–30434. doi: 10.1074/jbc.M305051200

Aird, W. C. (2003). The role of the endothelium in severe sepsis and multiple organ dysfunction syndrome. *Blood* 101, 3765–3777. doi: 10.1182/blood-2002-06-1887

Akbar, A., Yiangou, Y., Facer, P., Walters, J. R., Anand, P., and Ghosh, S. (2008). Increased capsaicin receptor TRPV1-expressing sensory fibres in irritable bowel syndrome and their correlation with abdominal pain. *Gut* 57, 923–929. doi: 10.1136/gut.2007.138982

Alexopoulou, L., Holt, A. C., Medzhitov, R., and Flavell, R. A. (2001). Recognition of double-stranded RNA and activation of NF-kappaB by Toll-like receptor 3. *Nature* 413, 732–738. doi: 10.1038/35099560

Alharazneh, A., Luk, L., Huth, M., Monfared, A., Steyger, P. S., Cheng, A. G., et al. (2011). Functional hair cell mechanotransducer channels are required for aminoglycoside ototoxicity. *PLOS ONE* 6:e22347. doi: 10.1371/journal.pone.0022347

Allan, S. M., and Rothwell, N. J. (2001). Cytokines and acute neurodegeneration. *Nat. Rev. Neurosci.* 2, 734–744. doi: 10.1038/35094583

Allegaert, K., Lahav, A., and Van Den Anker, J. N. (2016). A mechanism to explain ototoxicity in neonates exposed to bumetanide: lessons to help improve future product development in neonates. *Paediatr. Drugs* 18, 331–333. doi: 10.1007/s40272-016-0190-4

Al-Malky, G., Dawson, S. J., Sirimanna, T., Bagkeris, E., and Suri, R. (2015). High-frequency audiometry reveals high prevalence of aminoglycoside ototoxicity in children with cystic fibrosis. *J. Cyst. Fibros.* 14, 248–254. doi: 10.1016/j.jcf.2014.07.009

Alpizar, Y. A., Gees, M., Sanchez, A., Apetrei, A., Voets, T., Nilius, B., et al. (2013). Bimodal effects of cinnamaldehyde and camphor on mouse TRPA1. *Pflugers Arch.* 465, 853–864. doi: 10.1007/s00424-012-1204-x

Ando, M., and Takeuchi, S. (1999). Immunological identification of an inward rectifier K^+ channel (Kir4.1) in the intermediate cell (melanocyte) of the cochlear stria vascularis of gerbils and rats. *Cell Tissue Res.* 298, 179–183. doi: 10.1007/s004419900066

Arpornchayanon, W., Canis, M., Ihler, F., Settevendemie, C., and Strieth, S. (2013). TNF-alpha inhibition using etanercept prevents noise-induced hearing loss by improvement of cochlear blood flow in vivo. *Int. J. Audiol.* 52, 545–552. doi: 10.3109/14992027.2013.790564

Assmann, T. S., Brondani Lde, A., Boucas, A. P., Canani, L. H., and Crispim, D. (2015). Toll-like receptor 3 (TLR3) and the development of type 1 diabetes mellitus. *Arch. Endocrinol. Metab.* 59, 4–12. doi: 10.1590/2359-3997000000003

Atkinson, T. J. (2008). Toll-like receptors, transduction-effector pathways, and disease diversity: evidence of an immunobiological paradigm explaining all human illness? *Int. Rev. Immunol.* 27, 255–281. doi: 10.1080/08830180801959072

Bandell, M., Story, G. M., Hwang, S. W., Viswanath, V., Eid, S. R., Petrus, M. J., et al. (2004). Noxious cold ion channel TRPA1 is activated by pungent compounds and bradykinin. *Neuron* 41, 849–857. doi: 10.1016/S0896-6273(04)00150-3

Banke, T. G. (2011). The dilated TRPA1 channel pore state is blocked by amiloride and analogues. *Brain Res.* 1381, 21–30. doi: 10.1016/j.brainres.2011.01.021

Baratchi, S., Almazi, J. G., Darby, W., Tovar-Lopez, F. J., Mitchell, A., and Mcintyre, P. (2016). Shear stress mediates exocytosis of functional TRPV4 channels in endothelial cells. *Cell Mol. Life Sci.* 73, 649–666. doi: 10.1007/s00018-015-2018-8

Bautista, D., and Julius, D. (2008). Fire in the hole: pore dilation of the capsaicin receptor TRPV1. *Nat. Neurosci.* 11, 528–529. doi: 10.1038/nn0508-528

Bautista, D. M., Pellegrino, M., and Tsunozaki, M. (2013). TRPA1: a gatekeeper for inflammation. *Annu. Rev. Physiol.* 75, 181–200. doi: 10.1146/annurev-physiol-030212-183811

Becker, D., Blase, C., Bereiter-Hahn, J., and Jendrach, M. (2005). TRPV4 exhibits a functional role in cell-volume regulation. *J. Cell Sci.* 118, 2435–2440. doi: 10.1242/jcs.02372

Bitner-Glindzicz, M., Pembrey, M., Duncan, A., Heron, J., Ring, S. M., Hall, A., et al. (2009). Prevalence of mitochondrial 1555A→ G mutation in European children. *N. Engl. J. Med.* 360, 640–642. doi: 10.1056/NEJMc0806396

Blackwood, B. P., Hunter, C. J., and Grabowski, J. (2017). Variability in antibiotic regimens for surgical necrotizing enterocolitis highlights the need for new guidelines. *Surg. Infect.* 18, 215–220. doi: 10.1089/sur.2016.163

Bonnington, J. K., and McNaughton, P. A. (2003). Signalling pathways involved in the sensitisation of mouse nociceptive neurones by nerve growth factor. *J. Physiol.* 551, 433–446. doi: 10.1113/jphysiol.2003.039990

Borden, E. C., Sen, G. C., Uze, G., Silverman, R. H., Ransohoff, R. M., Foster, G. R., et al. (2007). Interferons at age 50: past, current and future impact on biomedicine. *Nat. Rev. Drug Discov.* 6, 975–990. doi: 10.1038/nrd2422

Cao, D. S., Zhong, L., Hsieh, T. H., Abooj, M., Bishnoi, M., Hughes, L., et al. (2012). Expression of transient receptor potential ankyrin 1 (TRPA1) and its role in insulin release from rat pancreatic beta cells. *PLOS ONE* 7:e38005. doi: 10.1371/journal.pone.0038005

Caterina, M. J., Schumacher, M. A., Tominaga, M., Rosen, T. A., Levine, J. D., and Julius, D. (1997). The capsaicin receptor: a heat-activated ion channel in the pain pathway. *Nature* 389, 816–824. doi: 10.1038/39807

Chakravarty, S., and Herkenham, M. (2005). Toll-like receptor 4 on nonhematopoietic cells sustains CNS inflammation during endotoxemia, independent of systemic cytokines. *J. Neurosci.* 25, 1788–1796. doi: 10.1523/JNEUROSCI.4268-04.2005

Chaudhuri, P., Rosenbaum, M. A., Sinharoy, P., Damron, D. S., Birnbaumer, L., and Graham, L. M. (2016). Membrane translocation of TRPC6 channels and endothelial migration are regulated by calmodulin and PI3 kinase activation. *Proc. Natl. Acad. Sci. U.S.A.* 113, 2110–2115. doi: 10.1073/pnas.1600371113

Chen, J., Kim, D., Bianchi, B. R., Cavanaugh, E. J., Faltynek, C. R., Kym, P. R., et al. (2009). Pore dilation occurs in TRPA1 but not in TRPM8 channels. *Mol. Pain* 5:3. doi: 10.1186/1744-8069-5-3

Cho, W. G., and Valtschanoff, J. G. (2008). Vanilloid receptor TRPV1-positive sensory afferents in the mouse ankle and knee joints. *Brain Res.* 1219, 59–65. doi: 10.1016/j.brainres.2008.04.043

Christensen, E. I., and Birn, H. (2002). Megalin and cubilin: multifunctional endocytic receptors. *Nat. Rev. Mol. Cell Biol.* 3, 256–266. doi: 10.1038/nrm778

Chung, M. K., Guler, A. D., and Caterina, M. J. (2008). TRPV1 shows dynamic ionic selectivity during agonist stimulation. *Nat. Neurosci.* 11, 555–564. doi: 10.1038/nn.2102

Coffin, A. B., Reinhart, K. E., Owens, K. N., Raible, D. W., and Rubel, E. W. (2009). Extracellular divalent cations modulate aminoglycoside-induced hair cell death in the zebrafish lateral line. *Hear. Res.* 253, 42–51. doi: 10.1016/j.heares.2009.03.004

Cohen, D. M. (2005). TRPV4 and the mammalian kidney. *Pflugers Arch.* 451, 168–175 doi: 10.1007/s00424-005-1456-9

Cohen-Salmon, M., Regnault, B., Cayet, N., Caille, D., Demuth, K., Hardelin, J. P., et al. (2007). Connexin30 deficiency causes instrastrial fluid-blood barrier disruption within the cochlear stria vascularis. *Proc. Natl. Acad. Sci. U.S.A.* 104, 6229–6234. doi: 10.1073/pnas.0605108104

Cross, C. P., Liao, S., Urdang, Z. D., Srikanth, P., Garinis, A. C., and Steyger, P. S. (2015). Effect of sepsis and systemic inflammatory response syndrome on neonatal hearing screening outcomes following gentamicin exposure. *Int. J. Pediatr. Otorhinolaryngol.* 79, 1915–1919. doi: 10.1016/j.ijporl.2015.09.004

Dai, C. F., Mangiardi, D., Cotanche, D. A., and Steyger, P. S. (2006). Uptake of fluorescent gentamicin by vertebrate sensory cells in vivo. *Hear. Res.* 213, 64–78. doi: 10.1016/j.heares.2005.11.011

Davis, J. B., Gray, J., Gunthorpe, M. J., Hatcher, J. P., Davey, P. T., Overend, P., et al. (2000). Vanilloid receptor-1 is essential for inflammatory thermal hyperalgesia. *Nature* 405, 183–187. doi: 10.1038/35012076

Didier, A., Droy-Lefaix, M. T., Aurousseau, C., and Cazals, Y. (1996). Effects of *Ginkgo biloba* extract (EGb 761) on cochlear vasculature in the guinea pig: morphometric measurements and laser Doppler flowmetry. *Eur. Arch. Otorhinolaryngol.* 253, 25–30. doi: 10.1007/BF00176698

Doherty, E. M., Fotsch, C., Bannon, A. W., Bo, Y., Chen, N., Dominguez, C., et al. (2007). Novel vanilloid receptor-1 antagonists: 2. Structure-activity relationships of 4-oxopyrimidines leading to the selection of a clinical candidate. *J. Med. Chem.* 50, 3515–3527. doi: 10.1021/jm070190p

Duscha, S., Boukari, H., Shcherbakov, D., Salian, S., Silva, S., Kendall, A., et al. (2014). Identification and evaluation of improved 4′-O-(alkyl) 4,5-disubstituted 2-deoxystreptamines as next-generation aminoglycoside antibiotics. *mBio* 5:e01827-14. doi: 10.1128/mBio.01827-14

Ehret, G. (1976). Development of absolute auditory thresholds in the house mouse (*Mus musculus*). *J. Am. Audiol. Soc.* 1, 179–184.

Engler, A., Aeschlimann, A., Simmen, B. R., Michel, B. A., Gay, R. E., Gay, S., et al. (2007). Expression of transient receptor potential vanilloid 1 (TRPV1) in synovial fibroblasts from patients with osteoarthritis and rheumatoid arthritis. *Biochem. Biophys. Res. Commun.* 359, 884–888. doi: 10.1016/j.bbrc.2007.05.178

Esterberg, R., Hailey, D. W., Rubel, E. W., and Raible, D. W. (2014). ER-mitochondrial calcium flow underlies vulnerability of mechanosensory hair cells to damage. *J. Neurosci.* 34, 9703–9719. doi: 10.1523/JNEUROSCI.0281-14.2014

Farrar, J. D., and Murphy, K. M. (2000). Type I interferons and T helper development. *Immunol. Today* 21, 484–489. doi: 10.1016/S0167-5699(00)01710-2

Farris, H. E., Leblanc, C. L., Goswami, J., and Ricci, A. J. (2004). Probing the pore of the auditory hair cell mechanotransducer channel in turtle. *J. Physiol.* 558, 769–792. doi: 10.1113/jphysiol.2004.061267

Farris, H. E., Wells, G. B., and Ricci, A. J. (2006). Steady-state adaptation of mechanotransduction modulates the resting potential of auditory hair cells, providing an assay for endolymph [Ca^{2+}]. *J. Neurosci.* 26, 12526–12536. doi: 10.1523/JNEUROSCI.3569-06.2006

Forge, A., and Schacht, J. (2000). Aminoglycoside antibiotics. *Audiol. Neurootol.* 5, 3–22. doi: 10.1159/000013861

Fortier, M. E., Kent, S., Ashdown, H., Poole, S., Boksa, P., and Luheshi, G. N. (2004). The viral mimic, polyinosinic:polycytidylic acid, induces fever in rats via an interleukin-1-dependent mechanism. *Am. J. Physiol. Regul. Integr. Comp. Physiol.* 287, R759–R766. doi: 10.1152/ajpregu.00293.2004

Fujioka, M., Okano, H., and Ogawa, K. (2014). Inflammatory and immune responses in the cochlea: potential therapeutic targets for sensorineural hearing loss. *Front. Pharmacol.* 5:287. doi: 10.3389/fphar.2014.00287

Fukuda, S., Harris, J. P., Keithley, E. M., Ishikawa, K., Kucuk, B., and Inuyama, Y. (1992). Spiral modiolar vein: its importance in viral load of the inner ear. *Ann. Otol. Rhinol. Laryngol. Suppl.* 157, 67–71. doi: 10.1177/0003489492101S1014

Gao, W., Xiong, Y., Li, Q., and Yang, H. (2017). Inhibition of toll-like receptor signaling as a promising therapy for inflammatory diseases: a journey from molecular to nano therapeutics. *Front. Physiol.* 8:508. doi: 10.3389/fphys.2017.00508

Garinis, A. C., Cross, C. P., Srikanth, P., Carroll, K., Feeney, M. P., Keefe, D. H., et al. (2017a). The cumulative effects of intravenous antibiotic treatments on hearing in patients with cystic fibrosis. *J. Cyst. Fibros.* 16, 401–409. doi: 10.1016/j.jcf.2017.01.006

Garinis, A. C., Kemph, A., Tharpe, A. M., Weitkamp, J. H., Mcevoy, C., and Steyger, P. S. (2017b). Monitoring neonates for ototoxicity. *Int. J. Audiol.* 10.1080/14992027.2017.1339130 [Epub ahead of print].

Garinis, A. C., Liao, S., Cross, C. P., Galati, J., Middaugh, J. L., Mace, J. C., et al. (2017c). Effect of gentamicin and levels of ambient sound on hearing screening outcomes in the neonatal intensive care unit: a pilot study. *Int. J. Pediatr. Otorhinolaryngol.* 97, 42–50. doi: 10.1016/j.ijporl.2017.03.025

Gavva, N. R., Tamir, R., Qu, Y., Klionsky, L., Zhang, T. J., Immke, D., et al. (2005). AMG 9810 [(E)-3-(4-t-butylphenyl)-N-(2,3-dihydrobenzo[b][1,4]dioxin-6-yl)acrylamide], a novel vanilloid receptor 1 (TRPV1) antagonist with antihyperalgesic properties. *J. Pharmacol. Exp. Ther.* 313, 474–484. doi: 10.1124/jpet.104.079855

Georgountzou, A., and Papadopoulos, N. G. (2017). Postnatal innate immune development: from birth to adulthood. *Front. Immunol.* 8:957. 10.3389/fimmu.2017.00957 doi: 10.3389/fimmu.2017.00957

Goel, M., and Schilling, W. P. (2010). Role of TRPC3 channels in ATP-induced Ca^{2+} signaling in principal cells of the inner medullary collecting duct. *Am. J. Physiol. Renal Physiol.* 299, F225–F233. doi: 10.1152/ajprenal.00670.2009

Guo, J., and Friedman, S. L. (2010). Toll-like receptor 4 signaling in liver injury and hepatic fibrogenesis. *Fibrogenesis Tissue Repair* 3:21. doi: 10.1186/1755-1536-3-21

Hadjiminas, D. J., Mcmasters, K. M., Peyton, J. C., and Cheadle, W. G. (1994). Tissue tumor necrosis factor mRNA expression following cecal ligation and puncture or intraperitoneal injection of endotoxin. *J. Surg. Res.* 56, 549–555. doi: 10.1006/jsre.1994.1088

Hailey, D. W., Esterberg, R., Linbo, T. H., Rubel, E. W., and Raible, D. W. (2017). Fluorescent aminoglycosides reveal intracellular trafficking routes in mechanosensory hair cells. *J. Clin. Invest.* 127, 472–486. doi: 10.1172/JCI85052

Hamerman, J. A., Pottle, J., Ni, M., He, Y., Zhang, Z. Y., and Buckner, J. H. (2016). Negative regulation of TLR signaling in myeloid cells–implications for autoimmune diseases. *Immunol. Rev.* 269, 212–227. doi: 10.1111/imr.12381

Hanson, S. M., Sansom, M. S., and Becker, E. B. (2015). Modeling suggests TRPC3 hydrogen bonding and not phosphorylation contributes to the ataxia phenotype of the moonwalker mouse. *Biochemistry* 54, 4033–4041. doi: 10.1021/acs.biochem.5b00235

Hartmannsgruber, V., Heyken, W. T., Kacik, M., Kaistha, A., Grgic, I., Harteneck, C., et al. (2007). Arterial response to shear stress critically depends on endothelial TRPV4 expression. *PLOS ONE* 2:e827. doi: 10.1371/journal.pone.0000827

Hepper, P. G., and Shahidullah, B. S. (1994). Development of fetal hearing. *Arch. Dis. Child.* 71, F81–F87. doi: 10.1136/fn.71.2.F81

Hiel, H., Erre, J. P., Aurousseau, C., Bouali, R., Dulon, D., and Aran, J. M. (1993). Gentamicin uptake by cochlear hair cells precedes hearing impairment during chronic treatment. *Audiology* 32, 78–87. doi: 10.3109/00206099309072930

Hirose, K., Discolo, C. M., Keasler, J. R., and Ransohoff, R. (2005). Mononuclear phagocytes migrate into the murine cochlea after acoustic trauma. *J. Comp. Neurol.* 489, 180–194. doi: 10.1002/cne.20619

Hirose, K., Hartsock, J. J., Johnson, S., Santi, P., and Salt, A. N. (2014a). Systemic lipopolysaccharide compromises the blood-labyrinth barrier and increases entry of serum fluorescein into the perilymph. *J. Assoc. Res. Otolaryngol.* 15, 707–719. doi: 10.1007/s10162-014-0476-6

Hirose, K., Li, S. Z., Ohlemiller, K. K., and Ransohoff, R. M. (2014b). Systemic lipopolysaccharide induces cochlear inflammation and exacerbates the synergistic ototoxicity of kanamycin and furosemide. *J. Assoc. Res. Otolaryngol.* 15, 555–570. doi: 10.1007/s10162-014-0458-8

Hofer, S., Bopp, C., Hoerner, C., Plaschke, K., Faden, R. M., Martin, E., et al. (2008). Injury of the blood brain barrier and up-regulation of icam-1 in polymicrobial sepsis. *J. Surg. Res.* 146, 276–281. doi: 10.1016/j.jss.2007.07.021

Hofmann, T., Obukhov, A. G., Schaefer, M., Harteneck, C., Gudermann, T., and Schultz, G. (1999). Direct activation of human TRPC6 and TRPC3 channels by diacylglycerol. *Nature* 397, 259–263. doi: 10.1038/16711

Hsu, C. C., Bien, M. Y., Huang, Y. T., Ruan, T., Kou, Y. R., and Lin, Y. S. (2009). N-arachidonyl dopamine sensitizes rat capsaicin-sensitive lung vagal afferents via activation of TRPV1 receptors. *Respir. Physiol. Neurobiol.* 167, 323–332. doi: 10.1016/j.resp.2009.06.007

Hu, H., Bandell, M., Petrus, M. J., Zhu, M. X., and Patapoutian, A. (2009). Zinc activates damage-sensing TRPA1 ion channels. *Nat. Chem. Biol.* 5, 183–190. doi: 10.1038/nchembio.146

Imaizumi, T., Shimada, T., Matsumiya, T., Yoshida, H., Watanabe, S., Tsuruga, K., et al. (2016a). Interferon-stimulated gene 15, a Type I interferon-dependent transcript, is involved in a negative feedback loop in innate immune reactions in human mesangial cells. *Nephron* 132, 144–152. doi: 10.1159/000443934

Imaizumi, T., Yano, C., Numata, A., Tsugawa, K., Hayakari, R., Matsumiya, T., et al. (2016b). Interferon (IFN)-induced protein 35 (IFI35), a Type I interferon-dependent transcript, upregulates inflammatory signaling pathways by activating toll-like receptor 3 in human mesangial cells. *Kidney Blood Press. Res.* 41, 635–642. doi: 10.1159/000447932

Ishibashi, T., Takumida, M., Akagi, N., Hirakawa, K., and Anniko, M. (2009). Changes in transient receptor potential vanilloid (TRPV) 1, 2, 3 and

4 expression in mouse inner ear following gentamicin challenge. *Acta Otolaryngol.* 129, 116–126. doi: 10.1080/00016480802032835

Jara-Oseguera, A., Llorente, I., Rosenbaum, T., and Islas, L. D. (2008). Properties of the inner pore region of TRPV1 channels revealed by block with quaternary ammoniums. *J. Gen. Physiol.* 132, 547–562. doi: 10.1085/jgp.200810051

Ji, R. R., Samad, T. A., Jin, S. X., Schmoll, R., and Woolf, C. J. (2002). p38 MAPK activation by NGF in primary sensory neurons after inflammation increases TRPV1 levels and maintains heat hyperalgesia. *Neuron* 36, 57–68. doi: 10.1016/S0896-6273(02)00908-X

Jiang, M., Johnson, A., Karasawa, T., Kachelmeier, A., and Steyger, P. S. (2015). "Role of transient receptor potential vanilloid 1 (TRPV1) in the cellular uptake of aminoglycosides," in *Proceedings of the ARO Midwinter Meeting Abstracts 38, PS-582*, Baltimore, MD.

Jiang, M., Karasawa, T., and Steyger, P. S. (2017). Aminoglycoside-induced cochleotoxicity: a review. *Front. Cell. Neurosci.* 11:308. doi: 10.3389/fncel.2017.00308

Jordt, S. E., Bautista, D. M., Chuang, H. H., Mckemy, D. D., Zygmunt, P. M., Hogestatt, E. D., et al. (2004). Mustard oils and cannabinoids excite sensory nerve fibres through the TRP channel ANKTM1. *Nature* 427, 260–265. doi: 10.1038/nature02282

Julius, D., and Basbaum, A. I. (2001). Molecular mechanisms of nociception. *Nature* 413, 203–210. doi: 10.1038/35093019

Juskewitch, J. E., Knudsen, B. E., Platt, J. L., Nath, K. A., Knutson, K. L., Brunn, G. J., et al. (2012). LPS-induced murine systemic inflammation is driven by parenchymal cell activation and exclusively predicted by early MCP-1 plasma levels. *Am. J. Pathol.* 180, 32–40. doi: 10.1016/j.ajpath.2011.10.001

Kadurugamuwa, J. L., Clarke, A. J., and Beveridge, T. J. (1993). Surface action of gentamicin on *Pseudomonas aeruginosa*. *J. Bacteriol.* 175, 5798–5805. doi: 10.1128/jb.175.18.5798-5805.1993

Kalinec, G. M., Lomberk, G., Urrutia, R. A., and Kalinec, F. (2017). Resolution of cochlear inflammation: novel target for preventing or ameliorating drug-, noise- and age-related hearing loss. *Front. Cell. Neurosci.* 11:192. doi: 10.3389/fncel.2017.00192

Kaplanski, G., Granel, B., Vaz, T., and Durand, J. M. (1998). Jarisch-Herxheimer reaction complicating the treatment of chronic Q fever endocarditis: elevated TNFalpha and IL-6 serum levels. *J. Infect.* 37, 83–84. doi: 10.1016/S0163-4453(98)91120-3

Karasawa, T., Wang, Q., Fu, Y., Cohen, D. M., and Steyger, P. S. (2008). TRPV4 enhances the cellular uptake of aminoglycoside antibiotics. *J. Cell Sci.* 121, 2871–2879. doi: 10.1242/jcs.023705

Karashima, Y., Prenen, J., Talavera, K., Janssens, A., Voets, T., and Nilius, B. (2010). Agonist-induced changes in Ca^{2+} permeation through the nociceptor cation channel TRPA1. *Biophys. J.* 98, 773–783. doi: 10.1016/j.bpj.2009.11.007

Kaur, T., Mukherjea, D., Sheehan, K., Jajoo, S., Rybak, L. P., and Ramkumar, V. (2011). Short interfering RNA against STAT1 attenuates cisplatin-induced ototoxicity in the rat by suppressing inflammation. *Cell Death Dis.* 2, e180. doi: 10.1038/cddis.2011.63

Kawai, T., and Akira, S. (2010). The role of pattern-recognition receptors in innate immunity: update on Toll-like receptors. *Nat. Immunol.* 11, 373–384. doi: 10.1038/ni.1863

Kawashima, Y., Geleoc, G. S., Kurima, K., Labay, V., Lelli, A., Asai, Y., et al. (2011). Mechanotransduction in mouse inner ear hair cells requires transmembrane channel-like genes. *J. Clin. Invest.* 121, 4796–4809. doi: 10.1172/JCI60405

Keithley, E. M., and Harris, J. P. (1996). Late sequelae of cochlear infection. *Laryngoscope* 106, 341–345. doi: 10.1097/00005537-199603000-00019

Keithley, E. M., Woolf, N. K., and Harris, J. P. (1989). Development of morphological and physiological changes in the cochlea induced by cytomegalovirus. *Laryngoscope* 99, 409–414. doi: 10.1288/00005537-198904000-00010

Kim, J. J., and Sears, D. D. (2010). TLR4 and insulin resistance. *Gastroenterol. Res. Pract.* 2010:212563 doi: 10.1155/2010/212563

Kirkwood, N. K., O'Reilly, M., Derudas, M., Kenyon, E. J., Huckvale, R., Van Netten, S. M., et al. (2017). d-Tubocurarine and berbamine: alkaloids that are permeant blockers of the hair cell's mechano-electrical transducer channel and protect from aminoglycoside toxicity. *Front. Cell. Neurosci.* 11:262. doi: 10.3389/fncel.2017.00262

Kishimoto, T. (2010). IL-6: from its discovery to clinical applications. *Int. Immunol.* 22, 347–352. doi: 10.1093/intimm/dxq030

Kitahara, T., Li, H. S., and Balaban, C. D. (2005). Changes in transient receptor potential cation channel superfamily V (TRPV) mRNA expression in the mouse inner ear ganglia after kanamycin challenge. *Hear. Res.* 201, 132–144. doi: 10.1016/j.heares.2004.09.007

Koivisto, A., Chapman, H., Jalava, N., Korjamo, T., Saarnilehto, M., Lindstedt, K., et al. (2014). TRPA1: a transducer and amplifier of pain and inflammation. *Basic Clin. Pharmacol. Toxicol.* 114, 50–55. doi: 10.1111/bcpt.12138

Koo, J. W., Quintanilla-Dieck, L., Jiang, M., Liu, J., Urdang, Z. D., Allensworth, J. J., et al. (2015). Endotoxemia-mediated inflammation potentiates aminoglycoside-induced ototoxicity. *Sci. Transl. Med.* 7, 298ra118. doi: 10.1126/scitranslmed.aac5546

Koo, J. W., Wang, Q., and Steyger, P. S. (2011). Infection-mediated vasoactive peptides modulate cochlear uptake of fluorescent gentamicin. *Audiol. Neurootol.* 16, 347–358. doi: 10.1159/000322851

Kwan, K. Y., Allchorne, A. J., Vollrath, M. A., Christensen, A. P., Zhang, D. S., Woolf, C. J., et al. (2006). TRPA1 contributes to cold, mechanical, and chemical nociception but is not essential for hair-cell transduction. *Neuron* 50, 277–289. doi: 10.1016/j.neuron.2006.03.042

Lawton, S. K., Xu, F., Tran, A., Wong, E., Prakash, A., Schumacher, M., et al. (2017). N-Arachidonoyl dopamine modulates acute systemic inflammation via nonhematopoietic TRPV1. *J. Immunol.* 199, 1465–1475 doi: 10.4049/jimmunol.1602151

Levy, O. (2005). Innate immunity of the human newborn: distinct cytokine responses to LPS and other Toll-like receptor agonists. *J. Endotoxin Res.* 11, 113–116. doi: 10.1177/09680519050110020701

Li, H., Kachelmeier, A., Furness, D. N., and Steyger, P. S. (2015). Local mechanisms for loud sound-enhanced aminoglycoside entry into outer hair cells. *Front. Cell. Neurosci.* 9:130. doi: 10.3389/fncel.2015.00130

Li, H., and Steyger, P. S. (2011). Systemic aminoglycosides are trafficked via endolymph into cochlear hair cells. *Sci. Rep.* 1:159. doi: 10.1038/srep00159

Li, H., Wang, Q., and Steyger, P. S. (2011). Acoustic trauma increases cochlear and hair cell uptake of gentamicin. *PLOS ONE* 6:e19130. doi: 10.1371/journal.pone.0019130

Li, X., Shi, X., Qiao, Y., Xu, K., Zeng, L., Wang, C., et al. (2014). Observation of permeability of blood-labyrinth barrier during cytomegalovirus-induced hearing loss. *Int. J. Pediatr. Otorhinolaryngol.* 78, 995–999. doi: 10.1016/j.ijporl.2014.03.013

Liedtke, W., Choe, Y., Marti-Renom, M. A., Bell, A. M., Denis, C. S., Sali, A., et al. (2000). Vanilloid receptor-related osmotically activated channel (VR-OAC), a candidate vertebrate osmoreceptor. *Cell* 103, 525–535. doi: 10.1016/S0092-8674(00)00143-4

Lien, E., and Zipris, D. (2009). The role of Toll-like receptor pathways in the mechanism of type 1 diabetes. *Curr. Mol. Med.* 9, 52–68. doi: 10.2174/156652409787314453

Lima, C. X., Souza, D. G., Amaral, F. A., Fagundes, C. T., Rodrigues, I. P., Alves-Filho, J. C., et al. (2015). Therapeutic effects of treatment with anti-TLR2 and anti-TLR4 monoclonal antibodies in polymicrobial sepsis. *PLOS ONE* 10:e0132336. doi: 10.1371/journal.pone.0132336

Lin, D. W., and Trune, D. R. (1997). Breakdown of stria vascularis blood-labyrinth barrier in C3H/lpr autoimmune disease mice. *Otolaryngol. Head Neck Surg.* 117, 530–534. doi: 10.1016/S0194-5998(97)70026-3

Ma, X., Cheng, K. T., Wong, C. O., O'neil, R. G., Birnbaumer, L., Ambudkar, I. S., et al. (2011). Heteromeric TRPV4-C1 channels contribute to store-operated Ca^{2+} entry in vascular endothelial cells. *Cell Calcium* 50, 502–509. doi: 10.1016/j.ceca.2011.08.006

MacArthur, C. J., Hausman, F., Kempton, J. B., Sautter, N., and Trune, D. R. (2013). Inner ear tissue remodeling and ion homeostasis gene alteration in murine chronic otitis media. *Otol. Neurotol.* 34, 338–346. doi: 10.1097/MAO.0b013e31827b4d0a

MacArthur, C. J., Hefeneider, S. H., Kempton, J. B., and Trune, D. R. (2006). C3H/HeJ mouse model for spontaneous chronic otitis media. *Laryngoscope* 116, 1071–1079. doi: 10.1097/01.mlg.0000224527.41288.c4

Mahmoudi, L., Niknam, R., Mousavi, S., Ahmadi, A., Honarmand, H., Ziaie, S., et al. (2013). Optimal aminoglycoside therapy following the sepsis: how much is too much? *Iran. J. Pharm. Res.* 12, 261–269.

Majkova, Z., Toborek, M., and Hennig, B. (2010). The role of caveolae in endothelial cell dysfunction with a focus on nutrition and environmental toxicants *J. Cell Mol. Med.* 14, 2359–2370. doi: 10.1111/j.1582-4934.2010.01064.x

Marcotti, W., Van Netten, S. M., and Kros, C. J. (2005). The aminoglycoside antibiotic dihydrostreptomycin rapidly enters mouse outer hair cells through the mechano-electrical transducer channels. *J. Physiol.* 567, 505–521. doi: 10.1113/jphysiol.2005.085951

Marcus, D. C., Wu, T., Wangemann, P., and Kofuji, P. (2002). KCNJ10 (Kir4.1) potassium channel knockout abolishes endocochlear potential. *Am. J. Physiol. Cell Physiol.* 282, C403–C407. doi: 10.1152/ajpcell.00312.2001

Martin, N. L., and Beveridge, T. J. (1986). Gentamicin interaction with *Pseudomonas aeruginosa* cell envelope. *Antimicrob. Agents Chemother.* 29, 1079–1087. doi: 10.1128/AAC.29.6.1079

Martino, D., Holt, P., and Prescott, S. (2012). A novel role for interleukin-1 receptor signaling in the developmental regulation of immune responses to endotoxin. *Pediatr. Allergy Immunol.* 23, 567–572. doi: 10.1111/j.1399-3038.2012.01287.x

McMahon, S. B., and Wood, J. N. (2006). Increasingly irritable and close to tears: TRPA1 in inflammatory pain. *Cell* 124, 1123–1125. doi: 10.1016/j.cell.2006.03.006

McNamara, F. N., Randall, A., and Gunthorpe, M. J. (2005). Effects of piperine, the pungent component of black pepper, at the human vanilloid receptor (TRPV1). *Br. J. Pharmacol.* 144, 781–790. doi: 10.1038/sj.bjp.0706040

Mendoza, S. A., Fang, J., Gutterman, D. D., Wilcox, D. A., Bubolz, A. H., Li, R., et al. (2010). TRPV4-mediated endothelial Ca^{2+} influx and vasodilation in response to shear stress. *Am. J. Physiol. Heart Circ. Physiol.* 298, H466–H476. doi: 10.1152/ajpheart.00854.2009

Mergler, S., Garreis, F., Sahlmuller, M., Reinach, P. S., Paulsen, F., and Pleyer, U. (2011). Thermosensitive transient receptor potential channels in human corneal epithelial cells. *J. Cell. Physiol.* 226, 1828–1842. doi: 10.1002/jcp.22514

Miller, R. J., Jung, H., Bhangoo, S. K., and White, F. A. (2009). Cytokine and chemokine regulation of sensory neuron function. *Handb. Exp. Pharmacol.* 417–449. doi: 10.1007/978-3-540-79090-7_12

Miman, M. C., Ozturan, O., Iraz, M., Erdem, T., and Olmez, E. (2002). Amikacin ototoxicity enhanced by *Ginkgo biloba* extract (EGb 761). *Hear. Res.* 169, 121–129. doi: 10.1016/S0378-5955(02)00385-4

Mio, K., Ogura, T., Kiyonaka, S., Hiroaki, Y., Tanimura, Y., Fujiyoshi, Y., et al. (2007). The TRPC3 channel has a large internal chamber surrounded by signal sensing antennas. *J. Mol. Biol.* 367, 373–383. doi: 10.1016/j.jmb.2006.12.043

Miyao, M., Firestein, G. S., and Keithley, E. M. (2008). Acoustic trauma augments the cochlear immune response to antigen. *Laryngoscope* 118, 1801–1808. doi: 10.1097/MLG.0b013e31817e2c27

Moiseenkova-Bell, V. Y., Stanciu, L. A., Serysheva, I. I., Tobe, B. J., and Wensel, T. G. (2008). Structure of TRPV1 channel revealed by electron cryomicroscopy. *Proc. Natl. Acad. Sci. U.S.A.* 105, 7451–7455. doi: 10.1073/pnas.0711835105

Myrdal, S. E., Johnson, K. C., and Steyger, P. S. (2005). Cytoplasmic and intra-nuclear binding of gentamicin does not require endocytosis. *Hear. Res.* 204, 156–169. doi: 10.1016/j.heares.2005.02.002

Myrdal, S. E., and Steyger, P. S. (2005). TRPV1 regulators mediate gentamicin penetration of cultured kidney cells. *Hear. Res.* 204, 170–182. doi: 10.1016/j.heares.2005.02.005

Nagai, J., and Takano, M. (2014). Entry of aminoglycosides into renal tubular epithelial cells via endocytosis-dependent and endocytosis-independent pathways. *Biochem. Pharmacol.* 90, 331–337. doi: 10.1016/j.bcp.2014.05.018

Nagai, J., Tanaka, H., Nakanishi, N., Murakami, T., and Takano, M. (2001). Role of megalin in renal handling of aminoglycosides. *Am. J. Physiol. Renal Physiol.* 281, F337–F344.

Nemzek, J. A., Hugunin, K. M., and Opp, M. R. (2008). Modeling sepsis in the laboratory: merging sound science with animal well-being. *Comp. Med.* 58, 120–128.

Numata, T., Kiyonaka, S., Kato, K., Takahashi, N., and Mori, Y. (2011). "Activation of TRP channels in mammalian systems," in *TRP Channels*, ed. M. X. Zhu (Boca Raton, FL: CRC Press), 43–90.

Odell, A. F., Scott, J. L., and Van Helden, D. F. (2005). Epidermal growth factor induces tyrosine phosphorylation, membrane insertion, and activation of transient receptor potential channel 4. *J. Biol. Chem.* 280, 37974–37987. doi: 10.1074/jbc.M503646200

Oh, G. S., Kim, H. J., Choi, J. H., Shen, A., Kim, C. H., Kim, S. J., et al. (2011). Activation of lipopolysaccharide-TLR4 signaling accelerates the ototoxic potential of cisplatin in mice. *J. Immunol.* 186, 1140–1150. doi: 10.4049/jimmunol.1002183

Ohlemiller, K. K., Wright, J. S., and Dugan, L. L. (1999). Early elevation of cochlear reactive oxygen species following noise exposure. *Audiol. Neurootol.* 4, 229–236. doi: 10.1159/000013846

O'Neill, L. A., Golenbock, D., and Bowie, A. G. (2013). The history of Toll-like receptors - redefining innate immunity. *Nat. Rev. Immunol.* 13, 453–460. doi: 10.1038/nri3446

Osterman, M. J. K., Martin, J. A., Mathews, T. J., and Hamilton, B. E. (2011). Expanded data from the new birth certificate. *Natl. Vital Stat. Rep.* 59, 1–29.

O'Sullivan, M. E., Perez, A., Lin, R., Sajjadi, A., Ricci, A. J., and Cheng, A. G. (2017). Towards the prevention of aminoglycoside-related hearing loss. *Front. Cell. Neurosci.* 11:325. doi: 10.3389/fncel.2017.00325

Petho, G., Izydorczyk, I., and Reeh, P. W. (2004). Effects of TRPV1 receptor antagonists on stimulated iCGRP release from isolated skin of rats and TRPV1 mutant mice. *Pain* 109, 284–290. doi: 10.1016/j.pain.2004.01.038

Pickles, J. O. (2012). *An Introduction to the Physiology of Hearing.* Bingley: Emerald Group Publishing.

Pillarisetti, N., Williamson, E., Linnane, B., Skoric, B., Robertson, C. F., Robinson, P., et al. (2011). Infection, inflammation, and lung function decline in infants with cystic fibrosis. *Am. J. Respir. Crit. Care Med.* 184, 75–81. doi: 10.1164/rccm.201011-1892OC

Planells-Cases, R., Valente, P., Ferrer-Montiel, A., Qin, F., and Szallasi, A. (2011). Complex regulation of TRPV1 and related thermo-TRPs: implications for therapeutic intervention. *Adv. Exp. Med. Biol.* 704, 491–515. doi: 10.1007/978-94-007-0265-3_27

Poltorak, A., He, X., Smirnova, I., Liu, M. Y., Van Huffel, C., Du, X., et al. (1998). Defective LPS signaling in C3H/HeJ and C57BL/10ScCr mice: mutations in Tlr4 gene. *Science* 282, 2085–2088. doi: 10.1126/science.282.5396.2085

Quick, K., Zhao, J., Eijkelkamp, N., Linley, J. E., Rugiero, F., Cox, J. J., et al. (2012). TRPC3 and TRPC6 are essential for normal mechanotransduction in subsets of sensory neurons and cochlear hair cells. *Open Biol.* 2:120068. doi: 10.1098/rsob.120068

Quintanilla-Dieck, L., Larrain, B., Trune, D., and Steyger, P. S. (2013). Effect of systemic lipopolysaccharide-induced inflammation on cytokine levels in the murine cochlea: a pilot study. *Otolaryngol. Head Neck Surg.* 149, 301–303. doi: 10.1177/0194599813491712

Reilly, C. A., Taylor, J. L., Lanza, D. L., Carr, B. A., Crouch, D. J., and Yost, G. S. (2003). Capsaicinoids cause inflammation and epithelial cell death through activation of vanilloid receptors. *Toxicol. Sci.* 73, 170–181. doi: 10.1093/toxsci/kfg044

Remington, J. S. (2011). *Infectious Diseases of the Fetus and Newborn Infant.* Philadelphia, PA: Saunders.

Richardson, G. P., Forge, A., Kros, C. J., Fleming, J., Brown, S. D., and Steel, K. P. (1997). Myosin VIIA is required for aminoglycoside accumulation in cochlear hair cells. *J. Neurosci.* 17, 9506–9519.

Roy, S., Ryals, M. M., Van Den Bruele, A. B., Fitzgerald, T. S., and Cunningham, L. L. (2013). Sound preconditioning therapy inhibits ototoxic hearing loss in mice. *J. Clin. Invest.* 123, 4945–4949. doi: 10.1172/JCI71353

Rugiero, F., and Wood, J. N. (2009). The mechanosensitive cell line ND-C does not express functional thermoTRP channels. *Neuropharmacology* 56, 1138–1146. doi: 10.1016/j.neuropharm.2009.03.012

Sagwa, E. L., Ruswa, N., Mavhunga, F., Rennie, T., Leufkens, H. G., and Mantel-Teeuwisse, A. K. (2015). Comparing amikacin and kanamycin-induced hearing loss in multidrug-resistant tuberculosis treatment under programmatic conditions in a Namibian retrospective cohort. *BMC Pharmacol. Toxicol.* 16:36. doi: 10.1186/s40360-015-0036-7

Sartor, R. B. (2006). Mechanisms of disease: pathogenesis of Crohn's disease and ulcerative colitis. *Nat. Clin. Pract. Gastroenterol. Hepatol.* 3, 390–407. doi: 10.1038/ncpgasthep0528

Schafers, M., and Sorkin, L. (2008). Effect of cytokines on neuronal excitability. *Neurosci. Lett.* 437, 188–193. doi: 10.1016/j.neulet.2008.03.052

Schmidt, M., Dubin, A. E., Petrus, M. J., Earley, T. J., and Patapoutian, A. (2009). Nociceptive signals induce trafficking of TRPA1 to the plasma membrane. *Neuron* 64, 498–509. doi: 10.1016/j.neuron.2009.09.030

Schmitz, C., Hilpert, J., Jacobsen, C., Boensch, C., Christensen, E. I., Luft, F. C., et al. (2002). Megalin deficiency offers protection from renal aminoglycoside accumulation. *J. Biol. Chem.* 277, 618–622. doi: 10.1074/jbc.M109959200

Schumann, R. R., Leong, S. R., Flaggs, G. W., Gray, P. W., Wright, S. D., Mathison, J. C., et al. (1990). Structure and function of lipopolysaccharide binding protein. *Science* 249, 1429–1431. doi: 10.1126/science.2402637

Sharif Naeini, R., Witty, M. F., Seguela, P., and Bourque, C. W. (2006). An N-terminal variant of Trpv1 channel is required for osmosensory transduction. *Nat. Neurosci.* 9, 93–98. doi: 10.1038/nn1614

Shenep, J. L., and Mogan, K. A. (1984). Kinetics of endotoxin release during antibiotic therapy for experimental gram-negative bacterial sepsis. *J. Infect. Dis.* 150, 380–388. doi: 10.1093/infdis/150.3.380

Sheth, S., Mukherjea, D., Rybak, L., and Ramkumar, V. (2017). Mechanisms of cisplatin-induced ototoxicity and otoprotection. *Front. Cell. Neurosci.* 11:338. doi: 10.3389/fncel.2017.00338

Shimazu, R., Akashi, S., Ogata, H., Nagai, Y., Fukudome, K., Miyake, K., et al. (1999). MD-2, a molecule that confers lipopolysaccharide responsiveness on Toll-like receptor 4. *J. Exp. Med.* 189, 1777–1782. doi: 10.1084/jem.189.11.1777

Singla, S., Predescu, D., Bardita, C., Wang, M., Zhang, J., Balk, R. A., et al. (2011). Pro-inflammatory endothelial cell dysfunction is associated with intersectin-1s down-regulation. *Respir. Res.* 12:46. doi: 10.1186/1465-9921-12-46

Sisignano, M., Park, C. K., Angioni, C., Zhang, D. D., Von Hehn, C., Cobos, E. J., et al. (2012). 5,6-EET is released upon neuronal activity and induces mechanical pain hypersensitivity via TRPA1 on central afferent terminals. *J. Neurosci.* 32, 6364–6372. doi: 10.1523/JNEUROSCI.5793-11.2012

Smith, P. L., Maloney, K. N., Pothen, R. G., Clardy, J., and Clapham, D. E. (2006). Bisandrographolide from *Andrographis paniculata* activates TRPV4 channels. *J. Biol. Chem.* 281, 29897–29904. doi: 10.1074/jbc.M605394200

Sokabe, T., and Tominaga, M. (2010). The TRPV4 cation channel: a molecule linking skin temperature and barrier function. *Commun. Integr. Biol.* 3, 619–621. doi: 10.4161/cib.3.6.13461

Song, L., Mcgee, J., and Walsh, E. J. (2006). Frequency- and level-dependent changes in auditory brainstem responses (ABRS) in developing mice. *J. Acoust. Soc. Am.* 119, 2242–2257. doi: 10.1121/1.2180533

Stepanyan, R. S., Indzhykulian, A. A., Velez-Ortega, A. C., Boger, E. T., Steyger, P. S., Friedman, T. B., et al. (2011). TRPA1-mediated accumulation of aminoglycosides in mouse cochlear outer hair cells. *J. Assoc. Res. Otolaryngol.* 12, 729–740. doi: 10.1007/s10162-011-0288-x

Strotmann, R., Harteneck, C., Nunnenmacher, K., Schultz, G., and Plant, T. D. (2000). OTRPC4, a nonselective cation channel that confers sensitivity to extracellular osmolarity. *Nat. Cell Biol.* 2, 695–702. doi: 10.1038/35036318

Sullivan, M. N., Gonzales, A. L., Pires, P. W., Bruhl, A., Leo, M. D., Li, W., et al. (2015). Localized TRPA1 channel Ca^{2+} signals stimulated by reactive oxygen species promote cerebral artery dilation. *Sci. Signal.* 8, ra2. doi: 10.1126/scisignal.2005659

Takahashi, K., and Ohta, T. (2017). Membrane translocation of transient receptor potential ankyrin 1 induced by inflammatory cytokines in lung cancer cells. *Biochem. Biophys. Res. Commun.* 490, 587–593. doi: 10.1016/j.bbrc.2017.06.082

Takeuchi, O., and Akira, S. (2009). Innate immunity to virus infection. *Immunol. Rev.* 227, 75–86. doi: 10.1111/j.1600-065X.2008.00737.x

Talavera, K., Gees, M., Karashima, Y., Meseguer, V. M., Vanoirbeek, J. A., Damann, N., et al. (2009). Nicotine activates the chemosensory cation channel TRPA1. *Nat. Neurosci.* 12, 1293–1299. doi: 10.1038/nn.2379

Tan, Y., Zanoni, I., Cullen, T. W., Goodman, A. L., and Kagan, J. C. (2015). Mechanisms of toll-like receptor 4 endocytosis reveal a common immune-evasion strategy used by pathogenic and commensal bacteria. *Immunity* 43, 909–922. doi: 10.1016/j.immuni.2015.10.008

Tang, H. Y., Hutcheson, E., Neill, S., Drummond-Borg, M., Speer, M., and Alford, R. L. (2002). Genetic susceptibility to aminoglycoside ototoxicity: how many are at risk? *Genet. Med.* 4, 336–345. doi: 10.1097/00125817-200209000-00004

Tauris, J., Christensen, E. I., Nykjaer, A., Jacobsen, C., Petersen, C. M., and Ovesen, T. (2009). Cubilin and megalin co-localize in the neonatal inner ear. *Audiol. Neurootol.* 14, 267–278. doi: 10.1159/000199446

Tauseef, M., Knezevic, N., Chava, K. R., Smith, M., Sukriti, S., Gianaris, N., et al. (2012). TLR4 activation of TRPC6-dependent calcium signaling mediates endotoxin-induced lung vascular permeability and inflammation. *J. Exp. Med.* 209, 1953–1968. doi: 10.1084/jem.20111355

Thorneloe, K. S., Sulpizio, A. C., Lin, Z., Figueroa, D. J., Clouse, A. K., Mccafferty, G. P., et al. (2008). N-((1S)-1-{[4-((2S)-2-{[(2,4-dichlorophenyl)sulfonyl]amino}-3-hydroxypropanoyl)-1-piperazinyl]carbonyl}-3-methylbutyl)-1-benzothiophene-2-carboxamide (GSK1016790A), a novel and potent transient receptor potential vanilloid 4 channel agonist induces urinary bladder contraction and hyperactivity: part I. *J. Pharmacol. Exp. Ther.* 326, 432–442. doi: 10.1124/jpet.108.139295

Tran Ba Huy, P., Bernard, P., and Schacht, J. (1986). Kinetics of gentamicin uptake and release in the rat. Comparison of inner ear tissues and fluids with other organs. *J. Clin. Invest.* 77, 1492–1500. doi: 10.1172/JCI112463

Trune, D. R. (1997). Cochlear immunoglobulin in the C3H/lpr mouse model for autoimmune hearing loss. *Otolaryngol. Head Neck Surg.* 117, 504–508. doi: 10.1016/S0194-5998(97)70022-6

Utech, M., Mennigen, R., and Bruewer, M. (2010). Endocytosis and recycling of tight junction proteins in inflammation. *J. Biomed. Biotechnol.* 2010:484987. doi: 10.1155/2010/484987

Vellani, V., Mapplebeck, S., Moriondo, A., Davis, J. B., and Mcnaughton, P. A. (2001). Protein kinase C activation potentiates gating of the vanilloid receptor VR1 by capsaicin, protons, heat and anandamide. *J. Physiol.* 534, 813–825. doi: 10.1111/j.1469-7793.2001.00813.x

Vriens, J., Watanabe, H., Janssens, A., Droogmans, G., Voets, T., and Nilius, B. (2004). Cell swelling, heat, and chemical agonists use distinct pathways for the activation of the cation channel TRPV4. *Proc. Natl. Acad. Sci. U.S.A.* 101, 396–401. doi: 10.1073/pnas.0303329101

Vu, A. A., Nadaraja, G. S., Huth, M. E., Luk, L., Kim, J., Chai, R., et al. (2013). Integrity and regeneration of mechanotransduction machinery regulate aminoglycoside entry and sensory cell death. *PLOS ONE* 8:e54794. doi: 10.1371/journal.pone.0054794

Wang, Q., Kachelmeier, A., and Steyger, P. S. (2010). Competitive antagonism of fluorescent gentamicin uptake in the cochlea. *Hear. Res.* 268, 250–259. doi: 10.1016/j.heares.2010.06.008

Wood, M. B., and Zuo, J. (2017). The contribution of immune infiltrates to ototoxicity and cochlear hair cell loss. *Front. Cell. Neurosci.* 11:106. doi: 10.3389/fncel.2017.00106

Wu, W. J., Sha, S. H., Mclaren, J. D., Kawamoto, K., Raphael, Y., and Schacht, J. (2001). Aminoglycoside ototoxicity in adult CBA, C57BL and BALB mice and the Sprague-Dawley rat. *Hear. Res.* 158, 165–178. doi: 10.1016/S0378-5955(01)00303-3

Yamada, T., Ogi, K., Sakashita, M., Kanno, M., Kubo, S., Ito, Y., et al. (2017). Toll-like receptor ligands induce cytokine and chemokine production in human inner ear endolymphatic sac fibroblasts. *Auris Nasus Larynx* 44, 398–403. doi: 10.1016/j.anl.2016.10.007

Yamasaki, M., Komune, S., Shimozono, M., Matsuda, K., and Haruta, A. (2000). Development of monovalent ions in the endolymph in mouse cochlea. *ORL J. Otorhinolaryngol. Relat. Spec.* 62, 241–246. doi: 10.1159/000027753

Yang, C. J., Lee, N. Y., Lin, Y. H., Lee, H. C., Ko, W. C., Liao, C. H., et al. (2010). Jarisch-Herxheimer reaction after penicillin therapy among patients with syphilis in the era of the hiv infection epidemic: incidence and risk factors. *Clin. Infect. Dis.* 51, 976–979. doi: 10.1086/656419

Yoon, P. J., Price, M., Gallagher, K., Fleisher, B. E., and Messner, A. H. (2003). The need for long-term audiologic follow-up of neonatal intensive care unit (NICU) graduates. *Int. J. Pediatr. Otorhinolaryngol.* 67, 353–357. doi: 10.1016/S0165-5876(02)00400-7

Yun, J. H., Park, S. W., Kim, K. J., Bae, J. S., Lee, E. H., Paek, S. H., et al. (2017). Endothelial STAT3 activation increases vascular leakage through downregulating tight junction proteins: implications for diabetic retinopathy. *J. Cell. Physiol.* 232, 1123–1134. doi: 10.1002/jcp.25575

Zarember, K. A., and Godowski, P. J. (2002). Tissue expression of human Toll-like receptors and differential regulation of Toll-like receptor mRNAs in leukocytes in response to microbes, their products, and cytokines. *J. Immunol.* 168, 554–561. doi: 10.4049/jimmunol.168.2.554

Zhang, W., Dai, M., Fridberger, A., Hassan, A., Degagne, J., Neng, L., et al. (2012). Perivascular-resident macrophage-like melanocytes in the inner ear are essential for the integrity of the intrastrial fluid-blood barrier. *Proc. Natl. Acad. Sci. U.S.A.* 109, 10388–10393. doi: 10.1073/pnas.1205210109

Zhang, X., Huang, J., and Mcnaughton, P. A. (2005). NGF rapidly increases membrane expression of TRPV1 heat-gated ion channels. *EMBO J.* 24, 4211–4223. doi: 10.1038/sj.emboj.7600893

Zheng, J., Dai, C., Steyger, P. S., Kim, Y., Vass, Z., Ren, T., et al. (2003). Vanilloid receptors in hearing: altered cochlear sensitivity by vanilloids and expression of TRPV1 in the organ of corti. *J. Neurophysiol.* 90, 444–455. doi: 10.1152/jn.00919.2002

Zheng, X., Zinkevich, N. S., Gebremedhin, D., Gauthier, K. M., Nishijima, Y., Fang, J., et al. (2013). Arachidonic acid-induced dilation in human coronary arterioles: convergence of signaling mechanisms on endothelial TRPV4-mediated Ca^{2+} entry. *J. Am. Heart Assoc.* 2:e000080. doi: 10.1161/JAHA.113.000080

5

Mechanisms of Cisplatin-Induced Ototoxicity and Otoprotection

Sandeep Sheth[1], *Debashree Mukherjea*[2], *Leonard P. Rybak*[1,2] *and Vickram Ramkumar*[1]*

[1] *Department of Pharmacology, Southern Illinois University School of Medicine, Springfield, IL, United States,* [2] *Department of Surgery (Otolaryngology), Southern Illinois University School of Medicine, Springfield, IL, United States*

Edited by:
Lisa Cunningham,
National Institutes of Health (NIH),
United States

Reviewed by:
Allison B. Coffin,
Washington State University,
United States
Andy Groves,
Baylor College of Medicine,
United States
Evangelia Tserga,
Karolinska Institute (KI), Sweden

***Correspondence:**
Vickram Ramkumar
vramkumar@siumed.edu

Evidence of significant hearing loss during the early days of use of cisplatin as a chemotherapeutic agent in cancer patients has stimulated research into the causes and treatment of this side effect. It has generally been accepted that hearing loss is produced by excessive generation of reactive oxygen species (ROS) in cell of the cochlea, which led to the development of various antioxidants as otoprotective agents. Later studies show that ROS could stimulate cochlear inflammation, suggesting the use of anti-inflammatory agents for treatment of hearing loss. In this respect, G-protein coupled receptors, such as adenosine A_1 receptor and cannabinoid 2 receptors, have shown efficacy in the treatment of hearing loss in experimental animals by increasing ROS scavenging, suppressing ROS generation, or by decreasing inflammation. Inflammation could be triggered by activation of transient receptor potential vanilloid 1 (TRPV1) channels in the cochlea and possibly other TRP channels. Targeting TRPV1 for knockdown has also been shown to be a useful strategy for ensuring otoprotection. Cisplatin entry into cochlear hair cells is mediated by various transporters, inhibitors of which have been shown to be effective for treating hearing loss. Finally, cisplatin-induced DNA damage and activation of the apoptotic process could be targeted for cisplatin-induced hearing loss. This review focuses on recent development in our understanding of the mechanisms underlying cisplatin-induced hearing loss and provides examples of how drug therapies have been formulated based on these mechanisms.

Keywords: cisplatin, ototoxicity, otoprotection, oxidative stress, apoptosis, antioxidants, anti-inflammatory agents

CISPLATIN OTOTOXICITY

Cisplatin is a widely used and effective drug for the treatment of solid tumors ranging from ovarian, lung, head, and neck to testicular cancer. Dose limiting side effects, such as ototoxicity, neurotoxicity, and nephrotoxicity, are generally encountered with a majority of patients treated with cisplatin-based chemotherapy. Methods to increase diuresis, such as hydration, have been shown to reduce nephrotoxicity. However, to date no effective FDA approved treatment for ototoxicity is available. Cisplatin-induced hearing loss is primarily in the high frequency range. It is bilateral and permanent and severely affects the quality of life for cancer patients. The incidence of cisplatin-induced hearing loss in children ranges from 22 to 77% (Knight et al., 2005; Kushner et al., 2006; Coradini et al., 2007). This range reflects hearing loss observed with the different doses and duration of cisplatin treatment in addition to the different age groups of the patients who were treated. Accordingly, children show greater risk for developing hearing loss following cisplatin treatment than adults

(Knight et al., 2005; Kushner et al., 2006; Gurney et al., 2007). Hearing loss is especially difficult for children who are undergoing treatment for brain tumors, such as neuroblastoma. It could affect early speech development and hamper social integration. Development of effective therapies for treating hearing loss is therefore of primary importance.

Several approaches have been undertaken over the past two decades to treat cisplatin ototoxicity. These include the use of localized or systemic administration of antioxidants or drugs which activate endogenous antioxidant systems. Cisplatin induces apoptosis of hair cells through activation of mitochondrial pathway which can be targeted to inhibit cell death. Another approach involves using anti-inflammatory agents which target the pro-inflammatory mechanisms associated with cisplatin treatment in the cochlea. Recent insights into the entry processes of cisplatin in hair cells and other cells in the cochlea should stimulate the development of drugs which specifically block entry of drugs into these cells without affecting cisplatin entry into cancer cells. This report reviews the currently accepted mechanisms underlying cisplatin-induced damage or death to cochlear cells and highlights how these mechanisms could guide the future development of effective otoprotective agents.

COCHLEAR ROS GENERATION AND ANTIOXIDANT DEFENSE SYSTEM

The normal function of the cochlea requires its high metabolic activity in areas such as the stria vascularis, spiral ligament, and spiral prominence (Salt et al., 1987; Ryan, 1988). This high metabolic activity leads to leakage of electrons from the mitochondrial respiratory chain which can react with oxygen (O_2) to form superoxide ($O_2^{-\bullet}$). Environmental stimuli which increase the metabolic activity of the cochlea, such as loud noise, are expected to increase oxidative stress in the cochlea. The metabolic demand on the cochlea renders it very sensitive to hypoxic events and ischemia-reperfusion injuries (Seidman et al., 1991). Ototoxic drugs, such as cisplatin have been shown to increase the generation of reactive oxygen species (ROS) (Clerici and Yang, 1996; Kopke et al., 1997) by either stimulating enzyme systems linked to this process or by inactivating antioxidant systems (Church et al., 1995; Rybak et al., 1995). Rats injected with cisplatin demonstrate reduced cochlear glutathione (GSH) and antioxidant enzyme activities (Ravi et al., 1995). A primary target of cisplatin for generation of ROS is the NOX3 NADPH oxidase system (Banfi et al., 2004). NOX3 is induced by cisplatin and knockdown of this enzyme by *trans*-tympanic delivery of siRNA protects against cisplatin-induced ototoxicity (Mukherjea et al., 2010). Since NOX3 is localized primarily to the cochlea, systemic administration of inhibitors of NOX3 could effectively reduce enzyme activity and treat hearing loss. Another active ROS generating system in the cochlea is xanthine oxidase. This enzyme converts hypoxanthine (a metabolite derived from the breakdown of adenosine by adenosine deaminase) to uric acid. Inhibition of this enzyme by allopurinol contributes to reductions in cisplatin-induced ototoxicity and nephrotoxicity when administered with ebselen, a glutathione peroxidase (GSH.Px) mimetic (Lynch et al., 2005).

The cochlea possesses an efficient antioxidant defense system. This includes antioxidants such as vitamin C, vitamin E, and low molecular weight thiols, such as GSH (Kopke et al., 1999). Studies in the guinea pig cochlea show that the highest levels of GSH are present in the basal and intermediate cells of the stria vascularis and in cells of the spiral ligament (Usami et al., 1996). This distribution matches well with the distribution of glutathione *S*-transferase (el Barbary et al., 1993), an enzyme which conjugates and detoxifies xenobiotics (such as cisplatin). Increased levels of glutathione *S*-transferase in cancer cells can aid in the inactivation of cisplatin and contribute to resistance to cisplatin in the cochlea. In addition, the cochlea expresses several antioxidant enzymes, which include superoxide dismutase (SOD), GSH.Px, and catalase (CAT). SOD catalyzes the conversion of $O_2^{-\bullet}$ to H_2O_2 and O_2 while CAT converts H_2O_2 to O_2 and H_2O. GSH.Px reduces H_2O_2 and possibly other peroxides. The enzyme GSH.Px also catalyzes the conversion of reduced GSH to its oxidized form (GSSG), in the process of detoxifying H_2O_2. In addition, glutathione reductase (GR) is important for the defense against ROS by aiding in the regeneration of GSH from GSSG (**Figure 1**). Two forms of SOD are expressed in the cochlea. A Cu/Zn isoform of SOD is localized in the cytosol, while a Mn-regulated isoform (Mn-SOD) is localized to the mitochondria (Yao and Rarey, 1996). Mn-SOD is localized to metabolically active sites in the cochlea such as stria vascularis, spiral ligament, spiral prominence, spiral limbus, and organ of Corti (Lai et al., 1996). Activities of SOD were higher in the subcellular fractions of stria vascularis and spiral ligament compared to the organ of Corti (Pierson and Gray, 1982; Yao and Rarey, 1996). High activities of other antioxidant enzymes were also observed in the lateral wall tissues compared to the rest of the cochlea, suggesting their roles in mitigating oxidative stress in these regions (Pierson and Gray, 1982). In the absence of this ROS detoxification system, ROS can produce cellular damage by lipid peroxidation, with increased levels of the lipid peroxide, malondialdehyde, and 4-hydroxynonenal.

INCREASED ROS GENERATION CONTRIBUTES TO CISPLATIN-INDUCED HEARING LOSS

Exposure of explants to ROS induces bleb formation and changes in length of outer hair cells which were attenuated by co-administration of the antioxidant, deferoxamine, or antioxidant enzymes (Clerici et al., 1995). Infusion of ROS into the guinea pig ear led to increased compound action potential (CAP) threshold amplitudes, which were reduced by co-administration of antioxidant or antioxidant enzymes (Clerici and Yang, 1996). Furthermore, it was observed that cochleae obtained from cisplatin-treated animals showed depletion of GSH and reduced activities of antioxidant enzymes, such as SOD, CAT, GSH.Px, and GR along with increased evidence of lipid peroxidation (Rybak et al., 2000). This reduction in antioxidant capacity in the cochlea could result from: (1) covalent binding of cisplatin

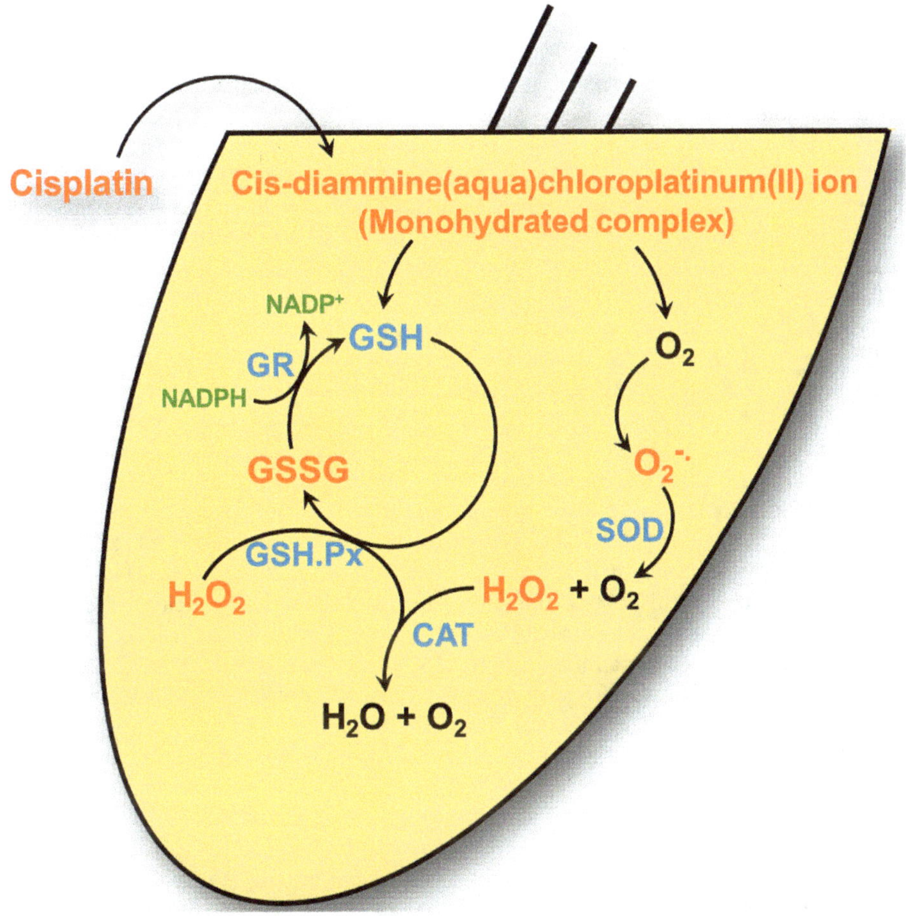

FIGURE 1 | Cisplatin's interaction with the cochlear antioxidant defense system. Cisplatin is converted to a *cis*-diammine(aqua)chloroplatinum(II) (a monohydrate cisplatin complex) upon entering the cell cytoplasm. These reactive platinum species can react with molecular oxygen (O_2) to generate superoxide (O_2^{-}•) which is detoxified by superoxide dismutase (SOD) to hydrogen peroxide (H_2O_2) and oxygen. Hydrogen peroxide is further detoxified by catalase to water (H_2O) and oxygen. Cisplatin reactive intermediates readily bind to and oxidizes the antioxidant reduced glutathione (GSH) to oxidized glutathione (GSSG). Glutathione peroxidase (GSH.Px) consumes GSH to produce GSSG in the process of converting H_2O_2 into H_2O. Glutathione reductase (GR) reduces GSSG to GSH by using the reduced from of nicotinamide adenine dinucleotide phosphate ($NADP^+$), NAPDH, as cofactor.

to sulfhydryl groups within the antioxidant enzymes, causing enzyme inactivation; (2) loss of metal cofactors, such as copper and selenium, which are vital for activity of SOD and GSH.Px; (3) increased ROS which could exhaust antioxidant enzymes; and/or (4) depletion of cochlear antioxidant enzyme cofactors, such as GSH and NADPH, which are essential for GSH.Px and GR activities, respectively (for review see Rybak et al., 2000). The increased oxidative stress within the cochlea could increase lipid peroxidation of membranes, inactivate essential cellular enzymes and membrane transporters, and disrupt ion channel function. The ultimate effect of increased ROS generation is to promote apoptotic and necrotic cell death. These data suggest that ROS plays a critical role in cisplatin-induced ototoxicity and that its inhibition could ameliorate hearing loss.

As discussed below, one important result of increased oxidative stress is induction of inflammatory processes in the cochlea. The importance of managing ROS in mediating otoprotection is underscored by the observation that polymorphisms of glutathione *S*-transferase gene increase susceptibility to cisplatin hearing loss (Oldenburg et al., 2007). In this report, it was shown that patients inheriting the 105Ile/105Ile-GSTP1 or 105Val/105Ile-GSTP1 alleles had greater hearing loss than those inheriting the 105Val/105Val-GSTP1 alleles (Oldenburg et al., 2007).

TARGETING OXIDATIVE STRESS FOR TREATING CISPLATIN-INDUCED HEARING LOSS

The cochlea is endowed with a number of distinct cellular mechanisms which could contribute to otoprotection. These include various endogenous antioxidant enzymes and antioxidants (detailed above), heat shock proteins, kidney injury molecule-1, anti-apoptotic proteins, transcription factors such as nuclear factor erythroid 2-related factor 2 (Nrf2) and signal transducer and activator of transcription (STAT) proteins, and a number of hormone and G-protein-coupled receptors (Ford et al., 1997; Oh et al., 2000; Mukherjea et al., 2006; So et al., 2006; Borse et al., 2017). Therefore, it is very surprising that these mechanisms are not able to effectively protect against cisplatin ototoxicity. However, it is possible that over the course of cisplatin treatment in animal models and humans that these protective systems become overwhelmed and are no longer able to manage the toxicity. It is believed that exogenously administered antioxidants or other drugs can boost the local protective mechanism to ensure otoprotection.

Early studies were directed at examining the effects of drugs which reduce oxidative stress for treating hearing loss. Studies performed in animals indicated that antioxidants protected against cisplatin-induced hearing loss. Many of these antioxidants are thiol compounds which have high affinities for platinum. This forms the basis for their protection against cisplatin toxicity but also could account for the antitumor interference with cisplatin. Studies showed that *N*-acetyl cysteine (NAC) protected against cisplatin-ototoxicity in rats (Dickey et al., 2008) and guinea pigs (Choe et al., 2004). Sodium thiosulfate (STS) was also effective against cisplatin-induced hearing loss (Otto et al., 1988). However, systemic administration of this drug led to formation of cisplatin–STS complex, which reduced the levels of cisplatin in circulation needed for effective antitumor therapy (Wimmer et al., 2004). Thus, local application of STS into the cochlea would be required to provide effective otoprotection (Wimmer et al., 2004), as was shown previously (Wang et al., 2003). Several studies have shown that D-methionine, another sulfur-containing compound, protects against cisplatin-induced hearing loss when administered by both the systemic and local routes (Campbell et al., 1996; Korver et al., 2002). At the cellular level, the otoprotection mediated by this compound was associated with its ability to increase the activity of intrinsic antioxidant enzymes (Campbell et al., 2003). Other antioxidants which show promise against cisplatin-induced hearing loss include ebselen, lipoic acid, diethyldithiocarbamate, and 4-methylthiobenzoic acid (Rybak et al., 1999). Similarly, high doses of amifostine provided otoprotection in hamsters but its use was associated with neurotoxicity (Church et al., 2004).

Contrary to the pre-clinical findings, studies performed in humans showed that STS protected against cisplatin-induced nephrotoxicity (Goel et al., 1989) but was ineffective against cisplatin-induced hearing loss (Zuur et al., 2007). Amifostine was also ineffective as an otoprotectant in patients with metastatic melanoma (Ekborn et al., 2002) and in children suffering from neuroblastoma or germ cell tumors and were on a chemotherapeutic regimen including cisplatin (Marina et al., 2005; Sastry and Kellie, 2005). However, later studies showed that higher doses of amifostine were able to provide significant otoprotection (Fouladi et al., 2008).

Several G-protein-coupled receptors have been characterized in the cochlea, activation of which confer protection against cisplatin-induced hearing loss. Immunolabeling studies show distribution of the A_1 adenosine receptors (A_1ARs) in the stria vascularis, spiral ganglion cells, and organ of Corti (Vlajkovic et al., 2009). In the organ of Corti, the greatest distribution of A_1AR is in the inner hair cells, Deiter's cells and lower levels in the outer hair cells. Expression of A_1AR was also observed in mouse organ of Corti-derived cell lines including the UB/OC-1 cells (Kaur et al., 2016) and HEI-OC1 cells (unpublished data). Localized application of A_1AR agonist resulted in an increase in the activities of the antioxidative enzymes GSH.Px and SOD (Ford et al., 1997). Furthermore, A_1AR agonist also reduced the cisplatin-mediated increase in malondialdehyde levels in the cochlea resulting in protection against cisplatin-induced hair cell damage and hearing loss (Whitworth et al., 2004). No significant benefits was observed following activation of the A_{2a}AR and A_3AR (Whitworth et al., 2004) which are also distributed in the cochlea (Vlajkovic et al., 2009). Systemic administration of the adenosine amine congener (ADAC) was shown to protect against cisplatin ototoxicity, presumably by activating the A_1AR (Gunewardene et al., 2013). Recent data support an anti-inflammatory role of A_1AR activation in the cochlea mediated by suppression of the NOX3 isoform of NADPH oxidase and suppression of STAT1-mediated inflammatory pathway (Kaur et al., 2016). STAT1 activation plays an integral role in cisplatin ototoxicity, as inhibition or knockdown of this transcription factor reduced cisplatin-induced hearing loss (Schmitt et al., 2009; Kaur et al., 2011; Mukherjea et al., 2011). A recent study from our laboratory has further documented an essential role of STAT1 in mediating cisplatin-induced hearing loss, as inhibition of this factor by a green tea extract and a known STAT1 inhibitor, epigallocatechin-3-gallate (EGCG), provided otoprotection (Borse et al., 2017). In a rodent model, EGCG protected against cisplatin-induced hearing loss without compromising cisplatin antitumor efficacy (Borse et al., 2017) (see model depicted in **Figure 2**). *In vitro* studies performed in HEI-OC1 cells demonstrate that cannabinoid 2 receptor (CB2) agonists reduce cisplatin-induced cell killing (Jeong et al., 2007). CB2 are also expressed in the stria vascularis, inner hair cells and spiral ganglion cells of the cochlea from adult albino rats (Martin-Saldana et al., 2016). Recent studies from our laboratories support an otoprotective role of CB2 activation in the cochlea, which is mediated at least in part, through inhibition of STAT1 (Ghosh et al., 2016; unpublished data). Thus, the protective action of CB2 could share a similar mechanism as observed by A_1AR, namely inhibition of STAT1.

Additional studies from our laboratory implicated transient receptor potential vanilloid 1 (TRPV1) channels in cisplatin-mediated ototoxicity (Mukherjea et al., 2008). In a rat model, we showed knockdown of these channels by *trans*-tympanic administration of short interfering (si) RNA protected against cisplatin-induced hearing loss and damage to the outer hair cells (Mukherjea et al., 2008) (**Figure 3**). Protection was likely mediated by reducing the expression of a downstream target of TRPV1, such as NOX3, activation of which promotes ROS generation and STAT1 activation, as indicated above. STAT1 can promote both the inflammatory and pro-apoptotic actions of cisplatin in the cochlea (Kaur et al., 2011). This study suggests that inhibition of TRPV1 or NOX3 could serve as useful approaches for reducing cisplatin ototoxicity.

Characterization of cisplatin-induced cell death in HEI-OC1 cells showed induction of apoptosis by increased lipid

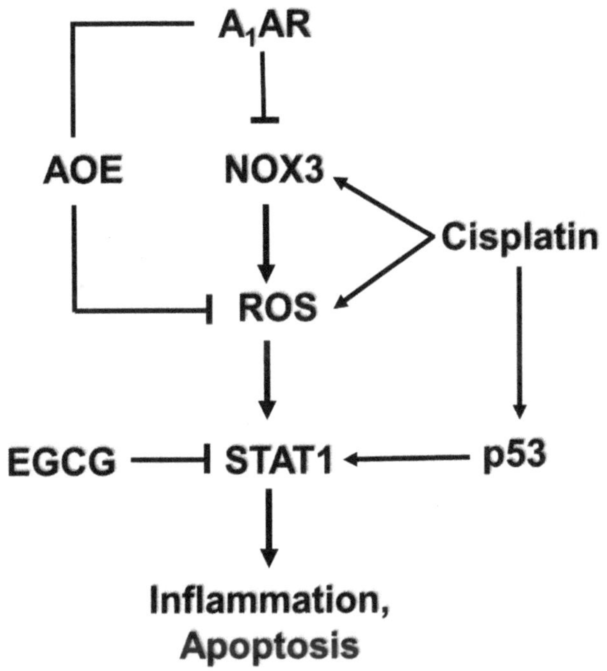

FIGURE 2 | Mechanism of cisplatin-induced hearing loss and A_1 adenosine receptor (A_1AR)-dependent otoprotection. Cisplatin mediates NOX3 activation and reactive oxygen species (ROS) generation. The generation of ROS promotes signal transducer and activator of transcription 1 (STAT1) activation which stimulates the inflammatory process. Activated STAT1 association with active p53 promotes the apoptosis of cochlear cells. The otoprotective effects of A_1AR activation is mediated by reducing oxidative stress in the cochlea by activating antioxidant enzymes (AOE) and/or by suppressing the induction of NOX3. EGCG, a known inhibitor of STAT1, has been shown to protect against cisplatin-induced hearing loss.

peroxidation and altered mitochondrial permeability transition. It was shown that the calcium-channel blocker, flunarizine, attenuated cisplatin-induced cell death (So et al., 2006). The mechanism underlying the otoprotective action of flunarizine appears to involve activation of Nrf2 and increased expression of hemeoxygenase-1 (HO-1) (So et al., 2006). Flunarizine also exhibited an anti-inflammatory role, as evidenced from its ability to inhibit the ERK1/2 MAP kinase-nuclear factor (NF)-κB-dependent pathway (So et al., 2008).

MITOCHONDRIAL TARGETS OF CISPLATIN-INDUCED OTOTOXICITY

Bcl-2 Family

The Bcl-2 family of proteins consists of members that form the mitochondrial apoptotic pathway and function as regulators of cell death and cell survival. Among its members, Bcl-2 and Bcl-xL promote cell survival, whereas Bax, Bak, Bcl-XS, Bid, Bad, and Bim induce apoptosis (Siddiqui et al., 2015). The balance between the pro-apoptotic and anti-apoptotic proteins is crucial for the well-being of the cell. However, cellular damage caused by noxious stimuli can tilt this balance in favor of apoptosis. This process is initiated when pro-apoptotic protein such as Bax and Bid translocate from the cytoplasm to the mitochondria. This triggers a sequence of events leading to the permeabilization of the outer mitochondrial membrane, which results in the loss of mitochondrial membrane potential, generation of ROS, and release of cytochrome c from mitochondria into the cytoplasm (Siddiqui et al., 2015).

Several studies have implicated the mitochondrial pathways in the apoptosis of auditory cells after cisplatin treatment. Mongolian gerbils administered cisplatin showed deterioration in the responses of both distortion product otoacoustic emissions (DPOAE) and the endocochlear potential as compared with age-matched controls (Alam et al., 2000). The cisplatin-induced hearing loss was correlated with increased levels of Bax and decreased expression of Bcl-2 in the cells of organ of Corti, spiral ganglion and the lateral wall, as determined by immunohistochemistry. Moreover, cisplatin significantly elevated the ratio of Bax to Bcl-2, an important indicator of apoptosis, in the three representative regions in all turns of the cochlea. Similarly, cochlear hair cells from cisplatin-treated guinea pigs demonstrated apoptosis which was linked to the activation and redistribution of cytosolic Bax and the release of cytochrome c from the mitochondria (Wang et al., 2004). In another study conducted in HEI/OC1 cells, cisplatin-induced apoptosis through mitochondrial pathway which involved truncation of Bid, mitochondrial translocation of Bax, and release of cytochrome c (Devarajan et al., 2002). Recently, cisplatin treatment in UB/OC-1 cells significantly increased expression of *Bax*, but reduced the levels of *Bcl-xL* (Borse et al., 2017). Treatment with EGCG, a known inhibitor of STAT1, reversed these cisplatin-mediated effects on the expression of *Bax* and *Bcl-xL* (Borse et al., 2017) and protected against hearing loss (**Figure 4**). These data indicate that cisplatin induces apoptosis through activation of mitochondrial pathway and that inhibiting elements of this pathway could alleviate hearing loss.

Caspases

Stress signals from the mitochondria also regulate the cleavage of pro-caspase-9 into its active form, caspase-9 (Hengartner, 2000). Activated caspase-9 can then cleave and activate the downstream effector caspase, caspase-3, resulting in apoptotic destruction of the cell. Caspase-3 is also activated by caspase-8, which is an initiator caspase activated by plasma membrane death receptors (Salvesen and Dixit, 1997). Cisplatin induces apoptosis of auditory hair cells and cochlear cell lines via activation of initiator caspase-9 and its effector caspase-3. Cisplatin-induced activation of caspase-9 and caspase-3 was also seen in HEI/OC1 (Devarajan et al., 2002; Chung et al., 2008) cells and UB/OC1 cells (Borse et al., 2017). Wang et al. (2004) reported the activation of caspase-9 and caspase-3, but not caspase-8, in cochlear hair cells of pigmented guinea pigs treated with cisplatin. Furthermore, intracochlear perfusion of specific inhibitors of caspase-9 and caspase-3 protected against cisplatin-induced hair cell death and hearing loss in these animals (Wang et al., 2004). In another study, treatment of neonatal rat organ of Corti explants with caspase-1- and caspase-3-specific inhibitors and a general caspase inhibitor protected more than 80% of the auditory hair

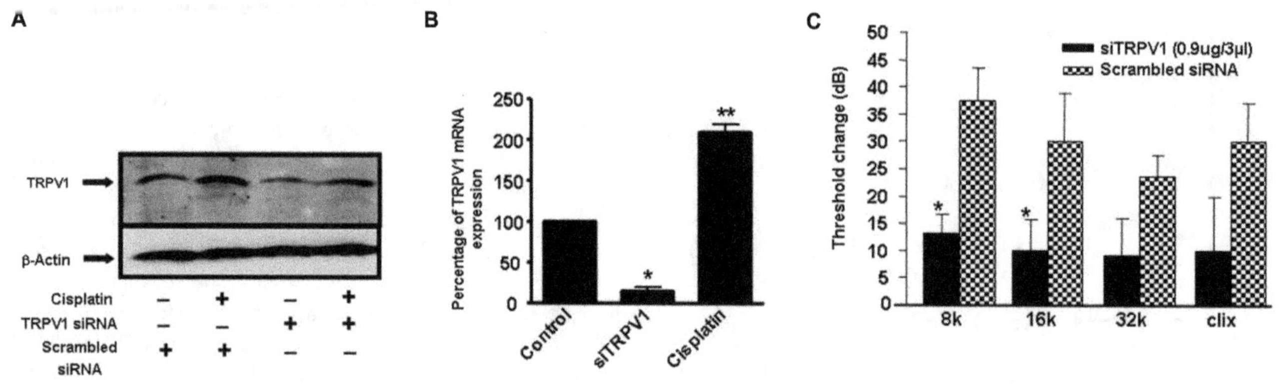

FIGURE 3 | Round window administration of siRNA against *TRPV1* protects against cisplatin-induced ototoxicity in rats. **(A)** Round window application of *TRPV1* siRNA reduced both, basal and cisplatin-stimulated TRPV1 protein levels in the cochlea, assessed 24 h following cisplatin administration. **(B)** *TRPV1* siRNA suppressed *TRPV1* expression in the rat cochlea. **(C)** Functional studies show that *TRPV1* siRNA (0.9 μg) administered by round window application protected against cisplatin-induced elevations in hearing thresholds at all frequencies tested and for click stimuli. Cisplatin (13 mg/kg i.p.) was administered 48 h following siRNA or a scrambled siRNA sequence and post-treatment ABRs were determined after an additional 72 h period. $^{*}p < 0.05$ versus scrambled siRNA-treated cochleae and $^{**}p < 0.05$ versus TRPV1 siRNA ($n = 5$). This figure was adapted from Mukherjea et al. (2008), with permission.

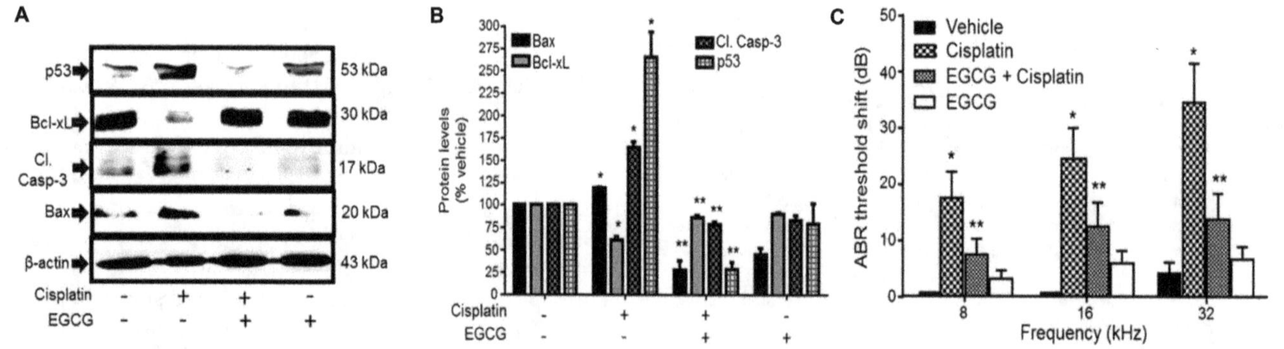

FIGURE 4 | Epigallocatechin-3-gallate (EGCG) inhibited cisplatin-induced apoptosis and hearing loss. **(A)** UB/OC-1 cells pretreated with either vehicle or EGCG (100 μM) followed by cisplatin (20 μM) for 24 h were analyzed for pro-apoptotic proteins, such as p53, cleaved caspase-3 and Bax and anti-apoptotic protein, Bcl-xL. The expression of pro-apoptotic proteins was substantially reduced by EGCG while the reductions in Bcl-xL were attenuated. **(B)** The bar graph represents results from **A** after normalization with β-actin bands and are presented as the mean ± SEM. $^{*}p < 0.05$ versus vehicle and $^{**}p < 0.05$ versus vehicle + cisplatin ($n = 4$). **(C)** Pre-treatment ABR thresholds were recorded in Wistar rats, which were then treated with oral EGCG (100 mg/kg body weight). Cisplatin (11 mg/kg) was administered intraperitoneally 24 h later and animals were continued on daily oral EGCG treatments for additional 3 days. Post-treatment ABRs were performed on day 4. Daily oral administration of EGCG protected from cisplatin-induced ABR threshold shifts at all frequencies tested. $^{*}p < 0.05$ versus vehicle and $^{**}p < 0.05$ versus vehicle + cisplatin ($n = 4$). This figure was adapted from Borse et al. (2017), with permission.

cells from cisplatin-induced apoptosis (Liu et al., 1998). Unlike other caspases, caspase-1 is not linked with the induction of apoptosis in cells. Caspase-1 is studied for its role in initiating inflammatory immune responses through formation of inflammasomes. Activation of caspase-1 was recently reported to induce hearing loss after cytomegalovirus (CMV) infection in the inner ear through upregulation of its downstream inflammatory factors, such as interleukin-1β and interleukin-18 (Shi et al., 2015). Therefore, it is possible that caspase-1-specific inhibitor may protect from cisplatin ototoxicity by inhibiting cisplatin-induced inflammation in the cochlea.

Several mechanisms underlying cisplatin-induced caspase activation has been proposed. For example, cisplatin-induced apoptosis and caspase-3 activation in HEI/OC1 cells was reduced after treatment with NF-κB inhibitors, Bay 11-7085 and SN-50 (Chung et al., 2008). This finding indicates that NF-κB is activated by cisplatin and plays a pro-apoptotic role in HEI/OC1 cell death. Cisplatin-induced apoptosis and activation of caspase-3, -8, and -9 were also inhibited by activation of CB2 receptors (Jeong et al., 2007), which are present in the cochlear cells and upregulated by cisplatin (Martin-Saldana et al., 2016). Cisplatin-mediated expression of cleaved-caspase-3 in UB/CO1 cells was inhibited by treatment with EGCG through inhibition of STAT1 (Borse et al., 2017). Taken together, loss of auditory cells as a result of cisplatin-induced apoptosis involves activation of caspases as a final common pathway activated by different upstream signaling pathways described above. Inhibition of one or more of these signaling pathways could effectively rescue hair cell loss and restore hearing.

p53

The general mechanism of action of cisplatin in tumor cells is that it forms crosslinks with the purine bases of the DNA, causing DNA damage. The overwhelming DNA damage caused by formation of DNA adducts interferes with the DNA replication and repair mechanisms, which subsequently induces apoptosis (Dasari and Tchounwou, 2014). The apoptotic signal is initiated by activation (through phosphorylation) of p53, a tumor suppressor gene and an important mediator of DNA damage-induced apoptosis. Accumulating evidence suggest that in response to stress signal, a fraction of activated p53 rapidly translocates to the mitochondria, where it interacts with the various pro- and anti-apoptotic members of Bcl-2 family to either activate or inhibit them, respectively (Vaseva and Moll, 2009). In the mitochondria, p53 also induces loss of mitochondrial membrane potential, cytochrome c release and caspase-3 activation, triggering apoptosis (Marchenko et al., 2000). These findings were consistent with those in p53-deficient cells, where Bax translocation, cytochrome c release, and caspase-3 activation were downregulated, confirming that p53 acts upstream of mitochondrial apoptotic regulators (Morris et al., 2001). Interestingly, overexpression of anti-apoptotic

TABLE 1 | Potential drug targets for treatment of cisplatin ototoxicity.

Drug targets	Mechanism(s)	Reference
GPCRs		
Adenosine A_1 receptor (A_1AR)	(1) Enhance endogenous antioxidant defense system	Ford et al., 1997; Whitworth et al., 2004
	(2) Suppression of NOX3/STAT1 inflammatory pathway	Kaur et al., 2016
Cannabinoid 2 receptor (CB2)	Anti-apoptotic	Jeong et al., 2007
Pro-inflammatory markers		
Transient receptor potential vanilloid 1 (TRPV-1)	(1) Marker for oxidative stress and inflammation in the cochlea	Mukherjea et al., 2008
	(2) Facilitates entry of cisplatin?	
Tumor necrosis factor-α (TNF-α)	Pro-inflammatory cytokine induced by cisplatin	So et al., 2007
Signal transducer and activator of transcription-1 (STAT1)	Pro-inflammatory transcription factor	Schmitt et al., 2009
Nuclear factor-κB (NF-κB)	Pro-inflammatory/pro-apoptotic transcription factor	Chung et al., 2008; So et al., 2008
Transporters		
Organic cation transporter 2 (OCT2)	Involved in cellular uptake mechanisms for cisplatin	Ciarimboli et al., 2010
Copper transport 1 (Ctr1)	Facilitates cisplatin entry into cells	More et al., 2010
Mechano-electrical transduction (MET) channel	Facilitates cisplatin entry into zebrafish lateral line	Thomas et al., 2013
Antioxidant defense system		
NOX3	Responsible for ROS generation in the cochlea	Banfi et al., 2004
Superoxide dismutase (SOD)	Detoxifies superoxide anion into H_2O_2 and O_2	Ravi et al., 1995
Catalase (CAT)	Breaks down H_2O_2 into H_2O and O_2	Ravi et al., 1995
Glutathione (GSH)	Endogenous antioxidant molecule	Usami et al., 1996
Glutathione peroxidase (GSH.Px)	Catalyzes breakdown of H_2O_2 into H_2O and O_2 by using GSH	Ravi et al., 1995
Glutathione reductase (GR)	Converts oxidized glutathione (GSSG) to reduced GSH	Ravi et al., 1995
Glutathione *S*-transferase (GST)	Conjugates GSH with xenobiotics	el Barbary et al., 1993
Heme oxygenase-1 (HO-1)	Induced in response to oxidative stress	So et al., 2006
Nuclear factor erythroid 2-related factor 2 (Nrf2)	Regulator of cellular resistance to oxidants	So et al., 2006
Kidney injury molecule-1 (KIM-1)	Marker for oxidative stress in the cochlea	Mukherjea et al., 2006
Vitamin E	Antioxidant molecule	Kalkanis et al., 2004
N-acetyl cysteine (NAC)	Antioxidant molecule	Choe et al., 2004; Dickey et al., 2008
Sodium thiosulfate (STS)	Antioxidant molecule	Otto et al., 1988
D-Methionine (D-Met)	Antioxidant molecule	Campbell et al., 1996; Korver et al., 2002
Amifostine	Free radical scavenger	Church et al., 2004
Ebselen	Glutathione peroxidase mimetic	Rybak et al., 1999; Lynch et al., 2005
Allopurinol	Xanthine oxidase inhibitor	Lynch et al., 2005
Miscellaneous		
Heat shock protein 70 (HSP70)	Molecular chaperones important for protein folding	Roy et al., 2013; Baker et al., 2015
Signal transducer and activator of transcription-3 (STAT3)	Cytoprotection	Borse et al., 2017
Pifithrin-α	p53 inhibitor	Zhang et al., 2003; Benkafadar et al., 2017
Epigallocatechin-3-gallate (EGCG)	STAT1 inhibitor	Borse et al., 2017
Transcription-coupled repair (TCR)	Nucleotide excision repair (NCR) mechanism for damaged DNA	Rainey et al., 2016

Bcl 2 or Bcl xL prevented stress signal-mediated mitochondrial accumulation of p53 and apoptosis, suggesting a feedback loop between p53 and mitochondrial apoptotic regulators (Marchenko et al., 2000).

The role of p53 in the regulation of cisplatin-induced apoptosis in the auditory system has been investigated. Application of the p53 inhibitor, pifithrin-α, to cochlear organotypic cultures exposed to cisplatin attenuated hair cell damage (Zhang et al., 2003; Benkafadar et al., 2017). The protection was associated with reduction in the expression of *p53*, *caspase-1*, and *caspase-3* (Zhang et al., 2003). The validity of these *in vitro* results was tested in hair cells derived from p53-deficient mice, which exhibited resistance to cisplatin-induced apoptosis (Benkafadar et al., 2017) and reduced caspase-3 activation (Cheng et al., 2005a,b). Although systemic inhibition of p53 protects against cisplatin-induced ototoxicity, this treatment strategy would interfere with the anti-cancer efficacy of cisplatin, restricting its use for treatment in humans. To overcome this problem, Benkafadar et al. (2017) demonstrated that intra-tympanic application of pifithrin-α protects auditory function without compromising the chemotherapeutic efficacy of systemically administered cisplatin. They further showed that systemic administration of pifithrin-α even sensitizes TP53-mutant tumors to cisplatin. These results illustrate the role of p53 as an important regulator of cisplatin-induced apoptosis in auditory hair cells.

CISPLATIN TARGETS DNA IN THE COCHLEA

Previous studies have shown that platinated DNA accumulates in the nuclei of outer hair cells, supporting cells, marginal cells of the stria vascularis and cells in the spiral ligament (van Ruijven et al., 2005). Other studies have also shown DNA adduct in spiral ganglion neurons following cisplatin administration. The cochlear cells express DNA repair enzymes which can reduce the level of DNA adduct formed over time. These repair enzymes, known as nucleotide excision repair (NER) enzymes, are classified as transcriptional-coupled repair (TCR) enzymes or global DNA repair (GDR) enzymes which differ in their targets. Defective TCR function is observed in Cockayne syndrome which is characterized by progressive hearing loss. Outer hair cells from Cockayne syndrome group A (*Csa*$^{-}$/$^{-}$) and group B (*Csb*$^{-}$/$^{-}$) mice were hypersensitive to cisplatin. In contrast, *Xpc*$^{-}$/$^{-}$ mice which were deficient in global genome repair enzymes showed normal sensitivity to cisplatin (Rainey et al., 2016). This study implicates DNA damage as one mechanism of cisplatin-induced loss of outer hair cells and hearing loss and suggests that TCR plays a primary role in protecting hair cells from cisplatin-induced hearing loss. The effects of eight single-nucleotide polymorphisms in excision repair cross-complementing group 1, 2, 4, and 5 (*ERCC1*, *ERCC2*, *ERCC4*, and *ERCC5*) genes and xeroderma pigmentosum complementary group C and A (*XPC* and *XPA*) genes were assessed in patients with osteosarcoma who were treated with cisplatin. These studies showed that polymorphisms in DNA repair gene, *XPC*, was associated with increased cisplatin-induced ototoxicity in cancer patients. Increased ototoxicity was associated with the CC genotype of *XPC* Lys939Gln (Caronia et al., 2009).

UPTAKE OF CISPLATIN INTO THE COCHLEA

One of the major entry ports for cisplatin in the cochlea is the mammalian copper transport 1 (Ctrl). Ctrl is highly expressed in the cochlea where it is localized to outer hair cells, inner hair cells, stria vascularis, and spiral ganglion neurons and contributes to drug entry and cell apoptosis. Decreasing cisplatin entry by intra-tympanic administration of copper sulfate, a substrate of Ctrl, protects against hearing loss induced by cisplatin (More et al., 2010). Cisplatin entry into cochlear cells is also mediated by organic cation transporter (OCT). Three isoforms of this protein exists, OCT1-3, which are present mainly in the kidneys and liver. Expression of OCT2 has also been detected in the organ of Corti and stria vascularis (Ciarimboli et al., 2010). Inhibition of these transporters with cimetidine protects against cisplatin-induced nephrotoxicity and ototoxicity. *OCT* knockout mice exhibit reduced toxicity to cisplatin. Single-nucleotide polymorphism in *OCT-2* gene protects against ototoxicity in children (Lanvers-Kaminsky et al., 2015). Several studies have reported that the entry of aminoglycosides into cochlear hair cells is mediated by mechanotransducer (MET) channels (Gale et al., 2001; Marcotti et al., 2005; Dai et al., 2006; Wang and Steyger, 2009; Alharazneh et al., 2011). In fact, changes in the structure of aminoglycosides which limits their entry through MET channels are less ototoxic (Huth et al., 2015). Cisplatin has also shown to block MET channels in chick cochlear hair cells (Kimitsuki et al., 1993). Recent studies have indicated that cisplatin-induced damage to hair cells in the zebrafish is dependent on functional MET channels (Thomas et al., 2013). These investigators showed that inhibition of mechanotransduction channels by quinine or EGTA protected against cisplatin-induced hair cell death. Furthermore, these investigators showed that zebrafish mutants which lacked mechanotransduction channels were also resistant to cisplatin-induced hair cell death. These studies suggest that mechanotransduction channels are a major contributor to the entry of cisplatin into hair cells, at least in the zebrafish. Interestingly, chemical inhibition of Ctrl and OCT-2 did not provide significant protection against killing of lateral line hair cells in zebrafish (Thomas et al., 2013). Preliminary data from our lab indicate a similar pathway of entry of transplatin, the inactive isomer of cisplatin, which protects against cisplatin ototoxicity (Dhukhwa et al., 2017). These studies suggest that MET channels could serve as an additional entry ports for cisplatin into cochlear hair cells. Several other ion channels might also contribute to aminoglycoside uptake into hair cells. In addition to TRPV1, several TRP channels including TRPV4, TRPA1, TRPC3, and TRPML3 are expressed in the cochlea (Cuajungco et al., 2007; Asai et al., 2010). These channels have been shown to allow entry of aminoglycoside into kidney cells (Myrdal and Steyger, 2005). The potential role of these channels in mediating the entry of aminoglycosides and cisplatin into hair cells has not yet been established.

Megalin is a low-density lipoprotein which is highly expressed in the kidney and in the stria vascularis of the cochlea which accumulate high levels of platinum DNA adducts. Patients who showed cisplatin-induced hearing impairment demonstrate a higher frequency of megalin gene polymorphism compared to those with no hearing loss after cisplatin therapy. These findings implicate *megalin* gene polymorphisms in susceptibility to cisplatin ototoxicity (Riedemann et al., 2008). In the kidneys, megalin has been shown to bind β_2-microglobulin, cytochrome c, retinal binding proteins, and polybasic antibiotics (such as gentamicin). These investigators show that the accumulation of cisplatin in the renal proximal tubules is mediated by binding of cisplatin-metallothionein complex to megalin (Klassen et al., 2004). The expression of *megalin* in the stria vascularis might similarly allow the accumulation of cisplatin into the stria vascularis.

CONCLUSION

Studies described above have identified a number of different mechanisms which mediated cisplatin ototoxicity and provide the basis for rational drug design to treat this debilitating condition. While most of the drugs which target these mechanisms have shown promise, efficacy studies are still in the experimental animal stage (see **Table 1** for list of drugs/drug targets). These studies need to be extended in human clinical trials for final validation. The routes of drug administration would be a major issue, as systemic administration of these drugs could compromise cisplatin chemotherapeutic efficacy. In this regard, the use of a number of cisplatin transporters (namely Ctrl and OCT2) and antioxidants would have the greatest likelihood of interfering with cisplatin antitumor efficacy (as discussed above). Localized delivery of these drugs into the cochlea would eliminate potential systemic toxicities but would require an additional minor surgical procedure to accomplish this goal. This would allow the use of a majority of the agents listed in this table for protection against hearing loss. Several of these drugs are currently in clinical use or in clinical trials for other indications. These include TNF-α antagonists which are used for the treatment of chronic inflammatory diseases (Aggarwal et al., 2012) and EGCG which is in various clinical trials for the treatment of cancer (Singh et al., 2011). These agents which are effective systemically could serve as initial candidates for treating cisplatin-induced hearing loss and other forms of hearing loss. Other drugs which could be advanced quickly into clinical use are MET channel blockers, such as bulky aminoglycoside antibiotics, which demonstrate low potential for ototoxicity (Huth et al., 2015). Continued research in this area would uncover new mechanisms underlying cisplatin-induced hearing loss and validate novel targets and drugs to treat this condition.

AUTHOR CONTRIBUTIONS

SS and VR conceived and together outlined this review. SS and VR wrote the manuscript. DM and LR critiqued and revised the manuscript.

ACKNOWLEDGMENTS

The authors would like to acknowledge the NIH grant support (NCI RO1 CA166907, NIDCD RO1-DC 002396 and RO3 DC011621) for work described in the review which were performed in the authors laboratories.

REFERENCES

Aggarwal, B. B., Gupta, S. C., and Kim, J. H. (2012). Historical perspectives on tumor necrosis factor and its superfamily: 25 years later, a golden journey. *Blood* 119, 651–665. doi: 10.1182/blood-2011-04-325225

Alam, S. A., Ikeda, K., Oshima, T., Suzuki, M., Kawase, T., Kikuchi, T., et al. (2000). Cisplatin-induced apoptotic cell death in Mongolian gerbil cochlea. *Hear. Res.* 141, 28–38. doi: 10.1016/S0378-5955(99)00211-7

Alharazneh, A., Luk, L., Huth, M., Monfared, A., Steyger, P. S., Cheng, A. G., et al. (2011). Functional hair cell mechanotransducer channels are required for aminoglycoside ototoxicity. *PLOS ONE* 6:e22347. doi: 10.1371/journal.pone.0022347

Asai, Y., Holt, J. R., and Geleoc, G. S. (2010). A quantitative analysis of the spatiotemporal pattern of transient receptor potential gene expression in the developing mouse cochlea. *J. Assoc. Res. Otolaryngol.* 11, 27–37. doi: 10.1007/s10162-009-0193-8

Baker, T. G., Roy, S., Brandon, C. S., Kramarenko, I. K., Francis, S. P., Taleb, M., et al. (2015). Heat shock protein-mediated protection against Cisplatin-induced hair cell death. *J. Assoc. Res. Otolaryngol.* 16, 67–80. doi: 10.1007/s10162-014-0491-7

Banfi, B., Malgrange, B., Knisz, J., Steger, K., Dubois-Dauphin, M., and Krause, K. H. (2004). NOX3, a superoxide-generating NADPH oxidase of the inner ear. *J. Biol. Chem.* 279, 46065–46072. doi: 10.1074/jbc.M403046200

Benkafadar, N., Menardo, J., Bourien, J., Nouvian, R., Francois, F., Decaudin, D., et al. (2017). Reversible p53 inhibition prevents cisplatin ototoxicity without blocking chemotherapeutic efficacy. *EMBO Mol. Med.* 9, 7–26. doi: 10.15252/emmm.201606230

Borse, V., Al Aameri, R. F. H., Sheehan, K., Sheth, S., Kaur, T., Mukherjea, D., et al. (2017). Epigallocatechin-3-gallate, a prototypic chemopreventative agent for protection against cisplatin-based ototoxicity. *Cell Death Dis.* 8:e2921. doi: 10.1038/cddis.2017.314

Campbell, K. C., Meech, R. P., Rybak, L. P., and Hughes, L. F. (2003). The effect of D-methionine on cochlear oxidative state with and without cisplatin administration: mechanisms of otoprotection. *J. Am. Acad. Audiol.* 14, 144–156.

Campbell, K. C., Rybak, L. P., Meech, R. P., and Hughes, L. (1996). D-methionine provides excellent protection from cisplatin ototoxicity in the rat. *Hear. Res.* 102, 90–98. doi: 10.1016/S0378-5955(96)00152-9

Caronia, D., Patino-Garcia, A., Milne, R. L., Zalacain-Diez, M., Pita, G., Alonso, M. R., et al. (2009). Common variations in ERCC2 are associated with response to cisplatin chemotherapy and clinical outcome in osteosarcoma patients. *Pharmacogenomics J.* 9, 347–353. doi: 10.1038/tpj.2009.19

Cheng, A. G., Cunningham, L. L., and Rubel, E. W. (2005a). Mechanisms of hair cell death and protection. *Curr. Opin. Otolaryngol. Head Neck Surg.* 13, 343–348.

Cheng, A. G., Morrison, R. S., and Rubel, E. W. (2005b). *p53 Mediates Cisplatin-Induced Hair Cell Death In Vitro.* Mt Royal, NJ: Association for Research in Otolaryngology, 211.

Choe, W. T., Chinosornvatana, N., and Chang, K. W. (2004). Prevention of cisplatin ototoxicity using transtympanic N-acetylcysteine and lactate. *Otol. Neurotol.* 25, 910–915. doi: 10.1097/00129492-200411000-00009

Chung, W. H., Boo, S. H., Chung, M. K., Lee, H. S., Cho, Y. S., and Hong, S. H. (2008). Proapoptotic effects of NF-kappaB on cisplatin-induced cell death in auditory cell line. *Acta Otolaryngol.* 128, 1063–1070. doi: 10.1080/00016480701881811

Church, M. W., Blakley, B. W., Burgio, D. L., and Gupta, A. K. (2004). WR-2721 (Amifostine) ameliorates cisplatin-induced hearing loss but causes neurotoxicity in hamsters: dose-dependent effects. *J. Assoc. Res. Otolaryngol.* 5, 227–237. doi: 10.1007/s10162-004-4011-z

Church, M. W., Kaltenbach, J. A., Blakley, B. W., and Burgio, D. L. (1995). The comparative effects of sodium thiosulfate, diethyldithiocarbamate, fosfomycin and WR-2721 on ameliorating cisplatin-induced ototoxicity. *Hear. Res.* 86, 195–203. doi: 10.1016/0378-5955(95)00066-D

Ciarimboli, G., Deuster, D., Knief, A., Sperling, M., Holtkamp, M., Edemir, B., et al. (2010). Organic cation transporter 2 mediates cisplatin-induced oto- and nephrotoxicity and is a target for protective interventions. *Am. J. Pathol.* 176, 1169–1180. doi: 10.2353/ajpath.2010.090610

Clerici, W. J., DiMartino, D. L., and Prasad, M. R. (1995). Direct effects of reactive oxygen species on cochlear outer hair cell shape in vitro. *Hear. Res.* 84, 30–40. doi: 10.1016/0378-5955(95)00010-2

Clerici, W. J., and Yang, L. (1996). Direct effects of intraperilymphatic reactive oxygen species generation on cochlear function. *Hear. Res.* 101, 14–22. doi: 10.1016/S0378-5955(96)00126-8

Coradini, P. P., Cigana, L., Selistre, S. G., Rosito, L. S., and Brunetto, A. L. (2007). Ototoxicity from cisplatin therapy in childhood cancer. *J. Pediatr. Hematol. Oncol.* 29, 355–360. doi: 10.1097/MPH.0b013e318059c220

Cuajungco, M. P., Grimm, C., and Heller, S. (2007). TRP channels as candidates for hearing and balance abnormalities in vertebrates. *Biochim. Biophys. Acta* 1772, 1022–1027. doi: 10.1016/j.bbadis.2007.01.002

Dai, C. F., Mangiardi, D., Cotanche, D. A., and Steyger, P. S. (2006). Uptake of fluorescent gentamicin by vertebrate sensory cells in vivo. *Hear. Res.* 213, 64–78. doi: 10.1016/j.heares.2005.11.011

Dasari, S., and Tchounwou, P. B. (2014). Cisplatin in cancer therapy: molecular mechanisms of action. *Eur. J. Pharmacol.* 740, 364–378. doi: 10.1016/j.ejphar.2014.07.025

Devarajan, P., Savoca, M., Castaneda, M. P., Park, M. S., Esteban-Cruciani, N., Kalinec, G., et al. (2002). Cisplatin-induced apoptosis in auditory cells: role of death receptor and mitochondrial pathways. *Hear. Res.* 174, 45–54. doi: 10.1016/S0378-5955(02)00634-2

Dhukhwa, A., Mukherjea, D., Ghosh, S., Sheehan, K., Borse, V., Sheth, S., et al. (2017). *Transplatin, A Novel Treatment for Cisplatin Ototoxicity.* Mt Royal, NJ: Association for Research in Otolaryngology, 402

Dickey, D. T., Muldoon, L. L., Doolittle, N. D., Peterson, D. R., Kraemer, D. F., and Neuwelt, E. A. (2008). Effect of N-acetylcysteine route of administration on chemoprotection against cisplatin-induced toxicity in rat models. *Cancer Chemother. Pharmacol.* 62, 235–241. doi: 10.1007/s00280-007-0597-2

Ekborn, A., Laurell, G., Johnstrom, P., Wallin, I., Eksborg, S., and Ehrsson, H. (2002). D-Methionine and cisplatin ototoxicity in the guinea pig: D-methionine influences cisplatin pharmacokinetics. *Hear. Res.* 165, 53–61. doi: 10.1016/S0378-5955(02)00277-0

el Barbary, A., Altschuler, R. A., and Schacht, J. (1993). Glutathione S-transferases in the organ of Corti of the rat: enzymatic activity, subunit composition and immunohistochemical localization. *Hear. Res.* 71, 80–90. doi: 10.1016/0378-5955(93)90023-T

Ford, M. S., Maggirwar, S. B., Rybak, L. P., Whitworth, C., and Ramkumar, V. (1997). Expression and function of adenosine receptors in the chinchilla cochlea. *Hear. Res.* 105, 130–140. doi: 10.1016/S0378-5955(96)00204-3

Fouladi, M., Chintagumpala, M., Ashley, D., Kellie, S., Gururangan, S., Hassall, T., et al. (2008). Amifostine protects against cisplatin-induced ototoxicity in children with average-risk medulloblastoma. *J. Clin. Oncol.* 26, 3749–3755. doi: 10.1200/JCO.2007.14.3974

Gale, J. E., Marcotti, W., Kennedy, H. J., Kros, C. J., and Richardson, G. P. (2001). FM1-43 dye behaves as a permeant blocker of the hair-cell mechanotransducer channel. *J. Neurosci.* 21, 7013–7025.

Ghosh, S., Mukherjea, D., Sheehan, K., Tupal, S., Borse, V., Dhukhwa, A., et al. (2016). *Expression, Regulation and Function of Cannabinoid Receptor 2 in the Cochlea.* Mt Royal, NJ: Association for Research in Otolaryngology, 52.

Goel, R., Cleary, S. M., Horton, C., Kirmani, S., Abramson, I., Kelly, C., et al. (1989). Effect of sodium thiosulfate on the pharmacokinetics and toxicity of cisplatin. *J. Natl. Cancer Inst.* 81, 1552–1560. doi: 10.1093/jnci/81.20.1552

Gunewardene, N., Guo, C. X., Wong, A. C. Y., Thorne, P. R., and Vlajkovic, S. M. (2013). Adenosine amine congener ameliorates cisplatin-induced hearing loss. *World J. Otorhinolaryngol.* 3, 100–107. doi: 10.5319/wjo.v3.i3.100

Gurney, J. G., Tersak, J. M., Ness, K. K., Landier, W., Matthay, K. K., Schmidt, M. L., et al. (2007). Hearing loss, quality of life, and academic problems in long-term neuroblastoma survivors: a report from the Children's Oncology Group. *Pediatrics* 120, e1229–e1236. doi: 10.1542/peds.2007-0178

Hengartner, M. O. (2000). The biochemistry of apoptosis. *Nature* 407, 770–776. doi: 10.1038/35037710

Huth, M. E., Han, K. H., Sotoudeh, K., Hsieh, Y. J., Effertz, T., Vu, A. A., et al. (2015). Designer aminoglycosides prevent cochlear hair cell loss and hearing loss. *J. Clin. Invest.* 125, 583–592. doi: 10.1172/JCI77424

Jeong, H. J., Kim, S. J., Moon, P. D., Kim, N. H., Kim, J. S., Park, R. K., et al. (2007). Antiapoptotic mechanism of cannabinoid receptor 2 agonist on cisplatin-induced apoptosis in the HEI-OC1 auditory cell line. *J. Neurosci. Res.* 85, 896–905. doi: 10.1002/jnr.21168

Kalkanis, J. G., Whitworth, C., and Rybak, L. P. (2004). Vitamin E reduces cisplatin ototoxicity. *Laryngoscope* 114, 538–542. doi: 10.1097/00005537-200403000-00028

Kaur, T., Borse, V., Sheth, S., Sheehan, K., Ghosh, S., Tupal, S., et al. (2016). Adenosine A1 receptor protects against cisplatin ototoxicity by suppressing the NOX3/STAT1 inflammatory pathway in the cochlea. *J. Neurosci.* 36, 3962–3977. doi: 10.1523/JNEUROSCI.3111-15.2016

Kaur, T., Mukherjea, D., Sheehan, K., Jajoo, S., Rybak, L. P., and Ramkumar, V. (2011). Short interfering RNA against STAT1 attenuates cisplatin-induced ototoxicity in the rat by suppressing inflammation. *Cell Death Dis.* 2:e180. doi: 10.1038/cddis.2011.63

Kimitsuki, T., Nakagawa, T., Hisashi, K., Komune, S., and Komiyama, S. (1993). Cisplatin blocks mechano-electric transducer current in chick cochlear hair cells. *Hear. Res.* 71, 64–68. doi: 10.1016/0378-5955(93)90021-R

Klassen, R. B., Crenshaw, K., Kozyraki, R., Verroust, P. J., Tio, L., Atrian, S., et al. (2004). Megalin mediates renal uptake of heavy metal metallothionein complexes. *Am. J. Physiol. Renal Physiol.* 287, F393–F403. doi: 10.1152/ajprenal.00233.2003

Knight, K. R., Kraemer, D. F., and Neuwelt, E. A. (2005). Ototoxicity in children receiving platinum chemotherapy: underestimating a commonly occurring toxicity that may influence academic and social development. *J. Clin. Oncol.* 23, 8588–8596. doi: 10.1200/JCO.2004.00.5355

Kopke, R., Allen, K. A., Henderson, D., Hoffer, M., Frenz, D., and Van de Water, T. (1999). A radical demise. toxins and trauma share common pathways in hair cell death. *Ann. N. Y. Acad. Sci.* 884, 171–191. doi: 10.1111/j.1749-6632.1999.tb08641.x

Kopke, R. D., Liu, W., Gabaizadeh, R., Jacono, A., Feghali, J., Spray, D., et al. (1997). Use of organotypic cultures of Corti's organ to study the protective effects of antioxidant molecules on cisplatin-induced damage of auditory hair cells. *Am. J. Otol.* 18, 559–571.

Korver, K. D., Rybak, L. P., Whitworth, C., and Campbell, K. M. (2002). Round window application of D-methionine provides complete cisplatin otoprotection. *Otolaryngol. Head Neck Surg.* 126, 683–689. doi: 10.1067/mhn.2002.125299

Kushner, B. H., Budnick, A., Kramer, K., Modak, S., and Cheung, N. K. (2006). Ototoxicity from high-dose use of platinum compounds in patients with neuroblastoma. *Cancer* 107, 417–422. doi: 10.1002/cncr.22004

Lai, M. T., Ohmichi, T., Egusa, K., Okada, S., and Masuda, Y. (1996). Immunohistochemical localization of manganese superoxide dismutase in the rat cochlea. *Eur. Arch. Otorhinolaryngol.* 253, 273–277. doi: 10.1007/BF00171142

Lanvers-Kaminsky, C., Sprowl, J. A., Malath, I., Deuster, D., Eveslage, M., Schlatter, E., et al. (2015). Human OCT2 variant c.808G > T confers protection effect against cisplatin-induced ototoxicity. *Pharmacogenomics* 16, 323–332. doi: 10.2217/pgs.14.182

Liu, W., Staecker, H., Stupak, H., Malgrange, B., Lefebvre, P., and Van De Water, T. R. (1998). Caspase inhibitors prevent cisplatin-induced apoptosis of auditory sensory cells. *Neuroreport* 9, 2609–2614. doi: 10.1097/00001756-199808030-00034

Lynch, E. D., Gu, R., Pierce, C., and Kil, J. (2005). Reduction of acute cisplatin ototoxicity and nephrotoxicity in rats by oral administration of allopurinol and ebselen. *Hear. Res.* 201, 81–89. doi: 10.1016/j.heares.2004.08.002

Marchenko, N. D., Zaika, A., and Moll, U. M. (2000). Death signal-induced localization of p53 protein to mitochondria. A potential role in apoptotic signaling. *J. Biol. Chem.* 275, 16202–16212. doi: 10.1074/jbc.275.21.16202

Marcotti, W., van Netten, S. M., and Kros, C. J. (2005). The aminoglycoside antibiotic dihydrostreptomycin rapidly enters mouse outer hair cells through the mechano-electrical transducer channels. *J. Physiol.* 567(Pt 2), 505–521. doi: 10.1113/jphysiol.2005.085951

Marina, N., Chang, K. W., Malogolowkin, M., London, W. B., Frazier, A. L., Womer, R. B., et al. (2005). Amifostine does not protect against the ototoxicity of high-dose cisplatin combined with etoposide and bleomycin in pediatric germ-cell tumors: a Children's Oncology Group study. *Cancer* 104, 841–847. doi: 10.1002/cncr.21218

Martin-Saldana, S., Trinidad, A., Ramil, E., Sanchez-Lopez, A. J., Coronado, M. J., Martinez-Martinez, E., et al. (2016). Spontaneous cannabinoid receptor 2 (CB2) expression in the cochlea of adult albino rat and its up-regulation after cisplatin treatment. *PLOS ONE* 11:e0161954. doi: 10.1371/journal.pone.0161954

Meyers, J. R., MacDonald, R. B., Duggan, A., Lenzi, D., Standaert, D. G., Corwin, J. T., et al. (2003). Lighting up the senses: FM1-43 loading of sensory cells through nonselective ion channels. *J. Neurosci.* 23, 4054–4065.

More, S. S., Akil, O., Ianculescu, A. G., Geier, E. G., Lustig, L. R., and Giacomini, K. M. (2010). Role of the copper transporter, CTR1, in platinum-induced ototoxicity. *J. Neurosci.* 30, 9500–9509. doi: 10.1523/JNEUROSCI.1544-10.2010

Morris, E. J., Keramaris, E., Rideout, H. J., Slack, R. S., Dyson, N. J., Stefanis, L., et al. (2001). Cyclin-dependent kinases and P53 pathways are activated independently and mediate Bax activation in neurons after DNA damage. *J. Neurosci.* 21, 5017–5026.

Mukherjea, D., Jajoo, S., Kaur, T., Sheehan, K. E., Ramkumar, V., and Rybak, L. P. (2010). Transtympanic administration of short interfering (si)RNA for the NOX3 isoform of NADPH oxidase protects against cisplatin-induced hearing loss in the rat. *Antioxid. Redox Signal.* 13, 589–598. doi: 10.1089/ars.2010.3110

Mukherjea, D., Jajoo, S., Sheehan, K., Kaur, T., Sheth, S., Bunch, J., et al. (2011). NOX3 NADPH oxidase couples transient receptor potential vanilloid 1 to signal transducer and activator of transcription 1-mediated inflammation and hearing loss. *Antioxid. Redox Signal.* 14, 999–1010. doi: 10.1089/ars.2010.3497

Mukherjea, D., Jajoo, S., Whitworth, C., Bunch, J. R., Turner, J. G., Rybak, L. P., et al. (2008). Short interfering RNA against transient receptor potential vanilloid 1 attenuates cisplatin-induced hearing loss in the rat. *J. Neurosci.* 28, 13056–13065. doi: 10.1523/JNEUROSCI.1307-08.2008

Mukherjea, D., Whitworth, C. A., Nandish, S., Dunaway, G. A., Rybak, L. P., and Ramkumar, V. (2006). Expression of the kidney injury molecule 1 in the rat cochlea and induction by cisplatin. *Neuroscience* 139, 733–740. doi: 10.1016/j.neuroscience.2005.12.044

Myrdal, S. E., and Steyger, P. S. (2005). TRPV1 regulators mediate gentamicin penetration of cultured kidney cells. *Hear. Res.* 204, 170–182. doi: 10.1016/j.heares.2005.02.005

Oh, S. H., Yu, W. S., Song, B. H., Lim, D., Koo, J. W., Chang, S. O., et al. (2000). Expression of heat shock protein 72 in rat cochlea with cisplatin-induced acute ototoxicity. *Acta Otolaryngol.* 120, 146–150. doi: 10.1080/000164800750000793

Oldenburg, J., Kraggerud, S. M., Cvancarova, M., Lothe, R. A., and Fossa, S. D. (2007). Cisplatin-induced long-term hearing impairment is associated with specific glutathione s-transferase genotypes in testicular cancer survivors. *J. Clin. Oncol.* 25, 708–714. doi: 10.1200/JCO.2006.08.9599

Otto, W. C., Brown, R. D., Gage-White, L., Kupetz, S., Anniko, M., Penny, J. E., et al. (1988). Effects of cisplatin and thiosulfate upon auditory brainstem responses of guinea pigs. *Hear. Res.* 35, 79–85. doi: 10.1016/0378-5955(88)90042-1

Pierson, M. G., and Gray, B. H. (1982). Superoxide dismutase activity in the cochlea. *Hear. Res.* 6, 141–151. doi: 10.1016/0378-5955(82)90050-8

Rainey, R. N., Ng, S. Y., Llamas, J., van der Horst, G. T., and Segil, N. (2016). Mutations in cockayne syndrome-associated genes (Csa and Csb) predispose to cisplatin-induced hearing loss in mice. *J. Neurosci.* 36, 4758–4770. doi: 10.1523/JNEUROSCI.3890-15.2016

Ravi, R., Somani, S. M., and Rybak, L. P. (1995). Mechanism of cisplatin ototoxicity: antioxidant system. *Pharmacol. Toxicol.* 76, 386–394. doi: 10.1111/j.1600-0773.1995.tb00167.x

Riedemann, L., Lanvers, C., Deuster, D., Peters, U., Boos, J., Jurgens, H., et al. (2008). Megalin genetic polymorphisms and individual sensitivity to the ototoxic effect of cisplatin. *Pharmacogenomics J.* 8, 23–28. doi: 10.1038/sj.tpj.6500455

Roy, S., Ryals, M. M., Van den Bruele, A. B., Fitzgerald, T. S., and Cunningham, L. L. (2013). Sound preconditioning therapy inhibits ototoxic hearing loss in mice. *J. Clin. Invest.* 123, 4945–4949. doi: 10.1172/JCI71353

Ryan, A. F. (1988). "Circulation of the inner ear. II. The relationship between metabolism and blood flow in the cochlea," in *Physiology of the Ear*, eds A. F. Jahn and J. Santos-Sacchi (New York, NY: Raven Press), 317–325.

Rybak, L. P., Husain, K., Morris, C., Whitworth, C., and Somani, S. (2000). Effect of protective agents against cisplatin ototoxicity. *Am. J. Otol.* 21, 513–520.

Rybak, L. P., Ravi, R., and Somani, S. M. (1995). Mechanism of protection by diethyldithiocarbamate against cisplatin ototoxicity: antioxidant system. *Fundam. Appl. Toxicol.* 26, 293–300. doi: 10.1006/faat.1995.1100

Rybak, L. P., Whitworth, C., and Somani, S. (1999). Application of antioxidants and other agents to prevent cisplatin ototoxicity. *Laryngoscope* 109, 1740–1744. doi: 10.1097/00005537-199911000-00003

Salt, A. N., Melichar, I., and Thalmann, R. (1987). Mechanisms of endocochlear potential generation by stria vascularis. *Laryngoscope* 97(8 Pt 1), 984–991.

Salvesen, G. S., and Dixit, V. M. (1997). Caspases: intracellular signaling by proteolysis. *Cell* 91, 443–446. doi: 10.1016/S0092-8674(00)80430-4

Sastry, J., and Kellie, S. J. (2005). Severe neurotoxicity, ototoxicity and nephrotoxicity following high-dose cisplatin and amifostine. *Pediatr. Hematol. Oncol.* 22, 441–445. doi: 10.1080/08880010590964381

Schmitt, N. C., Rubel, E. W., and Nathanson, N. M. (2009). Cisplatin-induced hair cell death requires STAT1 and is attenuated by epigallocatechin gallate. *J. Neurosci.* 29, 3843–3851. doi: 10.1523/JNEUROSCI.5842-08.2009

Seidman, M. D., Quirk, W. S., Nuttall, A. L., and Schweitzer, V. G. (1991). The protective effects of allopurinol and superoxide dismutase-polyethylene glycol on ischemic and reperfusion-induced cochlear damage. *Otolaryngol. Head Neck Surg.* 105, 457–463. doi: 10.1177/019459989110500318

Shi, X., Dong, Y., Li, Y., Zhao, Z., Li, H., Qiu, S., et al. (2015). Inflammasome activation in mouse inner ear in response to MCMV induced hearing loss. *J. Otol.* 10, 143–149. doi: 10.1016/j.joto.2015.12.001

Siddiqui, W. A., Ahad, A., and Ahsan, H. (2015). The mystery of BCL2 family: Bcl-2 proteins and apoptosis: an update. *Arch. Toxicol.* 89, 289–317. doi: 10.1007/s00204-014-1448-7

Singh, B. N., Shankar, S., and Srivastava, R. K. (2011). Green tea catechin, epigallocatechin-3-gallate (EGCG): mechanisms, perspectives and clinical applications. *Biochem. Pharmacol.* 82, 1807–1821. doi: 10.1016/j.bcp.2011.07.093

So, H., Kim, H., Kim, Y., Kim, E., Pae, H. O., Chung, H. T., et al. (2008). Evidence that cisplatin-induced auditory damage is attenuated by downregulation of pro-inflammatory cytokines via Nrf2/HO-1. *J. Assoc. Res. Otolaryngol.* 9, 290–306. doi: 10.1007/s10162-008-0126-y

So, H., Kim, H., Lee, J. H., Park, C., Kim, Y., Kim, E., et al. (2007). Cisplatin cytotoxicity of auditory cells requires secretions of proinflammatory cytokines via activation of ERK and NF-kappaB. *J. Assoc. Res. Otolaryngol.* 8, 338–355. doi: 10.1007/s10162-007-0084-9

So, H. S., Kim, H. J., Lee, J. H., Lee, J. H., Park, S. Y., Park, C., et al. (2006). Flunarizine induces Nrf2-mediated transcriptional activation of heme oxygenase-1 in protection of auditory cells from cisplatin. *Cell Death Differ.* 13, 1763–1775. doi: 10.1038/sj.cdd.4401863

Thomas, A. J., Hailey, D. W., Stawicki, T. M., Wu, P., Coffin, A. B., Rubel, E. W., et al. (2013). Functional mechanotransduction is required for cisplatin-induced hair cell death in the zebrafish lateral line. *J. Neurosci.* 33, 4405–4414. doi: 10.1523/JNEUROSCI.3940-12.2013

Usami, S., Hjelle, O. P., and Ottersen, O. P. (1996). Differential cellular distribution of glutathione–an endogenous antioxidant–in the guinea pig inner ear. *Brain Res.* 743, 337–340. doi: 10.1016/S0006-8993(96)01090-6

van Ruijven, M. W., de Groot, J. C., Hendriksen, F., and Smoorenburg, G. F. (2005). Immunohistochemical detection of platinated DNA in the cochlea of cisplatin-treated guinea pigs. *Hear. Res.* 203, 112–121. doi: 10.1016/j.heares.2004.12.007

Vaseva, A. V., and Moll, U. M. (2009). The mitochondrial p53 pathway. *Biochim. Biophys. Acta* 1787, 414–420. doi: 10.1016/j.bbabio.2008.10.005

Vlajkovic, S. M., Housley, G. D., and Thorne, P. R. (2009). Adenosine and the auditory system. *Curr. Neuropharmacol.* 7, 246–256. doi: 10.2174/157015909789152155

Wang, J., Ladrech, S., Pujol, R., Brabet, P., Van De Water, T. R., and Puel, J. L. (2004). Caspase inhibitors, but not c-Jun NH2-terminal kinase inhibitor treatment, prevent cisplatin-induced hearing loss. *Cancer Res.* 64, 9217–9224. doi: 10.1158/0008-5472.CAN-04-1581

Wang, J., Lloyd Faulconbridge, R. V., Fetoni, A., Guitton, M. J., Pujol, R., and Puel, J. L. (2003). Local application of sodium thiosulfate prevents cisplatin-induced hearing loss in the guinea pig. *Neuropharmacology* 45, 380–393. doi: 10.1016/S0028-3908(03)00194-1

Wang, Q., and Steyger, P. S. (2009). Trafficking of systemic fluorescent gentamicin into the cochlea and hair cells. *J. Assoc. Res. Otolaryngol.* 10, 205–219. doi: 10.1007/s10162-009-0160-4

Whitworth, C. A., Ramkumar, V., Jones, B., Tsukasaki, N., and Rybak, L. P. (2004). Protection against cisplatin ototoxicity by adenosine agonists. *Biochem. Pharmacol.* 67, 1801–1807. doi: 10.1016/j.bcp.2004.01.010

Wimmer, C., Mees, K., Stumpf, P., Welsch, U., Reichel, O., and Suckfull, M. (2004). Round window application of D-methionine, sodium thiosulfate, brain-derived neurotrophic factor, and fibroblast growth factor-2 in cisplatin-induced ototoxicity. *Otol. Neurotol.* 25, 33–40. doi: 10.1097/00129492-200401000-00007

Yao, X., and Rarey, K. E. (1996). Detection and regulation of Cu/Zn-SOD and Mn-SOD in rat cochlear tissues. *Hear. Res.* 96, 199–203. doi: 10.1016/0378-5955(96)00050-0

Zhang, M., Liu, W., Ding, D., and Salvi, R. (2003). Pifithrin-alpha suppresses p53 and protects cochlear and vestibular hair cells from cisplatin-induced apoptosis. *Neuroscience* 120, 191–205. doi: 10.1016/S0306-4522(03)00286-0

Zuur, C. L., Simis, Y. J., Lansdaal, P. E., Hart, A. A., Rasch, C. R., Schornagel, J. H., et al. (2007). Risk factors of ototoxicity after cisplatin-based chemo-irradiation in patients with locally advanced head-and-neck cancer: a multivariate analysis. *Int. J. Radiat. Oncol. Biol. Phys.* 68, 1320–1325. doi: 10.1016/j.ijrobp.2007.01.042

6

Towards the Prevention of Aminoglycoside-Related Hearing Loss

Mary E. O'Sullivan [1], Adela Perez [1], Randy Lin [1], Autefeh Sajjadi [1], Anthony J. Ricci [1,2] and Alan G. Cheng [1]**

[1]Department of Otolaryngology-Head and Neck Surgery, Stanford University School of Medicine, Stanford, CA, United States, [2]Department of Molecular and Cellular Physiology, Stanford University School of Medicine, Stanford, CA, United States

Edited by:
Jian Zuo,
St. Jude Children's Research Hospital, United States

Reviewed by:
Andy Groves,
Baylor College of Medicine, United States
Wei Xiong,
School of Life Sciences, Tsinghua University, China

***Correspondence:**
Anthony J. Ricci
aricci@stanford.edu
Alan G. Cheng
aglcheng@stanford.edu

Aminoglycosides are potent antibiotics deployed worldwide despite their known side-effect of sensorineural hearing loss. The main etiology of this sensory deficit is death of inner ear sensory hair cells selectively triggered by aminoglycosides. For decades, research has sought to unravel the molecular events mediating sensory cell demise, emphasizing the roles of reactive oxygen species and their potentials as therapeutic targets. Studies in recent years have revealed candidate transport pathways including the mechanotransducer channel for drug entry into sensory cells. Once inside sensory cells, intracellular targets of aminoglycosides, such as the mitochondrial ribosomes, are beginning to be elucidated. Based on these results, less ototoxic aminoglycoside analogs are being generated and may serve as alternate antimicrobial agents. In this article, we review the latest findings on mechanisms of aminoglycoside entry into hair cells, their intracellular actions and potential therapeutic targets for preventing aminoglycoside ototoxicity.

Keywords: aminoglycoside antibiotics, mechanotransducer channel, ribosome, ototoxicity, mRNA misreading

INTRODUCTION

Aminoglycosides are critical antimicrobials with potent activities against gram negative bacteria (World Health Organization, 2011). Over 10 million doses are consumed annually in the United States (Van Boeckel et al., 2014). In developed countries, aminoglycoside administration is tightly regulated and generally confined to inpatient settings where indications for their use include endocarditis, urinary tract infection, sepsis and other severe infections (Avent et al., 2011). In contrast, in some developing countries, usage is less restricted and substantially more commonplace. Moreover, because of their affordable cost and low incidence of antibiotic resistance, aminoglycosides are often selected in these countries as a first line of treatment (Van Boeckel et al., 2014).

Aminoglycosides are a large family of water-soluble, polycationic molecules that exist as either three- or four-ringed compounds. More specifically, aminoglycosides contain a common neamine core, composed of a six-member aminocyclitol ring (ring II) glycosidically linked to a glucosaminopyranose (ring I). Substitutions attached at either position 5 or 6 on ring II give rise to different aminoglycoside molecules that are categorized as either 4, 5 or 4, 6 aminoglycosides. To date, over 25 aminoglycoside compounds have been purified or synthesized (NCBI PubChem Compound Database, 2017). Aminoglycosides that are more commonly used clinically include neomycin, tobramycin, gentamicin and amikacin (Arya, 2007; NCBI PubChem Compound Database, 2017).

A significant side effect of aminoglycoside administration is kidney damage (nephrotoxicity) and irreversible sensorineural hearing loss (ototoxicity). Nephrotoxicity is largely reversible, whilst hearing loss is permanent. Hearing loss occurs in a dose-dependent manner and the antibacterial efficacy, nephrotoxicity, and ototoxicity of these drugs correlate with aminoglycoside blood concentration (Lacy et al., 1998; Mingeot-Leclercq and Tulkens, 1999; Chen et al., 2013). Hence, aminoglycosides are typically administered in inpatient settings and therapeutic drug monitoring of aminoglycoside levels in the blood is routinely performed in most developed countries (Freeman et al., 1997; Smyth et al., 2005; Agency for Healthcare Research and Quality, 2012). Because aminoglycosides are not metabolized and excreted exclusively through the kidneys, drug monitoring is particularly important among patients with compromised kidney function.

Even when aminoglycoside blood concentrations are within the recommended therapeutic range, ototoxicity can still occur. Some studies have indicated that cumulative duration of therapy, rather than peak and trough levels of drugs, is predictive of ototoxicity (Beaubien et al., 1989; Cheng et al., 2009; Modongo et al., 2015). Moreover, in a subset of patients with the mitochondrial DNA mutation m.1555A>G, hearing loss can occur following a single dose (Usami et al., 1998). Individuals with this mutation may otherwise have hearing that is within normal limits unless they have been exposed to aminoglycosides (Bitner-Glindzicz et al., 2009; Rahman et al., 2012). These studies illustrate how patients' genotypes can influence the penetrance of aminoglycoside-related hearing loss. To date, four mutations in the mitochondrial genome and four genes in the nuclear genome are reported to be involved in aminoglycoside-related hearing loss, these will be returned to later in this review article (Li and Guan, 2002; Bykhovskaya et al., 2004a,b; Guan et al., 2006; Guan, 2011).

Estimates of the prevalence of ototoxicity in patients vary widely across the literature, ranging between 2%–25% for hearing deficits and 1%–10% for vestibular dysfunction (Ariano et al., 2008; Huth et al., 2015). For patients who require multiple courses of intravenous aminoglycoside antibiotics (e.g., treatment of tuberculosis and cystic fibrosis patients) estimates are higher and may exceed 50% (Duggal and Sarkar, 2007; Waters et al., 2015). This variability is likely due to a variety of factors such as the sensitivity of the audiometric tests, the patient population studied, their comorbid conditions, previous aminoglycoside treatment, the specific aminoglycoside used, its dosage and duration of treatment (Al-Malky et al., 2011, 2015; Seddon et al., 2012; Zimmerman and Lahav, 2013).

After aminoglycoside exposure, the main cochlear pathology underlying drug-induced hearing loss is sensory hair cell loss. Sensory hair cells are mechanoreceptors required for hearing and balance functions. In the cochlea, they are tonotopically arranged such that high frequency sounds stimulate hair cells in the basal region and low frequency in the apical region. Early on in the disease process when hearing loss typically begins in the high frequency, hair cell loss is found in the basal region (Fausti et al., 1992). However, hearing loss can progress into the mid- and low frequency ranges with corresponding hair cell loss in those regions in the cochlea. As such, research efforts have focused on defining the mechanisms of aminoglycoside trafficking into hair cells and the intracellular events leading to their demise.

In the mammalian cochlea, the apical surface of sensory hair cells are located in an extracellular fluid compartment filled with a unique endolymph solution, comprised of high potassium (K^+, replacing NaCl in normal extracellular fluid) and low calcium (Ca^{2+}, 20 μM as compared to 1.2 mM in normal extracellular fluid; Sterkers et al., 1982, 1984). Also unique to this compartment is a high endocochlear potential (+80 mV), which serves to drive positively charged ions into the hair cell. The endolymph compartment is bordered on the lateral wall of the cochlea by the stria vascularis, which is essential for endolymph maintenance and production (Sterkers et al., 1982; Salt and Plontke, 2005). The endocochlear potential, established by high concentration of K^+ ions (160 mM), is the major driver for sensory transduction. During sound stimulation, K^+ ions flow down an electrochemical gradient into hair cells through mechanically-gated channels located in sensory hair cell bundles. These unique, mechanically sensitive channels are non-selective cation carriers, allowing other large positively charged molecules, like aminoglycosides, to enter the hair cell.

Aminoglycosides were first discovered and used clinically in the 1940s, yet today and over 50 years later, preventative options remain largely limited to monitoring of dose and treatment duration. Decades of research have established fundamental knowledge and we refer the avid readers to other excellent reviews (Huth et al., 2011; Stawicki et al., 2015; Wong and Ryan, 2015). This review article will highlight two main research areas aminoglycoside transport and intracellular targets, as well as detailing novel mechanisms, and their respective potentials and limitations as therapeutic targets.

Targeting the Stria Vascularis to Prevent Ototoxicity

The stria vascularis houses the major blood-labyrinth barrier (BLB)–a highly specialized capillary network that controls exchanges between blood and the interstitial space in the cochlea. The BLB is one of the first sites of aminoglycoside entry from the blood into the inner ear, a concept first proposed by Hawkins (1973) (Dai and Steyger, 2008; Wang et al., 2010). The BLB is strongly influenced by physiological factors such as active and passive membrane functions, ion channels, blood flow, inflammation, free radicals and possibly noise exposure (Abbott and Blakley, 2007; Shi, 2016). This structure is capable of affecting the pharmacokinetics of aminoglycosides in the inner ear, supported by evidence that endotoxin-mediated inflammation enhances aminoglycoside trafficking across the BLB and potentiates cochlear uptake of aminoglycosides and permanent hearing loss in mice (Koo et al., 2015). Data also shows that melatonin exacerbates aminoglycoside ototoxicity *in vivo*, among its many roles in the body melatonin acts as a vasoconstrictor and vasodilator (Erdem et al., 2005).

Aminoglycosides conjugated to fluorescent labels have been developed and proven to be a powerful tool in the study of aminoglycoside trafficking from the blood into the endolymph. The most commonly used fluorescent aminoglycoside is gentamicin sulfate conjugated to the Texas red fluorophore, so called Gentamicin Texas Red (GTTR; Sandoval et al., 1998; Dai and Steyger, 2008). Notably, owing the variable chemical composition of compounds marketed as "Gentamicin Sulfate", GTTR is not one pure compound but contains a mixture of gentamicin compounds differing by methyl, amine and hydroxyl groups (Antec, 2014). Chemical limitations of the current synthesis method mean that the site to which the Texas red fluorophore is attached is unknown, moreover, it could be conjugated to one or more of the six amines on the structure of gentamicin (Sandoval et al., 1998; Dai and Steyger, 2008). Whilst the compound itself has purity and fluorophore-related limitations, the GTTR compound is an incredibly useful tool in tracing aminoglycoside transport in the cochlea.

Studies show that GTTR systemically administered is first found in strial capillaries before being distributed to the marginal cells in the stria vascularis and the endolymph (Dai and Steyger, 2008; Wang and Steyger, 2009). As noted earlier, aminoglycoside treatment is associated with nephrotoxicity and ototoxicity. Because of the commonality in genes expressed between the two tissues, it is hypothesized that agents that trigger a pathological change in one may similarly affect the other. In particular, there are similarities between the stria vascularis in the cochlea and the proximal tubules and loop of Henle of the kidney (Quick et al., 1973; Jentsch et al., 2004; Fahlke and Fischer, 2010). For example, both the stria vascularis and kidneys contain high levels of megalin, a vitamin D transporter that may play a role in aminoglycoside transport into the endolymph and megalin deficiency confers protection from aminoglycoside-induced nephrotoxicity (Mizuta et al., 1999; Schmitz et al., 2002). Closure or manipulation of vitamin D transporters or the stria vascularis as an entry pathway is not yet investigated but could serve as a mechanism to prevent aminoglycoside ototoxicity.

Targeting Mechanotransducer Channel Mediated Entry to Prevent Ototoxicity

As an otoprotective strategy, preventing aminoglycoside entry into hair cells has emerged as another research focus in recent years (Huth et al., 2015). Breakthroughs following this strategy stem from the knowledge pool gained on the mechanotransduction (MET) channel, an area we will briefly review below.

Aminoglycosides enter hair cells via the MET channel, a non-specific cation channel at the tips of the hair cell stereocilia that opens and closes in response to hair bundle deflection (Alharazneh et al., 2011; Vu et al., 2013; Marcotti et al., 2016). The molecular structure of this mechanically-gated channel has been the subject of much research and the protein composition of the MET channel in hair cells remains unclear (Fettiplace and Kim, 2014; Zhao and Müller, 2015). Nonetheless, studies have extensively characterized the biophysical properties of the MET channel and estimated its pore opening to be <1.70 nm and its narrowest portion at 1.25 nm (Farris et al., 2004; Marcotti et al., 2005). The MET channel pore dimension is thus large enough to accommodate the passage of dihydrostreptomycin, a four-ringed aminoglycoside whose end-on diameter was estimated at 0.8 nm (Marcotti et al., 2005). Whilst dihydrostreptomycin can fit through this pore, it also acts as a permeant channel blocker, i.e., it forms a temporary block that is reduced by high extracellular calcium, and is voltage dependent, decreasing at extreme positive and negative potentials (Gale et al., 2001; Ricci, 2002; Ricci et al., 2002; Marcotti et al., 2005). The ability of different aminoglycosides to serve as permeant blockers of the MET channel likely varies as a function of the chemical size and charge. An electrophysiology study showing a side-by-side comparison of aminoglycosides in terms of size and charge is lacking, only sisomicin and a novel derivative have been studied independently (Farris et al., 2004; Huth et al., 2015). Whether channel permeation by aminoglycosides correlates with the level of ototoxicity remains to be explored.

Aminoglycosides more readily enter hair cells in the base than the apex corresponding to larger transduction currents at the cochlear base, and the larger single channel conductance in basal outer hair cells (Ricci et al., 2003; Waguespack and Ricci, 2005; Beurg et al., 2006). This is also consistent with the findings that basal hair cells are more susceptible to damage by aminoglycosides and that patients experience hearing loss beginning at the high frequencies.

A number of critical experiments demonstrate the importance of the MET channel as a mechanism of aminoglycoside hair cell entry. First, using the GTTR compound, Alharazneh et al. (2011) found that aminoglycosides are rapidly taken up into hair cells within minutes in rat cochlear explants. Moreover a variety of MET channel blockers were observed to protect against hair cell loss *in vitro*, leading to the suggestion that channel blockers can be otoprotective. Blocking MET channels (e.g., with amiloride, quinine or curare) prevents aminoglycoside entry into hair cells and confers hair cell protection from various aminoglycosides (Alharazneh et al., 2011). However, the potential issue with using channel blockers for otoprotection is that many of the blockers used are toxic to humans and thus are not suitable as therapeutic agents. Second, the data indicating that calcium competes with aminoglycosides as a permeant blocker of the MET channel supports the role of MET channels in aminoglycoside entry (Ricci, 2002; Coffin et al., 2009). In mammalian studies, low calcium levels result in more robust drug uptake and toxicity and conversely, higher calcium levels, which decrease MET channel currents, were otoprotective (Ricci, 2002; Ricci et al., 2002; Vu et al., 2013). In other studies, decreased GTTR uptake is observed using high calcium in the extracellular solution, which also leads to a reduction in hair cell loss caused by aminoglycoside treatment in both the lateral line *in vivo* and cochlea *in vitro* (Coffin et al., 2009; Wang and Steyger, 2009; Ou et al., 2012). Thirdly, several genetic models with reduced or abolished MET channel function also demonstrate reduced aminoglycoside uptake and/or toxicity, such as those that result from Cadherin23 deletion, Myosin7a deletion, and Transmembrane channel-like proteins 1 and

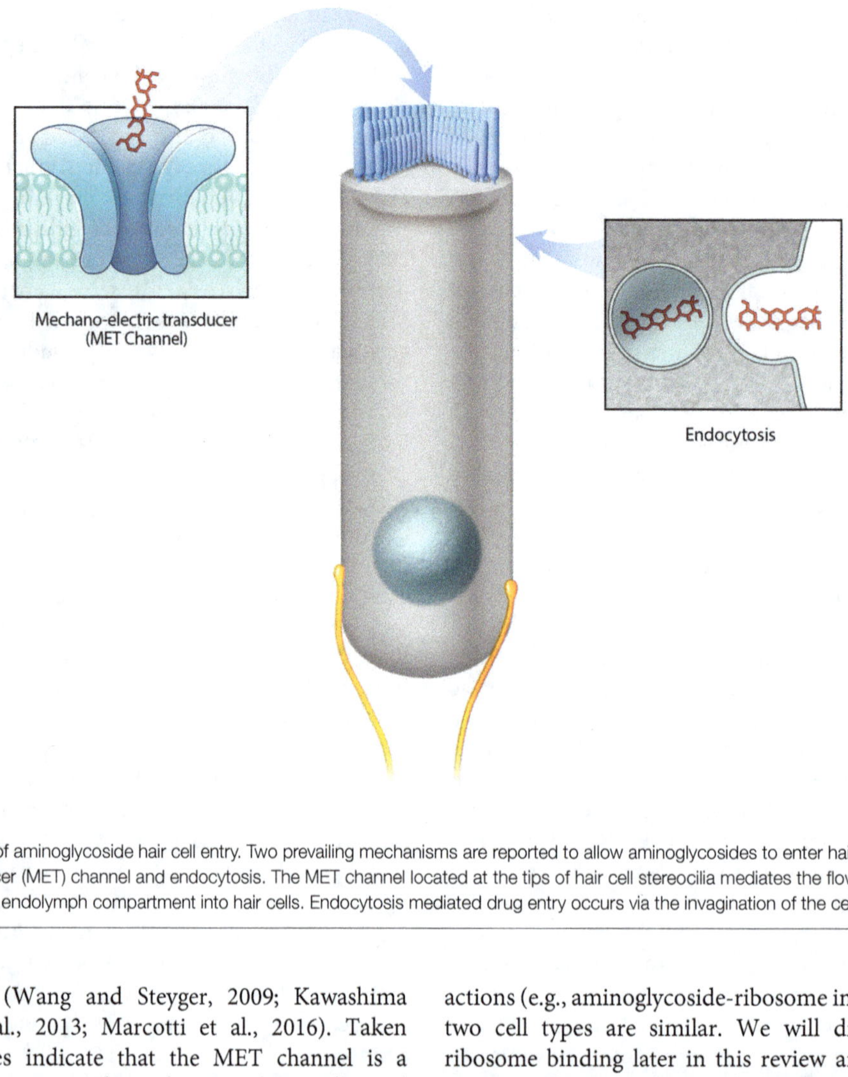

FIGURE 1 | Mechanisms of aminoglycoside hair cell entry. Two prevailing mechanisms are reported to allow aminoglycosides to enter hair cells—the mechano-electric transducer (MET) channel and endocytosis. The MET channel located at the tips of hair cell stereocilia mediates the flow of ions (including aminoglycosides) from the endolymph compartment into hair cells. Endocytosis mediated drug entry occurs via the invagination of the cell membrane.

2 double knockouts (Wang and Steyger, 2009; Kawashima et al., 2011; Vu et al., 2013; Marcotti et al., 2016). Taken together, these studies indicate that the MET channel is a major entry route for aminoglycosides into hair cells and that this mode of entry is required for hair cell toxicity (**Figure 1**).

Leveraging knowledge of the MET channel biophysical properties, Huth et al. (2015) designed a new version of modified aminoglycosides and found that sisomicin derivatives were less toxic to hair cells *in vitro* and *in vivo* than the parent aminoglycoside. When compared to sisomicin, the lead compound N1MS was found to permeate the MET channel to a lesser degree than the parent compound sisomicin by electrophysiological measurements (Kd = 65.0 $\pm$ 17.7 vs. 96.1 $\pm$ 9.9 μM, respectively; Huth et al., 2015). However, they found that altering aminoglycosides could decrease their antimicrobial activities, or in the case of N1MS, shift its spectrum of activities (Huth et al., 2015). While this study shows that it is possible to separate aminoglycoside entry into hair cells from entry into bacteria, more work is needed to gain insights into the relationship between aminoglycoside structure and antimicrobial actions, in particular bacterial uptake. While different mechanisms of aminoglycoside uptake likely exist between bacteria and sensory hair cells, it is possible intracellular actions (e.g., aminoglycoside-ribosome interactions) between the two cell types are similar. We will discuss aminoglycoside-ribosome binding later in this review article. In general, these recent studies provide proof-of-principal data that ototoxicity and antimicrobial activity can be separated and also that by preventing aminoglycoside entry via MET channels, ototoxicity is greatly reduced.

Targeting Alternative Entry Routes to Prevent Ototoxicity

Endocytosis is another route of entry for aminoglycosides into hair cells (**Figure 1**), however, relative to MET channel-mediated uptake it is slower (Hashino and Shero, 1995; Alharazneh et al., 2011). Immunogold-labeling and GTTR-based experiments show the presence of aminoglycosides in membrane-bound vesicles beneath the cell surface of hair cells (Hashino and Shero, 1995). The number of aminoglycoside-containing vesicles appears to increase over time with a subset increasing in size, presumably as a result of aggregation (Hashino and Shero, 1995). Recent live imaging studies reveal that both endocytic and non-endocytic uptake of aminoglycosides occur, and that both mechanisms can result in accumulation of drug in lysosomes (Nagai and Takano, 2014; Hailey et al., 2017). Lysosomes are the primary degradative compartment of eukaryotic cells (Giraldo et al., 2014; Perera and Zoncu, 2016). Notably, identification of compounds in vesicles does not causally link to the mechanism of uptake as entry via MET channels or endocytosis. Evidence supporting the role of endocytosis in aminoglycoside ototoxicity include observations made in the kidney where aminoglycosides are endocytosed and subsequently accumulate within lysosomes of renal proximal tubular cells, leading to cell death (Moestrup et al., 1995; Nagai and Takano, 2014).

In addition to the MET channels, other ion channels are implicated in mediating aminoglycoside entry into hair cells. One such family is the transient receptor potential (TRP) channels, which are large calcium-permeant, cationic channels (Myrdal and Steyger, 2005; Karasawa et al., 2008). While various channels are implicated in mediating aminoglycoside transport in renal tubular cells *in vitro*, their exact roles in mediating aminoglycoside ototoxicity are unclear (Myrdal and Steyger, 2005; Karasawa et al., 2008). For example, activated TRPA1 channels allow GTTR entry when the MET channel is blocked (Stepanyan et al., 2011). Since TRPA1 channels can be activated by lipid peroxidation products, it is proposed that it can amplify aminoglycoside uptake in addition to MET channel in damaged hair cells (Stepanyan et al., 2011). Another candidate modulator is the chloride/bicarbonate exchanger Slc4a1b, which mediates aminoglycoside uptake in the kidney (Stehberger et al., 2007; Alper, 2009) and in hair cells in the zebrafish lateral line (Hailey et al., 2017). Although the Slc family proteins are expressed in the stria vascularis in the mammalian cochlea, their exact roles in aminoglycoside transport are unknown and warrant further investigation (Stankovic et al., 1997).

As a strategy for preventing ototoxicity, targeting endocytosis and other ion channels is challenging as these pathways are not specific to hair cells, nor do these entry mechanisms appear to be the most predominant in the hair cell. Moreover, preventing endocytosis pharmacologically may have off-target effects. As we move further down the chain of events in aminoglycoside ototoxicity the issue of off-target effects becomes larger and the challenge of preventing damage becomes arguably greater.

Targeting Intracellular Mechanisms to Prevent Ototoxicity

A plethora of cellular structures and metabolic pathways are implicated in aminoglycoside ototoxicity. Building on a large body of literature on the roles of reactive oxygen species, recent studies aiming at unraveling these mechanisms at the organelle (mitochondria and endoplasmic reticulum (ER)) and other subcellular levels (ribosome, membrane lipids and potassium channel interactions) may open the door to preventing ototoxicity (Huth et al., 2015; Stawicki et al., 2015; Wong and Ryan, 2015). As it is difficult to distinguish between mechanisms that are primary and secondary in hair cell stress, we have grouped the mechanisms by target.

Once inside the hair cell, aminoglycosides rapidly fill the cytoplasm (Alharazneh et al., 2011). As cationic molecules, aminoglycosides are drawn to negatively charged molecules such as DNA, RNA, negatively charged phospholipids and cationic binding sites (basic residues) in proteins. In addition to building up in the cytoplasm, reports of ER and mitochondrial stress suggest that aminoglycosides accumulate within these organelles (**Figure 2**; Guan et al., 2000; Esterberg et al., 2014). These organelles are concentrated at two key functional zones in the hair cell, the apical region below the cuticular plate and hair bundle, and the basolateral region near the synaptic complex.

The mitochondrion is a dynamic, double membrane bound organelle that contains its own genome and translational apparatus (mitochondrial ribosome or mitoribosome; Anderson et al., 1981). The mtDNA is a closed circular molecule of 16,569 nucleotides that encodes proteins involved in oxidative phosphorylation (OXPHOS; Anderson et al., 1981). This organelle has many functions, most notably the production of ATP via OXPHOS, a pathway responsible for producing over 90% of cellular ATP. Other energetic mitochondrial functions are reviewed elsewhere (Wallace et al., 2010). On the other hand, the ER is one of the largest organelles in the eukaryotic cells (Oakes and Papa, 2015). It is a network of branching tubules and flattened sacs interconnected through enclosed spaces called the ER lumen, which plays major roles in protein folding and calcium regulation (Oakes and Papa, 2015).

Targeting the Ribosome to Prevent Ototoxicity

As in bacteria, an intracellular target for aminoglycosides in the mammalian cochlear hair cell is the ribosome. Ribosomes (~30% of eukaryotic cellular mass) decode genetic information and convert it into proteins (Kramer et al., 2009). Each cell contains up to 10^6 ribosomes and 5–9 amino acids are incorporated into proteins per second (Kramer et al., 2009). In bacteria, aminoglycosides bind to the small ribosomal subunit, where they disrupt the rate and accuracy of protein synthesis (Ogle and Ramakrishnan, 2005). In humans, a longstanding hypothesis of aminoglycoside ototoxicity is that hair cell dysfunction arises from a similar mechanism of action due to structural resemblances between eukaryotic and bacterial ribosomes (Hutchin et al., 1993; Prezant et al., 1993; Guan et al., 2000; Hobbie et al., 2006, 2008a,b; Greber et al., 2015).

Of the two types of ribosome (mitochondrial and cytoplasmic) in the eukaryotic cell, the mitoribosome was implicated in aminoglycoside ototoxicity in 1993 (Hutchin et al., 1993; Prezant et al., 1993). The strongest evidence supporting the role of the mitoribosome in aminoglycoside ototoxicity is antibiotic hypersensitivity in patients with the m.1555A>G mitochondrial DNA mutation (Hutchin et al., 1993; Prezant et al., 1993; Estivill et al., 1998). Patients with this mutation located adjacent to the aminoglycoside ribosomal binding site are particularly susceptible to aminoglycoside induced hearing loss. While the mitochondrial ribosomal transcript in eukaryotic cells normally differs from that in the bacteria, the m.1555A>G mutation re-establishes one of the evolutionarily lost bacterial-like base pairs in the mitoribosome (**Figure 3**). Consequently, the structure of mutant mitochondrial ribosomal transcript resembles that of the *E. coli* transcript, rendering the

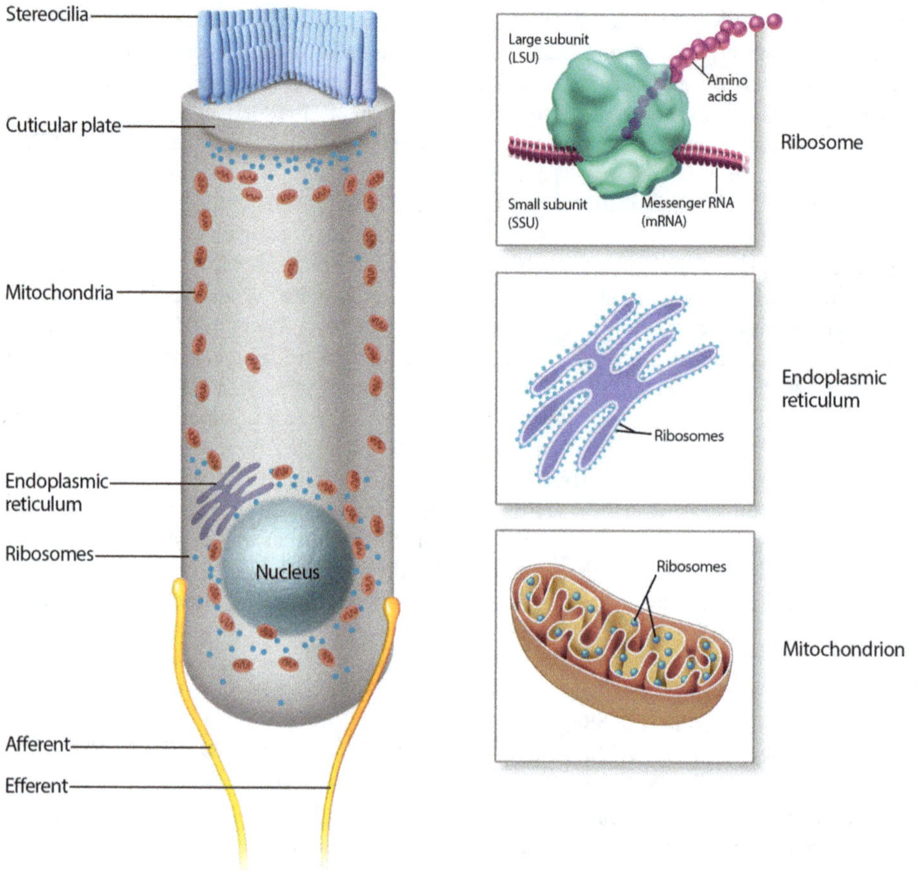

FIGURE 2 | Mechanisms of aminoglycoside intracellular action. Many intracellular mechanisms may be involved in cochlear hair cell death, including mitochondrial and cytosolic ribotoxicity, mitochondrial and endoplasmic reticulum (ER) calcium signaling, lipid interactions and reactive oxygen species (ROS) production.

mitochondrial decoding site more susceptible to aminoglycoside binding, resulting in translational impairment and possibly increased sensitivity to aminoglycoside toxicity (Hutchin et al., 1993; Böttger, 2010). In patients with the m.1555A>G mutation, hearing loss can occur following a single dose (Usami et al., 1998).

Functional studies also support the role of the mitoribosome in aminoglycoside ototoxicity. In human blood and skin-derived cell lines aminoglycoside treatment impairs mitochondrial protein synthesis (Guan et al., 2000; Giordano et al., 2002). Also a series of cell free assays using ribosomal constructs show that aminoglycosides have higher binding affinities for m.1555G ribosomes, which are less accurate at selecting the cognate tRNA when exposed to aminoglycosides (Hobbie et al., 2008b). Based on these results, it is hypothesized that cochlear hair cell death occurs when the level of translation decreases to below a certain threshold level (Guan et al., 2000; Giordano et al., 2002).

Furthermore, genetic studies lend additional support for mitoribosomal involvement by indicating that the variable penetrance of aminoglycoside-related hearing loss is due to the nuclear genetic background. Currently, four nuclear-encoded modifiers have been identified: mitochondrial transcription optimization 1 (MTO1); GTP binding protein 3 (GTPBP3); 5-methylaminomethyl-2-thiouridylate methyltransferase (TRMU); and mitochondrial transcription factor 1 (TFB1M; Li and Guan, 2002; Bykhovskaya et al., 2004a,b; Guan et al., 2006). GTPBP3, MTO1 and TRMU are hypothesized to alter the penetrance of aminoglycoside-related hearing loss by altering the accuracy of tRNA anti-codon mRNA codon interactions in the A-site (**Figure 3**; Li and Guan, 2002; Bykhovskaya et al., 2004b; Guan et al., 2006). The TFB1M enzyme modifies two, highly conserved, adjacent residues on the 3' end of the 16S rRNA (**Figure 3**), but it remains unclear how TFB1M modifies aminoglycoside-related hearing loss (Seidel-Rogol et al., 2003; Cotney et al., 2009; Metodiev et al., 2009; Raimundo et al., 2012; Sharoyko et al., 2014; Lee et al., 2015; O'Sullivan et al., 2015).

While the established model of aminoglycoside ototoxicity suggests that mitochondrial ribotoxicity triggers hearing loss, there is a growing body of evidence suggesting that the cytosolic ribosome may also be affected by aminoglycoside (Nudelman et al., 2010; Kandasamy et al., 2012; Francis et al., 2013; Shulman et al., 2014). The cytosolic ribosome is responsible for the synthesis of over 20,000 cytosolic proteins and its composition, origin and function are different from its mitochondrial and

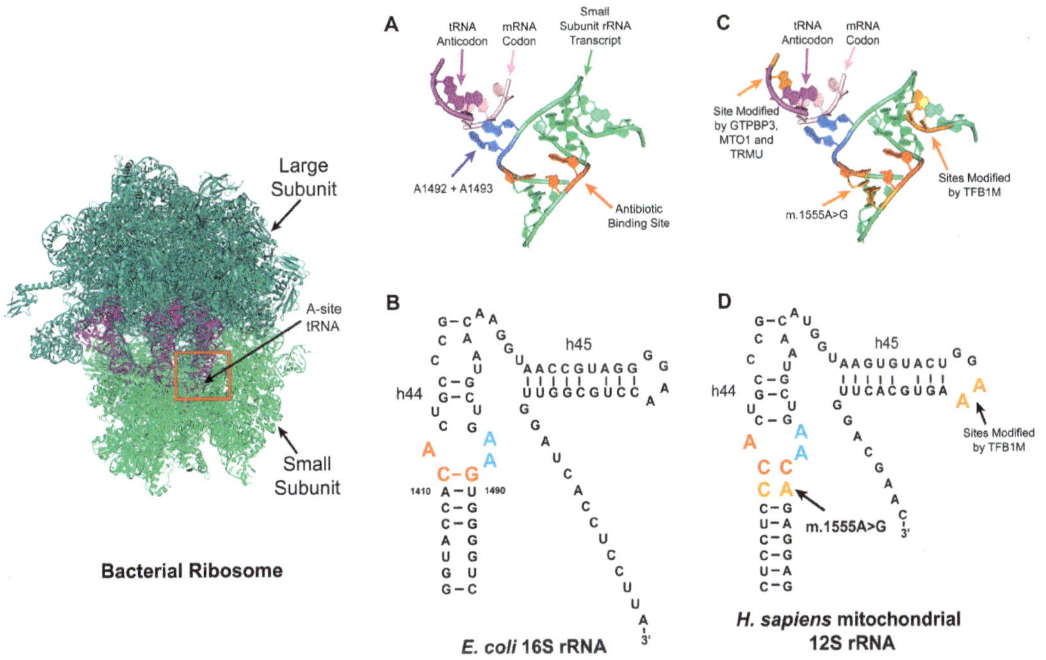

FIGURE 3 | Aminoglycoside ribosome binding. Aminoglycosides can bind to several sites on ribosomes, with the primary prokaryotic binding site reported to be a conserved pocket in the A-site (red box) formed by helix h44 of the 16S rRNA in the small ribosomal subunit. At this site, the correct tRNA anti-codon is matched with the correct mRNA codon. **(A,B)** Tertiary **(A)** and secondary **(B)** structures of the bacterial A-site. In bacteria, aminoglycosides bind to three conserved nucleotides A1408, C1409 and G1491 (red). **(C,D)** Schematic depicting the tertiary **(C)** and secondary **(D)** structures of the mitochondrial A-site. In the human mitochondrial ribosome, patients with the m.1555A>G mutation have a new base pair formed which makes it resemble the bacterial ribosome. Four nuclear genes are reported to modify the penetrance of aminoglycoside related hearing loss (TRMU, MTO1, GTPBP3 and TFB1M), the tRNA and rRNA nucleotides modified by these enzymes are shown in orange.

bacterial counterparts (Ramakrishnan, 2002; Greber et al., 2015; Khatter et al., 2015). Francis et al. (2013) showed that the degree of aminoglycoside toxicity correlates closely with the extent of inhibition of cytoplasmic protein synthesis using an *in vitro* model. A prime example of aminoglycoside cyto-ribosome interaction is the clinical application of aminoglycosides in "codon-read through" therapy as a treatment for genetic diseases such as Rett syndrome, cystic fibrosis and Duchenne muscular dystrophy (Burke and Mogg, 1985; Nudelman et al., 2010; Baradaran-Heravi et al., 2017). Here, the concept is that synthesis errors can suppress otherwise deleterious mutations, such as premature stop-codon mutations.

Current ribotoxicity paradigms indicate that aminoglycosides kill bacteria by binding to the bacterial ribosome causing mistranslation. It is reduced aminoglycoside affinities to the corresponding eukaryotic ribosome as well as differences in cell entry that provide the rationale for bacterial specificity of aminoglycosides. Several studies have characterized and developed aminoglycosides with lower affinities for the mitochondrial ribosome (Matt et al., 2012; Perez-Fernandez et al., 2014). For example, the veterinary aminoglycoside, apramycin, is less ototoxic to hair cells *in vitro* and *in vivo*, and the lower ototoxicity profile of this aminoglycoside can be attributed to the lower affinity of this drug for the binding pocket in the mitochondrial ribosome (Matt et al., 2012). To further the development of less ototoxic aminoglycosides, more detailed studies are needed to evaluate the contribution of mitochondrial and cytosolic translational inhibition in aminoglycoside ototoxicity as it is unclear which mechanism predominates *in vivo*.

In addition to modifying the aminoglycoside backbone to prevent ototoxicity, two other strategies may be employed to prevent the effects of aminoglycoside-induced ribotoxicity: increased ribosomal accuracy and increased tolerance by the cell for ribosomal errors. In the current model of ribosome related ototoxicity an increase in errors as a result of aminoglycosides triggers cellular dysfunction. Amino-acid mis-incorporations during translation naturally occur, one in every 1000–10,000 codons translated is mistranslated (Drummond and Wilke, 2009). Studies indicate that both bacterial and mammalian ribosomes have the potential to switch to hyper-accurate states (Ruusala et al., 1984; Lodmell and Dahlberg, 1997). Moreover, in cell lines carrying mitochondrial translational defects, amino acid supplementation is reported to increase the fidelity of mitochondrial translation and can rescue translation defects *in vitro* (Boczonadi et al., 2013).

Targeting the Other Intracellular Events to Prevent Ototoxicity

In addition to interaction with the mitochondrial and cytosolic ribosomes, many potentially overlapping cellular events likely occur upon aminoglycoside entry into the hair cell. We will briefly review these areas in this section.

Calcium Signaling

Calcium signaling is a key component in aminoglycoside induced cell death (Esterberg et al., 2013, 2014; Hailey et al., 2017). Calcium ions are important signaling molecules and in hair cells, precise regulation of Ca^{2+} concentrations is critical, e.g., Ca^{2+} defines the open probability of the MET channel (Ricci et al., 1998). Recent *in vivo* zebrafish experiments show Ca^{2+} levels are elevated in the ER following neomycin treatment and that the flow of Ca^{2+} between the ER and mitochondrion is a key event in aminoglycoside ototoxicity (Esterberg et al., 2013, 2014; Hailey et al., 2017). Esterberg et al. (2013) showed that in aminoglycoside-treated hair cells from the zebrafish lateral line, spikes in Ca^{2+} levels in the ER are followed by similar spikes in the mitochondria. Ca^{2+} spikes increase mitochondrial respiration, reactive oxygen species production and lead to a collapse in mitochondrial membrane potential, release of Ca^{2+} from these intracellular stores and subsequent cell death (Esterberg et al., 2013, 2014; Hailey et al., 2017).

Lysosomal Degradation

The lysosome controls the degradation and recycling of proteins and polysaccharides by intracellular autophagy (Giraldo et al., 2014; Perera and Zoncu, 2016). Damaged material is engulfed by autophagosomes via endocytic pathways, which then fuse with the lysosome and result in the recycling of amino acids and monosaccharides (Giraldo et al., 2014; Perera and Zoncu, 2016). Evidence for lysosomal involvement in ototoxicity arose from mechanisms associated with nephrotoxicity where aminoglycosides are known to be transported and accumulate within lysosomes of renal proximal tubular cells causing injury and necrosis (Moestrup et al., 1995). In aminoglycoside-treated hair cells, the antibiotic is also detectable in lysosomes (Hashino and Shero, 1995; Hashino et al., 1997, 2000; Steyger et al., 2003; Dai et al., 2006; Hailey et al., 2017). Interestingly, pharmacological inhibition of aminoglycoside uptake into lysosomes exacerbated hair cell death, implicating an important role of lysosomal degradation (Hailey et al., 2017).

Interactions with the Plasma Membrane, PIP2s and Potassium Channels

Aminoglycosides can also directly interact with membrane lipids. For example, they can induce rapid changes to the hair cell plasma membrane including phosphotidylserine externalization and membrane blebbing on the apical surface (Richardson and Russell, 1991; Goodyear et al., 2008). Aminoglycosides also bind to and alter the levels of phosphoinositides phosphatidylinositol-4,5-bisphosphate (PIP2) and phosphatidylinositol 1-3,4,5-trisphosphate (PIP3; Schacht, 1976; Gabev et al., 1989). As PIP2 controls transduction and adaptation by hair cells, this may in turn affect drug uptake and hair cell viability (Hirono et al., 2004). Biochemical studies demonstrate that several aminoglycoside members bind to negatively charged phospholipid bilayers and inhibit the activity of lysosomal enzymes (Brasseur et al., 1984, 1985). In bacteria, studies show that aminoglycosides also bind to lipid bilayers (Sautrey et al., 2016).

In the mammalian cochlea, the potassium channel KCNQ4 is highly expressed in outer hair cells and KCNQ4 mutations cause human hereditary hearing loss (Kubisch et al., 1999; Kharkovets et al., 2000, 2006). One proposed etiology of hearing loss is outer hair cell death caused by KCNQ4 deficiency (Kharkovets et al., 2000, 2006; Nouvian et al., 2003). As the activity of several KCNQ isoforms including KCNQ4 is linked to PIP2 metabolism aminoglycosides may indirectly cause KCNQ4 dysfunction by disrupting PIP2 homeostasis and in turn induce outer hair cell death (Li et al., 2005; Suh et al., 2006). In support of this possible mechanism, like the KCNQ4 deficient cochlea, aminoglycoside ototoxicity typically displays outer hair cell loss in a basal-to-apical gradient (Kubisch et al., 1999; Kharkovets et al., 2000, 2006).

Free Radical Production

Changes in free radicals contribute to signaling and cell death pathways. Free radicals encompass both reactive oxygen species (ROS) and reactive nitrogen species (RNS), and it is the odd number of electron(s) of a free radical that makes it unstable, short-lived and highly reactive (Forge and Schacht, 2000; Huth et al., 2011; Phaniendra et al., 2015). Both ROS and RNS are required for normal cellular function (e.g., intracellular signaling) and their damaging capabilities are tightly regulated by the antioxidant system. However, when the antioxidant defense system is overwhelmed, free-radical induced oxidative stress occurs damaging the integrity of various cellular components including lipids, proteins and DNA, thus contributing to cell death. Aminoglycoside-induced ROS production has been heavily studied. ROS are electrophilic molecules generated by the partial reduction of oxygen to form superoxide, hydrogen peroxide, and hydroxyl radicals. There are multiple sources of ROS in the cell, including mitochondria, peroxisomes, the ER, and NADPH oxidase enzymes (Brand, 2010; Phaniendra et al., 2015). In most cell types, the mitochondrial OXPHOS system is the largest contributor to intracellular oxidant production, with superoxide radicals being produced at two major sites during electron transport, namely Complex I (NADH dehydrogenase) and Complex III (ubiquinone cytochrome c reductase; Brand, 2010; Jastroch et al., 2010).

Aside from drug monitoring, efforts aimed at preventing aminoglycoside ototoxicity have focused on mitigating the damage effects of ROS since *in vivo* and *in vitro* studies show ROS production in cochlear hair cells following aminoglycoside treatment (Rybak and Whitworth, 2005; Shulman et al., 2014; Esterberg et al., 2016). Protection against aminoglycoside ototoxicity has also been demonstrated by a wide array of antioxidants (e.g., lipoic acid, Coenzyme Q10, N-acetylcysteine, vitamin E and salicylates; Rybak and Whitworth, 2005; Sha et al., 2006; Noack et al., 2017). A growing number of reports indicate that the mechanism of ROS generation and the role of ROS in aminoglycoside induced cell death may be more complicated than initially proposed (Francis et al., 2013; Majumder et al., 2015; Esterberg et al., 2016). For example, *in vitro* experiments show the depletion of glutathione (a major ROS scavenger) does not increase susceptibility to aminoglycoside induced cell death suggesting alternate roles for ROS (Majumder et al., 2015).

DISCUSSION

Aminoglycoside ototoxicity represents one of the most common, preventable forms of drug-related hearing loss worldwide. Studies in recent years have catapulted our understanding of this disease entity and revealed novel therapeutic approaches. Many unanswered questions remain thus impeding antibiotic/otoprotectant design and development. To help coordinate a targeted approach to tackle these questions, we will discuss key focus areas that can hopefully direct efforts to accelerate the prevention of aminoglycoside ototoxicity.

1. *How are novel aminoglycosides less ototoxic?* It remains incompletely understood how novel aminoglycosides that have been developed are less ototoxic (Matt et al., 2012; Perez-Fernandez et al., 2014; Huth et al., 2015). Not only will this shape the development of the next generation of safer aminoglycoside antibiotics but it will also be relevant to those using aminoglycosides for codon-read-through therapies for rare diseases (Baradaran-Heravi et al., 2017). Specifically, one will need to establish whether compounds with lower affinities for the mitochondrial ribosome also show less entry into hair cells (Matt et al., 2012; Perez-Fernandez et al., 2014). Conversely, understanding whether compounds less readily entering hair cells are also toxic to the human ribosome is equally important (Huth et al., 2015). For this work, an *in vitro* screening assay using cochleae from an m.1555A>G mouse model would be a powerful tool to assess the mitochondrial ribotoxicity of less toxic aminoglycosides, since hair cells with these mutations would be the most sensitive to compounds toxic to the mitochondrial ribosome. At present, this type of mouse model remains elusive owing to the limitations of mitochondrial DNA transformation (Holt and Jacobs, 2014).
2. *How do aminoglycosides travel from the blood to endolymph?* Our insights into how various medications including ototoxins such as aminoglycosides and the anti-neoplastic agent cisplatin traverse the blood-labyrinth-barrier is quite limited. This is in part due to our incomplete knowledge of candidate transporters expressed in the stria vascularis. Efforts by several laboratories to investigate gene expression and function should aid our understanding of aminoglycoside entry into the endolymph, an area that holds significant promise in preventing aminoglycoside ototoxicity (Dai and Steyger, 2008; Li et al., 2011; Shi, 2016).
3. *How do aminoglycosides enter hair cells and bacteria?* Strategies focused on modifying aminoglycosides to prevent entry into hair cells hypothesize that differences in aminoglycoside uptake likely exist between bacteria and sensory hair cells. In hair cells both the MET channel and endocytosis are potential entry pathways (**Figure 1**). In the bacteria the membrane transporters porins and mechanosensitive channels are reported to allow aminoglycoside entry into gram negative cells (Silver, 2016). Should entry in both cell types occur predominantly through channel-mediated pathways, electrophysiological studies showing the permeation properties of different aminoglycosides ranked in terms of size, charge and hydrophobicity would be particularly valuable for novel drug design. Electrophysiology studies are somewhat limited by the size of bacteria (0.8–2 μm) but techniques have been developed to record the activities of mechanosensitive channels in several bacterial species, including the MscS and MscL channels (Moe et al., 1998; Blount et al., 1999; Martinac et al., 2013).
4. *What are primary and secondary intracellular interactions?* Many intracellular targets/mediators in hair cells are reported to be involved in aminoglycoside ototoxicity. This complexity has presented challenges in defining the molecular mechanisms, their temporal sequence, and also candidate therapeutic targets. It is also unclear if redundancy may exist and if aminoglycosides have multiple intracellular targets, making the efficacy of singular-target approaches uncertain. Nonetheless, one of the attractive targets for aminoglycosides is the ribosome, as biochemical and molecular evidence strongly suggest their interaction. Recent advances in cryo-electron microscopy may soon reveal aminoglycosides binding to the cytosolic and mitochondrial ribosomes *in situ*, results from which may inform binding patterns and potentially drug design/development (Greber et al., 2015).
5. *What is the true prevalence of ototoxicity?* As discussed previously, the reported incidence of aminoglycoside-induced hearing loss varies widely and establishing the true prevalence of ototoxicity following aminoglycoside exposure is key. Estimates of ototoxicity in patients range between 2%–25% for hearing deficits and 1%–10% for vestibular dysfunction (Ariano et al., 2008). To move the development of therapeutic options forward (e.g., otoprotective compounds or less ototoxic antibiotics) and help guide public interventions, such fundamental knowledge is critical. For example, close to 100% of patients with the m.1555A>G mutation are reported to develop hearing loss following aminoglycoside exposure. However, for other patients, the incidence is significantly lower. In order to formulate a national policy on genetic testing for the mitochondrial m.1555A>G mutation in the context of aminoglycoside usage in neonatal intensive care, the contribution of m.1555A>G to deafness in neonates who are likely to have received multiple courses of aminoglycoside antibiotics is currently being assessed (Bitner-Glindzicz et al., 2014).

CONCLUSION

Tremendous genetic and functional work has shed light on the intricacies of aminoglycoside entry and action. This has facilitated the development of strategies with significant translational promise, in particular, the concept of modifying the aminoglycoside itself to prevent ototoxicity. The paradigm of modifying aminoglycoside antibiotics has been around for many years and nearly all antibiotics brought to market over the last 30 year have been variations on existing drugs (The Pew Charitable Trusts, 2016). However, it is only in recent years that this roadmap has been employed to reduce ototoxicity (Perez-Fernandez et al., 2014; Huth et al., 2015). In nature, aminoglycosides are modified by the living organisms (soil bacteria) that produce them. In industry, pharmaceutical companies have modified aminoglycosides (e.g., dibekacin, amikacin and netilmicin) synthetically to protect certain sites from aminoglycoside-modifying resistance enzymes and bolster antibacterial potency. Most recently, plazomicin, a semi-synthetic aminoglycoside with improved antibacterial efficacy has made it to a phase III clinical trials with readouts due in 2017 and 2018 (ClinicalTrials.gov, trial number NCT02486627 and NCT01970371). Should less ototoxic aminoglycosides with maintained or better antimicrobial potencies be developed, an accelerated track to clinical translation could be followed.

Going forward it is imperative that we continue to develop a better insight and scientific understanding of aminoglycoside entry and action, and that scientists modifying aminoglycosides to different ends continue to work together to develop compounds with better physiochemical properties. Whilst the development of life-saving antibiotics will always remain the priority, we owe it to our patients to continue to explore the possibility that a simple tag or chemical modification could limit the dramatic side effect that is aminoglycoside-related hearing loss—a global health problem.

AUTHOR CONTRIBUTIONS

MEO'S, AP, RL, AS, AGC and AJR: literature search; MEO'S, AGC and AJR: figure preparation and manuscript preparation.

ACKNOWLEDGMENTS

The authors thank C. Gralapp and H. DeMirci for assistance in figure preparation. This work was supported by Marie Skłodowska-Curie Actions Fellowship (MEO'S), the Stanford University Medical Scholars Research Program (AP), National Institutes of Health—RO1DC014720 (AJR and AGC) and RO1DC01910 (AGC).

REFERENCES

Abbott, N. J., and Blakley, B. (2007). "Specialised neural barriers," in *Strategies for Advancing Brain-Barriers Translational Research—Meeting Proceedings* (Stevenson, WA: International Brain Barriers Society), 1–36. Available online at: http://www.ibbsoc.org/PDFs/NeuralBarriers.pdf [Accessed October 11, 2017]

Agency for Healthcare Research and Quality. (2012). "Antibiotics for the prevention and treatment of early-onset neonatal infection," in *Agency for Healthcare Research and Quality, National Guideline Clearing House.* Available online at: https://www.guideline.gov/summaries/summary/38408/antibiotics-for-earlyonset-neonatal-infection-antibiotics-for-the-prevention-and-treatment-of-earlyonset-neonatal-infection?q=gentamicin

Alharazneh, A., Luk, L., Huth, M., Monfared, A., Steyger, P. S., Cheng, A. G., et al. (2011). Functional hair cell mechanotransducer channels are required for aminoglycoside ototoxicity. *PLoS One* 6:e22347. doi: 10.1371/journal.pone.0022347

Al-Malky, G., Dawson, S. J., Sirimanna, T., Bagkeris, E., and Suri, R. (2015). High-frequency audiometry reveals high prevalence of aminoglycoside ototoxicity in children with cystic fibrosis. *J. of Cyst. Fibros.* 14, 248–254. doi: 10.1016/j.jcf.2014.07.009

Al-Malky, G., Suri, R., Dawson, S. J., Sirimanna, T., and Kemp, D. (2011). Aminoglycoside antibiotics cochleotoxicity in paediatric cystic fibrosis (CF) patients: a study using extended high-frequency audiometry and distortion product otoacoustic emissions. *Int. J. Audiol.* 50, 112–122. doi: 10.3109/14992027.2010.524253

Alper, S. L. (2009). Molecular physiology and genetics of Na^+-independent SLC4 anion exchangers. *J. Exp. Biol.* 212, 1672–1683. doi: 10.1242/jeb.029454

Anderson, S., Bankier, A. T., Barrell, B. G., De Bruijn, M. H. L., Coulson, A. R., Drouin, J., et al. (1981). Sequence and organization of the human mitochondrial genome. *Nature* 290, 457–465. doi: 10.1038/290457a0

Antec. (2014). Gentamicin sulphate according to EP and USP method—application note aminoglycoside antibiotics. Available online at: https://antecscientific.com/downloads/notes/pharma/217_030_03%20-%20Gentamicin%20according%20EP%20and%20USP.pdf

Ariano, R. E., Zelenitsky, S. A., and Kassum, D. A. (2008). Aminoglycoside-induced vestibular injury: maintaining a sense of balance. *Annu. Pharmacother.* 42, 1282–1289. doi: 10.1345/aph.1l001

Arya, D. P. (Ed.). (2007). *Aminoglycoside Antibiotics: From Chemical Biology to Drug Discovery.* Hoboken, NJ: John Wiley and Sons.

Avent, M. L., Rogers, B. A., Cheng, A. C., and Paterson, D. L. (2011). Current use of aminoglycosides: indications, pharmacokinetics and monitoring for toxicity. *Intern. Med. J.* 41, 441–449. doi: 10.1111/j.1445-5994.2011.02452.x

Baradaran-Heravi, A., Niesser, J., Balgi, A. D., Choi, K., Zimmerman, C., South, A. P., et al. (2017). Gentamicin B1 is a minor gentamicin component with major nonsense mutation suppression activity. *Proc. Natl. Acad. Sci. U S A* 114, 3479–3484. doi: 10.1073/pnas.1620982114

Beaubien, A. R., Desjardins, S., Ormsby, E., Bayne, A., Carrier, K., Cauchy, M., et al. (1989). Incidence of amikacin ototoxicity: a sigmoid function of total drug exposure independent of plasma levels. *Am. J. Otolaryngol.* 10, 234–243. doi: 10.1016/0196-0709(89)90002-1

Beurg, M., Evans, M. G., Hackney, C. M., and Fettiplace, R. (2006). A large-conductance calcium-selective mechanotransducer channel in mammalian cochlear hair cells. *J. Neurosci.* 26, 10992–11000. doi: 10.1523/jneurosci.2188-06.2006

Bitner-Glindzicz, M., Pembrey, M., Duncan, A., Heron, J., Ring, S. M., Hall, A., et al. (2009). Prevalence of mitochondrial 1555A→G mutation in European children. *N. Engl. J. Med.* 360, 640–642. doi: 10.1056/NEJMc0806396

Bitner-Glindzicz, M., Rahman, S., Chant, K., and Marlow, N. (2014). Gentamicin, genetic variation and deafness in preterm children. *BMC Pediatr.* 14:66. doi: 10.1186/isrctn39982239

Blount, P., Sukharev, S. I., Moe, P. C., Martinac, B., and Kung, C. (1999). Mechanosensitive channels of bacteria. *Methods Enzymol.* 294, 458–482. doi: 10.1016/S0076-6879(99)94027-2

Boczonadi, V., Smith, P. M., Pyle, A., Gomez-Duran, A., Schara, U., Tulinius, M., et al. (2013). Altered 2-thiouridylation impairs mitochondrial translation in reversible infantile respiratory chain deficiency. *Hum. Mol. Genet.* 22, 4602–4615. doi: 10.1093/hmg/ddt309

Böttger, E. C. (2010). Mutant A1555G mitochondrial 12S rRNA and aminoglycoside susceptibility. *Antimicrob. Agents Chemother.* 54, 3073–3075. doi: 10.1128/aac.01819-09

Brand, M. D. (2010). The sites and topology of mitochondrial superoxide production. *Exp. Gerontol.* 45, 466–472. doi: 10.1016/j.exger.2010.01.003

Brasseur, R., Carlier, M. B., Laurent, G., Claes, P. J., Vanderhaeghe, H. J., Tulkens, P. M., et al. (1985). Interaction of streptomycin and streptomycylamine derivatives with negatively charged lipid layers: correlation between binding, conformation of complexes and inhibition of lysosomal phospholipase activities. *Biochem. Pharmacol.* 34, 1035–1047. doi: 10.1016/0006-2952(85)90607-0

Brasseur, R., Laurent, G., Ruysschaert, J. M., and Tulkens, P. (1984). Interactions of aminoglycoside antibiotics with negatively charged lipid layers:

biochemical and conformational studies. *Biochem. Pharmacol.* 33, 629–637. doi: 10.1016/0006-2952(84)90319-8

Burke, J. F., and Mogg, A. E. (1985). Suppression of a nonsense mutation in mammalian cells *in vivo* by the aminoglycoside anthiotics G-418 and paromomycin. *Nucleic Acids Res.* 13, 6265–6272. doi: 10.1093/nar/13.17.6265

Bykhovskaya, Y., Mengesha, E., Wang, D., Yang, H., Estivill, X., Shohat, M., et al. (2004a). Human mitochondrial transcription factor B1 as a modifier gene for hearing loss associated with the mitochondrial A1555G mutation. *Mol. Genet. Metab.* 82, 27–32. doi: 10.1016/j.ymgme.2004.01.020

Bykhovskaya, Y., Mengesha, E., Wang, D., Yang, H., Estivill, X., Shohat, M., et al. (2004b). Phenotype of non-syndromic deafness associated with the mitochondrial A1555G mutation is modulated by mitochondrial RNA modifying enzymes MTO1 and GTPBP3. *Mol. Genet. Metab.* 83, 199–206. doi: 10.1016/j.ymgme.2004.07.009

Chen, K. S., Bach, A., Shoup, A., and Winick, N. J. (2013). Hearing loss and vestibular dysfunction among children with cancer after receiving aminoglycosides. *Pediatr. Blood Cancer* 60, 1772–1777. doi: 10.1002/pbc.24631

Cheng, A. G., Johnston, P. R., Luz, J., Uluer, A., Fligor, B., Licameli, G. R., et al. (2009). Sensorineural hearing loss in patients with cystic fibrosis. *Otolaryngol. Head Neck Surg.* 141, 86–90. doi: 10.1016/j.otohns.2009.03.020

Coffin, A. B., Reinhart, K. E., Owens, K. N., Raible, D. W., and Rubel, E. W. (2009). Extracellular divalent cations modulate aminoglycoside-induced hair cell death in the zebrafish lateral line. *Hear. Res.* 253, 42–51. doi: 10.1016/j.heares.2009.03.004

Cotney, J., Mckay, S. E., and Shadel, G. S. (2009). Elucidation of separate, but collaborative functions of the rRNA methyltransferase-related human mitochondrial transcription factors B1 and B2 in mitochondrial biogenesis reveals new insight into maternally inherited deafness. *Hum. Mol. Genet.* 18, 2670–2682. doi: 10.1093/hmg/ddp208

Dai, C., Mangiardi, D., Cotanche, D., and Steyger, P. (2006). Uptake of fluorescent gentamicin by vertebrate sensory cells *in vivo*. *Hear. Res.* 213, 64–78. doi: 10.1016/j.heares.2005.11.011

Dai, C. F., and Steyger, P. S. (2008). A systemic gentamicin pathway across the stria vascularis. *Hear. Res.* 235, 114–124. doi: 10.1016/j.heares.2007.10.010

Drummond, D. A., and Wilke, C. O. (2009). The evolutionary consequences of erroneous protein synthesis. *Nat. Rev. Genet.* 10, 715–724. doi: 10.1038/nrg2662

Duggal, P., and Sarkar, M. (2007). Audiologic monitoring of multi-drug resistant tuberculosis patients on aminoglycoside treatment with long term follow-up. *BMC Ear Nose Throat Disord.* 7:5. doi: 10.1186/1472-6815-7-5

Erdem, T., Ozturan, O., Iraz, M., Miman, M. C., and Olmez, E. (2005). Dose-dependent dual effect of melatonin on ototoxicity induced by amikacin in adult rats. *Eur. Arch. Otorhinolaryngol.* 262, 314–321. doi: 10.1007/s00405-004-0793-1

Esterberg, R., Hailey, D. W., Coffin, A. B., Raible, D. W., and Rubel, E. W. (2013). Disruption of intracellular calcium regulation is integral to aminoglycoside-induced hair cell death. *J. Neurosci.* 33, 7513–7525. doi: 10.1523/jneurosci.4559-12.2013

Esterberg, R., Hailey, D. W., Rubel, E. W., and Raible, D. W. (2014). ER-mitochondrial calcium flow underlies vulnerability of mechanosensory hair cells to damage. *J. Neurosci.* 34, 9703–9719. doi: 10.1523/jneurosci.0281-14.2014

Esterberg, R., Linbo, T., Pickett, S. B., Wu, P., Ou, H. C., Rubel, E. W., et al. (2016). Mitochondrial calcium uptake underlies ROS generation during aminoglycoside-induced hair cell death. *J. Clin. Invest.* 126, 3556–3566. doi: 10.1172/jci84939

Estivill, X., Govea, N., Barceló, A., Perelló, E., Badenas, C., Romero, E., et al. (1998). Familial progressive sensorineural deafness is mainly due to the mtDNA A1555G mutation and is enhanced by treatment with aminoglycosides. *Am. J. Hum. Genet.* 62, 27–35. doi: 10.1086/301676

Fahlke, C., and Fischer, M. (2010). Physiology and pathophysiology of ClC-K/barttin channels. *Front. Physiol.* 1:155. doi: 10.3389/fphys.2010.00155

Farris, H. E., Leblanc, C. L., Goswami, J., and Ricci, A. J. (2004). Probing the pore of the auditory hair cell mechanotransducer channel in turtle. *J. Physiol.* 558, 769–792. doi: 10.3410/f.1006705.251756

Fausti, S. A., Henry, J. A., Schaffer, H. I., Olson, D. J., Frey, R. H., and Mcdonald, W. J. (1992). High-frequency audiometric monitoring for early detection of aminoglycoside ototoxicity. *J. Infect. Dis.* 165, 1026–1032. doi: 10.1093/infdis/165.6.1026

Fettiplace, R., and Kim, K. X. (2014). The physiology of mechanoelectrical transduction channels in hearing. *Physiol. Rev.* 94, 951–986. doi: 10.1152/physrev.00038.2013

Forge, A., and Schacht, J. (2000). Aminoglycoside antibiotics. *Audiol. Neurootol.* 5, 3–22. doi: 10.1159/000013861

Francis, S. P., Katz, J., Fanning, K. D., Harris, K. A., Nicholas, B. D., Lacy, M., et al. (2013). A novel role of cytosolic protein synthesis inhibition in aminoglycoside ototoxicity. *J. Neurosci.* 33, 3079–3093. doi: 10.3410/f.717997761.793474294

Freeman, C. D., Nicolau, D. P., Belliveau, P., and Nightingale, C. (1997). Once-daily dosing of aminoglycosides: review and recommendations for clinical practice. *J. Antimicrob. Chemother.* 39, 677–686. doi: 10.1093/jac/39.6.677

Gabev, E., Kasianowicz, J., Abbott, T., and Mclaughlin, S. (1989). Binding of neomycin to phosphatidylinositol 4,5-biphosphate (PIP_2). *Biochim. Biophys. Acta* 979, 105–112. doi: 10.1016/0005-2736(89)90529-4

Gale, J. E., Marcotti, W., Kennedy, H., Kros, C., and Richardson, G. (2001). FM1-43 dye behaves as a permeant blocker of the hair-cell mechanotransducer channel. *J. Neurosci.* 21, 7013–7025.

Giordano, C., Pallotti, F., Walker, W. F., Checcarelli, N., Musumeci, O., Santorelli, F., et al. (2002). Pathogenesis of the deafness-associated A1555G mitochondrial DNA mutation. *Biochem. Biophys. Res. Commun.* 293, 521–529. doi: 10.1016/S0006-291X(02)00256-5

Giraldo, A. M. V., Appelqvist, H., Ederth, T., and Öllinger, K. (2014). Lysosomotropic agents: impact on lysosomal membrane permeabilization and cell death. *Biochem. Soc. Trans.* 42, 1460–1464. doi: 10.1042/BST20140145

Goodyear, R. J., Gale, J. E., Ranatunga, K. M., Kros, C. J., and Richardson, G. P. (2008). Aminoglycoside-induced phosphatidylserine externalization in sensory hair cells is regionally restricted, rapid, and reversible. *J. Neurosci.* 28, 9939–9952. doi: 10.1523/jneurosci.1124-08.2008

Greber, B. J., Bieri, P., Leibundgut, M., Leitner, A., Aebersold, R., Boehringer, D., et al. (2015). The complete structure of the 55S mammalian mitochondrial ribosome. *Science* 348, 303–308. doi: 10.1126/science.aaa3872

Guan, M.-X. (2011). Mitochondrial 12S rRNA mutations associated with aminoglycoside ototoxicity. *Mitochondrion* 11, 237–245. doi: 10.1016/j.mito.2010.10.006

Guan, M.-X., Fischel-Ghodsian, N., and Attardi, G. (2000). A biochemical basis for the inherited susceptibility to aminoglycoside ototoxicity. *Hum. Mol. Genet.* 9, 1787–1793. doi: 10.1093/hmg/9.12.1787

Guan, M.-X., Yan, Q., Li, X., Bykhovskaya, Y., Gallo-Teran, J., Hajek, P., et al. (2006). Mutation in TRMU related to transfer RNA modification modulates the phenotypic expression of the deafness-associated mitochondrial 12S ribosomal RNA mutations. *Am. J. Hum. Genet.* 79, 291–302. doi: 10.1086/506389

Hailey, D. W., Esterberg, R., Linbo, T. H., Rubel, E. W., and Raible, D. W. (2017). Fluorescent aminoglycosides reveal intracellular trafficking routes in mechanosensory hair cells. *J. Clin. Invest.* 127, 472–486. doi: 10.1172/JCI85052

Hashino, E., and Shero, M. (1995). Endocytosis of aminoglycoside antibiotics in sensory hair cells. *Brain Res.* 704, 135–140. doi: 10.1016/0006-8993(95)01198-6

Hashino, E., Shero, M., and Salvi, R. J. (1997). Lysosomal targeting and accumulation of aminoglycoside antibiotics in sensory hair cells. *Brain Res.* 777, 75–85. doi: 10.1016/s0006-8993(97)00977-3

Hashino, E., Shero, M., and Salvi, R. J. (2000). Lysosomal augmentation during aminoglycoside uptake in cochlear hair cells. *Brain Res.* 887, 90–97. doi: 10.1016/s0006-8993(00)02971-1

Hawkins, E. (1973). Ototoxic mechanisms: a working hypothesis. *Audiology* 12, 383–393. doi: 10.3109/00206097309071652

Hirono, M., Denis, C. S., Richardson, G. P., and Gillespie, P. G. (2004). Hair cells require phosphatidylinositol 4,5-bisphosphate for mechanical transduction and adaptation. *Neuron* 44, 309–320. doi: 10.1016/j.neuron.2004.09.020

Hobbie, S. N., Akshay, S., Kalapala, S. K., Bruell, C. M., Shcherbakov, D., and Böttger, E. C. (2008a). Genetic analysis of interactions with eukaryotic rRNA identify the mitoribosome as target in aminoglycoside ototoxicity. *Proc. Natl. Acad. Sci. U S A* 105, 20888–20893. doi: 10.1073/pnas.0811258106

Hobbie, S. N., Bruell, C. M., Akshay, S., Kalapala, S. K., Shcherbakov, D., and Böttger, E. C. (2008b). Mitochondrial deafness alleles confer misreading of the genetic code. *Proc. Natl. Acad. Sci. U S A* 105, 3244–3249. doi: 10.1073/pnas.0707265105

Hobbie, S. N., Bruell, C., Kalapala, S., Akshay, S., Schmidt, S., Pfister, P., et al. (2006). A genetic model to investigate drug-target interactions at the ribosomal decoding site. *Biochimie* 88, 1033–1043. doi: 10.1016/j.biochi.2006.04.008

Holt, I. J., and Jacobs, H. T. (2014). Unique features of DNA replication in mitochondria: a functional and evolutionary perspective. *Bioessays* 36, 1024–1031. doi: 10.1002/bies.201400052

Hutchin, T., Haworth, L., Higashi, K., Fischel-Ghodsian, N., Stoneking, M., Saha, N., et al. (1993). A molecular basis for human hypersensitivity of aminoglyscoside antibiotics. *Nucleic Acids Res.* 21, 4174–4179. doi: 10.1093/nar/21.18.4174

Huth, M., Ricci, A., and Cheng, A. (2011). Mechanisms of aminoglycoside ototoxicity and targets of hair cell protection. *Int. J. Otolaryngol.* 2011:937861. doi: 10.1155/2011/937861

Huth, M. E., Han, K.-H., Sotoudeh, K., Hsieh, Y.-J., Effertz, T., Vu, A. A., et al. (2015). Designer aminoglycosides prevent cochlear hair cell loss and hearing loss. *J. Clin. Invest.* 125, 583–592. doi: 10.1172/JCI77424

Jastroch, M., Divakaruni, A. S., Mookerjee, S., Treberg, J. R., and Brand, M. D. (2010). Mitochondrial proton and electron leaks. *Essays Biochem.* 47, 53–67. doi: 10.1042/bse0470053

Jentsch, T. J., Hübner, C. A., and Fuhrmann, J. C. (2004). Ion channels: function unravelled by dysfunction. *Nat. Cell Biol.* 6, 1039–1047. doi: 10.1038/ncb1104-1039

Kandasamy, J., Atia-Glikin, D., Shulman, E., Shapira, K., Shavit, M., Belakhov, V., et al. (2012). Increased selectivity toward cytoplasmic versus mitochondrial ribosome confers improved efficiency of synthetic aminoglycosides in fixing damaged genes: a strategy for treatment of genetic diseases caused by nonsense mutations. *J. Med. Chem.* 55, 10630–10643. doi: 10.1021/jm3012992

Karasawa, T., Wang, Q., Fu, Y., Cohen, D. M., and Steyger, P. S. (2008). TRPV4 enhances the cellular uptake of aminoglycoside antibiotics. *J. Cell Sci.* 121, 2871–2879. doi: 10.1242/jcs.023705

Kawashima, Y., Géléoc, G. S., Kurima, K., Labay, V., Lelli, A., Asai, Y., et al. (2011). Mechanotransduction in mouse inner ear hair cells requires transmembrane channel-like genes. *J. Clin. Invest.* 121, 4796–4809. doi: 10.3410/f.13372023.14859074

Kharkovets, T., Dedek, K., Maier, H., Schweizer, M., Khimich, D., Nouvian, R., et al. (2006). Mice with altered KCNQ4 K^+ channels implicate sensory outer hair cells in human progressive deafness. *EMBO J.* 25, 642–652. doi: 10.1038/sj.emboj.7600951

Kharkovets, T., Hardelin, J.-P., Safieddine, S., Schweizer, M., El-Amraoui, A., Petit, C., et al. (2000). KCNQ4, a K^+ channel mutated in a form of dominant deafness, is expressed in the inner ear and the central auditory pathway. *Proc. Natl. Acad. Sci. U S A* 97, 4333–4338. doi: 10.1073/pnas.97.8.4333

Khatter, H., Myasnikov, A. G., Natchiar, S. K., and Klaholz, B. P. (2015). Structure of the human 80S ribosome. *Nature* 520, 640–645. doi: 10.2210/pdb4ug0/pdb

Koo, J.-W., Quintanilla-Dieck, L., Jiang, M., Liu, J., Urdang, Z. D., Allensworth, J. J., et al. (2015). Endotoxemia-mediated inflammation potentiates aminoglycoside-induced ototoxicity. *Sci. Transl. Med.* 7:298ra118. doi: 10.1126/scitranslmed.aac5546

Kramer, G., Boehringer, D., Ban, N., and Bukau, B. (2009). The ribosome as a platform for co-translational processing, folding and targeting of newly synthesized proteins. *Nat. Struct. Mol. Biol.* 16, 589–597. doi: 10.1038/nsmb.1614

Kubisch, C., Schroeder, B. C., Friedrich, T., Lütjohann, B., El-Amraoui, A., Marlin, S., et al. (1999). KCNQ4, a novel potassium channel expressed in sensory outer hair cells, is mutated in dominant deafness. *Cell* 96, 437–446. doi: 10.1016/s0092-8674(00)80556-5

Lacy, M. K., Nicolau, D. P., Nightingale, C. H., and Quintiliani, R. (1998). The pharmacodynamics of aminoglycosides. *Clin. Infect. Dis.* 27, 23–27. doi: 10.1086/514620

Lee, S., Rose, S., Metodiev, M. D., Becker, L., Vernaleken, A., Klopstock, T., et al. (2015). Overexpression of the mitochondrial methyltransferase TFB1M in the mouse does not impact mitoribosomal methylation status or hearing. *Neurosurgery* 24, 7286–7294. doi: 10.1093/hmg/ddv427

Li, H., Wang, Q., and Steyger, P. S. (2011). Acoustic trauma increases cochlear and hair cell uptake of gentamicin. *PLoS One* 6:e19130. doi: 10.1371/journal.pone.0019130

Li, X., and Guan, M.-X. (2002). A human mitochondrial GTP binding protein related to tRNA modification may modulate phenotypic expression of the deafness-associated mitochondrial 12S rRNA mutation. *Mol. Cell. Biol.* 22, 7701–7711. doi: 10.1128/mcb.22.21.7701-7711.2002

Li, Y., Gamper, N., Hilgemann, D. W., and Shapiro, M. S. (2005). Regulation of Kv7 (KCNQ) K^+ channel open probability by phosphatidylinositol 4,5-bisphosphate. *J. Neurosci.* 25, 9825–9835. doi: 10.1523/JNEUROSCI.2597-05.2005

Lodmell, J. S., and Dahlberg, A. E. (1997). A conformational switch in Escherichia coli 16S ribosomal RNA during decoding of messenger RNA. *Science* 277, 1262–1267. doi: 10.1126/science.277.5330.1262

Majumder, P., Duchen, M. R., and Gale, J. E. (2015). Cellular glutathione content in the organ of Corti and its role during ototoxicity. *Front. Cell. Neurosci.* 9:143. doi: 10.3389/fncel.2015.00143

Marcotti, W., Corns, L. F., Goodyear, R. J., Rzadzinska, A. K., Avraham, K. B., Steel, K. P., et al. (2016). The acquisition of mechano-electrical transducer current adaptation in auditory hair cells requires myosin VI. *J. Physiol.* 594, 3667–3681. doi: 10.1113/JP272220

Marcotti, W., Van Netten, S. M., and Kros, C. J. (2005). The aminoglycoside antibiotic dihydrostreptomycin rapidly enters mouse outer hair cells through the mechano-electrical transducer channels. *J. Physiol.* 567, 505–521. doi: 10.3410/f.1026826.323564

Martinac, B., Rohde, P. R., Cranfield, C. G., and Nomura, T. (2013). Patch clamp electrophysiology for the study of bacterial ion channels in giant spheroplasts of *E. coli*. *Methods Mol. Biol.* 966, 367–380. doi: 10.1007/978-1-62703-245-2_23

Matt, T., Ng, C. L., Lang, K., Sha, S.-H., Akbergenov, R., Shcherbakov, D., et al. (2012). Dissociation of antibacterial activity and aminoglycoside ototoxicity in the 4-monosubstituted 2-deoxystreptamine apramycin. *Proc. Natl. Acad. Sci. U S A* 109, 10984–10989. doi: 10.1073/pnas.1204073109

Metodiev, M. D., Lesko, N., Park, C. B., Cámara, Y., Shi, Y., Wibom, R., et al. (2009). Methylation of 12S rRNA is necessary for *in vivo* stability of the small subunit of the mammalian mitochondrial ribosome. *Cell Metab.* 9, 386–397. doi: 10.1016/j.cmet.2009.03.001

Mingeot-Leclercq, M.-P., and Tulkens, P. M. (1999). Aminoglycosides: nephrotoxicity. *Antimicrob. Agents Chemother.* 43, 1003–1012.

Mizuta, K., Saito, A., Watanabe, T., Nagura, M., Arakawa, M., Shimizu, F., et al. (1999). Ultrastructural localization of megalin in the rat cochlear duct. *Hear. Res.* 129, 83–91. doi: 10.1016/s0378-5955(98)00221-4

Modongo, C., Pasipanodya, J. G., Zetola, N. M., Williams, S. M., Sirugo, G., and Gumbo, T. (2015). Amikacin concentrations predictive of ototoxicity in multidrug-resistant tuberculosis patients. *Antimicrob. Agents Chemother.* 59, 6337–6343. doi: 10.1128/aac.01050-15

Moe, P. C., Blount, P., and Kung, C. (1998). Functional and structural conservation in the mechanosensitive channel MscL implicates elements crucial for mechanosensation. *Mol. Microbiol.* 28, 583–592. doi: 10.1046/j.1365-2958.1998.00821.x

Moestrup, S. K., Cui, S., Vorum, H., Bregengård, C., Bjørn, S., Norris, K., et al. (1995). Evidence that epithelial glycoprotein 330/megalin mediates uptake of polybasic drugs. *J. Clin. Invest.* 96, 1404–1413. doi: 10.1172/jci118176

Myrdal, S. E., and Steyger, P. S. (2005). TRPV1 regulators mediate gentamicin penetration of cultured kidney cells. *Hea. Res.* 204, 170–182. doi: 10.1016/j.heares.2005.02.005

Nagai, J., and Takano, M. (2014). Entry of aminoglycosides into renal tubular epithelial cells via endocytosis-dependent and endocytosis-independent pathways. *Biochem. Pharmacol.* 90, 331–337. doi: 10.1016/j.bcp.2014.05.018

NCBI PubChem Compound Database. (2017). National center for biotechnology information. PubChem compound database. Available online at: https://pubchem.ncbi.nlm.nih.gov/

Noack, V., Pak, K., Jalota, R., Kurabi, A., and Ryan, A. F. (2017). An antioxidant screen identifies candidates for protection of cochlear hair cells from gentamicin toxicity. *Front. Cell. Neurosci.* 11:242. doi: 10.3389/fncel.2017.00242

Nouvian, R., Ruel, J., Wang, J., Guitton, M. J., Pujol, R., and Puel, J. L. (2003). Degeneration of sensory outer hair cells following pharmacological blockade of cochlear KCNQ channels in the adult guinea pig. *Eur. J. Neurosci.* 17, 2553–2562. doi: 10.1046/j.1460-9568.2003.02715.x

Nudelman, I., Glikin, D., Smolkin, B., Hainrichson, M., Belakhov, V., and Baasov, T. (2010). Repairing faulty genes by aminoglycosides: development of new derivatives of geneticin (G418) with enhanced suppression of diseases-causing nonsense mutations. *Bioorg. Med. Chem.* 18, 3735–3746. doi: 10.1016/j.bmc.2010.03.060

O'Sullivan, M., Rutland, P., Lucas, D., Ashton, E., Hendricks, S., Rahman, S., et al. (2015). Mitochondrial m.1584A 12S m62A rRNA methylation in families with m.1555A>G associated hearing loss. *Hum. Mol. Genet.* 24, 1036–1044. doi: 10.1093/hmg/ddu518

Oakes, S. A., and Papa, F. R. (2015). The role of endoplasmic reticulum stress in human pathology. *Annu. Rev. Pathol.* 10, 173–194. doi: 10.1146/annurev-pathol-012513-104649

Ogle, J. M., and Ramakrishnan, V. (2005). Structural insights into translational fidelity. *Annu. Rev. Biochem.* 74, 129–177. doi: 10.1146/annurev.biochem.74.061903.155440

Ou, H. C., Keating, S., Wu, P., Simon, J. A., Raible, D. W., and Rubel, E. W. (2012). Quinoline ring derivatives protect against aminoglycoside-induced hair cell death in the zebrafish lateral line. *J. Assoc. Res. Otolaryngol.* 13, 759–770. doi: 10.1007/s10162-012-0353-0

Perera, R. M., and Zoncu, R. (2016). The lysosome as a regulatory hub. *Annu. Rev. Cell Dev. Biol.* 32, 223–253. doi: 10.1146/annurev-cellbio-111315-125125

Perez-Fernandez, D., Shcherbakov, D., Matt, T., Leong, N. C., Kudyba, I., Duscha, S., et al. (2014). 4′-O-substitutions determine selectivity of aminoglycoside antibiotics. *Nat. Commun.* 5:3112. doi: 10.1038/ncomms4112

Phaniendra, A., Jestadi, D. B., and Periyasamy, L. (2015). Free radicals: properties, sources, targets, and their implication in various diseases. *Indian J. Clin. Biochem.* 30, 11–26. doi: 10.1007/s12291-014-0446-0

Prezant, T. R., Agapian, J. V., Bohlman, M. C., Bu, X., Öztas, S., Qiu, W.-Q., et al. (1993). Mitochondrial ribosomal RNA mutation associated with both antibiotic-induced and non-syndromic deafness. *Nat. Genet.* 4, 289–294. doi: 10.1136/jmg.30.10.885

Quick, C. A., Fish, A., and Brown, C. (1973). The relationship between cochlea and kidney. *Laryngoscope* 83, 1469–1482. doi: 10.1288/00005537-197309000-00007

Rahman, S., Ecob, R., Costello, H., Sweeney, M. G., Duncan, A. J., Pearce, K., et al. (2012). Hearing in 44–45 year olds with m.1555A>G, a genetic mutation predisposing to aminoglycoside-induced deafness: a population based cohort study. *BMJ Open* 2:e000411. doi: 10.1136/bmjopen-2011-000411

Raimundo, N., Song, L., Shutt, T. E., Mckay, S. E., Cotney, J., Guan, M.-X., et al. (2012). Mitochondrial stress engages E2F1 apoptotic signaling to cause deafness. *Cell* 148, 716–726. doi: 10.3410/f.14263963.15777086

Ramakrishnan, V. (2002). Ribosome structure and the mechanism of translation. *Cell* 108, 557–572. doi: 10.1016/s0092-8674(02)00619-0

Ricci, A. (2002). Differences in mechano-transducer channel kinetics underlie tonotopic distribution of fast adaptation in auditory hair cells. *J. Neurophysiol.* 87, 1738–1748. doi: 10.1152/jn.00574.2001

Ricci, A. J., Crawford, A. C., and Fettiplace, R. (2002). Mechanisms of active hair bundle motion in auditory hair cells. *J. Neurosci.* 22, 44–52.

Ricci, A., Wu, Y., and Fettiplace, R. (1998). The endogenous calcium buffer and the time course of transducer adaptation in auditory hair cells. *J. Neurosci.* 18, 8261–8277.

Ricci, A. J., Crawford, A. C., and Fettiplace, R. (2003). Tonotopic variation in the conductance of the hair cell mechanotransducer channel. *Neuron* 40, 983–990. doi: 10.3410/f.1016611.201037

Richardson, G. P., and Russell, I. J. (1991). Cochlear cultures as a model system for studying aminoglycoside induced ototoxicity. *Hear. Res.* 53, 293–311. doi: 10.1016/0378-5955(91)90062-e

Ruusala, T., Andersson, D., Ehrenberg, M., and Kurland, C. G. (1984). Hyper-accurate ribosomes inhibit growth. *EMBO J.* 3, 2575–2580.

Rybak, L. P., and Whitworth, C. A. (2005). Ototoxicity: therapeutic opportunities. *Drug Discov. Today* 10, 1313–1321. doi: 10.1016/s1359-6446(05)03552-x

Salt, A. N., and Plontke, S. K. (2005). Local inner-ear drug delivery and pharmacokinetics. *Drug Discov. Today* 10, 1299–1306. doi: 10.1016/s1359-6446(05)03574-9

Sandoval, R., Leiser, J., and Molitoris, B. A. (1998). Aminoglycoside antibiotics traffic to the Golgi complex in LLC-PK1 cells. *J. Am. Soc. Nephrol.* 9, 167–174.

Sautrey, G., El Khoury, M., Dos Santos, A. G., Zimmermann, L., Deleu, M., Lins, L., et al. (2016). Negatively charged lipids as a potential target for new amphiphilic aminoglycoside antibiotics: a biophsyical study. *J. Biol. Chem.* 291, 13864–13874. doi: 10.1074/jbc.m115.665364

Schacht, J. (1976). Inhibition by neomycin of polyphosphoinositide turnover in subcellular fractions of guinea-pig cerebral cortex *in vitro*. *J. Neurochem.* 27, 1119–1124. doi: 10.1111/j.1471-4159.1976.tb00318.x

Schmitz, C., Hilpert, J., Jacobsen, C., Boensch, C., Christensen, E. I., Luft, F. C., et al. (2002). Megalin deficiency offers protection from renal aminoglycoside accumulation. *J. Biol. Chem.* 277, 618–622. doi: 10.1074/jbc.m109959200

Seddon, J. A., Godfrey-Faussett, P., Jacobs, K., Ebrahim, A., Hesseling, A. C., and Schaaf, H. S. (2012). Hearing loss in patients on treatment for drug-resistant tuberculosis. *Eur. Respir. J.* 40, 1277–1286. doi: 10.1183/09031936.00044812

Seidel-Rogol, B. L., Mcculloch, V., and Shadel, G. S. (2003). Human mitochondrial transcription factor B1 methylates ribosomal RNA at a conserved stem-loop. *Nat. Genetics* 33, 23–24. doi: 10.1038/ng1064

Sha, S.-H., Qiu, J.-H., and Schacht, J. (2006). Aspirin to prevent gentamicin-induced hearing loss. *N. Engl. J. Med.* 354, 1856–1857. doi: 10.1056/nejmc053428

Sharoyko, V. V., Abels, M., Sun, J., Nicholas, L. M., Mollet, I. G., Stamenkovic, J. A., et al. (2014). Loss of TFB1M results in mitochondrial dysfunction that leads to impaired insulin secretion and diabetes. *Hum. Mol. Genet.* 23, 5733–5749. doi: 10.1093/hmg/ddu288

Shi, X. (2016). Pathophysiology of the cochlear intrastrial fluid-blood barrier. *Hear. Res.* 338, 52–63. doi: 10.1016/j.heares.2016.01.010

Shulman, E., Belakhov, V., Wei, G., Kendall, A., Meyron-Holtz, E. G., Ben-Shachar, D., et al. (2014). Designer aminoglycosides that selectively inhibit cytoplasmic rather than mitochondrial ribosomes show decreased ototoxicity a strategy for the treatment of genetic diseases. *J. Biol. Chem.* 289, 2318–2330. doi: 10.1074/jbc.m113.533588

Silver, L. L. (2016). A Gestalt approach to Gram-negative entry. *Bioorg. Med. Chem.* 24, 6379–6389. doi: 10.1016/j.bmc.2016.06.044

Smyth, A., Tan, K. H., Hyman-Taylor, P., Mulheran, M., Lewis, S., Stableforth, D., et al. (2005). Once versus three-times daily regimens of tobramycin treatment for pulmonary exacerbations of cystic fibrosis—the TOPIC study: a randomised controlled trial. *Lancet* 365, 573–578. doi: 10.1016/S0140-6736(05)17906-9

Stankovic, K. M., Brown, D., Alper, S. L., and Adams, J. C. (1997). Localization of pH regulating proteins H^+ ATPase and Cl^- HCO_3^- exchanger in the guinea pig inner ear. *Hear. Res.* 114, 21–34. doi: 10.1016/s0378-5955(97)00072-5

Stawicki, T. M., Esterberg, R., Hailey, D. W., Raible, D. W., and Rubel, E. W. (2015). Using the zebrafish lateral line to uncover novel mechanisms of action and prevention in drug-induced hair cell death. *Front. Cell. Neurosci.* 9:46. doi: 10.3389/fncel.2015.00046

Stehberger, P. A., Shmukler, B. E., Stuart-Tilley, A. K., Peters, L. L., Alper, S. L., and Wagner, C. A. (2007). Distal renal tubular acidosis in mice lacking the AE1 (band3) Cl^-/HCO_3^- exchanger (*slc4a1*). *J. Am. Soc. Nephrol.* 18, 1408–1418. doi: 10.1681/ASN.2006101072

Stepanyan, R. S., Indzhykulian, A. A., Vélez-Ortega, A. C., Boger, E. T., Steyger, P. S., Friedman, T. B., et al. (2011). TRPA1-mediated accumulation of aminoglycosides in mouse cochlear outer hair cells. *J. Assoc. Res. Otolaryngol.* 12, 729–740. doi: 10.1007/s10162-011-0288-x

Sterkers, O., Ferrary, E., and Amiel, C. (1984). Inter-and intracompartmental osmotic gradients within the rat cochlea. *Am. J. Physiol.* 247, F602–F606.

Sterkers, O., Saumon, G., Huy, P. T. B., and Amiel, C. (1982). K, Cl, and H2O entry in endolymph, perilymph, and cerebrospinal fluid of the rat. *Am. J. Physiol.* 243, F173–F180.

Steyger, P. S., Peters, S., Rehling, J., Hordichok, A., and Dai, C. (2003). Uptake of gentamicin by bullfrog saccular hair cells *in vitro*. *J. Assoc. Res. Otolaryngol.* 4, 565–578. doi: 10.1007/s10162-003-4002-5

Suh, B.-C., Inoue, T., Meyer, T., and Hille, B. (2006). Rapid chemically induced changes of PtdIns (4,5) P_2 gate KCNQ ion channels. *Science* 314, 1454–1457. doi: 10.1126/science.1131163

The Pew Charitable Trusts. (2016). *A Scientific Roadmap for Antibiotic Discovery—Antibiotic Resistance Report*. Washington, DC: The Pew Charitable Trusts. Available online at: http://www.pewtrusts.org/en/research-and-analysis/reports/2016/05/a-scientific-roadmap-for-antibiotic-discovery [Accessed October 11, 2017]

Usami, S.-I., Abe, S., Shinkawa, H., and Kimberling, W. J. (1998). Sensorineural hearing loss caused by mitochondrial DNA mutations: special reference to the A1555G mutation. *J. Commun. Disord.* 31, 423–435. doi: 10.1016/s0021-9924(98)00014-8

Van Boeckel, T. P., Gandra, S., Ashok, A., Caudron, Q., Grenfell, B. T., Levin, S. A., et al. (2014). Global antibiotic consumption 2000 to 2010: an analysis of national pharmaceutical sales data. *Lancet Infect. Dis.* 14, 742–750. doi: 10.1016/s1473-3099(14)70780-7

Vu, A. A., Nadaraja, G. S., Huth, M. E., Luk, L., Kim, J., Chai, R., et al. (2013). Integrity and regeneration of mechanotransduction machinery regulate aminoglycoside entry and sensory cell death. *PLoS One* 8:e54794. doi: 10.1371/journal.pone.0054794

Waguespack, J., and Ricci, A. (2005). Aminoglycoside ototoxicity: permeant drugs cause permanent hair cell loss. *J. Physiol.* 567, 359–360. doi: 10.1113/jphysiol.2005.094474

Wallace, D. C., Fan, W., and Procaccio, V. (2010). Mitochondrial energetics and therapeutics. *Annu. Rev. Pathol.* 5, 297–348. doi: 10.1146/annurev.pathol.4.110807.092314

Wang, Q., and Steyger, P. S. (2009). Trafficking of systemic fluorescent gentamicin into the cochlea and hair cells. *J. Assoc. Res. Otolaryngol.* 10, 205–219. doi: 10.1007/s10162-009-0160-4

Wang, Q., Kachelmeier, A., and Steyger, P. S. (2010). Competitive antagonism of fluorescent gentamicin uptake in the cochlea. *Hear. Res.* 268, 250–259. doi: 10.1016/j.heares.2010.06.008

Waters, V., Stanojevic, S., Klingel, M., Chiang, J., Sonneveld, N., Kukkar, R., et al. (2015). Prolongation of antibiotic treatment for cystic fibrosis pulmonary exacerbations. *J. Cyst. Fibros.* 14, 770–776. doi: 10.1016/j.jcf.2015.07.010

Wong, A. C., and Ryan, A. F. (2015). Mechanisms of sensorineural cell damage, death and survival in the cochlea. *Front. Aging Neurosci.* 7:58. doi: 10.3389/fnagi.2015.00058

World Health Organization. (2011). *Critically Important Antimicrobials for Human Medicine.* Geneva: WHO Document Production Services

Zhao, B., and Müller, U. (2015). The elusive mechanotransduction machinery of hair cells. *Curr. Opin. Neurobiol.* 34, 172–179. doi: 10.1016/j.conb.2015.08.006

Zimmerman, E., and Lahav, A. (2013). Ototoxicity in preterm infants: effects of genetics, aminoglycosides, and loud environmental noise. *J. Perinatol.* 33, 3–8. doi: 10.1038/jp.2012.105

7

Magnetic Nanoparticle Mediated Steroid Delivery Mitigates Cisplatin-Induced Hearing Loss

Bharath Ramaswamy[1,2], *Soumen Roy*[3], *Andrea B. Apolo*[4], *Benjamin Shapiro*[1,5,6]* and *Didier A. Depireux*[5,6,7]

[1] *Fischell Department of Bioengineering, University of Maryland, College Park, MD, United States,* [2] *Pfizer Inc., New York, NY, United States,* [3] *Sensory Cell Biology, National Institute on Deafness and Other Communication Disorders (NIDCD), National Institutes of Health (NIH), Bethesda, MD, United States,* [4] *Genitourinary Malignancies Branch, Center for Cancer Research, National Cancer Institute, National Institutes of Health (NIH), Bethesda, MD, United States,* [5] *Institute for Systems Research, University of Maryland, College Park, MD, United States,* [6] *Otomagnetics, Rockville, MD, United States,* [7] *Department of Otorhinolaryngology/Head and Neck Surgery, University of Maryland School of Medicine, Baltimore, MD, United States*

Edited by:
Jian Zuo,
St. Jude Children's Research Hospital, United States

Reviewed by:
Jung-Bum Shin,
University of Virginia, United States
Shikha Tarang,
Creighton University, United States

****Correspondence:***
Benjamin Shapiro
benshap@umd.edu

Cisplatin (cis-diamminedichloroplatinum) is widely used as a chemotherapeutic drug for genitourinary, breast, lung and head and neck cancers. Though effective in inducing apoptosis in cancer cells, cisplatin treatment causes severe hearing loss among patients. Steroids have been shown to mitigate cisplatin-induced hearing loss. However, steroids may interfere with the anti-cancer properties of cisplatin if administered systemically, or are rapidly cleared from the middle and inner ear and hence lack effectiveness when administered intra-tympanically. In this work, we deliver prednisolone-loaded nanoparticles magnetically to the cochlea of cisplatin-treated mice. This magnetic delivery method substantially reduced hearing loss in treated animals at high frequency compared to control animals or animals that received intra-tympanic methylprednisolone. The method also protected the outer hair cells from cisplatin-mediated ototoxicity.

Keywords: cisplatin, ototoxicity, magnetic nanoparticles, drug delivery, hair cells

INTRODUCTION

Cisplatin (cis-diamminedichloroplatinum) and other platinum based drugs are the antineoplastic drugs of choice for various genitourinary cancers, certain forms of breast cancers, and as radiosensitizers for most head and neck cancers. However, these platinum-based drugs are very toxic to the kidneys (Miller et al., 2010), the inner ear (Rademaker-Lakhai et al., 2006), and sometimes the peripheral nervous system (Gregg et al., 1992). While the nephrotoxicity may be mitigated by hyper-hydrating patients in the hours before and during cisplatin injections, addressing ototoxicity in cisplatin-treated patients remains an unmet medical need.

Cisplatin induced hearing loss occurs in adults with an average incidence of 62% (Marshak et al., 2014). Among pediatric patients, significant sensorineural hearing loss is observed in 90.5% of patients at 8 kHz (Allen et al., 1998). The ototoxic effect of cisplatin is noticeable, with hearing loss within hours or days after the first cisplatin injection (Rybak et al., 2009). It is also cumulative, and the cumulative effect implies particular vulnerability in pediatric populations as repeated treatments, even separated by years, eventually lead to complete hearing loss, which may in turn lead to pervasive developmental delays including speech, cognitive and social developmental challenges.

The molecular mechanisms underlying the ototoxicity of cisplatin remain under debate. The various mechanisms include generation of reactive oxygen species and the depletion of antioxidant enzymes such as superoxide dismutase (DeWoskin and Riviere, 1992), catalase, glutathione peroxidase and glutathione reductase (Rybak et al., 2009). Overall, cisplatin causes damage to the organ of Corti, the stria vascularis and spiral ganglion cells, possibly through different molecular mechanisms (Lee et al., 2004; Monzack et al., 2015).

Steroids have been shown to reduce cisplatin-induced hearing loss, presumably by counteracting the effect of the reactive oxygen species induced by cisplatin administration (Himeno et al., 2002; Marshak et al., 2014). Though commonly used, pre-clinical studies indicate steroids may interfere with cisplatin's efficacy, plus prolonged use of systemic steroids is undesirable due to additive toxicities (Wooldridge et al., 2001; Fardet and Fève, 2014; Morin and Fardet, 2015; Ranganath et al., 2015). Thus, it has been proposed that local administration of steroids into the middle ear, subsequently diffusing into the cochlea via the round window membrane at the base of the cochlea, could be used to protect hearing. However, administration of a liquid steroid into the middle ear results in a rapid elimination of the drug from the cochlea as well as a very steep drug gradient from the base to the apex of the cochlea (Bird et al., 2007; Salt and Plontke, 2009). The liquid formulation in the middle ear is also rapidly eliminated via the Eustachian tube as soon as the patient stands up and swallows.

This paper describes results for protecting hearing from cisplatin by magnetically delivering steroids into the cochlea. In prior animal studies we showed that application of our magnetic injection device could be used to transport drug-eluting bio-compatible nanoparticles from the middle ear to the inner ear. Once inside the inner ear, the drug payload is released from the nanoparticles, providing a significant therapeutic effect (Shapiro et al., 2014a,b). In this paper, we show that magnetic steroid delivery to the inner ear can be used to protect hearing in mice receiving systemic cisplatin regimens. Previously both dexamethasone and prednisolone had been used for their otoprotective effect against cisplatin (Marshak et al., 2014; Özel et al., 2016). We employed prednisolone-loaded magnetic nanoparticles deposited intra-tympanically into the middle ear, and then applied a magnetic field that transported the nanoparticles through the window membranes into the inner ear where they released the steroid in therapeutic amounts. In the mouse model employed in this study, this steroid delivery method effectively mitigated the cisplatin-induced rise in hearing threshold of the animals at high frequencies and protected the outer hair cells in the basal cochlear region from the ototoxic effect of cisplatin.

MATERIALS AND METHODS

Animals

The study was conducted on CBA/CAJ mice (10 weeks old) of both sexes (23–27 gm body weight) from the Jackson Laboratory (Bar Harbor, ME). All animal studies were conducted in accordance with the policies and recommendations of the National Institute of Health Guide for the Care and Use of Laboratory Animals, and under approval from the Institutional Animal Care and Use Committee of the University of Maryland.

Anesthesia

The mice were anesthetized via intraperitoneal injections of ketamine 100 mg/kg and xylazine 20 mg/kg supplemented as necessary and were placed on a warming pad (Deltaphase isothermal pad, Braintree Scientific, MA) to maintain body temperature at 37°C.

Study Design

The overall study design is shown in **Table 1**. The mouse cisplatin administration protocol (Roy et al., 2013) involves multiple cisplatin cycles spread over time (as is the case for patients), and it reliably elicits hearing loss but leads to less than 10% animal mortality. Compared to this protocol, we halved the duration of the last chemotherapy cycle in an effort to further reduce animal mortality. Hearing of all mice was first tested by auditory brainstem response (ABR) measurements. Then, all mice were pre-hydrated with two subcutaneous doses of 1 mL of sterile normal saline (Hospiral, IL) separated by 8 h, and 24 h before starting each cisplatin cycle, to protect their kidneys against nephrotoxicity. Cisplatin was administered intraperitoneally at 4 mg/kg daily for 4 days on and 10 days off (14-day cycles for the first 2 cycles) plus a 16-day (3rd) cycle (2 days on and 14 days off) (**Table 1**). During the recovery periods, the animals were hydrated with 1 mL of normal saline twice per day for 5 days or more based on animal's weight and health. After the third cycle, hearing was measured by post-treatment ABR. Then the mice were sacrificed and prepared for cytocochleograms as described below.

The animals were divided into four different groups, with $N = 6$ mice per group for group A, B and D and $N = 4$ mice for group C. For all groups, ear treatment was administered 1 day before the second and third cisplatin cycles respectively. Group A mice received 1.8 µL of intra-tympanic saline into their left ears. Group B mice received 1.8 µL of intra-tympanic methylprednisolone (Pharmacia&Upjohn, NJ) at a concentration of 40 mg/ml (close to the clinical dosage used in humans) into their left ears. Group C mice received 1.8 µL of 300 nm diameter magnetic nanoparticles without prednisolone into their left ears. Group D mice received 1.8 µL of 300 nm diameter magnetic nanoparticles that were loaded with prednisolone sodium phosphate at a concentration of 82 µg/mL (the maximum drug loading these particles could carry), also into their left ears. Both unloaded and prednisolone loaded particles were labeled with Texas red fluorescent dye for easy visualization in tissue samples (Chemicell, Berlin, Germany). A 0.5 Tesla magnet (5 × 2.5 × 2.5 cm, K&J Magnetics, PA) was then placed contralateral near the right eye of each animal in group C and group D for 20 min to pull the nanoparticles from the middle ear into the inner ear. For all animals in all groups, the right ears remained as untreated same-animal controls.

Auditory Brainstem Response

The hearing thresholds of the animals in all groups were measured by performing auditory brain stem response (ABR) assays before and after the cisplatin treatment and recovery

TABLE 1 | Animal groups and schedule for our cisplatin and ear treatment study.

	Group A: Saline control	**Group B: Intra-tympanic methyl-prednisolone**	**Group C: Magnetic delivery of nanoparticles without prednisolone**	**Group D: Magnetic delivery of nanoparticles with prednisolone**
Number of animals	***N* = 6**	***N* = 6**	***N* = 4**	***N* = 6**
Day 0	Pre-treatment auditory brainstem response recording			
Day 1–4	4 mg/kg of cisplatin per day	4 mg/kg of cisplatin per day	4 mg/kg of cisplatin per day	4 mg/kg of cisplatin per day
Day 5–14	Recovery period with 2 mL/day of subcutaneous saline injection			
Day 15	Left ear saline injection	Left ear methyl-prednisolone injection	Left ear nanoparticle injection + magnet exposure for 20 min	Left ear nanoparticle injection + magnet exposure for 20 min
Day 16–19	4 mg/kg of cisplatin per day	4 mg/kg of cisplatin per day	4 mg/kg of cisplatin per day	4 mg/kg of cisplatin per day
Day 20–29	Recovery period with 2 mL/day of subcutaneous saline injection			
Day 30	Left ear saline injection	Left ear methyl-prednisolone injection	Left ear nanoparticle injection + magnet exposure for 20 min	Left ear nanoparticle injection + magnet exposure for 20 min
Day 31–32	4 mg/kg of cisplatin per day	4 mg/kg of cisplatin per day	4 mg/kg of cisplatin per day	4 mg/kg of cisplatin per day
Day 33–46	Recovery period with 2 mL/day of subcutaneous saline injection			
Day 47	Post-treatment auditory brainstem response recording			
Day 50	Termination and cochlear preparations			

periods. The mice were anesthetized and placed inside a sound booth (Industrial Acoustics, NY). Two recording electrodes (RLSND110-1.5, Rhythmlink International) were inserted postero-ventral to the auricular area of the left and right ears. A reference electrode was placed at the apex of the head. A ground reference electrode was placed subcutaneously in the lumbar area. Using our ABR recording system (Tucker Davis Technologies, FL), the animals were then presented in free field with 600 sweeps of 5 ms long bursts (shaped with 1 ms onset and offset sinusoidal ramps) at varying intensities beginning at a 94 dB sound pressure level (SPL) and proceeding in 5 dB decrements down to a 14 dB SPL. The electrophysiological signals were recorded for 10 ms. These cycles of sound intensities were repeated for different sound frequencies (8, 16, and 32 kHz). Hearing threshold at each frequency was determined as the lowest intensity at which a definite cochlear response could be identified (waves I & II). **Figure 1B** shows sample traces at 16 KHz for various SPLs and the corresponding hearing threshold. The percentage hearing loss of each animal at a specific frequency was defined as the ratio of the change in thresholds after the treatment compared to pre-treatment thresholds. Hence 0% represents no loss in hearing at that frequency (pre and post hearing thresholds were identical), while 100% represents no measurable response or a measurable response only at the highest sound pressure level of 94 dB.

Cytocochleogram

The cochleas from the different groups were dissected to study the pathophysiology of the cisplatin treatment on the organ of Corti, as well as any effect of the otoprotective treatments. The animals were euthanized using carbon dioxide and the cochleas rapidly isolated. The cochleas were continuously perfused with ice cold 4% paraformaldehyde into the round window membrane and out of a small hole pierced in the apex of the cochlea, and then placed in paraformaldehyde overnight at 4°C. This was followed by 3X wash with 1X PBS at pH 7.4 and decalcification in 0.5 M EDTA for 3–4 days. After washing the cochleas three times using 1X PBS, they were micro-dissected into three turns (Basal, Middle, Apical) using an ophthalmic knife (MANI Ophthalmics, Tochigi, Japan). The tectorial membrane was removed. Cochlear outer and inner hair cell layers were stained using Alexa Fluor 488 Phalloidin (1:800 in 1X PBS + 0.5% Tween, Life Technologies) for 45 min. The turns were mounted on a glass slide using Fluoromount-G with DAPI (Electron Microscopy Sciences). Images of each cochlear turn were taken at 40X magnification using an LSM 710 confocal microscope (Zeiss) in z-stack mode. The outer hair cells in these images were counted for the presence of nuclei and cell membranes over a 200 μm distance of the different cochlear turns using Zen 2010 software (Zeiss) and the assessments were made blind to avoid biases.

RESULTS

In our experiments, the hearing thresholds of the animals in the different groups were determined after the completion of the cisplatin treatment by using ABR assays. The hearing loss experienced by the animal at a particular frequency was determined by the ratio of change in threshold post-treatment to the initial hearing threshold at the same frequency. After systemic cisplatin treatment, this threshold increase is known to occur first at high frequencies, progressing to the lower frequencies as treatment continues, eventually reaching speech frequencies (Rybak et al., 2009; Chirtes and Albu, 2014).

In our study, for untreated (right) ears the hearing loss was greatest at high frequency (at 32 kHz), as compared to at 16 and

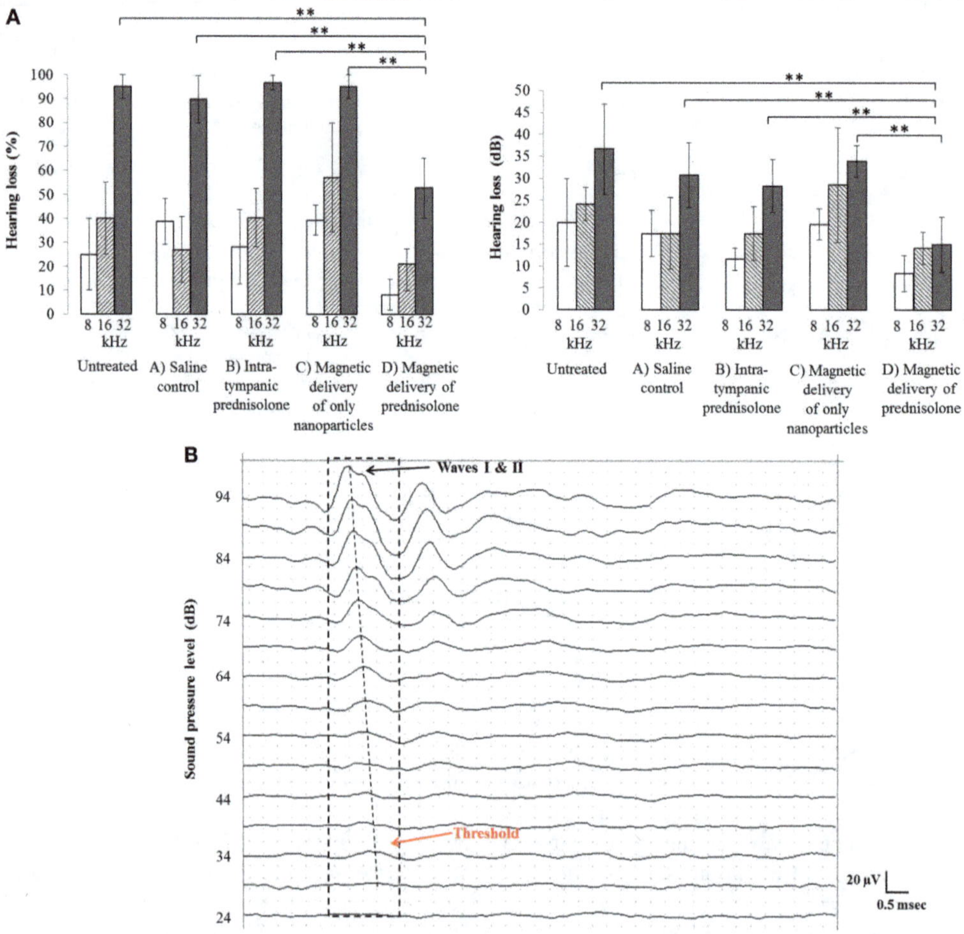

FIGURE 1 | (A) Comparison of hearing loss between the four animal groups for the injected left ears and corresponding untreated right ears. Percent hearing loss at each frequency (Left) and the corresponding hearing loss in dB (Right), per group, are shown. Treated ears that received magnetic nanoparticles showed significantly less hearing loss (group D bars), as compared to the only nanoparticle group (group C bars, $^{**}p < 0.05$), the intra-tympanic methyl-prednisolone group (group B bars, $^{**}p < 0.05$), and the saline control group (group A bars, $^{**}p < 0.05$), especially at the high frequency of 32 KHz. Hearing loss remained similar at high frequency across all groups for untreated ears. **(B)** A sample ABR trace containing the waves I and II (dotted black box) at 16 KHz has been shown, to demonstrate the threshold measurement (note that positive voltage is up, the convention for animal ABRs). The threshold for this animal is at 34 dB beyond which the waves I and II are completely attenuated.

8 kHz (**Figure 1A**). In treated (left) ears at 32 kHz, the magnetic delivery group D ears experienced substantially less hearing loss (53 ± 12%) compared to ears that received saline (group A, 93 ± 7%) or to intra-tympanic methylprednisolone (group B, 97 ± 3%) or to only magnetic nanoparticles (group C, 95 ± 5%). The error bars indicate the standard deviation observed in the measurements. As evident in **Figure 1A** at 32 kHz, the difference in means between group D and the other groups was much larger than the variance within each group. According to a standard t-test, magnetic delivery achieved a statistically significant reduction in high frequency hearing loss for the magnetically treated group D (magnetic delivery of prednisolone) ears, as compared to control group A, B, and C ears which exhibited almost complete hearing loss at high frequencies ($^{**}p < 0.05$). Overall, the prednisolone loaded nanoparticles mitigated cisplatin induced ototoxicity at high frequencies, with 95% statistical significance. At 8 and 16 kHz, magnetic delivery also seemed to reduce the degree of hearing loss, but at these lower frequencies a statistical significance of 95% was not reached, in part because cisplatin caused less hearing loss in mice at these lower frequencies (see the 8 and 16 kHz bars in **Figure 1A**). A greater effect at high frequencies may also be because the drug coated nanoparticles have easier access to the basal layer of the cochlea, which corresponds to high frequencies of hearing.

Cisplatin is known to induce apoptosis in the three rows of outer hair cells starting at the outer row and progressing to the inner row (Kujawa and Liberman, 2006). There have also been reports of damage to the inner hair cells of the organ of Corti, cuticular plate and stria vascularis (Chirtes and Albu, 2014). These ototoxic effects have been consistently shown to progress from the basal, high frequency region of the cochlea to the apical, low frequency region with continuing cisplatin treatment. We extracted cytocochleograms to evaluate the effect of magnetic delivery in protecting hair cells. The cochleas were micro-dissected post-treatment and the organ of Corti examined in the different turns after staining the hair cells. Sample cytocochleograms are shown for the basal cochlear region (from the window membrane to the distal end of the cochlea) in **Figure 2**. Hair cell preservation is evident in the magnetically treated cochlea (**Figure 2D**) compared to groups that received intra-tympanic saline or methyl prednisolone injections. Magnetically delivered nanoparticles can be seen among the hair cells in the cochlea (red fluorescence in **Figure 2D**).

The number of outer hair cells in each cochlear micro-sections was counted and compared between the cochleas receiving magnetic treatment, receiving intra-tympanic saline, and receiving methyl-prednisolone injections. The outer hair cell density observed for control animals (no cisplatin and no ear treatments) vs. from ears of animals that received cisplatin plus one of the three types of ear treatments (saline, intra-tympanic methylprednisolone, or magnetic delivery of prednisolone) is shown in **Table 2**. A significant decrease in hair cells was observed for the saline ears (72% decrease) and intra-tympanic methyl prednisolone ears (33% decrease). In contrast, cochleas from treated ears in the magnetic delivery group displayed a small loss of 9% of hair cells in the basal region compared to control (no cisplatin) animals. This indicates that in the magnetic delivery of prednisolone

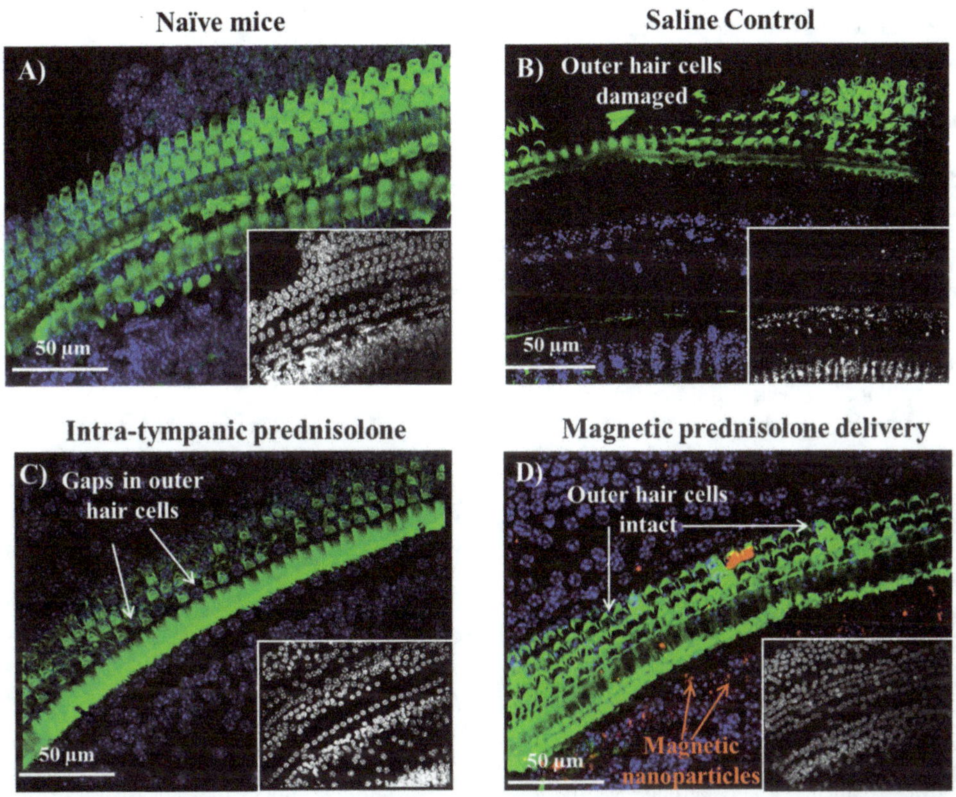

FIGURE 2 | Sample cytocochleograms of the basal cochlear region of different groups. The outer hair cells were stained for actin with Alexa Fluor 488 Phalloidin (green) and the various cell nuclei were stained using DAPI counterstain (blue). **(A)** Left ear from a naïve animal that did not receive any cisplatin treatment or otoprotection. For animals that were administered cisplatin: **(B)** Left ear that received saline; **(C)** Left ear that received intra-tympanic methyl-prednisolone; and **(D)** Left ear that received magnetic delivery of prednisolone. The images of the DAPI stained nuclei for all the groups have been shown in the image insets of **(A–D)** correspondingly. (A version of this figure has also appeared in an invited feature article in The Hearing Journal, July 2017 issue.)

TABLE 2 | Comparison of outer hair cell density for cochleas in naïve mice ($N = 6$), vs. in mice that received the three ear treatment types (also $N = 6$ for each group). The second row lists the percent decrease in hair cell density compared to the no cisplatin naïve group. In the magnetically treated group D, hair cell density decreased by just 9% compared to substantially greater hair loss in the other groups.

	Naïve mice: no cisplatin or ear treatment	Treated ears : cisplatin + intra-tympanic saline	Treated ears: cisplatin + intra-tympanic methyl prednisolone	Treated ears: cisplatin + magnetic delivery of prednisolone	Untreated ears: cisplatin, but no ear treatment
Outer hair cell density (number per 200 µm)	75 ± 2	21 ± 5	50 ± 7	68 ± 4	26 ± 9
% decrease in hair cell density	N/A	72%	33%	9%	65%

group, the outer hair cells in the basal cochlear region were preserved.

DISCUSSION

The benefit of magnetic delivery is that it actively and directly transports drug into the cochlea, in contrast to intra-tympanic administration where drug diffuses passively into the cochlea from the middle ear. Although it was not possible to measure the amount of steroid delivered into mouse cochleas in this study (the mouse perilymph sample volume was too small to enable mass spectrometry measurement of prednisolone concentrations), in initial adult human cadaver studies we have observed significantly greater delivery of steroid to the cochlea with magnetic delivery as compared to intra-tympanic administration without magnetic fields and particles. Improved delivery to the cochlea, and also to the vestibular system, is of interest not only for protection of hearing from chemotherapy, but also for other conditions of the inner ear such as sudden and noise-induced hearing loss, for presbycusis, for tinnitus, and for Ménière's disease. This study achieved efficacy by delivering prednisolone, a generic off-the-shelf steroid. However, magnetic nanoparticles can be loaded with many other therapies. Magnetic delivery of new and emerging therapies (novel compounds, growth factors, gene therapy) is anticipated to yield even greater benefits than delivery of a generic drug. Conversely, even the best new drug or therapy will not be effective if it does not reach the cochlea in sufficient quantities to be therapeutic.

The cisplatin regimens that were administered to the animals caused hearing loss primarily at high frequencies. In human patients also, hearing loss due to cisplatin is known to occur first at higher frequencies and then to progress to lower frequencies as treatment continues (Rybak et al., 2009; Chirtes and Albu, 2014). Magnetic delivery of prednisolone acted primarily to protect this high frequency hearing, as evident in the right panel of **Figure 1A** where the 32 kHz hearing loss for untreated ears and group A-C ears was reduced in group D ears. Greater protection at high frequency may be due both to the fact that there was more hearing to be saved at higher than at lower frequencies, and perhaps also because particles are delivered through the window membranes first to the base of the cochlea (which is where high frequency hearing resides). Intra-tympanic prednisolone treatment without magnetic particles did decrease cochlear outer hair cell loss (**Figure 2C**), but high frequency hearing was still lost in this group (**Figure 1**, group B). Such a mismatch between outer hair cell loss and hearing loss has been observed previously in the literature (Kujawa and Liberman, 2006) and may be due to other factors such as damage to spiral ganglion neurons or stria vascularis cells.

CONCLUSIONS

Cisplatin administration is known to be ototoxic, likely by the production of reactive oxygen species in the inner ear and by depletion of the inherent antioxidant system of the cochlea, leading to apoptosis of hair cells in the organ of Corti, spiral ganglion cells, and marginal cells of the stria vascularis (Boulikas and Vougiouka, 2003; Chirtes and Albu, 2014). Steroids such as dexamethasone and prednisolone are thought to reduce the production of free radicals in the inner ear and decrease the formation of inflammatory molecules and could protect hearing from cisplatin (Marshak et al., 2014; Okano, 2014; Özel et al., 2016). However, prolonged systemic administration of steroids may reduce the anti-cancer efficacy of cisplatin and is also undesirable due to added toxicity (Wooldridge et al., 2001; Herr et al., 2003; Zhang et al., 2006; Fardet and Fève, 2014; Morin and Fardet, 2015; Ranganath et al., 2015), which has led to studies on local intra-tympanic administration of steroids to protect hearing (Herr et al., 2003). Compared to intra-tympanic administration, magnetic forces can better deliver therapy directly to the cochlea and can confer a stronger therapeutic effect. In this animal study we observed that magnetic delivery of steroid protected hair cells more effectively and concomitantly reduced the degree of cisplatin-induced hearing loss; as compared to no treatment, to intra-tympanic steroid administration, and to magnetic delivery of nanoparticles without attached steroid.

AUTHOR CONTRIBUTIONS

All authors contributed to the research presented in this article. BR conducted the experiments. SR provided guidance on the cisplatin ototoxicity animal model. AA provided guidance for clinical needs. BS and DD provided guidance on design of experiments and the magnetic delivery system. All authors contributed to writing the article.

ACKNOWLEDGMENTS

We thank Dr. Lisa Cunningham for generous guidance in setting up the mouse model of cisplatin ototoxicity. We also thank Ms. Amy Beavan (University of Maryland Imaging core) for the access to the confocal microscopy facility. Funding is gratefully acknowledged from Action on Hearing Loss in the UK, from the Congressionally Directed Medical Research Program (CDMRP), from the National Institutes of Health (NIH), from the Maryland Innovation Initiative at the Maryland Technology Development Corporation (TEDCO) and the Maryland Industrial Partnerships (MIPS) program in the State of Maryland, as well as from the Sheikh Zayed Institute for Pediatric Surgical Innovation, Children's National Medical Center, in Washington DC.

REFERENCES

Allen, G. C., Tiu, C., Koike, K., Ritchey, A. K., Kurs-Lasky, M., and Wax, M. K. (1998). Transient-Evoked Otoacoustic Emissions in Children after Cisplatin Chemotherapy. *Otolaryngol. Head Neck Surg.* 118, 584–588.

Bird, P. A., Begg, E. J., Zhang, M., Keast, A. T., Murray, D. P., and Balkany, T. J. (2007). Intratympanic versus intravenous delivery of methylprednisolone to cochlear perilymph. *Otol. Neurotol.* 28, 1124–1130. doi: 10.1097/MAO.0b013e31815aee21

Boulikas, T., and Vougiouka, M. (2003). Cisplatin and platinum drugs at the molecular level (Review). *Oncol. Rep.* 10, 1663–1682. doi: 10.3892/or.10.6.1663

Chirtes, F., and Albu, S. (2014). Prevention and restoration of hearing loss associated with the use of cisplatin. *BioMed. Res. Int.* 2014:925485. doi: 10.1155/2014/925485

DeWoskin, R. S., and Riviere, J. E. (1992). Cisplatin-induced loss of kidney copper and nephrotoxicity is ameliorated by single dose diethyldithiocarbamate, but not mesna. *Toxicol. Appl. Pharmacol.* 112, 182–189. doi: 10.1016/0041-008X(92)90186-V

Fardet, L., and Fève, B. (2014). Systemic glucocorticoid therapy: a review of its metabolic and cardiovascular adverse events. *Drugs* 74, 1731–1745. doi: 10.1007/s40265-014-0282-9

Gregg, R. W., Molepo, J. M., Monpetit, V. J., Mikael, N. Z., Redmond, D., Gadia, M., et al. (1992). Cisplatin neurotoxicity: the relationship between dosage, time, and platinum concentration in neurologic tissues, and morphologic evidence of toxicity. *J Clin Oncol Off J Am Soc Clin Oncol.* 10, 795–803. doi: 10.1200/JCO.1992.10.5.795

Herr, I., Ucur, E., Herzer, K., Okouoyo, S., Ridder, R., Krammer, P. H., et al. (2003). Glucocorticoid cotreatment induces apoptosis resistance toward cancer therapy in carcinomas. *Cancer Res.* 63, 3112–3120.

Himeno, C., Komeda, M., Izumikawa, M., Takemura, K., Yagi, M., Weiping, Y., et al. (2002). Intra-cochlear administration of dexamethasone attenuates aminoglycoside ototoxicity in the guinea pig. *Hear Res.* 167, 61–70. doi: 10.1016/S0378-5955(02)00345-3

Kujawa, S. G., and Liberman, M. C. (2006). Acceleration of age-related hearing loss by early noise exposure: evidence of a misspent youth. *J. Neurosci.* 26, 2115–2123. doi: 10.1523/JNEUROSCI.4985-05.2006

Lee, J. E., Nakagawa, T., Kita, T., Kim, T. S., Iguchi, F., Endo, T., et al. (2004). Mechanisms of apoptosis induced by cisplatin in marginal cells in mouse stria vascularis. *ORL J. Otorhinolaryngol. Relat. Spec.* 66, 111–118. doi: 10.1159/000079329

Marshak, T., Steiner, M., Kaminer, M., Levy, L., and Shupak, A. (2014). Prevention of Cisplatin-induced hearing loss by intratympanic dexamethasone: a randomized controlled study. *Otolaryngol. Head Neck Surg.* 150, 983–990. doi: 10.1177/0194599814524894

Miller, R. P., Tadagavadi, R. K., Ramesh, G., and Reeves, W. B. (2010). Mechanisms of cisplatin nephrotoxicity. *Toxins* 2, 2490–2518. doi: 10.3390/toxins21 12490

Monzack, E. L., May, L. A., Roy, S., Gale, J. E., and Cunningham, L. L. (2015). Live imaging the phagocytic activity of inner ear supporting cells in response to hair cell death. *Cell Death Differ.* 22, 1995–2005. doi: 10.1038/cdd.2015.48

Morin, C., and Fardet, L. (2015). Systemic glucocorticoid therapy: risk factors for reported adverse events and beliefs about the drug. A cross-sectional online survey of 820 patients. *Clin. Rheumatol.* 34, 2119–2126. doi: 10.1007/s10067-015-2953-7

Okano, T. (2014). Immune system of the inner ear as a novel therapeutic target for sensorineural hearing loss. *Front. Pharmacol.* 5:205. doi: 10.3389/fphar.2014.00205

Özel, H. E., Özdogan, F., Gürgen, S. G., Esen, E., Genç, S., and Selçuk, A. (2016). Comparison of the protective effects of intratympanic dexamethasone and methylprednisolone against cisplatin-induced ototoxicity. *J. Laryngol. Otol.* 130, 225–234. doi: 10.1017/S0022215115003473

Rademaker-Lakhai, J. M., Crul, M., Zuur, L., Baas, P., Beijnen, J. H., Simis, Y. J. W., et al. (2006). Relationship between cisplatin administration and the development of ototoxicity. *J. Clin. Oncol.* 24, 918–924. doi: 10.1200/JCO.2006.10.077

Ranganath, P., Einhorn, L., Albany, C., Ranganath, P., Einhorn, L., and Albany, C. (2015). Management of chemotherapy induced Nausea and vomiting in patients on multiday cisplatin based combination chemotherapy. *BioMed. Res. Int.* 2015:e943618. doi: 10.1155/2015/943618

Roy, S., Ryals, M. M., Van den Bruele, A. B., Fitzgerald, T. S., and Cunningham, L. L. (2013). Sound preconditioning therapy inhibits ototoxic hearing loss in mice. *J. Clin. Invest.* 123, 4945–4949. doi: 10.1172/JCI71353

Rybak, L. P., Mukherjea, D., Jajoo, S., and Ramkumar, V. (2009). Cisplatin ototoxicity and protection: clinical and experimental studies. *Tohoku J. Exp. Med.* 219, 177–186. doi: 10.1620/tjem.219.177

Salt, A. N., and Plontke, S. K. (2009). Principles of Local Drug Delivery to the Inner Ear. *Audiol. Neurotol.* 14, 350–360. doi: 10.1159/000241892

Shapiro, B., Depireux, D. A., Sarwar, A., Nacev, A., Preciado, D., and Hausfeld, J. (2014a). *Pre-Clinical Development of Magnetic Delivery of Therapy to Middle and Inner Ears, 23rd Edn, Vol. 23.* ENT & Audiology News.

Shapiro, B., Kulkarni, S., Nacev, A., Sarwar, A., Preciado, D., and Depireux, D. A. (2014b). Shaping magnetic fields to direct therapy to ears and eyes. *Annu Rev Biomed Eng.* 16, 455–481. doi: 10.1146/annurev-bioeng-071813-105206

Wooldridge, J. E., Anderson, C. M., and Perry, M. C. (2001). Corticosteroids in advanced cancer. *Oncol (Williston Park)* 15, 225–234; discussion 234–236.

Zhang, C., Beckermann, B., Kallifatidis, G., Liu, Z., Rittgen, W., Edler, L., et al. (2006). Corticosteroids induce chemotherapy resistance in the majority of tumour cells from bone, brain, breast, cervix, melanoma and neuroblastoma. *Int. J. Oncol.* 29, 1295–1301. doi: 10.3892/ijo.29.5.1295

8

An Antioxidant Screen Identifies Candidates for Protection of Cochlear Hair Cells from Gentamicin Toxicity

Volker Noack[1], *Kwang Pak*[1,2], *Rahul Jalota*[1], *Arwa Kurabi*[1] *and Allen F. Ryan*[1,2]*

[1] *Department of Surgery and Otolaryngology, School of Medicine, University of California, San Diego, La Jolla, CA, United States,* [2] *VA San Diego Healthcare System, San Diego, CA, United States*

Edited by:
Peter S. Steyger, Oregon Health and Science University, United States

Reviewed by:
Su-Hua Sha, Medical University of South Carolina, United States
Debashree Mukherjea, Southern Illinois University School of Medicine, United States

***Correspondence:**
Allen F. Ryan
afryan@ucsd.edu

Reactive oxygen species are important elements in ototoxic damage to hair cells (HCs), appearing early in the damage process. Higher levels of natural antioxidants are positively correlated with resistance to ototoxins and many studies have shown that exogenous antioxidants can protect HCs from damage. While a very wide variety of antioxidants with different characteristics and intracellular targets exist, most ototoxicity studies have focused upon one or a few well-characterized compounds. Relatively little research has attempted to determine the comparative efficacy of large variety of different antioxidants. This has been in part due to the lack of translation between cell culture and *in vivo* measures of efficacy. To circumvent this limitation, we used an *in vitro* assay based on micro-explants from the basal and middle turns of the neonatal mouse organ of Corti to screen a commercial redox library of diverse antioxidant compounds for their ability to protect mammalian HCs from a high dose of the ototoxic antibiotic gentamicin. The library included several antioxidants that have previously been studied as potential treatments for HC damage, as well as many antioxidants that have never been applied to ototoxicity. The micro-explants were treated with 200 μM gentamicin alone, gentamicin plus one of three dosages of a redox compound, the highest dosage of compound alone, or were untreated. HC counts were determined before the gentamicin insult and at 1, 2, and 3 days afterward to evaluate the HC survival. From a total of 81 antioxidant compounds, 13 exhibited significant protection of HCs. These included members of a variety of antioxidant classes with several novel antioxidants, not previously tested on HCs, appearing to alleviate the damaging gentamicin effect. Some compounds previously shown to be protective of HCs were correspondingly protective in this *in vitro* screen, while others were not. Finally, one of the three pro-oxidant compounds included in the library as well as six antioxidants exhibited evidence of toxicity in the absence of gentamicin. The results demonstrate the wide variability in the ability of antioxidants to protect HCs from high-dose gentamicin damage, and identify promising candidate leads for further study as potential drug targets.

Highlights

- A medium-throughput assay based on micro-explants of the organ of Corti was developed to screen mammalian cochlear hair cells for protection from damage by ototoxins.
- Eighty one antioxidants and 3 pro-oxidants were evaluated for hair cell protection from high-dose gentamicin.
- Thirteen antioxidants were significantly protective, while 6 proved to be damaging.
- The use of a common assay permitted an evaluation of the relative capacity of different antioxidants for the protection of hair cells.

Keywords: inner ear, sensory cell, redox, ototoxicity, damage prevention, hair cell, screen

INTRODUCTION

Ototoxicity, hearing loss and vestibular disorders are significant side effects of a number of valuable medications. This includes important categories of drugs used to treat life-threatening illnesses, such as aminoglycoside antibiotics and platinum-based anti-neoplastic agents. Hearing loss due to aminoglycosides is estimated to occur in almost 50% of patients (Fausti et al., 1992), while the incidence of hearing loss following cisplatin or carboplatin treatment can be as high as 75–100% (McKeage, 1995; Rybak et al., 2009). The potential for ototoxicity can limit the use of these drugs. If their use is unavoidable, it can result in hearing loss up to and including complete deafness. Vestibular disorders are also a common side effect (Schacht et al., 2012).

The most vulnerable elements of the inner ear to ototoxic drugs are the sensory HCs (Wong and Ryan, 2015). The cellular mechanisms that underlie HC damage are incompletely understood. However, there is extensive evidence that ototoxins induce the formation of ROS as an early step in the damage course. ROS formation precedes visible damage to the cell by up to 24 h (h) (Choung et al., 2009), consistent with an early role. The antioxidant glutathione increases in HCs from the base to the apex of the cochlea (Sha et al., 2001a), while sensitivity to ototoxins decreases from base to apex (e.g., Ryan and Dallos, 1975). In animals, treatment with antioxidants or the upregulation of antioxidant genes has been convincingly shown to delay or prevent ototoxin-induced HC loss (e.g., Garetz et al., 1994a,b; Rybak et al., 1999; Sha et al., 2001b).

This success in animal experiments has led to a limited number of clinical trials that have evaluated the effects of antioxidant treatment on ototoxic or noise-induced HC and hearing loss. Kocyigit et al. (2015) reported that NAC provided a degree of protection against amikacin ototoxicity at the highest frequencies tested. A trial of NAC in military trainees undergoing firearms training also showed some degree of protection (Lindblad et al., 2011). In contrast, a recent trial of NAC versus placebo treatment prior to stapedectomy, where drilling noise and surgical trauma can produce sensorineural hearing loss, showed an equivalent level of hearing loss (~10 dB) in both groups, and thus was unable to demonstrate a protective effect (Bagger-Sjöbäck et al., 2015). Kramer et al. (2006) found no effect of NAC on temporary threshold shift induced by loud music.

The reasons for the variability in clinical trial results are unclear. However, the degree of experimental control in clinical trials is much less than that in animal studies. Another possibility is that the antioxidant dose actually reaching the cochlea after systemic administration may be non-optimal. Moreover, different antioxidants can exert their effects via several distinct mechanisms and targets. This includes scavenging the radical species that initiate peroxidation, quenching singlet oxygen, chelating metals, breaking free radical chain reactions, reducing the concentration of O_2, preventing oxidation of proteins or DNA, and/or stimulating endogenous antioxidant enzymes (Lü et al., 2010). Because antioxidants may employ one or more of several mechanisms, differences in their effectiveness may vary with differences in the cellular processes involved.

It should also be noted that while many antioxidants have been tested for their ability to protect HCs, there are many other compounds with antioxidant properties. Moreover, few studies have compared HC protection by antioxidants in a standardized model, so that relative effectiveness can be estimated. For the reasons noted above, differences in their potential for HC protection seem likely. Hence, a comparative screen of a large number of antioxidants using a standardized model of HC damage could identify novel antioxidants with protective properties and might also provide evidence regarding differences in protective efficacy.

To address these issues, we screened a commercial library of antioxidants in a single model of aminoglycoside-induced HC damage. Micro-explants from the neonatal murine oC were exposed to a high dose of the ototoxic aminoglycoside gentamicin to elicit oxidative stress. We used a transgenic mouse line in which HCs express GFP under the control of a HC-specific promoter (Masuda et al., 2011). This allowed for visualization of HC loss over the course of gentamicin treatment in culture. HC loss was compared between micro-explants without any treatment, with gentamicin treatment alone, or with gentamicin and antioxidant co-treatment. This allowed us to determine the relative efficacy of the 81 different antioxidants and 3 pro-oxidants to influence HC viability.

Abbreviations: BHA, butylated hydroxyanisole; BHT, butylated hydroxytoluene; DTT, dithiotreitol; GFP, green florescent protein; HCs, hair cells; NAC, *N*-acetyl cysteine; NFκB, nuclear factor kappa B; oC, organ of Corti; OH, hydroxyl; ROS, reactive oxygen species.

MATERIALS AND METHODS

Animals

Experiments were performed on transgenic animals in which eGFP was selectively expressed in HCs under the control of a *pou4f3* promoter construct (Masuda et al., 2011). All experiments were performed to National Institutes of Health guidelines and approved by the Institutional Animal Care and Use Committee of the VA San Diego Medical Center.

Micro-Explant Preparation

The oC was dissected from the cochleas of postnatal day 3–5 *pou4f3*/eGFP mouse pups. The apical region of each epithelium, which is relatively insensitive to aminoglycoside toxicity, was discarded. The basal and middle regions of the epithelium were divided using a diamond scalpel into micro-explants consisting of approximately 20 inner HCs and the 60 associated outer HCs. Micro-explants were individually plated in each well of a flat-bottom 96 well plates in media consisting of DMEM F-12 (Gibco) plus 30 U/ml Penicillin and 5% FBS, maintained in a humidified tissue culture incubator (37°C, 5% CO_2).

Redox Library Screening

Screening was performed using the Screen-Well Redox Library (BML-2835, Enzo Life Sciences, Farmingdale, NY, United States). The library consists of 81 antioxidant and 3 pro-oxidant compounds. The library represents a variety of classes of compounds, including some that have been shown previously to protect HCs from damage. This includes glutathione (Garetz et al., 1994a), α-lipoic acid (Rybak et al., 1999), α-tocopherol (Fetoni et al., 2003), D-methionine and ebselen (Kopke et al., 1997). Many pharmacological compounds that had not been previously applied to HC protection were also present, providing the opportunity to identify new protective compounds discovery and repurposing. The compounds present in the library are listed in Supplementary Table 1. Test compounds were initially dissolved in DMSO and diluted in culture media with the total amount of DMSO adjusted to a final concentration of 0.1%.

Each experimental oC micro-explant was pretreated for 24 h with one of the library compounds at concentration of 10, 100, or 1000 μM, performed in triplicate wells. The next day, the media were withdrawn, fresh media containing 200 μM gentamicin plus the pharmacological compound with the appropriate concentration was added, and the micro-explants were cultured for 72 h. Untreated (negative) controls were maintained in media alone and positive controls were treated with 200 μM gentamicin alone. Media for both control groups contained 0.1% DMSO, to match the experimental groups. Compounds were screened in duplicated 96-well plates with seven compounds per plate, plus controls. The size of the testing plates and performance of experiments on different days and with different media or gentamicin batches required replication of both control conditions on each plate, for comparison with the results from the compounds evaluated on that plate.

Green florescent protein-positive HCs were imaged by fluorescence microcopy on each day of treatment, and survival curves were generated for each compound and condition. HC counts, including both inner and outer HCs, were evaluated in ImageJ, and normalized as percentages to the number of HCs present on D1, prior to the start of gentamicin treatment. Any micro-explants that did not attach and flatten in the well by D1 were excluded (usually less than 3% per plate), because HC counts could not be accurately quantified at that time. There were sufficient wells on each plate that three micro-explants per condition could almost always be accommodated even with some unattached samples.

Statistical Analysis

Statistical analysis was performed using GraphPad Prism 6, StatView 5, using the Kruskal–Wallis non-parametric ANOVA to detect treatment effects. Individual condition comparisons were performed using the Mann–Whitney *U* test, with correction for multiple comparisons. For purposes of the figures, standard deviations were calculated from the non-normalized HC counts.

Validation

Redox compound "hits" were identified in the initial round of screening as deviating significantly from the controls. Following this initial identification, repeat plates were prepared in an identical manner for all hits, for a total N of 6 micro-explants. Statistical analysis was then repeated. Hits that demonstrated a repeatable effect in the following round were considered to be confirmed.

RESULTS

Control Micro-Explants and Gentamicin Cytotoxicity

Imaging of GFP-positive HCs in control wells typically showed HC survival similar to that illustrated in **Figure 1**. Untreated (negative control) micro-explants maintained only in culture media showed near-complete HC survival from D1-D3, with some HC loss on D4. In contrast, HCs treated with 200 μM gentamicin (positive control) showed significant losses by D1, and severe losses by D2 and D3. HC counts from negative and positive control micro-explants in each plate were generated, converted to percent survival relative to Day 1 (D1, just prior to gentamicin exposure), and averaged across all plates. The results are illustrated in **Figure 2**. Negative controls showed high levels of HC survival on both D2 (96%) and D3 (93%). By D4, negative control micro-explants showed somewhat reduced HC survival (71%). Positive control micro-explants showed significantly reduced survival on D2, after 24 h exposure to gentamicin (53%), and significantly lower survival on D3 after 48 h gentamicin exposure (14%). D4 gentamicin showed continued loss of GFP-positive cells (8%). As expected, Kruskal–Wallis non-parametric ANOVA and Mann–Whitney *post hoc* tests showed a highly significant difference between negative and positive controls from D2–D4 ($p < 0.0001$). It should be noted that variation in controls was noted, as can been seen in later figures. In particular, some negative controls showed HC loss on D3 greater than the average

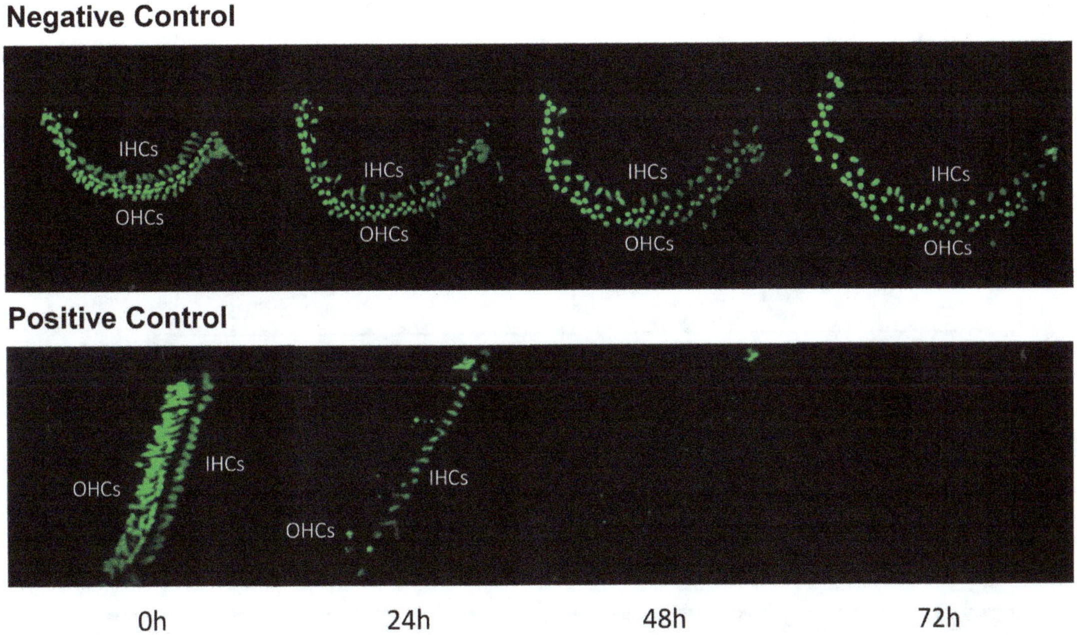

FIGURE 1 | Control cultures. Montage of a typical negative control oC micro-explant **(top)** and a 200 μM gentamicin-treated positive-control micro-explant **(bottom)**, illustrating GFP-positive HCs from D1 (just prior to addition of gentamicin to the positive controls) to D4. In the negative control, there is modest loss of HCs, primarily on D3 and D4. In the positive control, HC loss is significant by D2 and near-total on D3 and D4.

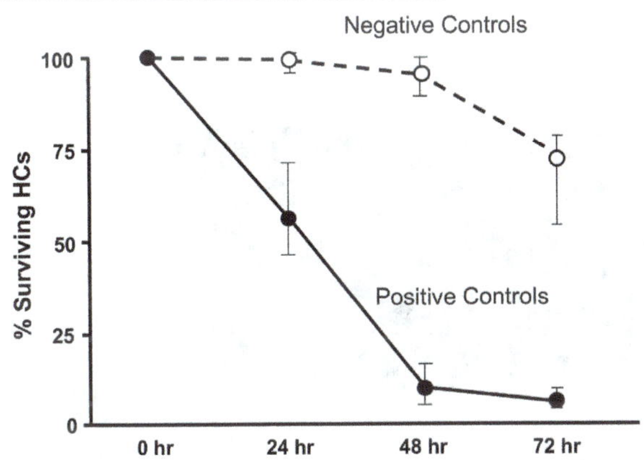

FIGURE 2 | Control culture cell counts. All of the positive and negative control oC micro-explants from all plates were counted and the results pooled to illustrate the control survival curves between D1 and D4. Data points represent medians, and error bars present the interquartile range.

range, while some positive controls showed HC loss on D1 that was less than the average range. This is reflected in the greater variation shown in **Figure 2** for those time points. However, data were always compared statistically to positive controls from the same plate, which were generated with the same batches of media and gentamicin.

Library Results

Of the 81 antioxidants and 3 pro-oxidants in the redox library, 68 antioxidants and 2 pro-oxidants had no effect on either untreated or gentamicin-treated micro-explants. Two examples of antioxidants with no effect are illustrated in **Figures 3, 4.** Micro-explants treated with the highest concentration of each antioxidant (1000 μM) exhibited HC counts very similar to that seen for negative control micro-explants cultured in media alone. Micro-explants treated with three concentrations of each antioxidant plus 200 μM gentamicin showed HC counts that were similar to that observed with gentamicin alone.

Thirteen antioxidants exhibited statistically significant protection of HCs in micro-explants treated with both the compound and gentamicin. The results for these compounds are illustrated in **Figure 5**, arranged in order of degree of HC protection. Seratrodast and idebenone exhibited the strongest protection from gentamicin toxicity, which was complete at 1000 μM, the highest dosage tested, and, also, significant at 100 μM. However, idebenone alone appeared to reduce HC survival on D4. Resveretrol, BHA, α-lipoic acid, hinokitiol, BHT, dithiotreitol and MC-186 were strongly protective at some gentamicin exposure times and antioxidant dose concentrations. However, at the highest concentration tested, MC-186 significantly enhanced early HC loss due to gentamicin. Procysteine and trolox were more modestly protective at some times and concentrations, while thiourea and thymoquinone were protective only at 24 h, and only for the lowest antioxidant concentrations. Examples of two micro-explants that were protected by antioxidants are presented in **Figure 6.**

The pro-oxidant β-lapachone and the antioxidants disuliram, ferulic acid ethylester, gossypol, gentisisc acid and caffeic acid were significantly toxic to HCs in the absence of gentamicin, although none significantly worsened gentamicin-induced HC

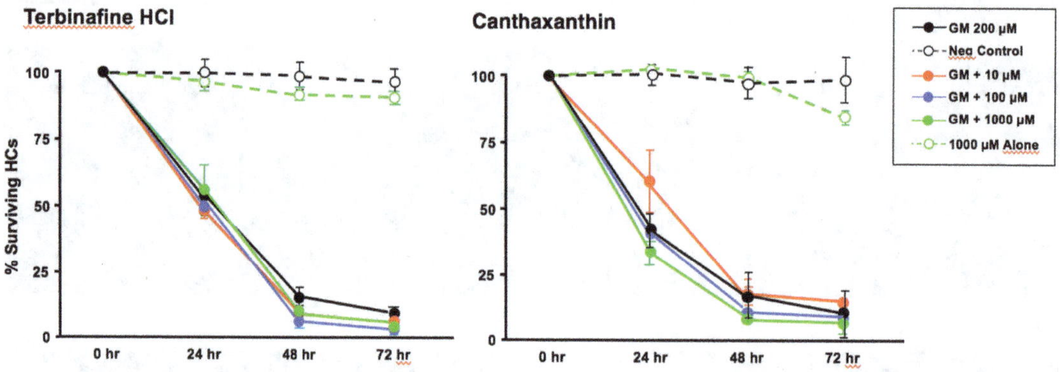

FIGURE 3 | Normalized D1-4 HC survival curves for two antioxidants (canthatraxin and terbinafine HCl) that had no significant effect on normal or gentamicin-treated micro-explants. HC survival with 1000 μM of the compound alone (open green circles) was not significantly different from an untreated, negative control micro-explant (open black circles). Treatment with the compound at 10 μM (solid red circles), 100 μM (solid blue) or 1000 μM (solid green) plus 200 μM gentamicin was not significantly different from 200 μM gentamicin alone (solid black). *N* = 6 micro-explants per data point.

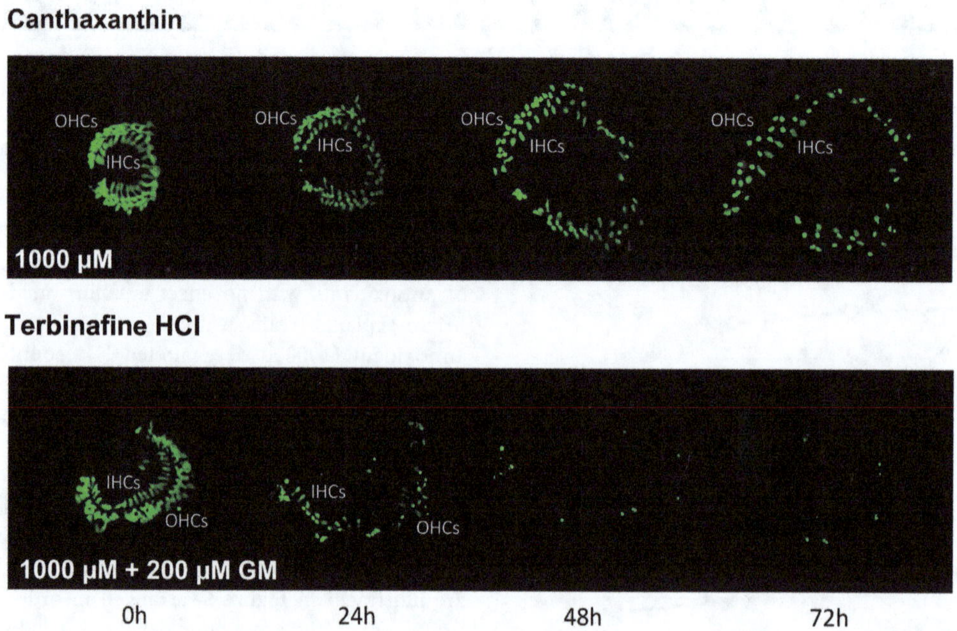

FIGURE 4 | Montages illustrating representative oC micro-explants treated with 1000 μM canthatraxin alone, or 100 μM terbinafine HCl plus 200 μM gentamicin, for 72 h.

damage. HC survival curves for the pro-oxidant and two damaging antioxidants are presented in **Figure 7**. Image montages demonstrating the HC toxicity after treatment with lapachone alone, or ferulic acid ethylester alone, for 72 h, is seen in **Figure 8**.

DISCUSSION

Summary

We have developed an assay based on micro-explants of the neonatal mouse oC to screen a variety of antioxidants for their ability to alter aminoglycoside damage to mammalian cochlear HCs *in vitro*. All significantly positive "hits" were confirmed by re-screening. This resulted in the identification of 13 out of 81 antioxidants that offered significant protection against gentamicin-induced HC damage. In addition, we identified several antioxidants that showed evidence of toxicity in our assay, even in the absence of gentamicin. Some of the protective antioxidants identified in the screen have been studied previously and a protective role identified *in vitro* or *in vivo*. The HC protective role of others is identified here for the first time. The screen also provides comparative information on the protective capacity of antioxidants, under the conditions tested, with some antioxidants offering significant superior protection.

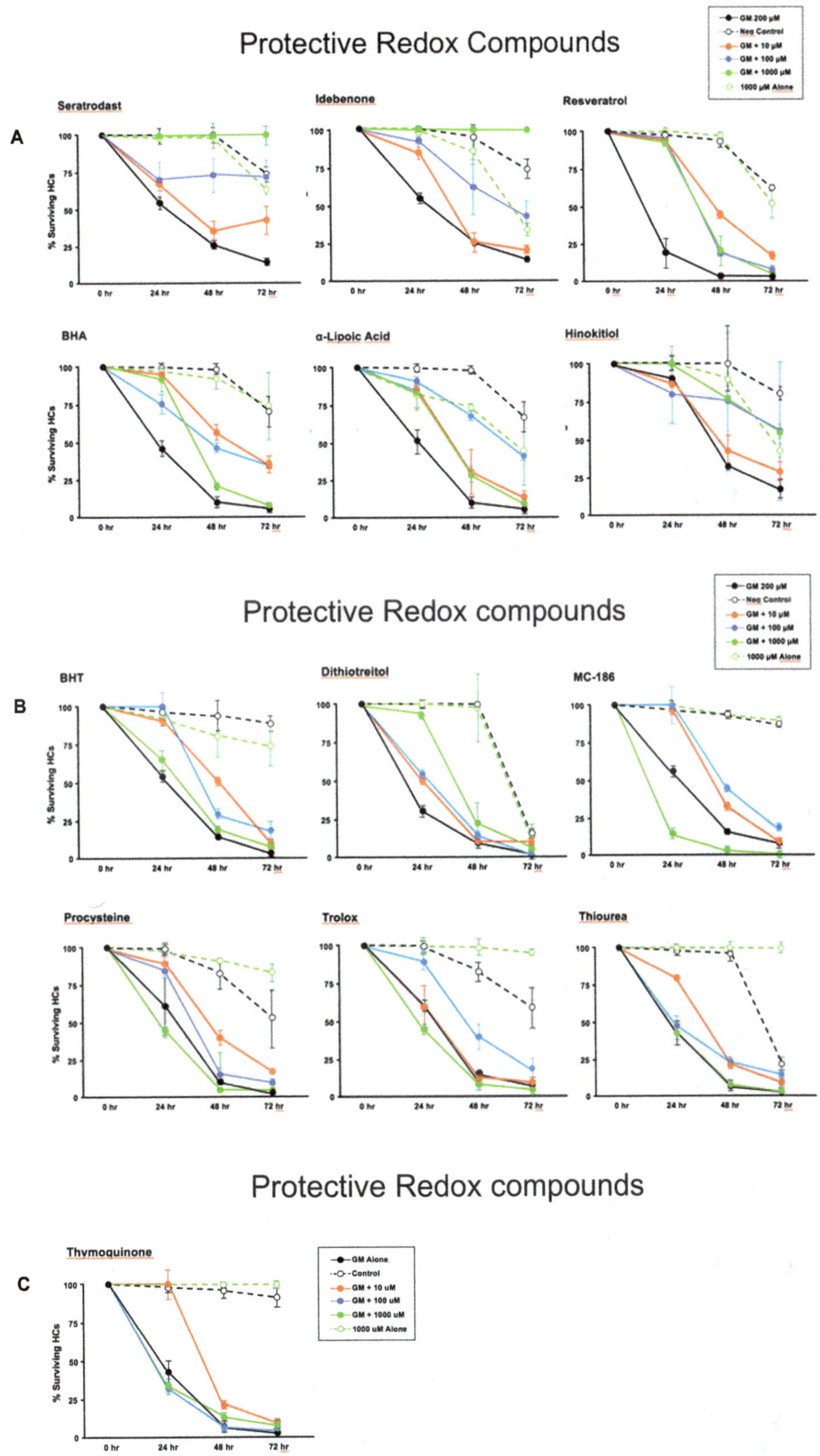

FIGURE 5 | (A–C) Normalized D1–4 HC survival curves for 13 compounds that showed significant protection from gentamicin. The data also illustrate the variability seen in positive in negative controls. This variability necessitated the use of separate controls for each plate in our assay. $N = 6$ micro-explants/data point.

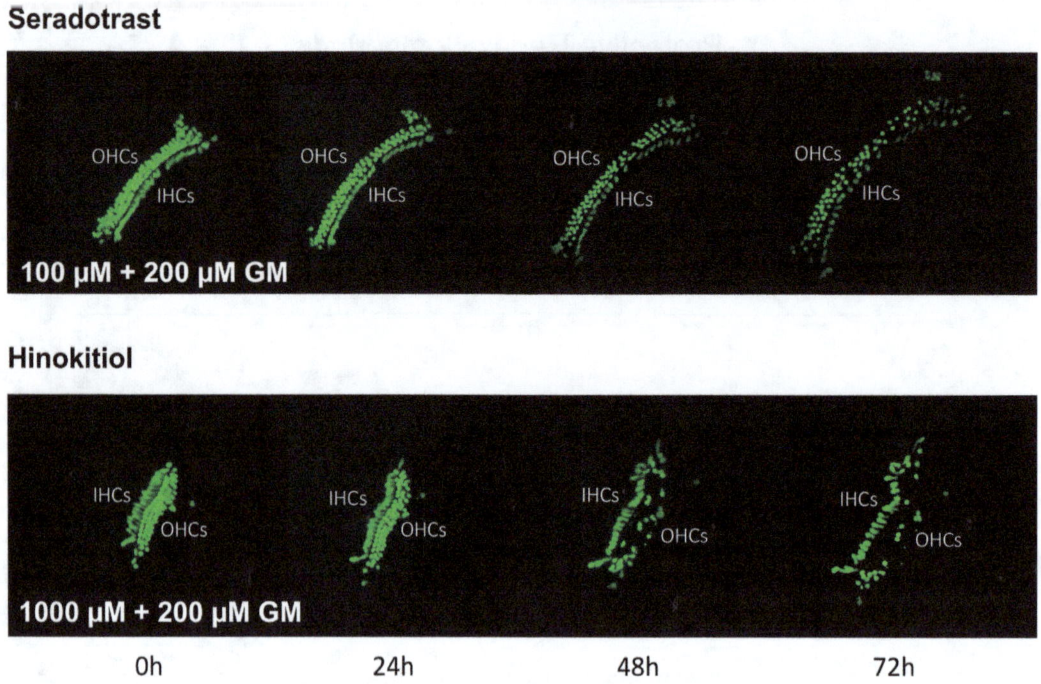

FIGURE 6 | Montages illustrating representative micro-explants treated with 100 μM seratrodast plus 200 μM gentamicin or 1000 μM hinokitiol plus 200 μM gentamicin, for 72 h.

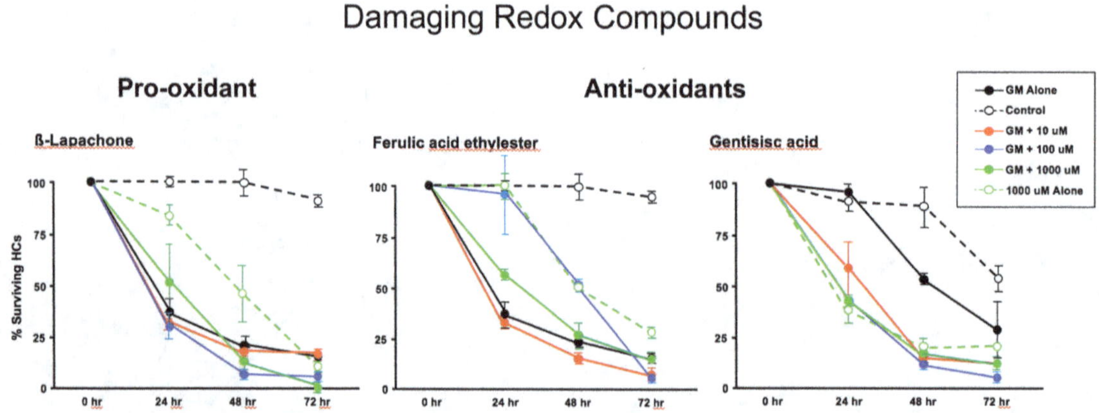

FIGURE 7 | Normalized D1–4 HC survival curves for 1 pro-oxidant (β-lapachone) and 2 representative antioxidants (ferulic acid ethylester and gentisisc acid). When each of these compounds was applied to micro-explants in the absence of concurrent gentamicin, far more HC damage was observed than in untreated (negative controls) micro-explants. *N* = 6 micro-explants/data point.

Mammalian Organ of Corti Micro-Explant Assay

Many assays for the evaluation of compounds on HCs have been developed. The assay presented here, like any preclinical assay, has both advantages and disadvantages. A key advantage of the micro-explant screening assay is that it employs mammalian HCs rather than HCs from different animal classes or mammalian cell lines. This is important since mammalian HCs, and especially cochlear HCs, are quite different from the HCs of different animal classes such as birds or fish. The outer HC, the most vulnerable element in the mammalian cochlea, is not present in other classes of animals. HCs are of course quite different from mammalian cell lines. Thus, it might be argued that an assay based on the mammalian oC gives results more applicable to humans.

Another advantage of the model is the ability to evaluate the effects of a much larger number of compounds than can be achieved with an *in vivo* mammalian model. This is because several explants can be generated from each murine oC. While the assay is by no means high-throughput, it would allow the screening of a few hundred compounds. Because the assay is

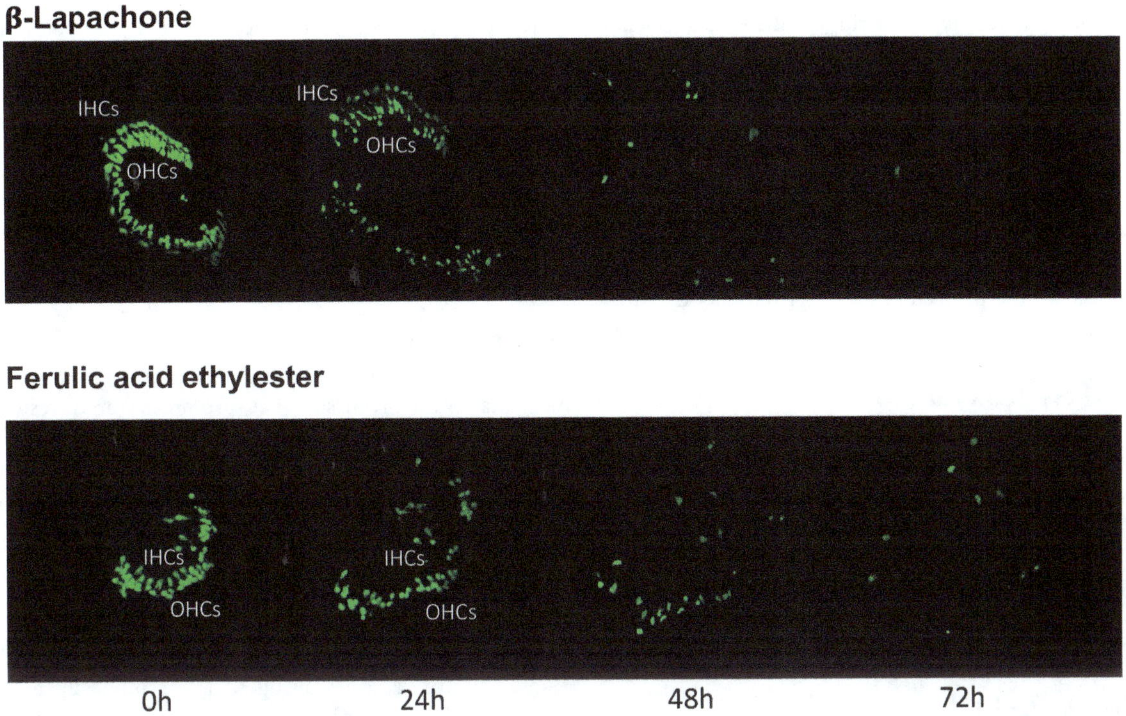

FIGURE 8 | Montages illustrating representative oC micro-explants treated with 1000 μM β-lapachone alone, or 1000 μM ferulic acid ethylester alone, for 72 h, illustrating HC toxicity without gentamicin.

uniform, it allows not only hit identification, but also information on relative effectiveness. Thus, we found that seratrodast and idebenone were the most effective HC protectants under the conditions of this assay. Since seratrodast has not been studied as a HC protectant in the past, this compound, plus other novel antioxidants identified, deserve more extensive study.

Of course, there are also disadvantages to this assay system. Since adult HCs do not survive in culture, the assay is based on neonatal HCs that are not yet functionally mature. They may respond differently to gentamicin or to antioxidants than adult HCs. In addition, the number of compounds that can be tested is limited. Thus, screening very large compound libraries is beyond the capacity of our method. Similarly, including a very large number of conditions, such as a large range of gentamicin dosages, would be difficult when also varying compound concentrations. Finally, this is a screening assay, which as with all screens does not provide definitive data, but rather identifies candidates that warrant further study. These limitations must be considered when interpreting the results of the assay.

HC Protective Antioxidants

A relatively small number of antioxidants among those tested proved to be protective to HCs. The range of protection varied from nearly complete to modest. There was no single category of antioxidant that proved to be superior to others. Several different categories of antioxidants were represented in the protective compounds. Moreover, often some antioxidants of the same class were found to have no effect on HC survival, or even in a few cases to be harmful. Hence, the mechanism of protection is believed to be associated with their antioxidant capacity but is not fully understood.

Seratrodast

Seratrodast is a quinone antioxidant, and was one of the most protective compounds identified in the screen. It has not previously been studied as a protective agent for HCs. Seratrodast acts as a free radical scavenger. It is not only an antioxidant, but also a blocker of the thromboxane A2 receptor and is used in the treatment of asthma. While thromboxane A2 has been implicated in vascular disorders of the inner ear (e.g., Umemura et al., 1993), it has never been associated with ototoxicity. It therefore seems likely that the protective effects of seratrodast are related to its antioxidant properties.

Idebenone

Idebenone, is a quinone antioxidant and a synthetic analog of co-enzyme Q. It is a free radical scavenger that was also highly effective in protecting against high-dose gentamicin-induced HC damage in the assay. Sergi et al. (2006) found that systemically administered idebenone provided protection against noise-induced hearing loss in guinea pigs. Since this protection was not additive with that of α-tocopherol (vitamin E), it was assumed that their mechanisms of action were overlapping. There has been no previous study of idebenone as a HC protectant against ototoxins.

Resveratrol

Resveratrol is a naturally occurring stilbene polyphenolic antioxidant that acts as a free radical scavenger. It was very effective in protecting HCs from gentamicin toxicity. A number of studies have shown resveratrol to be protective against various forms of HC damage including cisplatin (Yumusakhuylu et al., 2012) and noise (Hanci et al., 2016) *in vivo*, as well as gentamicin *in vitro* treatment (Bonabi et al., 2008). In addition to its antioxidant properties, resveratrol has been shown to activate sirtuin-1 and to de-acetylate NFκB, and these properties have been implicated in the protection of HCs from anoxic damage (Wang et al., 2013).

Butylated Hydroxyanisole

Butylated hydroxyanisole is a phenolic antioxidant and potent free radical scavenger that is often used as a food additive to prevent oxidative damage, especially to lipids. It was a very effective HC protectant against high-dose gentamicin. BHA has not previously been studied as a HC protectant. Reports that BHA is a carcinogen at high levels have since been repudiated, but they led to limits on permissible BHA levels and a decline in BHA use in some foods from the 1990s (Hui, 2006).

DL-α-Lipoic Acid

DL-α-lipoic acid is a sulfur-containing antioxidant. It is a free radical scavenger and metal chelator that also enhances intracellular levels of glutathione (Shay et al., 2009). It was very protective of HCs against high-dose gentamicin. There have been numbers of studies of α-lipoic acid as a protective agent against cisplatin ototoxicity (see Rybak et al., 2009 for a review). Other animal studies have evaluated this compound as a protectant against age-related hearing loss (Ahn et al., 2008) and cochlear implant trauma (Chang et al., 2017).

Hinokitiol

Hinokitiol (β-thujaplicin) is a naturally occurring antioxidant, found in the heartwood of certain plants. It acts as a metal chelator and, also, enhances the activity of superoxide dismutase (Huang et al., 2015). It was found to be very protective in the assay. It has not been previously studied as a HC protectant. In addition to its antioxidant properties, hinokitiol has been shown to reduce inflammation via suppression of NFκB, and metalloproteinases, and to activate caspase 3. The former activities could contribute to its protective effect.

Butylated Hydroxytoluene

Butylated hydroxytoluene is a phenolic antioxidant and potent free radical scavenger that, like BHA, is a frequent food additive. It was moderately effective in the prevention of HC damage in the assay. It has not previously been studied as a HC protectant.

Dithiotreitol

Dithiotreitol is a thiol-containing, reducing agent that is a free radical scavenger and metal chelator. It was moderately protective in the assay. It has not previously been evaluated for its ability to protect HCs.

MC-186

MC-186 (MCI-186; edaravone) is a non-phenolic antioxidant. It is a potent free-radical and protein carbonyl scavenger and inhibitor of lipid peroxidation that is used in clinical trials for the treatment of chronic obstructive pulmonary disorder. It was moderately protective against high-dose gentamicin damage to HCs. Several previous studies have shown MC-186 to be protective against various forms of HC damage (e.g., Maetani et al., 2003; Horiike et al., 2004; Takemoto et al., 2004; Masuda et al., 2006).

Procysteine

Procysteine (L-2-Oxothiazolidine-4-carboxylic acid, OTC) is a glutathione precursor that promotes rapid restoration of intracellular glutathione levels following depletion by ROS. Procysteine has been shown to reduce threshold shifts and HC loss following noise exposure in guinea pigs (Yamasoba et al., 1998), and to protect HCs in zebrafish from ototoxins (Ton and Parng, 2005).

Trolox

Trolox is a water-soluble, short chain vitamin E analog. It is a potent free radical scavenger. It was modestly protective in the assay. It has previously been shown to slightly inhibit HC damage due to gentamicin *in vitro* (Garetz et al., 1994b) as well as cisplatin- (Teranishi and Nakashima, 2003) and noise-induced (Yamashita et al., 2005) cochlear damage *in vivo*.

Thiourea

Thiourea is a thiol-containing reducing agent and free radical scavenger. It was modestly protective in the assay. Thiourea is toxic when administered at high systemic dosages. It preferentially inhibits the peroxidase in the thyroid gland and thus inhibits thyroxine production. The reduced synthesis of thyroid hormone causes an increased pituitary secretion of thyreotropic hormone and so hyperplasia of the thyroid which, on continuous stimulation in animals, can lead to tumor formation and, in man, to various thyroid-treated illnesses (Peters et al., 1949). However, intracochlear thiourea has been found to protect against cisplatin-induced HC loss *in vivo* (Ekborn et al., 2003).

Thymoquinone

Thymoquinone is a quinone antioxidant. It was minimally effective in our assay, showing protection only after 24 h of gentamicin treatment, and only at the lowest dosage. It is therefore possible that this represents a false positive. However, thymoqunone has previously been shown to protect HCs against damage due to gentamicin (Sagit et al., 2014), cisplatin (Sagit et al., 2013), and noise (Aksoy et al., 2015) *in vivo*.

It should be noted that some of the antioxidants that failed to exhibit protection have been shown in previous studies to protect HCs and hearing. Consequently, their failure to provide protection in our assay was unanticipated and surprising. Nonetheless, there are many potential explanations for these differences. They may be related to the relatively high concentration of gentamicin employed in our assay (200 μM), which presumably provided a very strong oxidative stress response. Differences could also be related to the *in vitro* nature of our assay, specific culture conditions, redox compound effective concentrations, species differences between mice and other animal models or humans, or to the use of neonatal as opposed to adult HCs.

Antioxidants as HC Protectants

The range of protective and toxic responses observed in the assay illustrates the complexity of antioxidative compounds and their underlying mechanisms. Antioxidant effectiveness depends on several important intrinsic factors: permeability, activation energy, rate constants, molecular stability, oxidation–reduction potential, and solubility (Nawar, 1996). These functional factors are in turn closely related to the antioxidant molecular structure. Those antioxidants capable of interrupting the free radical chain reaction are usually the most effective (Brewer, 2011). They are characterized by aromatic or phenolic rings and act by donating a hydrogen atom to free radicals formed during oxidation. In the process, they transition into a radical form themselves; however, these radical intermediates are stable due to resonance delocalization of the extra electron within the aromatic ring and subsequent formation of stable quinones (Nawar, 1996). The most effective phenolic antioxidants have low oxidation-reduction potentials and OH groups in the *ortho*-position on the B phenolic ring. Phenolic antioxidants were well represented in our protective antioxidants. However, our two most effective antioxidants were quinone antioxidants. While they both possess an aromatic ring, the rings themselves are not characterized by OH groups, which lie elsewhere on the molecule.

As noted above, antioxidants also vary considerably in their mechanisms. These include scavenging the species that initiate peroxidation, quenching singlet oxygen, metal chelating, interrupting free radical chain reactions, and reducing oxygen concentrations (Badarinath et al., 2010). Antioxidants are not all equally powerful in reacting according to these varied mechanisms. For example, phenolic acids effectively trap free radicals but are not efficient metal chelators, while flavonoids can both scavenge free radicals and chelate metals efficiently (Brewer, 2011). Antioxidants can also differ in their ability to access the intracellular environment, and exhibit different half-lives. Finally, as noted above for some of the protective compounds, antioxidants can also have effects on cells that are not related to their antioxidant properties. This complexity makes the choice of antioxidants to employ difficult. The value of a broad screen, as employed here, is that no *a priori* knowledge of the properties of an antioxidant are required, and unexpected results may be obtained.

AUTHOR CONTRIBUTIONS

VN, AK, and AR designed, performed the experiments and wrote the manuscript. VN, KP, and RJ performed the studies.

ACKNOWLEDGMENT

Julie Lightner proofed the manuscript and provided valuable editorial assistance.

REFERENCES

Ahn, J. H., Kang, H. H., Kim, T. Y., Shin, J. E., and Chung, J. W. (2008). Lipoic acid rescues DBA mice from early-onset age-related hearing impairment. *Neuroreport* 19, 1265–1269. doi: 10.1097/WNR.0b013e328308b338

Aksoy, F., Dogan, R., Yenigun, A., Veyseller, B., Ozturan, O., and Ozturk, B. (2015). Thymoquinone treatment for inner-ear acoustic trauma in rats. *J. Laryngol. Otol.* 129, 38–45. doi: 10.1017/S0022215114002680

Badarinath, A. V., Rao, K. M., Chetty, C. M. S., Ramkanth, S., Rajan, T. V. S., and Gnanaprakash, K. (2010). A review on in-vitro antioxidant methods: comparisons, correlations and considerations. *Int. J. Pharmtech Res.* 2, 1276–1285.

Bagger-Sjöbäck, D., Strömbäck, K., Hakizimana, P., Plue, J., Larsson, C., Hultcrantz, M., et al. (2015). A randomized, double blind trial of N acetylcysteine for hearing protection during stapes surgery. *PLoS ONE* 10:e0115657. doi: 10.1371/journal.pone.0115657

Bonabi, S., Caelers, A., Monge, A., Huber, A., and Bodmer, D. (2008). Resveratrol protects auditory hair cells from gentamicin toxicity. *Ear Nose Throat J.* 87, 570–573.

Brewer, M. S. (2011). Natural antioxidants: sources, compounds, mechanisms of action, and potential applications. *Comp. Rev. Food Sci. Food Saf.* 10, 221–247. doi: 10.1111/j.1541-4337.2011.00156.x

Chang, M. Y., Gwon, T. M., Lee, H. S., Lee, J. H., Oh, S. H., Kim, S. J., et al. (2017). The effect of systemic lipoic acid on hearing preservation after cochlear implantation via the round window approach: a guinea pig model. *Eur. J. Pharmacol.* 799, 67–72. doi: 10.1016/j.ejphar.2017.01.042

Choung, Y. H., Taura, A., Pak, K., Choi, S. J., Masuda, M., and Ryan, A. F. (2009). Generation of highly-reactive oxygen species is closely related to hair cell damage in rat organ of Corti treated with gentamicin. *Neuroscience* 161, 214–226. doi: 10.1016/j.neuroscience.2009.02.085

Ekborn, A., Laurell, G., Ehrsson, H., and Miller, J. (2003). Intracochlear administration of thiourea protects against cisplatin-induced outer hair cell loss in the guinea pig. *Hear. Res.* 181, 109–115. doi: 10.1016/S0378-5955(03)00181-3

Fausti, S. A., Henry, J. A., Schaffer, H. I., Olson, D. J., Frey, R. H., and McDonald, W. J. (1992). High-frequency audiometric monitoring for early detection of aminoglycoside ototoxicity. *J. Infect. Dis.* 165, 1026–1032. doi: 10.1093/infdis/165.6.1026

Fetoni, A. R., Sergi, B., Scarano, E., Paludetti, G., Ferraresi, A., and Troiani, D. (2003). Protective effects of alpha-tocopherol against gentamicin-induced Oto-vestibulo toxicity: an experimental study. *Acta Otolaryngol.* 123, 192–197. doi: 10.1080/00016480310001484

Garetz, S. L., Altschuler, R. A., and Schacht, J. (1994a). Attenuation of gentamicin ototoxicity by glutathione in the guinea pig in vivo. *Hear. Res.* 77, 81–87.

Garetz, S. L., Rhee, D. J., and Schacht, J. (1994b). Sulfhydryl compounds and antioxidants inhibit cytotoxicity to outer hair cells of a gentamicin metabolite in vitro. *Hear. Res.* 77, 75–80.

Hanci, D., Ulusoy, S., Acar, M., Burukoglu, D., Kutlu, H. M., Bayar Muluk, N., et al. (2016). Potential protective effect of resveratrol on acoustic trauma: electron microscopy study. *Eur. Rev. Med. Pharmacol. Sci.* 20, 3469–3475.

Horiike, O., Shimogori, H., and Yamashita, H. (2004). Effect of edaravone on streptomycin-induced vestibulotoxicity in the guinea pig. *Laryngoscope* 114, 1630–1632. doi: 10.1097/00005537-200409000-00023

Huang, C. H., Jayakumar, T., Chang, C. C., Fong, T. H., Lu, S. H., Thomas, P. A., et al. (2015). Hinokitiol exerts anticancer activity through downregulation of MMPs 9/2 and enhancement of catalase and SOD enzymes: *in vivo* augmentation of lung histoarchitecture. *Molecules* 20, 17720–17734. doi: 10.3390/molecules201017720

Hui, Y. H. (2006). *Handbook of Food Science, Technology and Engineering*. Boca Raton, FL: CRC press.

Kocyigit, I., Vural, A., Unal, A., Sipahioglu, M. H., Yucel, H. E., Aydemir, S., et al. (2015). Preventing amikacin related ototoxicity with *N*-acetylcysteine in patients undergoing peritoneal dialysis. *Eur. Arch. Otorhinolaryngol.* 272, 2611–2620. doi: 10.1007/s00405-014-3207-z

Kopke, R. D., Liu, W., Gabaizadeh, R., Jacono, A., Feghali, J., Spray, D., et al. (1997). Use of organotypic cultures of Corti's organ to study the protective effects of antioxidant molecules on cisplatin-induced damage of auditory hair cells. *Am. J. Otol.* 18, 559–571.

Kramer, S., Dreisbach, L., Lockwood, J., Baldwin, K., Kopke, R., Scranton, S., et al. (2006). Efficacy of the antioxidant *N*-acetylcysteine (NAC) in protecting ears exposed to loud music. *J. Am. Acad. Audiol.* 17, 265–278. doi: 10.3766/jaaa.17.4.5

Lindblad, A. C., Rosenhall, U., Olofsson, A., and Hagerman, B. (2011). The efficacy of *N*-acetylcysteine to protect the human cochlea from subclinical hearing loss caused by impulse noise: a controlled trial. *Noise Health* 13, 392–401. doi: 10.4103/1463-1741.90293

Lü, J. M., Lin, P. H., Yao, Q., and Chen, C. (2010). Chemical and molecular mechanisms of antioxidants: experimental approaches and model systems. *J. Cell Mol. Med.* 14, 840–860. doi: 10.1111/j.1582-4934.2009.00897

Maetani, T., Hakuba, N., Taniguchi, M., Hyodo, J., Shimizu, Y., and Gyo, K. (2003). Free radical scavenger protects against inner hair cell loss after cochlear ischemia. *Neuroreport* 14, 1881–1884. doi: 10.1097/00001756-200310060-00025

Masuda, M., Dulon, D., Pak, K., Mullen, L. M., Li, Y., Erkman, L., et al. (2011). Regulation of *POU4F3* gene expression in hair cells by 5′, DNA in mice. *Neuroscience* 197, 48–64. doi: 10.1016/j.neuroscience.2011.09.033

Masuda, Y., Tanabe, T., Murata, Y., and Kitahara, S. (2006). Protective effect of edaravone in inner-ear barotrauma in guinea pigs. *J. Laryngol. Otol.* 120, 524–527. doi: 10.1017/S0022215106000855

McKeage, M. J. (1995). Comparative adverse effect profiles of platinum drugs. *Drug Saf.* 13, 228–244. doi: 10.2165/00002018-199513040-00003

Nawar, W. F. (1996). "Lipids," in *Food chemistry*, 3rd Edn, ed. O. Fennema (New York, NY: Marcel Dekker), 225–320.

Peters, J. P., Mann, E. B., Kidd, D. M., Enstrom, W. W., and Waters, L. C. (1949). Toxic effects of anti-thyroid drugs. *Yale J. Biol. Med.* 22, 139–145.

Ryan, A., and Dallos, P. (1975). Effect of absence of cochlear outer hair cells on behavioural auditory threshold. *Nature* 253, 44–46. doi: 10.1038/253044a0

Rybak, L. P., Husain, K., Whitworth, C., and Somani, S. M. (1999). Dose dependent protection by lipoic acid against cisplatin-induced ototoxicity in rats: antioxidant defense system. *Toxicol. Sci.* 47, 195–202. doi: 10.1093/toxsci/47.2.195

Rybak, L. P., Mukherjea, D., Jajoo, S., and Ramkumar, V. (2009). Cisplatin ototoxicity and protection: clinical and experimental studies. *Tohoku J. Exp. Med.* 219, 177–186. doi: 10.1620/tjem.219.177

Sagit, M., Korkmaz, F., Akcadag, A., and Somdas, M. A. (2013). Protective effect of thymoquinone against cisplatin-induced ototoxicity. *Eur. Arch. Otorhinolaryngol.* 270, 2231–2237. doi: 10.1007/s00405-012-2254-6

Sagit, M., Korkmaz, F., Gürgen, S. G., Kaya, M., Akcadag, A., and Ozcan, I. (2014). The protective role of thymoquinone in the prevention of gentamicin ototoxicity. *Am. J. Otolaryngol.* 35, 603–609. doi: 10.1016/j.amjoto.2014.07.002

Schacht, J., Talaska, A. E., and Rybak, L. P. (2012). Cisplatin and aminoglycoside antibiotics: hearing loss and its prevention. *Anat. Rec.* 295, 1837–1850. doi: 10.1002/ar.22578

Sergi, B., Fetoni, A. R., Paludetti, G., Ferraresi, A., Navarra, P., Mordente, A., et al. (2006). Protective properties of idebenone in noise-induced hearing loss in the guinea pig. *Neuroreport* 17, 857–861. doi: 10.1097/01.wnr.0000221834.18470.8c

Sha, S. H., Taylor, R., Forge, A., and Schacht, J. (2001a). Differential vulnerability of basal and apical hair cells is based on intrinsic susceptibility to free radicals. *Hear. Res.* 155, 1–8.

Sha, S. H., Zajic, G., Epstein, C. J., and Schacht, J. (2001b). Overexpression of copper/zinc-superoxide dismutase protects from kanamycin-induced hearing loss. *Audiol. Neurootol.* 6, 117–123.

Shay, K. P., Moreau, R. F., Smith, E. J., Smith, A. R., and Hagen, T. M. (2009). Alpha-lipoic acid as a dietary supplement: molecular mechanisms and therapeutic potential. *Biochim. Biophys. Acta* 1790, 1149–1160. doi: 10.1016/j.bbagen.2009.07.026

Takemoto, T., Sugahara, K., Okuda, T., Shimogori, H., and Yamashita, H. (2004). The clinical free radical scavenger, edaravone, protects cochlear hair cells from acoustic trauma. *Eur. J. Pharmacol.* 487, 113–116. doi: 10.1016/j.ejphar.2004.01.109

Teranishi, M. A., and Nakashima, T. (2003). Effects of trolox, locally applied on round windows, on cisplatin-induced ototoxicity in guinea pigs. *Int. J. Pediatr. Otorhinolaryngol.* 67, 133–139. doi: 10.1016/S0165-5876(02)00353-1

Ton, C., and Parng, C. (2005). The use of zebrafish for assessing ototoxic and otoprotective agents. *Hear. Res.* 208, 79–88. doi: 10.1016/j.heares.2005.05.005

Umemura, K., Asai, Y., Uematsu, T., and Nakashima, M. (1993). Role of thromboxane A2 in a microcirculation disorder of the rat inner ear. *Eur. Arch. Otorhinolaryngol.* 250, 342–344. doi: 10.1007/BF00188383

Wang, P., Du, B., Yin, W., Wang, X., and Zhu, W. (2013). Resveratrol attenuates CoCl2-induced cochlear hair cell damage through upregulation of Sirtuin1 and NF-κB deacetylation. *PLoS ONE* 8:e80854. doi: 10.1371/journal.pone.0080854

Wong, A. C., and Ryan, A. F. (2015). Mechanisms of sensorineural cell damage, death and survival in the cochlea. *Front. Aging Neurosci.* 7:58. doi: 10.3389/fnagi.2015.00058

Yamashita, D., Jiang, H.-Y., Le Prell, C. G., Schacht, J., and Miller, J. M. (2005). Post-exposure treatment attenuates noise-induced hearing loss. *Neuroscience* 134, 633–642. doi: 10.1016/j.neuroscience.2005.04.015

Yamasoba, T., Nuttall, A. L., Harris, C., Raphael, Y., and Miller, J. M. (1998). Role of glutathione in protection against noise-induced hearing loss. *Brain Res.* 784, 82–90. doi: 10.1016/S0006-8993(97)01156-6

Yumusakhuylu, A. C., Yazici, M., Sari, M., Binnetoglu, A., Kosemihal, E., Akdas, F., et al. (2012). Protective role of resveratrol against cisplatin induced ototoxicity in guinea pigs. *Int. J. Pediatr. Otorhinolaryngol.* 76, 404–408. doi: 10.1016/j.ijporl.2011.12.021

9

Histone Deacetylase Inhibitors are Protective in Acute but Not in Chronic Models of Ototoxicity

Chao-Hui Yang[1,2], *Zhiqi Liu*[3], *Deanna Dong*[3], *Jochen Schacht*[1], *Dev Arya*[4] *and Su-Hua Sha*[3]*

[1]Kresge Hearing Research Institute, Department of Otolaryngology, University of Michigan, Ann Arbor, MI, United States, [2]Department of Otolaryngology, Kaohsiung Chang Gung Memorial Hospital, Chang Gung University College of Medicine, Kaohsiung, Taiwan, [3]Department of Pathology and Laboratory Medicine, Medical University of South Carolina, Charleston, SC, United States, [4]Department of Chemistry, Clemson University, Clemson, SC, United States

Edited by:
Peter S. Steyger,
Oregon Health & Science University,
United States

Reviewed by:
Andy Groves,
Baylor College of Medicine,
United States
Kelvin Y. Kwan,
Rutgers University, The State University of New Jersey,
United States

***Correspondence:**
Su-Hua Sha
shasu@musc.edu

Previous studies have reported that modification of histones alters aminoglycoside-induced hair cell death and hearing loss. In this study, we investigated three FDA-approved histone deacetylase (HDAC) inhibitors (vorinostat/SAHA, belinostat, and panobinostat) as protectants against aminoglycoside-induced ototoxicity in murine cochlear explants and *in vivo* in both guinea pigs and CBA/J mice. Individually, all three HDAC inhibitors reduced gentamicin (GM)-induced hair cell loss in a dose-dependent fashion in explants. *In vivo*, however, treatment with SAHA attenuated neither GM-induced hearing loss and hair cell loss in guinea pigs nor kanamycin (KM)-induced hearing loss and hair cell loss in mice under chronic models of ototoxicity. These findings suggest that treatment with the HDAC inhibitor SAHA attenuates aminoglycoside-induced ototoxicity in an acute model, but not in chronic models, cautioning that one cannot rely solely on *in vitro* experiments to test the efficacy of otoprotectant compounds.

Keywords: ototoxicity, HDAC inhibitors, prevention of aminoglycoside-induced hearing loss, modification of histone acetylation, acute and chronic animal models

INTRODUCTION

Aminoglycoside antibiotics continue to be indispensable drugs for treatment of acute infections and for specific indications such as treatment of tuberculosis or Pseudomonas infections in patients with cystic fibrosis, owing to their broad antibacterial spectrum and efficacy against resistant bacterial strains. However, their use has been limited due to ototoxic and nephrotoxic side effects. A pathological feature of aminoglycoside-induced ototoxicity is loss of mechanosensory hair cells in the inner ear, resulting in hearing loss and vestibular dysfunction. Since mammalian cochlear sensory hair cells lack the ability to regenerate, the loss of or damage to sensory hair cells is permanent. Although there have been efforts to find potential therapies to mitigate these side effects, no established clinical therapies for prevention or amelioration are yet available.

Abbreviations: BUN, Blood urea nitrogen; Cr, Creatinine; DMSO, Dimethyl sulfoxide; ED50, Median effective dose; H4K8ac, Acetylation of histone H4 at lysine 8; HATs, Histone acetyltransferases; HD, Higher doses; HDACs, Histone deacetylases; IP, Intraperitoneal; LD, Lower doses; SQ, Subcutaneous; TD50, Median toxic dose; TI, Therapeutic index.

Gene expression can be modulated by epigenetic changes in response to physiological and metabolic demand or to environmental stimuli. For example, gene expression is silenced by condensing chromatin, methylating DNA, or deacetylating histones. Conversely, histones may be acetylated and chromatin will unravel to facilitate gene transcription. Two types of enzymes can modulate the acetylation status of histones: (1) Histone acetyltransferases (HATs) add acetyl groups to lysine residues on the histone tails, facilitating the binding of transcription factors to nucleosome DNA and activate transcription. (2) Histone deacetylases (HDACs) remove the acetyl groups, promoting chromatin condensation, and reduce transcription (Marks et al., 2001).

An imbalance of histone acetylation has been linked to a variety of diseases. For example, deficient histone acetylation is found in cancer and progressive neurodegenerative diseases, such as Parkinson and Alzheimer's diseases (Falkenberg and Johnstone, 2014). Our previous research has found that aminoglycoside antibiotics increased HDAC1, HDAC3 (class I HDACs) and HDAC4 (class II HDAC) in outer hair cells (OHCs) and reduced histone acetylation. The HDAC inhibitors trichostatin A and sodium butyrate rescued OHCs during acute aminoglycoside toxicity (Chen et al., 2009). These two drugs are highly toxic and rarely used in the clinic. However, in recent years, several less toxic HDAC inhibitors have been tested in clinical trials or are already approved by the FDA for the treatment of cancer. Among these, SAHA (vorinostat) attenuated hearing loss in mice caused by treatment with the combination of kanamycin (KM) and furosemide or by noise (Layman et al., 2015; Wen et al., 2015; Chen et al., 2016).

In order to provide basic information on the potential of HDAC inhibitors as therapeutic protectants, we evaluated three of these inhibitors (SAHA, belinostat, and panobinostat), which specifically inhibit HDAC subtypes I, II, and IV, for their likely protective effects during aminoglycoside challenge to organ of Corti explants. We then assessed the protective effects of SAHA *in vivo* both in guinea pigs and CBA/J mice in chronic hearing-loss models that we have previously established (Sha et al., 2001; Wu et al., 2001).

MATERIALS AND METHODS

Animals

For breeding, sexually mature male (6-week-old) and female (8-week-old) CBA/J mice were purchased from Harlan Sprague Dawley Incorporation (Indianapolis, IN, USA). For KM *in vivo* trials, male CBA/J mice at 4 weeks of age were purchased from Jackson Laboratory (Bar Harbor, ME, USA). Male Hartley guinea pigs (200–250 g) were purchased from Charles River (Wilmington, MA, USA). All animals were kept at 22 ± 1°C under a standard 12-h light/12-h dark schedule and had free access to water and a regular mouse (Harlan 2918) or guinea pig diet (#5025; 18.5% protein; Purina, St. Louis, MO, USA). All experimental protocols and all compounds used were approved either by the University of Michigan Committee on the Use and Care of Animals (UCUCA) or the Institutional Animal Care & Use Committee at the Medical University of South Carolina (MUSC). Animal care was under the supervision of the University of Michigan's Unit for Laboratory Animal Medicine (ULAM) or under the supervision of the Division of Laboratory Animal Resources at MUSC.

Organotypic Cultures of Post-Natal Murine Organ of Corti

The culture procedures have been described in detail (Chen et al., 2009). In brief, postnatal day 3 (p3) CBA/J pups were euthanized after antisepsis using 70% ethanol. Inner ears were extracted from surrounding tissue and immersed in cold Hank's balanced salt solution. The lateral wall tissues (stria vascularis and spiral ligament) and the auditory nerve bundle were micro-dissected from the organ of Corti. The explants were placed onto a prepared culture dish containing a 15-μL polymerized drop of rat tail collagen in 1 mL of culture medium consisting of Basal Medium Eagle, 1% serum-free supplement (Invitrogen, Carlsbad, CA, USA), 1% bovine serum albumin, 5 mg/mL glucose, and 10 U/mL penicillin G. After 4 h of incubation (37°C, 5% CO_2), an additional 1 mL of medium was added to submerge the explants.

Treatment of the Explants

Explants were incubated for 2 days to recover from dissection stress before administering HDAC inhibitors and gentamicin (GM; Sigma-Aldrich Co., St. Louis, MO, USA). The medium was then exchanged for new medium containing a final concentration of 4.5 μM GM with or without various concentrations of the HDAC inhibitors and incubated for 72 h. The stock solutions with 95 mM of SAHA/vorinostat (Cayman Chemical, Ann Arbor, MI, USA), 100 mM of belinostat (Selleckchem, Houson, TX, USA), and 100 mM of panobinostat (Cayman Chemical), were dissolved in 100% dimethyl sulfoxide (DMSO) and stored at −20°C. GM solution was made fresh from powder in culture medium at 0.2 mM and then diluted to the final concentration for each experiment.

Evaluation of Ototoxicity by Hair Cell Counts in Explants

Explants were fixed with 4% paraformaldehyde overnight at 4°C and permeabilized for 30 min with 3% Triton X-100 in phosphate-buffered saline (PBS) at room temperature (22–24°C). The specimens were then washed three times with PBS and incubated with rhodamine-phalloidin (Invitrogen) at a 1:100 dilution for 60 min at room temperature (22–24°C). After rinsing in PBS, the specimens were mounted on a slide with Gel-Mount^{TM} (BioMeda Corp., Foster City, CA, USA). The phalloidin-stained stereociliary bundles and circumferential F-actin rings on the cuticular plate of OHCs allowed the determination of cells that were present or missing. A clear "V" shape of stereocilia indicates the presence of OHCs. If the "V" shape is not visualized, we accept this as a damaged hair cells. Cell populations were assessed on a Leitz Orthoplan upright microscope equipped for epifluorescence, using a 50× oil-immersion objective. The right objective had a 0.19-mm calibrated scale imposed on the field for reference and all three rows of OHCs were oriented longitudinally within each 0.19-mm frame. Each successive 0.19-mm field was evaluated for the absence of OHCs beginning from the apex and moving down the organ of Corti to the base. The percentage of OHC loss was calculated.

Drug Administration to CBA/J Mice *in Vivo*

Male CBA/J mice at the age of 5 weeks received subcutaneous (SQ) injections of KM at 700 mg base/kg (dissolved in saline) twice per day (AM and PM). SAHA for administration was dissolved in 100% DMSO for stock solutions of 50 mg/mL and diluted with saline immediately before intraperitoneal (IP) injection, for a final dose of 50 mg/kg, given twice per day for 15 days. The concentration of DMSO vehicle control was 1 mL/kg body weight. All solutions were filtered with a syringe filter before injection. Body weight was measured before each injection.

Experimental Groups and Drug Administration to Pigmented Guinea Pigs *in Vivo*

Pigmented male guinea pigs initially weighing 200–250 g from Charles River were used in the *in-vivo* study. Experiments were begun 1 week after the guinea pigs arrived. To select safe doses of SAHA for protective studies, we conducted two separate sets of experiments to assess serum platelet concentrations. In the first set, pigmented guinea pigs received daily IP injections of SAHA at lower doses (LD; 2 mg/kg and 5 mg/kg) concurrent with SQ injections of 120 mg GM base/kg body weight daily for 2 weeks. In the second study, the higher doses (HD) of SAHA (15 mg/kg and 25 mg/kg) were used. The DMSO concentration was 1.1 g/kg, equal to the DMSO concentration used for the 25 mg/kg concentration of SAHA. Since the highest dose (25 mg/kg/day for 14 days) of SAHA significantly reduced serum platelet concentrations, the doses of SAHA used for the protective studies were 25 mg/kg or less. We then tested the protective ability of SAHA at LD (2 mg/kg and 5 mg/kg) and at HD of SAHA (15 mg/kg and 25 mg/kg) against GM-induced hearing loss concurrent with daily SQ injections of GM (dissolved in saline) at 120 mg base/kg for 14 days. SAHA was dissolved in 100% DMSO for stock solutions of 25 mg/mL and diluted with saline immediately before IP injections. All compound solutions were filtered with syringe filters before injection. Body weights were measured before each injection. If a guinea pig lost ~5% of its body weight, an additional 3–4 mL of saline was administrated subcutaneously.

Surface Preparations of Guinea Pig Cochlear Epithelia for Hair Cell Counts

The procedures for surface preparations of guinea pig cochlear epithelia were followed as previously described (Sha and Schacht, 1999b). After the last auditory brain stem response (ABR) measurement, guinea pigs from the second group of experiments were deeply anesthetized in a CO_2 chamber and decapitated. Cochleae were immediately removed and perfused with 4% paraformaldehyde in PBS at pH 7.4 and fixed overnight at 4°C. Micro-dissected surface preparations of the organ of Corti were permeabilized for 30 min with 0.5% Triton X-100 in PBS at room temperature (22–24°C) and stained with rhodamine phalloidin (Invitrogen) at a 1:100 dilution for 60 min at room temperature (22–24°C). After rinsing in PBS, the specimens were mounted on a slide with Gel-Mount^{TM} (BioMeda Corp.). OHC counts were conducted with microscopy as described above for mice.

Assessment of Guinea Pig Blood Urea Nitrogen (BUN), Creatinine, and Platelet Levels

Blood was obtained by nail clipping after light anesthesia of the guinea pigs by metofane inhalation after the last drug injections. Blood cells were separated by centrifugation at 1000× *g* for 15 min, and sera were stored at −20°C. Blood urea nitrogen (BUN), creatinine and platelet concentrations were determined using a Kodak Ektachem700XR Clinical Chemistry Analyzer (Clinical Products Division, Eastman Kodak, Rochester, NY, USA) and analyzed by Dr. Donald Giacherio, Chemical Pathology Laboratory, University of Michigan.

Auditory Brainstem Response (ABR)

ABRs were measured 3 days before and 3 weeks after drug treatments. Animals were anesthetized with IP injections of ketamine (100 mg/kg) and xylazine (10 mg/kg) for mice or ketamine (58.8 mg/kg), xylazine (2.4 mg/kg), and acepromazine (1.2 mg/kg) for guinea pigs. Body temperature was maintained near 37°C with a heating pad. ABRs were measured at 12 and 32 kHz for guinea pigs or 8, 16, and 32 kHz for mice in a sound-isolated and electrically shielded booth (Acoustic Systems, Austin, TX, USA). Sub-dermal electrodes were inserted at the vertex of the skull, under the left ear and under the right ear (ground). Tucker Davis Technology System III hardware and SigGen/Biosig software were used to present the stimuli monaurally (15 ms duration tone bursts with 1 ms rise-fall time) through a Beyer earphone attached to a customized plastic speculum inserted into the ear canal. Up to 1024 responses were averaged for each stimulus level. Thresholds (the lowest stimulus level with a reproducible response) were determined by reducing the intensity in 10-dB steps and then in 5-dB steps approaching the threshold until no organized response was detected. Thresholds were evaluated based on ABR wave I. Scores were given by an expert blinded to experimental conditions between the highest stimulus level without a response and the lowest stimulus level where an organized response was observed. All ABR measurements were conducted by the same experimenter.

Statistical Analysis

Data were analyzed using SYSTAT and GraphPad software for Windows. The group size (n) *in vivo* was determined by the variability of measurements and the magnitude of the differences between groups. Statistical methods used include one-way analysis of variance (ANOVA) with Tukey's multiple comparisons and unpaired t-tests. All tests were two-tailed and a p-value < 0.05 was considered statistically significant.

RESULTS

Toxicity of HDAC Inhibitors in Murine Cochlear Explants

In order to evaluate the protective potential of the three HDAC inhibitors on aminoglycoside-induced ototoxicity, we first determined their safety on auditory sensory hair cells using p3 murine organ of Corti explants. Explants were incubated for 2 days for recovery from the stress of dissection, followed by 72 h of incubation with or without inhibitors. Toxic effects were assessed by OHC loss. Control samples showed no loss of cells (**Figure 1A**) but all three HDAC inhibitors damaged OHCs in a dose-dependent manner. OHCs in the basal turn show changes in the orientation of the stereociliary bundles beginning with concentrations of 4 μM for SAHA, 3 μM for belinostat, and 20 nM for panobinostat. The toxic effects increased significantly with increasing concentrations and loss of OHCs reached 100% at 8 μM of SAHA, 5 μM of belinostat, and 50 nM of panobinostat ($p < 0.0001$). Statistical analysis using one-way ANOVA showed a significant dose-dependence of the toxic effect for SAHA ($F_{(4,12)} = 840.8$, $p < 0.0001$), as well as for belinostat ($F_{(3,9)} = 11{,}856$, $p < 0.0001$) and panobinostat ($F_{(3,9)} = 13{,}972$, $p < 0.0001$; **Figures 1B–D**; for detailed Tukey's multiple comparison test values see **Table 1**). The median toxic doses (TD50), defined as the concentrations leading to 50% OHC loss, for SAHA, belinostat and panobinostat were 5.5 μM, 3.5 μM, and 35 nM, respectively.

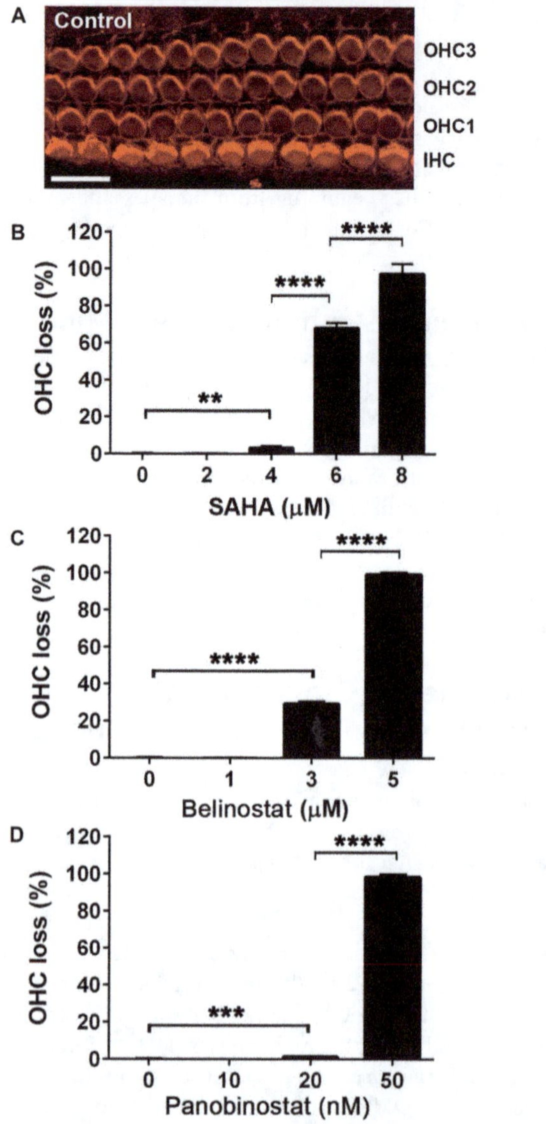

FIGURE 1 | Safety and toxicity of Histone deacetylase (HDAC) inhibitors in organ of Corti explants. **(A)** Image of a control p3 murine explant after culture for 5 days, stained with rhodamine phalloidin (red) to illustrate the preservation of three rows of outer hair cell (OHC) and one row of inner hair cells (IHCs) under the test conditions. Confocal images were taken from the basal turn. Scale bar = 10 μm. **(B–D)** Incubations in the presence of HDAC inhibitors for 72 h damaged hair cells of the basal turn in a dose-dependent manner. Data are presented as means ± SD, n = 3 or 4 at each concentration. $^{**}p < 0.01$, $^{***}p < 0.001$, $^{****}p < 0.0001$.

HDAC Inhibitors Protect Against Gentamicin-Induced Outer Hair Cell Loss in Murine Explants in a Dose-Dependent Manner

After having established the safe concentration range for the HDAC inhibitors, we explored their efficacy as protective agents against GM-induced OHC loss. In the 72-h incubations of explants, GM with the vehicle alone (DMSO) caused loss of OHCs in a base-to-apex gradient with a 40% overall loss at 4.5 μM. Co-incubation with SAHA (**Figure 2A**) proved protective, beginning at 0.5 μM SAHA and increasing in efficacy with increased doses, such that 2 μM SAHA completely protected from OHC loss ($F_{(3,24)} = 59.95$, $p < 0.001$; **Figure 2D**). Similarly, co-administration of belinostat (**Figure 2B**) or panobinostat (**Figure 2C**) with GM also reduced GM-induced OHC loss in a dose-dependent manner. GM-induced OHC loss was attenuated by co-administration of 0.1 μM belinostat and was totally prevented by 0.4 μM ($F_{(4,21)} = 29.2$, $p < 0.001$; **Figure 2E**). Additionally, with administration of panobinostat protection started at 5 nM and OHC loss was completely blocked by 15 nM panobinostat ($F_{(3,8)} = 81.19$, $p < 0.001$; **Figure 2F**). From the assessment of safe doses and the median effective (protective) doses (ED50) of the three HDAC inhibitors, we calculated the therapeutic index (TI = TD50/ED50) to be highest (safest) for belinostat and lowest for panobinostat (for detailed values see **Table 2**).

TABLE 1 | Tukey's multiple comparison test values for data in **Figure 1**.

HDAC inhibitors	Groups	*p* Value	*P* value summary
SAHA	0 vs. 4 μM	0.0089	**
	0 vs. 6 μM	<0.0001	***
	4 vs. 8 μM	<0.0001	****
	6 vs. 6 μM	0.0004	***
Belinostat	0 vs. 3 μM	<0.0001	****
	3 vs. 5 μM	<0.0001	****
Panobinostat	0 vs. 20 nM	0.0003	***
	20 vs. 50 nM	<0.0001	****

SAHA Does Not Prevent Kanamycin-Induced Hearing Loss in Mice *in Vivo*

In order to assess the protective potential of SAHA *in vivo* in a chronic ototoxicity model, we tested if SAHA treatment had protective effects against KM (700 mg base/kg body weight twice daily)-induced hearing loss in CBA/J mice. Consistent with our previous studies (Wu et al., 2001), treatment with KM for 15 days caused auditory threshold shifts of an average of 55 dB at 16 kHz ($p < 0.0001$) and 32 kHz ($p < 0.0001$). Treatment with SAHA at 50 mg/kg body weight twice daily did not attenuate KM-induced auditory threshold shifts (**Figure 3**). Typical ABR waveforms for each treated group are illustrated in **Supplementary Figure S1**.

The Effects of SAHA Treatment on Platelet Concentration in Guinea Pigs *in Vivo*

While the CBA/J mouse is a well-established model for chronic KM-induced ototoxicity, we wished to ascertain whether the lack of protection by SAHA might be species-dependent. We therefore tested if SAHA treatment had protective effects against GM-induced hearing loss in guinea pigs. To find safe doses to be used in guinea pigs *in vivo*, we first assessed serum platelet concentrations. Guinea pigs tolerated injections of SAHA at all concentrations of 5–25 mg/kg

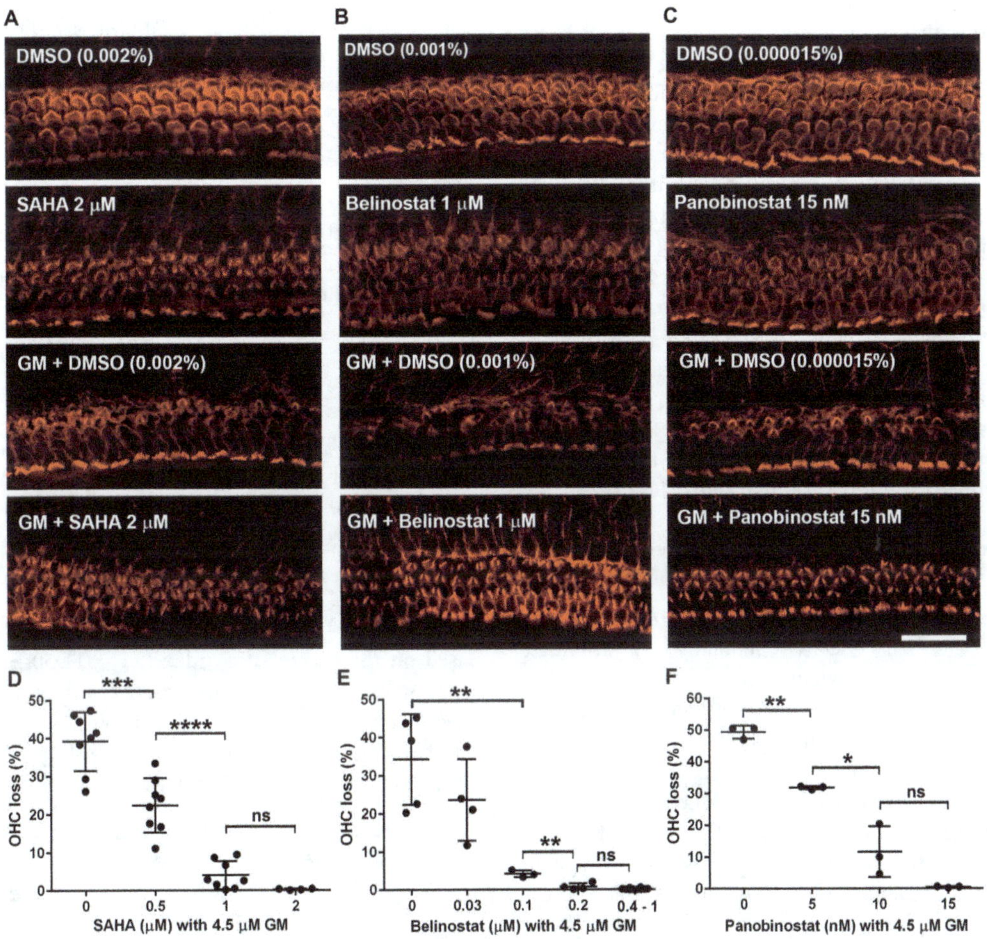

FIGURE 2 | HDAC inhibitors protect against gentamicin (GM)-induced hair cell loss in p3 murine explants. **(A–C)** Representative images show that administration of HDAC inhibitors (**A**: SAHA, **B**: belinostat, **C**: panobinostat) attenuated GM-induced sensory hair cell loss in the basal turn. Scale bar = 20 μm. **(D–F)** Quantification of HDAC inhibitors (**D**: SAHA, **E**: belinostat, **F**: panobinostat) prevented OHC loss from GM in a dose-dependent manner. Data are presented as individual points and means ± SD. *$p < 0.05$, **$p < 0.01$, ***$p < 0.001$, ****$p < 0.0001$, ns: not significant.

TABLE 2 | Therapeutic index (TI) of three HDAC inhibitors in murine explants.

HDAC inhibitors	TD_{50}	ED_{50}	TI (TD_{50}/ED_{50})
Vorinostat	5.5 μM	0.6 μM	9.2
Belinostat	3.5 μM	0.05 μM	70
Panobinostat	35 nM	9 nM	3.9

body weight concurrent with SQ injections of 120 mg GM base/kg body weight daily for 2 weeks with normal appearing fur and steadily increasing body weight. Blood samples were collected after the last injection. Renal function, assessed by BUN and creatinine (Cr) concentrations, was similar to that of control guinea pigs (detailed values see **Table 3**). However, the platelet concentration was significantly lower with the highest concentration of SAHA (25 mg/kg; $t_6 = 2.682$, $p = 0.037$) compared to GM alone treated groups (**Figure 4**).

SAHA Does Not Prevent Gentamicin-Induced Ototoxicity in Guinea Pigs *in Vivo*

Based on the experiments to assess safe doses of SAHA, we tested several doses of SAHA below 25 mg/kg body weight against 120 mg GM base/kg body weight daily for 2 weeks in guinea pigs *in vivo*. In agreement with our previous results, GM treatment induced significant auditory threshold shifts at high frequencies (**Figures 5A,B**) with an average shift of 40 dB at 12 kHz ($t_{10} = 3.128$, $p = 0.011$) and 60 dB at 32 kHz ($p < 0.0001$) and caused significant OHC loss in the basal turn ($F_{(1,4)} = 8.013$, $p = 0.047$; **Figures 5C,D**). Confirming the results from CBA/J mice, treatment with SAHA at a range of concentrations (LD: 2–5 mg/kg body weight or HD: 15–25 mg/kg body weight) did not attenuate GM-induced auditory threshold shifts at 12 ($F_{(2,19)} = 0.9708$, $p = 0.397$) and 32 kHz ($F_{(2,19)} = 0.03664$, $p = 0.964$) or loss of OHCs ($F_{(1,6)} = 0.849$, $p = 0.392$). DMSO (1.1 g/kg body weight) used as the solvent vehicle for SAHA did not affect GM-induced auditory threshold shifts (**Figure 5A**).

DISCUSSION

An intriguing line of evidence suggests that HDAC inhibitors could prove to be an effective modality to attenuate aminoglycoside-induced ototoxicity in acute models. The HDAC inhibitors trichostatin A and butyrate rescued hair cells from GM-induced damage in organotypic cultures of the cochlea (Chen et al., 2009), and butyrate also protected guinea pigs *in vivo* when locally applied to the middle ear (Wang et al., 2015). Systemic SAHA attenuated the acute effects of the ototoxic combination of KM and furosemide (Layman et al., 2015) and the trauma of exposure to excessive noise (Chen et al., 2016). The results presented here extend the palette of potential therapeutics to three clinically available HDAC inhibitors when studied in cochlear explants. *In vivo*, however, SAHA failed to reduce hair cell loss and threshold shifts induced by *chronic* aminoglycoside exposure both in mice and guinea pigs. This *in-vivo* result offers an

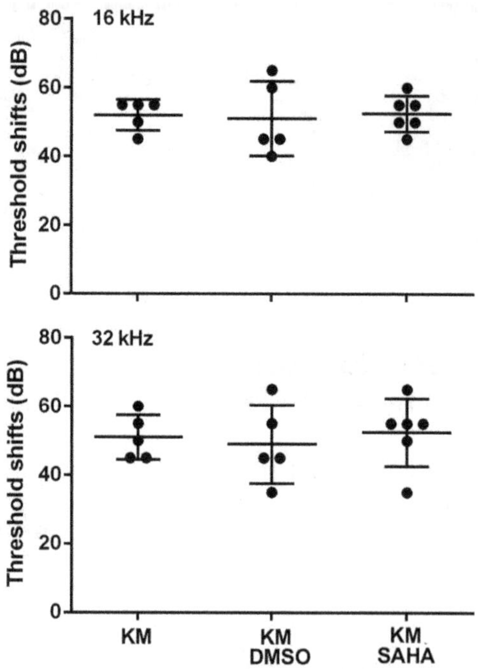

FIGURE 3 | Treatment with SAHA (50 mg/kg twice daily for 15 days) does not attenuate kanamycin (KM, 700 mg base/kg twice daily for 15 days)-induced auditory threshold shifts in CBA/J mice. Data are presented as individual points and means ± SD.

important caution because the chronic animal model better reflects clinical situations in which aminoglycosides tend to be administered for weeks, or even months in cases like tuberculosis.

In a chronic model the protective capability of the drug must be weighed against its potential side effects. Arguing for their safety, the chosen drugs are either FDA approved for treatment of cutaneous T-cell lymphoma (SAHA) or peripheral T-cell lymphoma (belinostat) or in a phase 3 trial for multiple myeloma (panobinostat). Indeed, although the median effective dose (ED50) varies, GM-induced OHC loss in explants is completely blocked by any of three HDAC inhibitors within non-toxic concentrations. However, as the explant studies also show, all three inhibitors tend to kill hair cells at higher concentrations. Based on the therapeutic index (TI = TD50/ED50), belinostat is the safest among the three HDAC inhibitors and might be selected for further *in-vivo* studies. We chose SAHA, however, based on published *in-vivo* data suggesting SAHA is suitable for prevention of inner ear trauma in mice (Layman et al.,

TABLE 3 | Guinea pigs renal function tests.

Groups	BUN	Cr	*n*
DMSO	17.8 ± 1.6	0.5 ± 0.19	5
SAHA (LD + HD)	17.5 ± 0.7	0.5 ± 0.007	2
GM + DMSO	16 ± 4.5	0.5 ± 0.22	4
GM + SAHA (LD)	17 ± 1.7	0.4 ± 0.06	6
GM + SAHA (HD)	17 ± 3.2	0.4 ± 0.08	5

LD: 2–5 mg/kg; HD: 15–25 mg/kg.

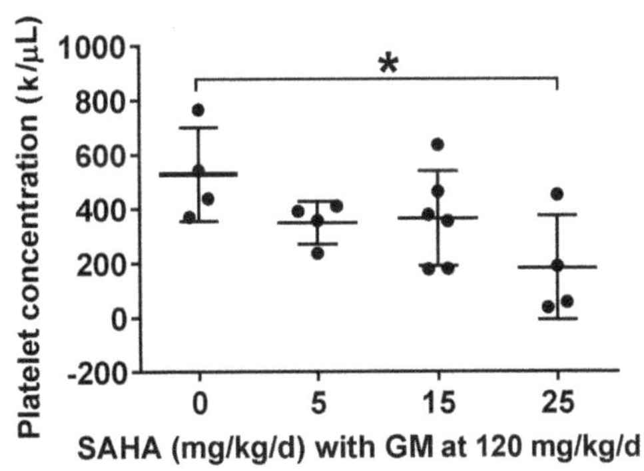

FIGURE 4 | Effects of SAHA treatment on platelet concentration. Treatment with SAHA for 2 weeks led to a decrease in platelet concentration, significant at 25 mg SAHA/kg with 120 mg GM base/kg in guinea pigs. Data are presented as individual points and means ± SD. $^{*}p < 0.05$.

2015; Chen et al., 2016). For example, administration of SAHA for 2 weeks at 100 mg/kg/day showed no ototoxicity in mice and IP injection of SAHA penetrates the mouse inner ear and crosses the blood-labyrinth barrier (Layman et al., 2015). SAHA also crosses the blood-brain barrier in a mouse model of Huntington's disease (Hockly et al., 2003) and thus can be expected to cross the blood-labyrinth barrier to the inner ear as well. We, therefore, tested SAHA in an established and reliable mouse model of chronic ototoxicity from 700 mg/kg KM twice per day for 2 weeks (Wu et al., 2001). Administration of SAHA at 100 mg/kg/day (dosed as SAHA at 50 mg/kg/twice daily concurrent with KM injections), however, did not prevent KM ototoxicity.

In order to challenge the robustness of our results and to rule out species-specific effects, we tested protection in the guinea pig, another well-established chronic model of GM-induced ototoxicity (Sha and Schacht, 1999b, 2000). In agreement with our previous data, treatment with GM at 120 mg/kg/day for 2 weeks resulted in significant elevations of auditory thresholds. Here again, administration of SAHA at low doses (2–5 mg/kg) or high doses (15–25 mg/kg/day) did not attenuate GM-induced auditory threshold shifts. Since the highest dose (25 mg/kg/day for 14 days) significantly reduced serum platelet concentrations, further increases in the dose of SAHA were considered to have no bearing for translational research.

The difference in the ability of SAHA to protect against inner ear insults in acute and chronic animal models of aminoglycoside-induced ototoxicity could be attributable to the vast differences between models used in the studies. In an acute model, as reported by Layman et al. (2015), the ototoxicity is induced by one SQ dose of KM with one dose of furosemide

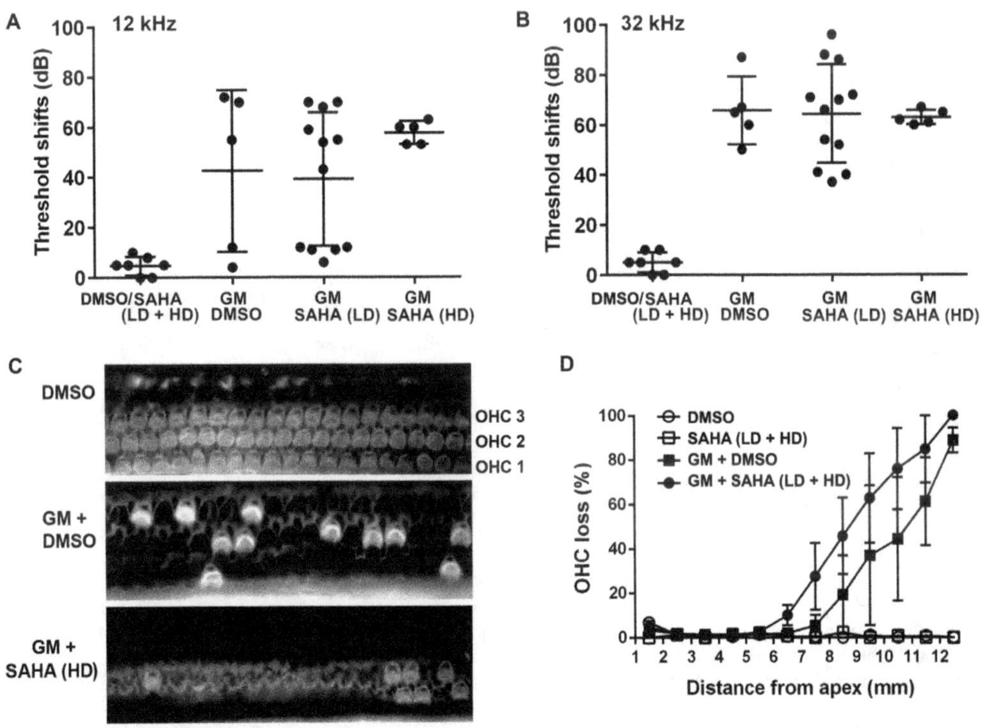

FIGURE 5 | Treatment with SAHA does not protect against GM-induced auditory threshold shifts and hair cell loss in pigmented guinea pigs *in vivo*. **(A,B)** Co-treatment with SAHA at low doses (2–5 mg/kg, LD) or high doses (15–25 mg/kg, HD) did not attenuate GM-induced (120 mg/kg, qd × 15 days) auditory threshold shifts at 12 kHz and 32 kHz. Data are presented as individual points and means ± SD. **(C)** Representative images illustrated OHC loss in the basal turn of surface preparations examined 1 week after 15 days of GM treatment. OHC1, 2 and 3 indicate the three rows of OHCs. Scale bar = 10 μm. **(D)** GM-induced OHC loss was not attenuated by treatment with SAHA in pigmented guinea pigs. Data are presented as means ± SD, n = 3–5 at each group.

via IP injection. In contrast, the chronic model of ototoxicity is induced by KM alone via SQ injection for 15 days twice per day. Although SAHA may cross the blood-labyrinth barrier to the inner ear, administration of furosemide or noise exposure may facilitate compounds crossing the blood-labyrinth barrier. Additionally, differences may be owed to the cell death pathways induced, as we previously reported that caspase-independent hair cell death predominates such chronic *in-vivo* models (Jiang et al., 2006). Such disparities may account for why some *in-vivo* models show a protective effect against aminoglycosides while others may not. Furthermore, such difference between acute and chronic models cautions that one cannot rely solely on *in-vitro* experiments to test the efficacy of otoprotectant compounds.

HDACs regulate acetylation of histone proteins at specific arginine and lysine residues, changing chromatin structure and altering gene expression. Acetylation tends to promote gene expression while inner ear insults such as aminoglycoside treatment or noise exposure promote histone deacetylation via HDACs. Among the four classes of mammalian HDACs identified (Dietz and Casaccia, 2010), class II has been recognized as having a pathogenic role in neurodegenerative diseases such as Alzheimer's disease (Falkenberg and Johnstone, 2014) and in HIV-infected neuronal cells (Atluri et al., 2014). In line with our previous and studies by others, the three HDAC inhibitors used in this study cover an even broader spectrum, acting as inhibitors of HDACs I, II, and VI (Chen et al., 2009, 2016; Layman et al., 2015).

The mechanism of the epigenetic effects of aminoglycosides remains unknown. Since aminoglycoside-induced ototoxicity is well documented to involve oxidative stress (Sha and Schacht, 1999a; Chen et al., 2013), it is reasonable to speculate that a pathway leading to the upregulation of HDAC involves oxidative stress, a condition that can lead to changes in genomic and epigenetic regulation of gene expression (Mikhed et al., 2015). In particular, gene expression mapping after ischemia-induced oxidative stress demonstrated cell-specific upregulation of HDAC 1, 2 and 3 in the brain (Baltan et al., 2011). Additionally, inner ear insults such as traumatic noise exposure induce oxidative stress (Ohlemiller et al., 1999; Yamashita et al., 2004; Yuan et al., 2015) and result in upregulation of HDAC 1, 2 and 3 in the inner ear of CBA/J mice (Chen et al., 2016).

In summary, this study highlights potential disparities between acute and chronic inner ear damage by demonstrating that treatment with the HDAC inhibitor SAHA attenuates aminoglycoside-induced ototoxicity *in vitro* but not *in vivo* in chronic animal models. Furthermore, our results suggest that the protective effects of other HDAC inhibitors against aminoglycoside-induced ototoxicity deserve careful exploration in animal models and more detailed studies, such as study of drug kinetics and permeability through the blood-labyrinth barrier, before these compounds are considered for clinical application.

AUTHOR CONTRIBUTIONS

C-HY performed *in vivo* and *in vitro* experiments. ZL conducted *in-vivo* experiments. DD conducted *in-vitro* experiments. JS designed research and commented on the manuscript. DA commented on the manuscript. S-HS designed research, analyzed data and wrote the article.

ACKNOWLEDGMENTS

The research project described was supported by grant R42GM097917 from the National Institute on General Medicine Sciences, National Institutes of Health, and P30 DC-005188 from the National Institute on Deafness and Other Communication Disorders, National Institutes of Health. We thank Thomas Schrepfer for conducting guinea pig hair cell counts and Andra Talaska for proofreading the manuscript.

SUPPLEMENTARY MATERIAL

FIGURE S1 | Typical ABR waveforms of CBA/J mice at 16 and 32 kHz. Baseline testing revealed normal ABRs measured before kanamycin (KM) treatment. The baseline thresholds at both 16 and 32 kHz were 25 dB SPL. I, II, III, IV and V indicate ABR waves I, II, III, IV and V. The images for KM, KM plus DMSO, and KM plus SAHA illustrate representative ABR waveforms measured 1 week after the end of 15 days of treatment.

REFERENCES

Atluri, V. S., Pilakka-Kanthikeel, S., Samikkannu, T., Sagar, V., Kurapati, K. R., Saxena, S. K., et al. (2014). Vorinostat positively regulates synaptic plasticity genes expression and spine density in HIV infected neurons: role of nicotine in progression of HIV-associated neurocognitive disorder. *Mol. Brain* 7:37. doi: 10.1186/1756-6606-7-37

Baltan, S., Bachleda, A., Morrison, R. S., and Murphy, S. P. (2011). Expression of histone deacetylases in cellular compartments of the mouse brain and the effects of ischemia. *Transl. Stroke Res.* 2, 411–423. doi: 10.1007/s12975-011-0087-z

Chen, J., Hill, K., and Sha, S. H. (2016). Inhibitors of histone deacetylases attenuate noise-induced hearing loss. *J. Assoc. Res. Otolaryngol.* 17, 289–302. doi: 10.1007/s10162-016-0567-7

Chen, F. Q., Schacht, J., and Sha, S. H. (2009). Aminoglycoside-induced histone deacetylation and hair cell death in the mouse cochlea. *J. Neurochem.* 108, 1226–1236. doi: 10.1111/j.1471-4159.2009.05871.x

Chen, F. Q., Zheng, H. W., Schacht, J., and Sha, S. H. (2013). Mitochondrial peroxiredoxin 3 regulates sensory cell survival in the cochlea. *PLoS One* 8:e61999. doi: 10.1371/journal.pone.0061999

Dietz, K. C., and Casaccia, P. (2010). HDAC inhibitors and neurodegeneration: at the edge between protection and damage. *Pharmacol. Res.* 62, 11–17. doi: 10.1016/j.phrs.2010.01.011

Falkenberg, K. J., and Johnstone, R. W. (2014). Histone deacetylases and their inhibitors in cancer, neurological diseases and immune disorders. *Nat. Rev. Drug Discov.* 13, 673–691. doi: 10.1038/nrd4360

Hockly, E., Richon, V. M., Woodman, B., Smith, D. L., Zhou, X., Rosa, E., et al. (2003). Suberoylanilide hydroxamic acid, a histone deacetylase inhibitor, ameliorates motor deficits in a mouse model of Huntington's disease. *Proc. Natl. Acad. Sci. U S A* 100, 2041–2046. doi: 10.1073/pnas.0437870100

Jiang, H., Sha, S.-H., Forge, A., and Schacht, J. (2006). Caspase-independent pathways of hair cell death induced by kanamycin *in vivo*. *Cell Death Differ.* 13, 20–30. doi: 10.1038/sj.cdd.4401706

Layman, W. S., Williams, D. M., Dearman, J. A., Sauceda, M. A., and Zuo, J. (2015). Histone deacetylase inhibition protects hearing against acute ototoxicity by activating the Nf-kappaB pathway. *Cell Death Discov.* 1:15012. doi: 10.1038/cddiscovery.2015.12

Marks, P., Rifkind, R. A., Richon, V. M., Breslow, R., Miller, T., and Kelly, W. K. (2001). Histone deacetylases and cancer: causes and therapies. *Nat. Rev. Cancer* 1, 194–202. doi: 10.1038/35106079

Mikhed, Y., Gorlach, A., Knaus, U. G., and Daiber, A. (2015). Redox regulation of genome stability by effects on gene expression, epigenetic pathways and DNA damage/repair. *Redox Biol.* 5, 275–289. doi: 10.1016/j.redox.2015.05.008

Ohlemiller, K. K., Wright, J. S., and Dugan, L. L. (1999). Early elevation of cochlear reactive oxygen species following noise exposure. *Audiol. Neurootol.* 4, 229–236. doi: 10.1159/000013846

Sha, S. H., and Schacht, J. (1999a). Formation of reactive oxygen species following bioactivation of gentamicin. *Free Radic. Biol. Med.* 26, 341–347. doi: 10.1016/s0891-5849(98)00207-x

Sha, S. H., and Schacht, J. (1999b). Salicylate attenuates gentamicin-induced ototoxicity. *Lab Invest.* 79, 807–813.

Sha, S. H., and Schacht, J. (2000). Antioxidants attenuate gentamicin-induced free radical formation *in vitro* and ototoxicity *in vivo*: D-methionine is a potential protectant. *Hear. Res.* 142, 34–40. doi: 10.1016/s0378-5955(00)00003-4

Sha, S. H., Zajic, G., Epstein, C. J., and Schacht, J. (2001). Overexpression of copper/zinc-superoxide dismutase protects from kanamycin-induced hearing loss. *Audiol. Neurootol.* 6, 117–123. doi: 10.1159/000046818

Wang, J., Wang, Y., Chen, X., Zhang, P. Z., Shi, Z. T., Wen, L. T., et al. (2015). Histone deacetylase inhibitor sodium butyrate attenuates gentamicin-induced hearing loss *in vivo*. *Am. J. Otolaryngol.* 36, 242–248. doi: 10.1016/j.amjoto.2014.11.003

Wen, L. T., Wang, J., Wang, Y., and Chen, F. Q. (2015). Association between histone deacetylases and the loss of cochlear hair cells: role of the former in noise-induced hearing loss. *Int. J. Mol. Med.* 36, 534–540. doi: 10.3892/ijmm.2015.2236

Wu, W. J., Sha, S. H., McLaren, J. D., Kawamoto, K., Raphael, Y., and Schacht, J. (2001). Aminoglycoside ototoxicity in adult CBA, C57BL and BALB mice and the Sprague-Dawley rat. *Hear. Res.* 158, 165–178. doi: 10.1016/s0378-5955(01)00303-3

Yamashita, D., Jiang, H. Y., Schacht, J., and Miller, J. M. (2004). Delayed production of free radicals following noise exposure. *Brain Res.* 1019, 201–209. doi: 10.1016/j.brainres.2004.05.104

Yuan, H., Wang, X., Hill, K., Chen, J., Lemasters, J., Yang, S. M., et al. (2015). Autophagy attenuates noise-induced hearing loss by reducing oxidative stress. *Antioxid. Redox Signal.* 22, 1308–1324. doi: 10.1089/ars.2014.6004

10

Activation of CHK1 in Supporting Cells Indirectly Promotes Hair Cell Survival

Azadeh Jadali [1,2,3]***, Yu-Lan M. Ying*** [4] ***and Kelvin Y. Kwan*** [1,2]*****

[1]Department of Cell Biology and Neuroscience, Rutgers University, Piscataway, NJ, USA, [2]Stem Cell Research Center and Keck Center for Collaborative Neuroscience, Rutgers University, Piscataway, NJ, USA, [3]3D Biotek, Bridgewater, NJ, USA, [4]Department of Otolaryngology—Head and Neck Surgery, Rutgers New Jersey Medical School, Newark, NJ, USA

Edited by:
Lisa Cunningham, National Institutes of Health (NIH), USA

Reviewed by:
Ertugrul Kilic, Istanbul Medipol University, Turkey
Su-Hua Sha, Medical University of South Carolina, USA

****Correspondence:***
Kelvin Y. Kwan
kwan@dls.rutgers.edu

The sensory hair cells of the inner ear are exquisitely sensitive to ototoxic insults. Loss of hair cells after exposure to ototoxic agents causes hearing loss. Chemotherapeutic agents such as cisplatin causes hair cell loss. Cisplatin forms DNA mono-adducts as well as intra- and inter-strand DNA crosslinks. DNA cisplatin adducts are repaired through the DNA damage response. The decision between cell survival and cell death following DNA damage rests on factors that are involved in determining damage tolerance, cell survival and apoptosis. Cisplatin damage on hair cells has been the main focus of many ototoxic studies, yet the effect of cisplatin on supporting cells has been largely ignored. In this study, the effects of DNA damage response in cochlear supporting cells were interrogated. Supporting cells play a major role in the development, maintenance and oto-protection of hair cells. Loss of supporting cells may indirectly affect hair cell survival or maintenance. Activation of the Phosphoinositide 3-Kinase (PI3K) signaling was previously shown to promote hair cell survival. To test whether activating PI3K signaling promotes supporting cell survival after cisplatin damage, cochlear explants from the neural subset (NS) Cre *Pten* conditional knockout mice were employed. Deletion of Phosphatase and Tensin Homolog (PTEN) activates PI3K signaling in multiple cell types within the cochlea. Supporting cells lacking PTEN showed increased cell survival after cisplatin damage. Supporting cells lacking PTEN also showed increased phosphorylation of Checkpoint Kinase 1 (CHK1) levels after cisplatin damage. Nearest neighbor analysis showed increased numbers of supporting cells with activated PI3K signaling in close proximity to surviving hair cells in cisplatin damaged cochleae. We propose that increased PI3K signaling promotes supporting cell survival through phosphorylation of CHK1 and increased survival of supporting cells indirectly increases hair cell survival after cisplatin damage.

Keywords: cisplatin, ototoxicity, cochlea, supporting cell, cell survival, PI3 kinase signaling, AKT, CHK1

INTRODUCTION

Sensorineural hearing loss caused by the exposure to loud sounds and ototoxic drugs results in the loss of sensory hair cells and spiral ganglion neurons of the inner ear. Cisplatin is a potent antitumor agent used for its wide clinical activity against many different types of tumors (Wang and Lippard, 2005). A side effect of cisplatin-induced hearing loss is the loss of cochlear hair cells (Rybak et al., 2009; Schacht et al., 2012). Systemic injection of cisplatin results in discernable cisplatin-DNA adducts in hair cells and supporting cells that reside in the organ of Corti (van Ruijven et al., 2005). Supporting cells have distinct morphology and specific anatomical locations within the organ of Corti. Dieters' cells reside below the outer hair cells (OHC), inner and outer pillar cells form the tunnel of Corti while Hensen's and Claudius cells are located in the outer sulcus. These cells contribute to the microarchitecture observed in the sensory epithelium (Monzack and Cunningham, 2013; Wan et al., 2013). In addition to maintaining the cytoarchitecture in the cochlea, supporting cells such as inner border cells and inner phalangeal play critical roles in development, maintenance and synaptogenesis of hair cells (Gómez-Casati et al., 2010; Mellado Lagarde et al., 2014). Supporting cells can phagocytose dying hair cells to clear up cellular debris in the sensory epithelium (Bird et al., 2010; Monzack et al., 2015). Supporting cells can protect hair cells from damage by secreting the Heat Shock Protein 70 (HSP70; May et al., 2013). Systemic application of cisplatin shows that supporting cells are structurally damaged and could contribute to delayed hair cell loss (Ramírez-Camacho et al., 2004). Furthermore, after cisplatin damage, phagocytosis of dead hair cells by supporting cells is impaired (Monzack et al., 2015). These studies suggest that supporting cells play distinct cellular roles to maintain proper cochlear function and may be targets of cisplatin damage.

Cytotoxicity after cisplatin exposure is caused by the formation of intra- and inter-strand DNA crosslinks as well as cisplatin DNA adducts (Wang and Lippard, 2005). DNA damage activates several signal transduction pathways that include Ataxia Telangiectasia and Rad3 Related Protein (ATR), p53, p73 and Mitogen-Activated Protein Kinase (MAPK) and results in either cell survival or apoptosis (Siddik, 2003). Checkpoint Kinase 1 (CHK1) is a key downstream target that is phosphorylated by ATR at serine residues 345 and 317 (Zhao and Piwnica-Worms, 2001). Phosphorylation of CHK1 increases kinase activity and initiates the DNA damage response by activating DNA damage repair, DNA damage checkpoints and cell death proteins (Zhang and Hunter, 2014). DNA damage-mediated apoptotic signals can be attenuated as observed in cisplatin resistant tumor cells. Cisplatin resistant cancer cells arise when propagation of the DNA damage signal to the apoptotic machinery is inhibited. These mechanisms include activation of the Phosphoinositide 3-Kinase (PI3K)/RAC-Alpha Serine Threonine Protein Kinase (PI3K/AKT) signaling, loss of p53 function and overexpression of anti-apoptotic factors such as B-cell leukemia/lymphoma 2 (BCL2) to promote cell survival (Siddik, 2003). In this study, we determined whether phosphorylation of CHK1 promotes cochlear supporting cell survival after cisplatin damage.

MATERIALS AND METHODS

Cell Culture

Immortalized multipotent otic progenitor (iMOP) cells were grown in suspension with DMEM/F12 (Life Technologies) containing B27 supplement (Life Technologies), 25 μg/ml carbenicillin and 20 ng/ml basic fibroblast growth factor (bFGF; Pepro Tech; Jadali et al., 2016). For differentiation experiments, cells were cultured for 3 or 7 days in the absence of bFGF depending on the experiment. iMOP cells were treated with LY294002 (LC laboratories), bpV(Hopic; Santa Cruz Biotechnology, Inc., Santa Cruz, CA, USA) or cisplatin (Sigma) at the specified concentrations. LY294002 and bpV(Hopic) were solubilized in dimethyl sulfoxide (DMSO) and added to medium as described. Cisplatin was dissolved into medium and warmed to 37°C to make a 1 mM stock solution. Cisplatin solution was diluted into culture medium at the described concentrations.

Proliferation and EdU Incorporation Assays

For 5-ethynyl-2′-deoxyuridine (EdU) labeling, the Click-iT EdU Alexa Fluor 488 assay kit (Life Technologies) was used. iMOP cells were pulsed with 1 μM EdU for 2 h. After EdU incorporation, cells were removed from culture, dissociated to generate single cells, fixed, labeled EdU with Alexafluor 488 by click chemistry, resuspended in 1× PBS containing 0.1% Tween 20 and mounted on a slide. Fluorescent images of labeled cells were taken using epifluorescence microscopy and the percentage of EdU positive cells in 1000 nuclei was determined.

Flow Cytometry and Apoptosis Assay

iMOP cells were differentiated for 3 days before they were treated with 50 μM cisplatin alone, or pre-treated with 25 μM LY294002 or 10 μM bpV(HOpic) for 1 h before treatment with 50 μM cisplatin. Apoptotic cells were analyzed 24 h after treatment with small molecules. To identify apoptotic cells, the Alexa Fluor 488 annexin V/PI dead cell apoptosis kit was used (Life Technologies) according to manufacturer's instructions. Cells labeled with Alexa Fluor 488 annexin V and/or PI and were quantified by flow cytometry using a Beckman Coulter Gallios flow cytometer with the appropriate filters.

Western Blot Analysis

Cells were lysed in lysis buffer (50 mM Tris/HCl, pH 7.5, 150 mM NaCl, 1 mM EDTA, 1 mM EGTA, 1% Triton X-100, and 10% glycerol containing phosphatase inhibitor (Thermo Scientific) and a mixture of protease inhibitors (Roche). Protein lysates (30 μg) were loaded and separated on 4%–12% Bis Tris Novax NuPAGE gradient gels (Life Technologies), transferred to PVDF membrane, and incubated in blocking buffer (phosphate-buffered saline (PBS), 0.1% Tween 20 and 5% nonfat dried milk) for 1 h. To detect proteins of interest, membranes were incubated overnight at 4°C with primary antibodies. Immunoreactive bands were detected by incubating with horseradish peroxidase-conjugated secondary antibodies, followed by application of chemiluminescence substrate (Pierce ECL, Thermo Fisher Scientific). Membranes were exposed to either X-ray film (RPI) or Amersham Hyperfilm ECL (GE Healthcare) for signal detection before film development. To detect multiple proteins using the same membrane, membranes were stripped and re-probed with the

TABLE 1 | Antibodies and Small Molecules.

Antibody/Small molecule	Company	Use	Dilution
AKT	Cell Signaling Technologies	Western blot	1:3000/1:1000
pAKT-Thr308	Cell Signaling Technologies	Western blot	1:1000
CHK1	Cell Signaling Technologies	Western blot	1:1000
pCHK1-Ser345	Cell Signaling Technologies	Western blot/Immunostaining	1:1000/1:100
ACTB	Santa Cruz Biotechnology	Western blot	1:1000
MYO7A	Proteus	Immunostaining	1:1000
Phalloidin-Alexafluor 647	Life Technologies	Immunostaining	1:400

appropriate primary antibodies. Quantification of the intensity from individual bands was done using Photoshop. Antibodies and dilutions of antibodies for Western blot are described in **Table 1**.

Cochlear Explant Cultures

Cochleae from P4–6 pups were dissected and cleaned of surrounding tissue and bone. The stria vascularis was trimmed and the Reissner's and the tectorial membrane peeled away to expose the sensory epithelium. To ensure that the explanted cochlea adhered to the bottom of the coverglass, the cochlea was cut into three individual pieces and adhered onto a 1.5 cover glass treated with 10 μg/ml poly-L-ornithine. Cochlear explants were cultured in DMEM/F12 containing 10% FBS, 2 mM L-Glutamine and 25 μg/ml carbenicillin. One day after plating, cochleae were treated with either 10 μM bpV(HOpic) or DMSO before addition of 20 μM cisplatin. Hair cells counts per 200 μm were divided into base, middle and apical regions of the cochlear explants and used to determine the percent of surviving hair cells along the tonotopic axis.

Immunofluorescence Staining

Conditions used for immunostaining of iMOP cells were previously described (Kwan et al., 2015). Cochlear explants were fixed in 4% formaldehyde with 1× PBS for 1 h, permeabilized in wash buffer (PBS and 0.1% Triton X-100) for 10 min, incubated in blocking buffer (PBS, 10% goat serum and 0.1% Triton X-100) for 1 h and incubated overnight with a 1:500 dilution of Myosin 7A (MYO7A; Proteus Biosciences) primary antibody in blocking buffer. For CHK1 labeling, antigen retrieval was accomplished by incubating fixed cochlea in 150 mM Tris-HCl at pH 9.0 for 5 min, followed by heating at 70°C for 15 min. Cochleae were rinsed in wash buffer before incubating overnight with a 1:100 dilution of pCHK1 (Cell Signaling) antibodies in blocking buffer. Detection of primary antibodies was done by removing the primary antibody solutions and washing the cochleae in wash buffer three times before incubating in 1:500 dilution of goat anti-rabbit Alexa Fluor 488 secondary antibody and 1:500 phalloidin Alexa Fluor 647 (Life Technologies) in blocking buffer for 2 h. Cochleae were rinsed and mounted on slides with prolong gold antifade mounting media (Life Technologies). Immunofluorescence images were obtained using a Zeiss 510 confocal microscope with a 40 × 1.3 NA water immersion objective. The average percent of MYO7A positive inner hair cells (IHC) and OHC were obtained by calculating the percentage of MYO7A cells along the cochlear axis from treated cochlear explants relative to untreated controls. Antibodies and dilutions of antibodies for immunostaining are described in **Table 1**.

Biohazardous Material

All biohazardous material such as LY294002, bpV (HOpic) and cisplatin were handled in a laminar flow hood and appropriately disposed after usage as recommended by Rutgers Environmental Health and Safety (REHS).

Animals

All mice were housed in the Nelson Labs animal facility in microisolator cages. Neural subset (NS) Cre *PTEN* mice in the B6;129S4 genetic background were previously described (Jadali and Kwan, 2016). This study was carried out in accordance with the recommendations of the Rutgers Animal Care and Facilities Committee (ACFC). The protocol was approved by the Rutgers University Institutional Animal Care and Use Committee (IACUC).

Statistical Analysis

All error bars shown in data are expressed as ± standard deviation (SD) of values obtained from independent experiments unless otherwise stated. The numbers (n) of independent experiments or individual wells from separate cultures are listed for experiments. Technical triplicates were included in each experiment. An unpaired two-tailed Student's t-test was used to determine statistical significance and associated with the appropriate p value. For all figures p values are defines as: $^{*}p < 0.05$, $^{**}p < 1 \times 10^{-2}$, $^{***}p < 1 \times 10^{-3}$ and $^{****}p < 1 \times 10^{-4}$ unless otherwise stated.

RESULTS

Differentiating iMOP Cells Express Hair Cell and Supporting Cell Markers

To identify signaling pathways that maintain hair cell survival, we used iMOP cells that can self-renew and differentiate into hair cells and supporting cells (Kwan et al., 2015). Differentiating iMOP cells were generated by withdrawing bFGF for 7 days, to promote cell cycle exit and differentiation (Jadali et al., 2016). To determine the proliferative capacity of proliferating or differentiating iMOP cultures, incorporation of the nucleotide analog EdU was used. As iMOP cells progress through the cell cycle and undergo DNA replication, EdU was incorporated into the DNA. Incorporation of EdU provides an index for proliferation. Proliferating iMOP cells and differentiating iMOP cells normally grow as clusters of cells, or otospheres. To allow for unambiguous cell counts, otospheres from iMOP cultures were dissociated, fixed and labeled with Hoechst after EdU incorporation. Proliferating iMOP cells showed EdU labeling in 37.9% ± 2.5 of Hoechst labeled nuclei (**Figure 1A**). Differentiating iMOP cells showed EdU labeling in 3.3% ± 1.2 of Hoechst labeled nuclei (**Figure 1B**). A significant 11.5 fold reduction ($p < 1 \times 10^{-4}$) in cells that have undergone DNA replication was observed in differentiating cells compared to proliferating cells. These results suggest that the vast majority of differentiating iMOP cells were no longer progressing through the cell cycle.

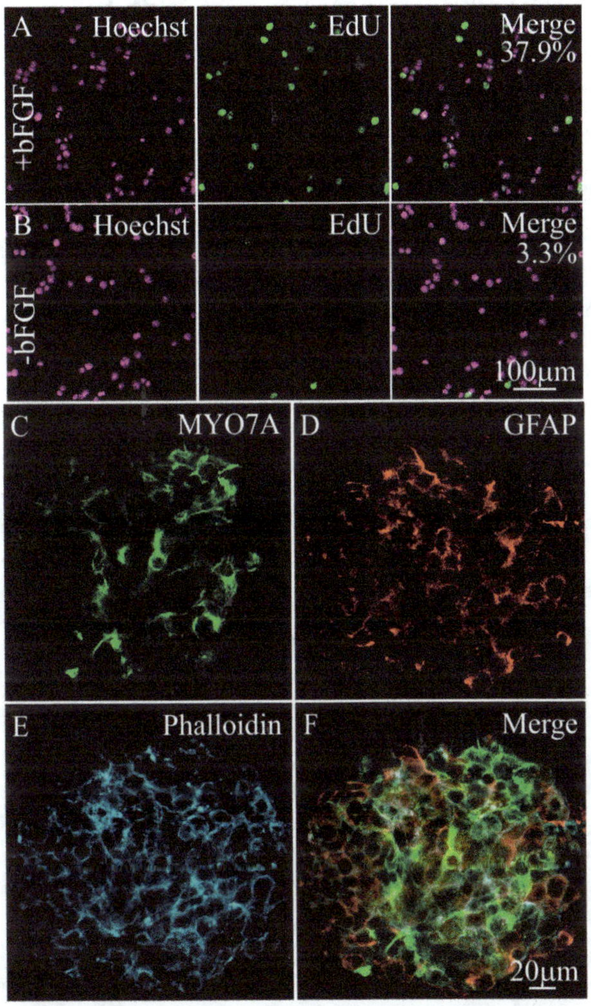

FIGURE 1 | Expression of hair cell and supporting cell markers in differentiating immortalized multipotent otic progenitor (iMOP) cells. Proliferating iMOP cells cultured in basic fibroblast growth factor (bFGF) were subjected to 5-ethynyl-2'-deoxyuridine (EdU) incorporation. **(A)** Hoechst labeled nuclei from proliferating iMOP cells show EdU incorporation in 37.9% of cells (n = 3). **(B)** Hoechst labeled nuclei from differentiating iMOP cells showed EdU incorporation in 3.3% of cells (n = 3). Differentiating iMOP cells express **(C)** MYO7A and **(D)** glial fibrillary acidic protein (GFAP) in **(E)** phalloidin marked otospheres. **(F)** Otospheres from differentiating iMOP cultures were used to test for the effects of cisplatin treatment.

To determine the extent of differentiation, otospheres from differentiating iMOP cultures were harvested, fixed and immmunostained with antibodies against MYO7A, a hair cell marker and glial fibrillary acidic protein (GFAP), a supporting cell marker. Differentiating iMOP cells showed MYO7A (**Figure 1C**) and GFAP (**Figure 1D**) labeling. Otospheres from differentiating iMOP cells also showed circumferential actin after phalloidin labeling (**Figure 1E**) that was reminiscent of actin filament distribution in the developing cochlea sensory epithelium. Differentiating iMOP cultures containing MYO7A and GFAP expressing cells were subsequently employed as a cellular platform to study the effects of cisplatin damage in hair cells and supporting cells (**Figure 1F**).

Activation of PI3K Promotes iMOP Cell Survival after Cisplatin Damage

Since PI3K signaling has been implicated in maintaining hair cell survival after aminoglycoside damage (Chung et al., 2006; Jadali and Kwan, 2016), we determined whether PI3K signaling was also involved in promoting supporting cell survival after cisplatin damage. To test how PI3K signaling affects cell survival, differentiating iMOP cells were treated with small molecules that activated or inhibited PI3K signaling. To activate PI3K/AKT signaling, we used the small molecule bpV(HOpic) that inhibits phosphatase tension homolog deleted on chromosome 10 (*PTEN*) and increase phosphatidylinositol-3,4,5-trisphosphate (PIP_3) levels. Excess PIP_3 at the cell membrane increases PI3K signaling (Cantley and Neel, 1999; Doillon et al., 1999; Schmid et al., 2004). As a control, the small molecule LY294002 was used as an inhibitor of PI3K activity (Vlahos et al., 1994). The concentrations of small molecules employed was previously identified from dose response curves (Jadali and Kwan, 2016). Activator or inhibitor of PI3K signaling was added before cisplatin-induced damage in differentiating iMOP cells and apoptotic cells were quantified by flow cytometry analysis. Differentiating iMOP cells were treated with cisplatin, harvested and subjected to dual labeling with propidium iodide (PI) and Alexafluor 488-conjugated annexin V. Treated samples were compared to DMSO treated controls. FACS analysis was employed to identify apoptotic cells labeled with PI and apoptotic marker annexin V (Vermes et al., 1995). The percentage of viable cells (PI- annexin V) in the lower left quadrant and the apoptotic cells (PI+ annexin V+) in the upper right quadrant of the FACS plot were quantified. In control, 64.2% viable cells and 28.7% apoptotic cells were observed (**Figure 2A**). Treatment with 50 μM cisplatin in differentiating iMOP cells resulted in 26.4% viable cells and 68.1% apoptotic cells (**Figure 2B**). These results suggest an increase in apoptotic cells after cisplatin treatment.

To test whether activation of the PI3K pathway would promote cell survival after cisplatin treatment, differentiating iMOP cells were cultured with 10 μM of bpV(HOpic) for 1 day before cisplatin treatment. Pre-treatment with bpV(HOpic)

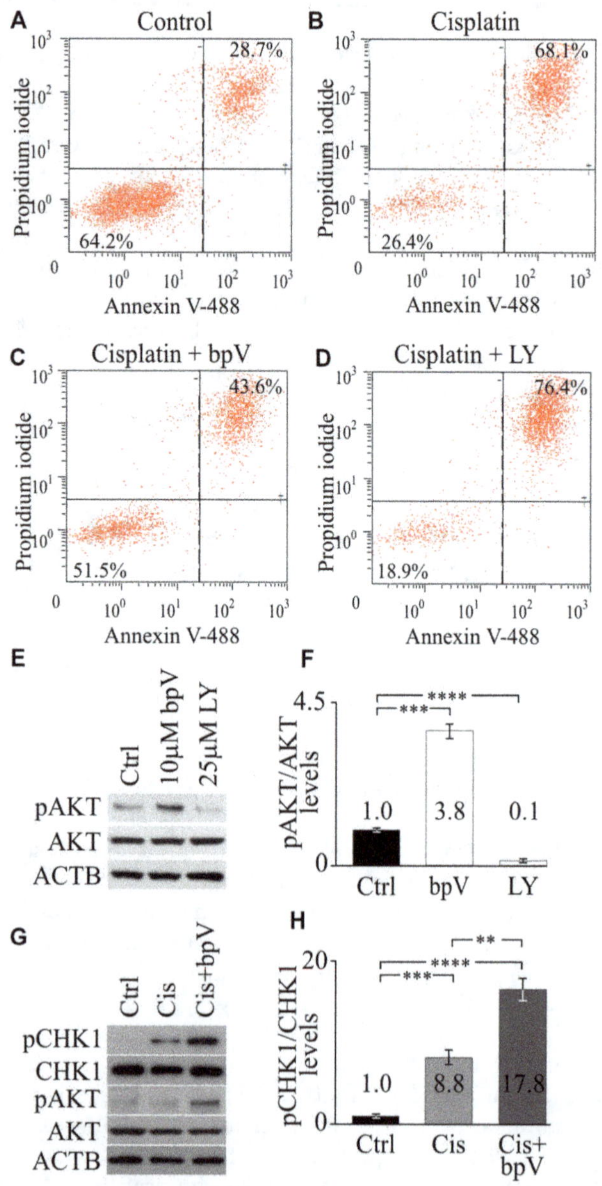

FIGURE 2 | Checkpoint Kinase 1 (CHK1) phosphorylation after activating phosphoinositide 3-kinase (PI3K) signaling. Propidium iodide (PI) and annexin V FACS analysis of **(A)** control dimethyl sulfoxide (DMSO), **(B)** cisplatin **(C)** cisplatin and bpV(HOpic) and **(D)** cisplatin and LY treated cells from representative plots. Average percentage of cells from viable (PI- annexin V-) and apoptotic (PI+ annexin V+) quandrants were displayed (n = 4). **(E)** Western blot of phospho-AKT (pAKT), total AKT and ACTB in control DMSO, 10 μM bpV(HOpic) or 25 μM LY294002 treated cells (n = 4). **(F)** Quantification of pAKT/AKT ratio from Western blots (n = 4). **(G)** Western blot of pCHK1, total phospho-CHK1 (CHK1), pAKT, total AKT and ACTB in control DMSO, 20 μM cisplatin, 20 μM cisplatin and 10 μM bpV(HOpic) treated cells (n = 4). **(H)** Quantification of pCHK1/CHK1 ratios from Western blots (n = 4). Statistical significance was determined using the Student's t-test and error bars are in standard deviation (SD).

resulted in 51.5% viable cells and 43.6% apoptotic cells (**Figure 2C**). Compared to cisplatin treatment alone, addition of bpV(HOpic) increased the percentage of viable cells. These results suggested that addition of bpV(HOpic) promotes cell survival even after exposure to cisplatin. To implicate the role of PI3K signaling in cell survival, LY294002, an inhibitor for PI3K activity was used. Differentiating iMOP cells were pretreated with 25 μM LY294002 before cisplatin treatment resulted in 18.9% viable cells and 76.4% apoptotic cells (**Figure 2D**). Inhibition of PI3K signaling increased the percentage of apoptotic cells. Together, these results suggest that activation of the PI3K signaling pathway may attenuate apoptosis and promote cell survival in differentiating iMOP cells.

Activation of PI3K Increases CHK1 Phosphorylation after Cisplatin Damage

To ensure that small molecules had the appropriate effect on PI3K signaling, phosphorylated RAC-alpha serine/threonine protein kinase (AKT) levels were employed as a measure of PI3K signaling activity. Western blot for phospho-AKT (pAKT), AKT and β-Actin (ACTB) was performed on cell lysates obtained from untreated control, 10 μM bpV(HOpic) treated and 25 μM LY294002 treated differentiating iMOP cultures (**Figure 2E**). ACTB served as a loading control. To quantify the amount of pAKT and total AKT, Western blot signals from the appropriate bands were quantified and the ratio of pAKT to AKT levels was determined. Signals were then normalized to untreated control and presented as fold change. After treatment with 10 μM bpV(HOpic), a significant 3.8 ± 0.32 fold increase in normalized pAKT levels was observed compared to control ($p < 1 \times 10^{-3}$). Treatment of differentiating iMOP cells with 25 μM LY294002 showed a significant 10 ± 0.02 fold decrease in normalized pAKT levels compared to control ($p < 1 \times 10^{-4}$; **Figure 2F**). These results suggested that 10 μM bpV(HOpic) and 25 μM LY294002 can be used to activate or inhibit PI3K signaling respectively in differentiating iMOP cells.

Following cisplatin damage, CHK1, an evolutionarily conserved protein kinase that regulates DNA damage repair is phosphorylated and activated by ATR (Zhao and Piwnica-Worms, 2001). ATR phosphorylates CHK1 at serine residues 317 and 345 in response to DNA damage (Zhao and Piwnica-Worms, 2001). Phosphorylation of CHK1 at Ser345 serves to localize CHK1 to the nucleus following DNA damage checkpoint activation (Jiang et al., 2003). To determine the effects of PI3K signaling in DNA damage response in differentiating iMOP cells, phosphorylation of CHK1 at Ser345 was determined by Western blot using phospho-specific antibodies. Differentiating iMOP cultures were treated with cisplatin to determine if phospho-CHK1 (pCHK1) levels increased relative to untreated control. To promote cell survival and determine the effects of activating PI3K signaling on pCHK1 levels, differentiating iMOP cultures were pretreated with 10 μM bpV(HOpic) before inducing cisplatin damage. Lysates from iMOP cultures were collected and used for Western blot analysis. ACTB was used as a loading control (**Figure 2G**). The ratio of pCHK1 and total CHK1 were used to determine normalized pCHK1 levels and represent the extent of DNA damage response. After treatment with 10 μM cisplatin alone, a significant 8.8 ± 1.0 fold increase in normalized pCHK1 levels was observed compared to untreated control ($p < 1 \times 10^{-3}$; **Figure 2H**). This suggests that cisplatin damage of differentiating iMOP cells activated the DNA damage response. To determine if activation of PI3K signaling alters pCHK1 levels, differentiating iMOP cultures were pretreated with bpV(HOpic) before cisplatin. Normalized pAKT levels were used as a measure of PI3K signaling activity. As observed in the Western blot, addition of bpV(HOpic) increased normalized pAKT levels 3.2 ± 0.2 fold relative to untreated control and increased 3.5 ± 0.5 fold relative to cisplatin treated cultures (**Figure 2G**). These results suggest that addition of bpV(HOpic) activates PI3K signaling. Pretreating iMOP cells with 10 μM bpV(HOpic) before incubating in 10 μM cisplatin resulted in a significant increase in pCHK1 levels (**Figure 2G**). Quantification of the Western blot showed a 17.8 ± 1.5 fold increase in normalized pCHK1 levels compared to untreated control ($p < 1 \times 10^{-4}$; **Figure 2H**). Comparing cisplatin treated sample to bpV(HOpic) and cisplatin treated samples, a significant 2.0 fold increase in normalized pCHK1 levels was observed ($p < 1 \times 10^{-2}$; **Figure 2H**). The results suggest that activation of PI3K signaling increases phosphorylation of CHK1 after cisplatin damage and could promote survival of differentiating iMOP cells.

Activation of PI3K Signaling Using bpV(HOpic) Promotes Hair Cell Survival after Cisplatin Damage

The above results suggested that activation of PI3K signaling could enhance CHK1 phosphorylation and promote a DNA damage response to increase cell survival. We previously showed that activation of PI3K signaling could promote hair cell survival (Jadali and Kwan, 2016). We wanted to extend our findings and determine if activation of the PI3K signaling can promote supporting cell survival in the cochlea when subjected to ototoxic damage. Since hair cell survival may depend on the oto-protective effect and maintenance of supporting cells (May et al., 2013; Mellado Lagarde et al., 2014), we used hair cells counts and hair cell organization as an indirect indicator for the presence of supporting cells after challenging cochlea explants with cisplatin.

To induce cochlear damage, murine cochlear explants were exposed to cisplatin. Cochleas were obtained from early post-natal day (P) 4–6 mice and cultured for a day to allow for recovery before addition of 10 μM bpV(HOpic). After bpV(HOpic) treatment, cochleae were exposed to 20 μM of cisplatin for 24 h before cisplatin and bpV(HOpic) were removed. Fresh medium without cisplatin or bpV(HOpic) was added to the cochlear cultures. The cochlear explants were allowed to recover for an additional 3 days, fixed and subjected to immunostaining (**Figure 3A**). Cochleae were immmunostained with antibodies against MYO7A to label IHC and OHC bodies while phalloidin highlighted the actin filled hair bundles and the actin filaments in the sensory epithelium (**Figure 3B**). In control untreated cochlear explants, the typical one row of IHC and

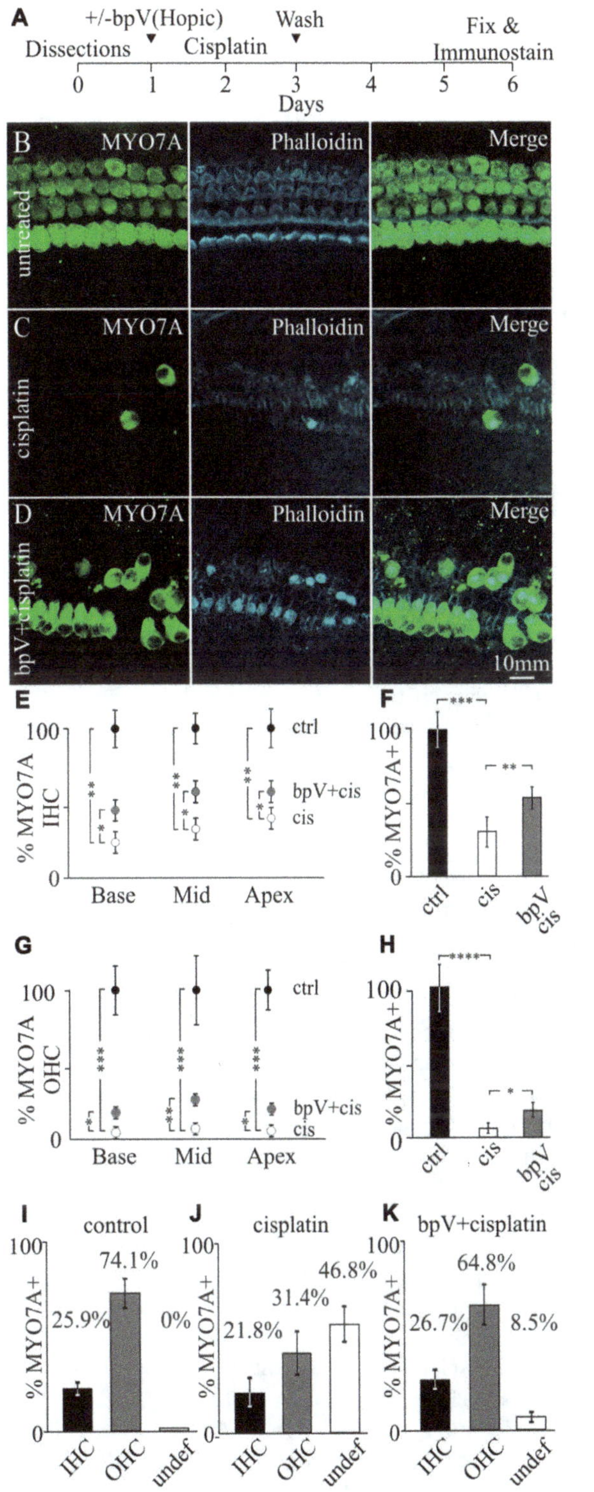

FIGURE 3 | Effects of bpV(HOpic) on hair cell survival after cisplatin damage. (A) Timeline of cochlear explant cultures describing the addition of 10 μM bpV(HOpic) 1 day before 10 μM cisplatin treatment and harvesting of explants for immunostaining. Immunofluorescence of MYO7A, phalloidin and merged images from **(B)** control cochlear explant (*n* = 4), **(C)** cochlear explant treated with cisplatin (*n* = 4) and **(D)** cochlear explant pretreated with

(Continued)

FIGURE 3 | Continued
10 μM bpV(HOpic) before cisplatin damage ($n = 4$). **(E)** Quantification of MYO7A inner hair cells (IHC) from the basal, middle and apical regions of cochlea explants in control (black), cisplatin (white) and bpV(HOpic)/cisplatin (gray; $n = 4$). **(F)** Average percent of IHC in control (black; $n = 4$), cisplatin (white; $n = 4$) and bpV(HOpic) and cisplatin (gray; $n = 4$) treated explants normalized to control. **(G)** Percentage of MYO7A outer hair cells (OHC) in control (black; $n = 4$), bpV(HOpic) and cisplatin (gray; $n = 4$) and cisplatin treated (white; $n = 4$) cochlear explants from the basal, middle and apical regions. **(H)** Average percent of OHC from control (black; $n = 4$), cisplatin (white; $n = 4$) and bpV(HOpic) and cisplatin (gray; $n = 4$) treated explants. Percentage of surviving IHC, OHC and undefined hair cells in **(I)** control, **(J)** cisplatin and **(K)** bpV(HOpic) and cisplatin treated cochlear explants. Statistical significance was determined using the Student's t-test and error bars are in SD.

three rows of OHC could be observed. The two types of hair cells are separated by the tunnel of Corti formed by inner and outer pillar cells. The heads of the pillar cells converge on the surface of the sensory epithelium and can be seen as phalloidin labeling between the IHCs and the first row of OHCs (**Figure 3B**). IHCs and OHCs were defined by their relative location to the heads of the pillar cells. Treatment of cochlear cultures with 20 μM cisplatin for 24 h resulted in the lack of MYO7A labeled hair cell bodies in the sensory epithelium along with the loss of phalloidin marked hair bundles (**Figure 3C**). Due to the disruption in the microarchitecture of the sensory epithelium, it was sometimes difficult to distinguish between IHCs and OHCs. Pretreatment of cochlear explants with 10 μM bpV(HOpic) displayed increased numbers of surviving MYO7A labeled hair cells with phalloidin marked hair bundles (**Figure 3D**). In some regions, the IHC and OHC organization could still be discerned.

Since cisplatin-induced toxicity has different effects on IHC and OHCs (Schacht et al., 2012), the percentages of the two different types of hair cells were separately quantified. Surviving IHCs and OHCs were distinguished based on their location relative to where the heads of the pillar cells were located. To determine the effects of IHC and OHC survival after bpV(HOpic) treatment, hair cells were counted along the length of the cochlea. The cochlea was partitioned into three segments, the base, middle and the apex. Surviving hair cells were then represented as a percentage of MYO7A labeled hair cells relative to untreated samples. Treatment of cisplatin showed a significant reduction of MYO7A labeled IHCs along the length of the cochlea relative to controls. The percentage of IHCs after cisplatin damage significantly dropped from 100% to 23.0 ± 5.2% in the base ($p < 1 \times 10^{-2}$), 32.3 ± 6.6% in the middle ($p < 1 \times 10^{-2}$) and 40.1 ± 5.7% in the apex ($p < 1 \times 10^{-2}$). After pretreatment with bpV(HOpic), the percentage of surviving IHCs compared to cisplatin treatment alone significantly increased to 44.8 ± 4.8% in the base ($p < 0.05$), 58.1 ± 6.5% in the middle ($p < 0.05$) and 56.8 ± 5.2% in the apex ($p < 0.05$; **Figure 3E**). On average, cisplatin treatment significantly decreased IHC levels from 100 ± 9.5% to 32.0 ± 4.4% ($p < 1 \times 10^{-3}$). Before cisplatin treatment, addition of bpV(HOpic) significantly increased the percentage of IHCs to 53.3 ± 4.2% ($p < 1 \times 10^{-2}$; **Figure 3F**). These results suggest that addition of bpV(HOpic) and activation of PI3K signaling increases IHC survival after cisplatin damage.

For OHCs, addition of cisplatin significantly decreased the percentage of MYO7A labeled OHCs from 100% to 3.7 ± 1.0% in the base, 6.7 ± 0.9% in the middle and 5.2 ± 1.3% in the apex. Pretreatment with bpV(HOpic) increased the percentage of surviving OHCs to 11.8 ± 2.8% in the base ($p < 0.05$), 20.2 ± 2.9% in the middle ($p < 1 \times 10^{-2}$) and 16.1 ± 2.8% in the apex ($p < 0.05$; **Figure 3G**). On average, cisplatin treatment significantly decreased percentage of OHCs from 100 ± 13.9% to 5.2 ± 1.94% ($p < 1 \times 10^{-4}$), while the addition of bpV(HOpic) significantly increased the percentage to 16.2 ± 2.7% ($p < 0.05$; **Figure 3H**). Although bpV(HOpic) promoted OHC survival, OHC loss was still more prominent than IHC loss as previously described (Schacht et al., 2012). Our results demonstrate that activation of PI3K signaling using bpV(HOpic) can increase both IHC and OHC survival after cisplatin-induced damage.

In addition to hair cell loss, we noticed that the microarchitecture of the sensory epithelium was altered and typical hair cell organization was disrupted. Some hair cells could not be unambiguously characterized as IHCs or OHCs. To quantify this effect, surviving IHCs or OHCs were characterized based on their location to the heads of pillar cells. Hair cells that could not be categorized were labeled as undefined. In untreated cells, 25.9 ± 1.5% and 74.1 ± 6.1% of hair cells corresponded to IHCs and OHCs respectively while no undefined hair cells were observed (**Figure 3I**). These percentages correlate well with the proportion of 1 IHC to 3 OHCs that are normally present in the cochlea. Treatment of cisplatin resulted in 21.8 ± 5.9% IHCs, 31.4 ± 8.5% OHCs with a large population, 46.8 ± 9.3% of undefined hair cells (**Figure 3J**). Addition of bpV(HOpic) before treatment with cisplatin resulted in 26.7 ± 3.8% IHCs, 64.8 ± 19.6% OHCs and 8.5 ± 2.8% undefined hair cells (**Figure 3K**). The data suggest that application of bpV(HOpic) to cochlear cultures could activate PI3K signaling in multiple cell types including supporting cells. After activating PI3K signaling, the cochlear cytoarchitecture is maintained in some regions of the sensory epithelium where IHCs can be distinguished from OHCs even after cisplatin damage. We hypothesize that activation of PI3K signaling increases survival of supporting cells by increasing CHK1 activity. Increased supporting cell survival helps provide oto-protection and maintain hair cell organization after cisplatin damage. To directly address whether activation of PI3K signaling increases phosphorylation of CHK1 promotes supporting cells survival after cisplatin damage, a genetic approach was employed.

Genetic Activation of PI3K Signaling in Supporting Cells

To genetically activate PI3K signaling, a *Pten* conditional knock out mouse model was used. PTEN normally dephosphorylates PIP_3 to PIP_2 and by ablating the *Pten* gene, PIP_3 levels increase to activate PI3K signaling (Cantley and Neel, 1999). To target cochlear cell types for Cre mediated excision of *Pten*, we used a neuronal-subset (NS) Cre recombinase mouse that was generated

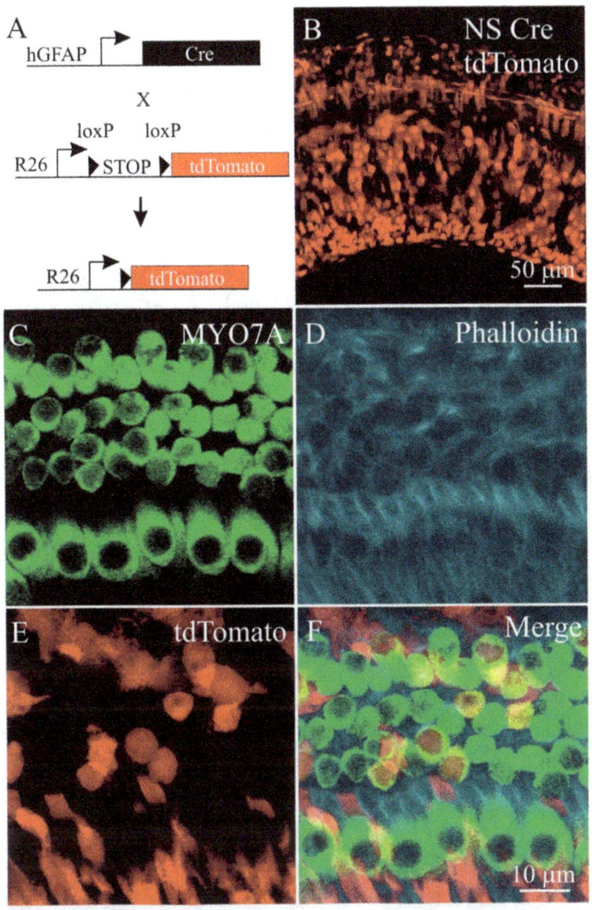

FIGURE 4 | Labeling cochlear cells using a neural subset (NS) Cre tdTomato reporter mouse. (A) Diagram of the NS Cre recombinase transgene using a fragment of the human GFAP (hGFAP) promoter driving Cre recombinase and a STOP floxed tdTomato reporter inserted in the ROSA26 (R26) locus. **(B)** tdTomato fluorescence from NS Cre tdTomato cochlea. Confocal section of the cochlear sensory epithelium labeled with **(C)** MYO7A, **(D)** phalloidin, **(E)** tdTomato from the NS Cre tdTomato reporter mouse. **(F)** Merged image ($n = 4$).

using a promoter fragment of the human *GFAP* promoter ablation to allow cell type specific knockout of *Pten* (Backman et al., 2001; Ljungberg et al., 2009). In these mice, expression of Cre recombinase under the ROSA26 promoter (R26) mediates excision of a loxP flanked STOP cassette and allows expression of the tdTomato red fluorescent protein (Madisen et al., 2010; **Figure 4A**). To confirm that NS Cre mice could mediate loxP excision in cochlear cell types, a NS Cre tdTomato reporter animal was generated to serve as a control. Fluorescent images of cochleae obtained from NS Cre tdTomato animals showed mosaic expression tdTomato fluorescence in many cochlear cell types (**Figure 4B**). To determine whether hair cells and supporting cells were labeled with tdTomato, cochlear explants were immmunostained using MYO7A antibodies (**Figure 4C**) and with phalloidin (**Figure 4D**). The tdTomato fluorescence (**Figure 4E**) marked MYO7A labeled hair cells as well as supporting cells that reside adjacent to both IHCs and OHCs (**Figure 4F**). Analysis of sparsely labeled cells allowed us to determine the direct effect of activating PI3K signaling in supporting cells. These observed effects are cell autonomous and independent of activating PI3K signaling in surrounding cell types.

Activation of PI3K Signaling Promotes Supporting Cell and Hair Cell Survival

Next, we tested whether activation of PI3K signaling increased CHK1 phosphorylation in supporting cells to promote cell survival after cisplatin damage. The *Pten* conditional knockout allele was introduced into the NS Cre tdTomato animals to generate NS Cre *Pten* cKO tdTomato (*Pten* cKO) animals. These animals allowed activation of PI3K signaling by *Pten* deletion and fluorescently marked cochlear supporting cells with tdTomato expression. To induce ototoxic damage, cochlear explants from NS Cre tdTomato (control) and *Pten* cKO animals were treated with cisplatin. Cisplatin was removed after 24 h and the cochlea explant was replenished with fresh medium without cisplatin. Explants were allowed to recover for an additional 3 days before being fixed and subjected to immunolabeling (**Figure 5A**). Explants were immunostained for MYO7A and phalloidin to mark the hair cell bodies and the hair bundle. In cisplatin treated control cochlea, few MYO7A labeled hair cells with phalloidin labeled hair bundles and tdTomato marked supporting cells were observed (**Figure 5B**). The merged image showed disorganized surviving hair cells in the sensory epithelium. In contrast, cisplatin treatment of *Pten* cKO cochlea showed the presence of more MYO7A labeled hair cells with phalloidin labeled hair bundles surrounded by tdTomato expressing supporting cells (**Figure 5C**). To determine if the increased numbers of tdTomato labeled supporting cells could be due to increased CHK1 phosphorylation after cisplatin damage and activation of PI3K signaling, *Pten* cKO cochleae were immmunostained for pCHK1 after cisplatin damage. Increased nuclear pCHK1 could be observed in tdTomato labeled cells after cisplatin damage (**Figure 5D**). Increased pCHK1 levels could activate the DNA damage response and improve supporting cell survival.

To ascertain whether increased pCHK1 levels could promote supporting cell survival, we determined the density of surviving supporting cells after cisplatin treatment in control and *Pten* cKO animals. To quantify the presence of supporting cells after cisplatin damage, MYO7A- tdTomato+ cells were counted. A significant increase of supporting cell density from 79.4 ± 2.3 to 198.3 ± 20.1 cells/0.1 mm^2 ($p < 1 \times 10^{-2}$) was observed when comparing controls to *Pten* cKO cochleae (**Figure 5E**). These results demonstrate that *Pten* deletion and subsequent activation of PI3K signaling increases the number of remaining supporting cells after cisplatin damage. As an internal control, MYO7A+ tdTomato+ hair cells were counted to determine whether activated PI3K signaling increases hair cell survival. A significant increase in the density of MYO7A+ tdTomato+ hair cells from 10.2 ± 5.3 to 56.8 ± 8.1 cells/0.1 mm^2 ($p < 1 \times 10^{-3}$) was observed when comparing controls to *Pten* cKO animals (**Figure 5F**). These results are consistent to previous

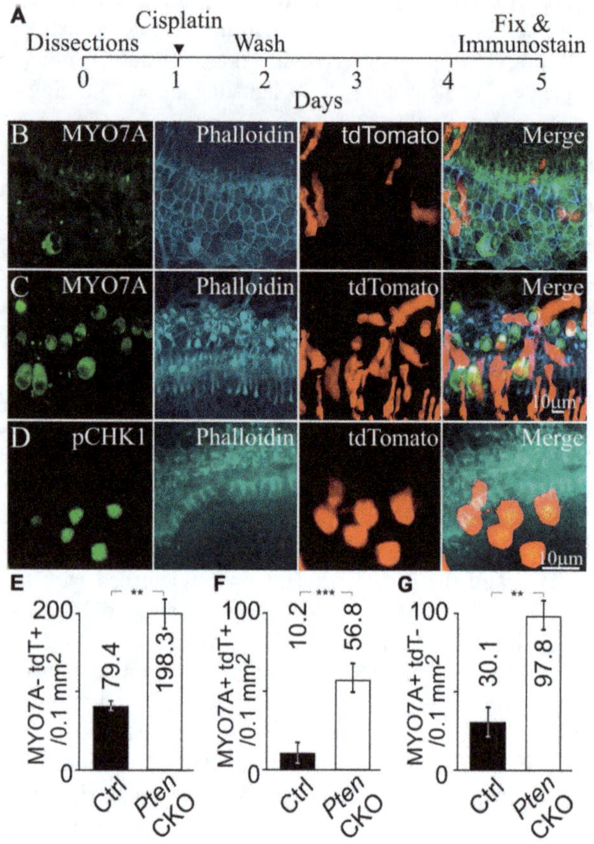

FIGURE 5 | Hair cell survival after genetic activation of PI3K signaling and cisplatin damage. (A) Timeline of cochlear explant cultures describing the addition of 10 μM cisplatin treatment for cochlear explants. MYO7A, phalloidin, tdTomato and merged fluorescent images from **(B)** NS Cre tdTomato (control) after cisplatin treatment (n = 4) and **(C)** NS Cre *Pten* cKO tdTomato (*Pten* cKO) cochleae after cisplatin treatment (n = 4). **(D)** pCHK1, phalloidin, tdTomato and merged fluorescent images from *Pten* cKO mouse after cisplatin damage. **(E)** Density (cells/0.1 mm^2) of MYO7A- tdTomato+ supporting cells in control (n = 4) and *Pten* cKO cochleae (n = 4). **(F)** Density of MYO7A+ tdTomato+ hair cells in control (n = 4) and *Pten* cKO cochleae (n = 4). **(G)** Density of MYO7A+ tdTomato- hair cells in control (n = 4) and *Pten* cKO cochleae (n = 4). Statistical significance was determined using the Student's t-test and error bars are in SD.

observations that activated PI3K signaling promotes hair cell survival (Jadali and Kwan, 2016). In addition, we also observed many MYO7A+ tdTomato- hair cells. A significant increase in the number of MYO7A+ tdTomato- hair cells from 30.1 ± 8.3 to 97.8 ± 8.1 cells/0.1 mm^2 ($p < 1 \times 10^{-2}$) was observed when comparing controls to *Pten* cKO animals (**Figure 5G**). These results suggest that hair cell survival could not be explained by a simple cell autonomous effect of activated PI3K signaling and increased pCHK1 levels. Since there was an increased density of supporting cells after cisplatin damage, one possibility was that the presence of more supporting cells may indirectly improve hair cell survival after cisplatin damage. To test this hypothesis, we determined whether there was an increased number of supporting cells in the proximity of surviving hair cells.

Surviving Hair Cells Reside in Close Proximity to Supporting Cells with Activated PI3K Signaling

To test if increased hair cell survival correlates to the increased density of neighboring supporting cells, cochlea from control and *Pten* cKO animals were treated with cisplatin and labeled with MYO7A and phalloidin. To reduce the complexity of the analysis, regions along the cochlea lacking tdTomato hair cells were used. In these regions, MYO7A and phalloidin marked surviving hair cells while tdTomato labeled supporting cells. Confocal stacks were used to generate 3D renderings of the region of interest to ensure that only tdTomato supporting cells were present (**Figure 6A**). Using the 3D confocal image, the image was collapsed to generate 2D masks of hair cells (green) and supporting cells (red; **Figure 6B**). Using the combined masks, individual surviving hair cells (green) were identified before determining whether a supporting cell (red) resides next to the hair cell. All remaining neighboring cells in the field of view were marked in blue. In controls, 16.3 ± 5.8% of MYO7A labeled hair cells reside adjacent to tdTomato supporting cells. In *Pten* cKO cochleae, 56.3 ± 8.3% of MYO7A labeled hair cells reside next to a PI3K activated tdTomato supporting cells (**Figure 6C**). A significant increase in the percentage of hair cells adjacent to supporting cells was observed in *Pten* cKO cochleae compared to controls ($p < 1 \times 10^{-2}$). These data show that many supporting cells with activated PI3K signaling

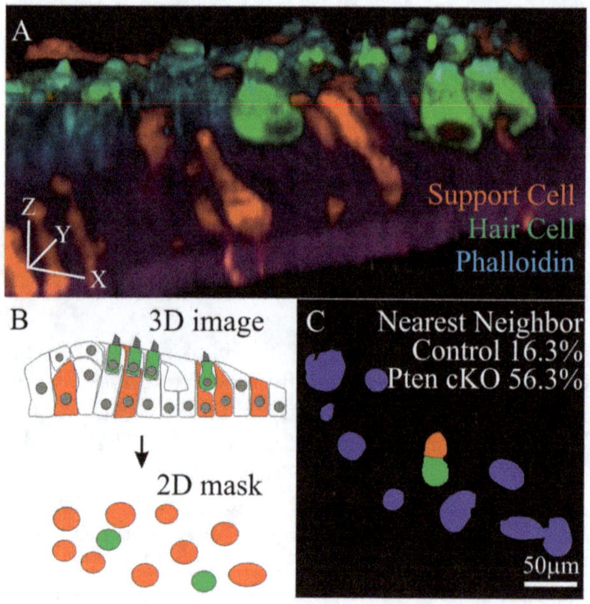

FIGURE 6 | Nearest neighbor analysis of supporting cell to surviving hair cells. (A) 3D rendering of a confocal stack with MYO7A and phalloidin labeled hair cells along with tdTomato labeled supporting cell **(B)** 3D images were compressed into a maximal intensity projection to generate a 2D mask for hair cells (green) and tdTomato labeled supporting cells (red). **(C)** Using the 2D masks, percent of surviving hair cells (green) that reside adjacent to supporting cells (red) were determined in control (n = 4) and *Pten* cKO cochleae (n = 4). All remaining cells in the field of view were labeled blue.

reside in close proximity to surviving hair cells after cisplatin damage.

Next, we wanted to determine if the distribution of tdTomato marked supporting cells to surviving MYO7A hair cells in control and *Pten* cKO cochleae were different. To determine the distance between supporting cells and hair cells, an individual hair cell was identified and the distance to all supporting cells in the field of view was measured. To accomplish this, the 2D masks generated from tdTomato expressing supporting cells (**Figure 7A**) and MYO7A labeled hair cells (**Figure 7B**) were used to identify the different cell types. The masks were merged into a single image to show the location of hair cells relative to supporting cells (**Figure 7C**). To determine the spatial distribution between the hair cells and supporting cells, a cellular "interaction analysis" was performed (Helmuth et al., 2010). Centroid determination was done to convert masks that represent individual cell bodies into single points that correspond to the center of the mask. The distance from each centroid corresponding to a hair cell was measured to the centroid of all other supporting cells in the field of view (**Figure 7D**). The distribution of distances between a single hair cell and supporting cells were measured and plotted as a histogram. The number of interactions and the average distance between hair cell and supporting cells were determined (**Figure 7E**). The distribution of tdTomato labeled supporting cell relative to surviving hair cells contains information about potential oto-protective effects of supporting cells. The distribution of supporting cells to hair cells would show a stronger "cellular interaction" if supporting cells promoted hair cell survival. The "cellular interactions" between hair cells and supporting cells can be modeled as an interaction potential between the two sets of centroids. Using the centroids obtained from the cell masks, the observed distances between hair cells and supporting cells represented a distribution pattern. From the distribution pattern, a probability density function q(d) of the observed nearest neighbor distances, was calculated to represent the likelihood of a "cellular interaction". The probability density function was then modeled as an interaction potential p(d), to describe the likelihood that the distribution was due to "cellular interactions" (**Figure 7F**). The interaction potential p(d) was used to described the "cellular interaction" strength, to determine if objects of a specific distribution had an effect on each other (**Figure 7G**). A significant increase in interaction strength between tdTomato labeled supporting cell and surviving hair cells was observed in control (1.29 ± 0.4) compared to *Pten* cKO (3.23 ± 0.5) cochleae ($p < 1 \times 10^{-2}$; **Figure 7H**). The increased interaction strength in *Pten* cKO cochlea relative to control suggests that the distribution of supporting cells with activated PI3K signaling are highly correlated to the increased numbers of surviving hair cells.

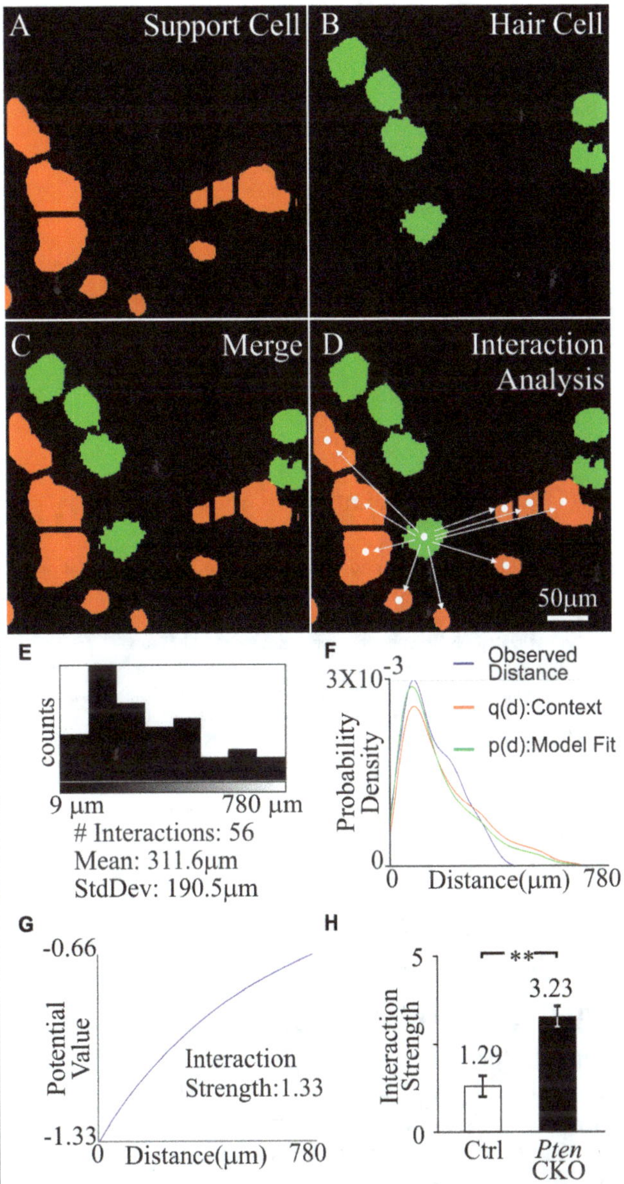

FIGURE 7 | Interaction strength of supporting cell and surviving hair cells. Region containing tdTomato+supporting cell and MYO7A+ tdTomato- hair cells were analyzed. **(A)** Supporting cell masks were generated from tdTomato labeled supporting cells (red). **(B)** Hair cell masks were generated from MYO7A labeled hair cells (green). **(C)** Merged image of supporting cell and hair cell masks. **(D)** Centroid of hair cell and supporting cells were generated from masks. Distance between an individual hair cell centroid to all supporting cell centroids in the field of view was determined. **(E)** Number of cell interactions within a field of view and the mean distance between the centroid of a hair cell to multiple supporting cells was displayed in the histogram. **(F)** The observed distances between a hair cell and supporting cells were fitted into probability density, p(d), and an interaction potential model, q(d). **(G)** Interaction strength between hair cell and supporting cells was calculated from the interaction potential q(d). **(H)** Comparison of the interaction strength between surviving hair cells and control supporting cells (n = 10) or surviving hair cells and *Pten* cKO supporting cells (n = 10) after cisplatin treatment. Statistical significance was determined using the Student's t-test and error bars in SD.

DISCUSSION

In this study, we showed increased phosphorylation of CHK1 after cisplatin damage and activation of PI3K signaling. Activation of CHK1 promotes survival of differentiating iMOP cells. Using cochlear explant cultures, increased phosphorylation of CHK1 after cisplatin damage and activation of PI3K signaling

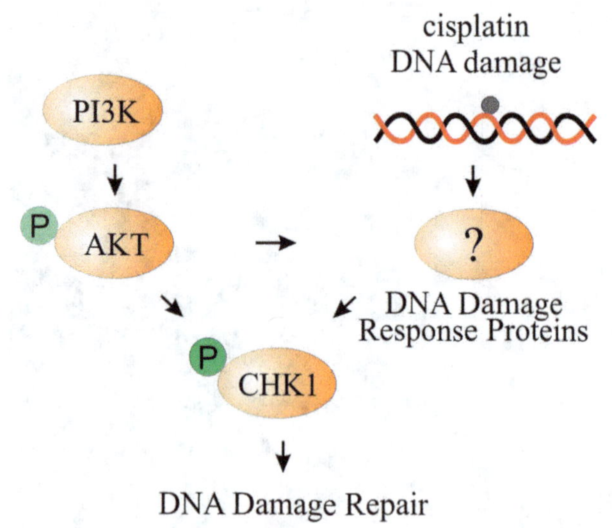

FIGURE 8 | Model of CHK1 phosphorylation through cisplatin damage and PI3K signaling. Activation of PI3K signaling either by bpV(HOpic) or *Pten* deletion results in increased AKT phosphorylation. DNA damage caused by cisplatin activates DNA damage response proteins that increase pCHK1 levels. Activated AKT can directly or indirectly increase pCHK1 levels by activating the DNA damage response proteins. Together, PI3K activation and cisplatin-induced DNA damage results in increased pCHK1 to promote supporting cell survival.

was observed in supporting cells. We propose that increased PI3K signaling activates AKT which could directly phosphorylate CHK1 or indirectly increase pCHK1 levels through DNA damage response proteins such as ATR. Activation of CHK1 allows supporting cells to repair cisplatin-induced DNA damage (**Figure 8**).

CHK1 Is Downstream of PI3K/AKT Signaling

Our results suggest that activating the PI3K/AKT signaling pathway increases phosphorylation of CHK1 after cisplatin damage in supporting cells. These results are similar to reports in other systems where CHK1 is phosphorylated by AKT (Jin et al., 2005; Kurosu et al., 2013). Phosphorylation of CHK1 serves as a checkpoint protein that arrests cells at the G2/M phase of the cell cycle after DNA damage (Liu et al., 2000; Takai et al., 2000) and has also been implicated in DNA damage response (Sorensen et al., 2005; Shimada et al., 2008). Since supporting cells are post-mitotic, pCHK1 in supporting cells may contribute to the DNA damage response after cisplatin damage. We propose that pCHK1 can promote survival of cochlear supporting cells. Using differentiating iMOP cells, we showed that cisplatin-induced DNA damage results in phosphorylation of CHK1 at serine 345 using phospho-specific antibodies. Phosphorylation of serine 345 is essential for nuclear localization of CHK1 and response to DNA damage (Niida et al., 2007). Increased PI3K signaling as shown by increased pAKT in iMOP cells contributes to the phosphorylation of CHK1. *In vivo*, activation of PI3K signaling in tdTomato labeled supporting cells increased nuclear pCHK1 levels compared to surrounding cells. We propose that the additive effects of CHK1 phosphorylation may help enhance DNA damage response and increase supporting cell survival after cisplatin damage.

AKT in Cochlear Supporting Cell Survival

AKT (AKT1) belongs to a family of serine/threonine kinases that act downstream of PI3K and participates in a variety of cellular processes to play a critical role in cell survival (Datta et al., 1999). All three AKT isozymes are expressed in the cochlea (Brand et al., 2015). Mounting evidence shows that the PI3K/AKT signaling pathway plays a role in hair cell survival after exposure to ototoxic drugs. Inhibiting PI3K signaling in cochlear explants while treating with gentamicin showed increased hair cell loss compared to gentamicin exposure alone (Chung et al., 2006). Another study demonstrates that dexamethasone protects HCs against TNFα-initiated apoptosis by activating the PI3K/AKT signaling pathway (Haake et al., 2009). Exposure to simvastatin in cochlear explants activates AKT signaling and protects hair cells from gentamicin toxicity (Brand et al., 2011). These studies suggest that activation of PI3K/AKT signaling promotes hair cell survival. In addition to promoting hair cell survival, activation of PI3K signaling may also promote survival of supporting cells as observed by the increased density of supporting cells in *Pten* cKO cochleae compared to controls after cisplatin treatment. We propose that activation of PI3K/AKT signaling contributes to supporting cell survival by CHK1 phosphorylation.

In cancer cells, several studies have established the involvement of AKT in contributing to cell survival by their acquired cisplatin resistance. These cancers cells include samples from ovarian, uterine, small-cell lung cancer, non-small-cell lung cancer and hepatoblastoma. Studies from these different cell lines and cancer cells suggest that cisplatin-induced DNA damage results in AKT phosphorylation of the pro-apoptotic factor Bcl2-associated agonist of cell death (BAD) at Ser136 to suppress cell death and promote cell survival (Datta et al., 1997; Hayakawa et al., 2000). In ovarian cancer cells, cisplatin-induced DNA damage results in activation of AKT and phosphorylation of X-linked inhibitor of apoptosis (XIAP). AKT phosphorylation of XIAP prevents XIAP ubiquitination and degradation in response to cisplatin to promote cell survival (Dan et al., 2004). In small-cell lung cancer cells, AKT phosphorylates the anti-apoptotic protein survivin to protect cells against cisplatin-induced cell death (Belyanskaya et al., 2005). In all, AKT phosphorylation of key molecules such as BAD, XIAP or survivin promotes cell survival after cisplatin damage. We propose that CHK1 is another downstream target of AKT in both iMOP cells and cochlear supporting cells after cisplatin damage.

Increased Supporting Cell Survival Maintains Cochlear Cytoarchitecture and Indirectly Promotes Hair Cell Survival

We noticed that after cisplatin damage, many hair cells could not be defined as either IHCs or OHCs due to the altered microarchitecture of the sensory epithelium. We propose that disorganization of hair cells may be due to supporting cell loss. Increased survival of supporting cells after activating PI3K signaling helps maintains hair cell organization in the sensory epithelium. In addition to changes in the cytoarchitecture of the sensory epithelium, supporting cell loss may indirectly contribute to hair cell loss. Our study showed increased density of PI3K activated supporting cells that reside in the vicinity of surviving hair cells compared to controls. The increased presence of supporting cells may provide additional oto-protection to hair cells. One mechanism for oto-protection is the release of HSP70 by supporting cells onto nearby hair cells (May et al., 2013). Another potential mechanism of oto-protection is cell-cell signlaing between hair cells and supporting cells. The ERBB signaling pathway is an example that cell types in the cochlea are constantly communicating with each other through cell-cell signaling. ERBB signaling has been observed between SGNs and supporting cells and presence of this signaling pathway is essential for survival of SGNs (Stankovic et al., 2004). Cell-cell signaling between supporting cells and hair cells may be another cellular mechanism that normally maintains hair cell viability. Ablation of inner border cells and inner phalangeal cells that flank IHCs causes loss of IHC and significantly impairs hearing in adult mice (Mellado Lagarde et al., 2014). The study suggests that cellular contact between supporting cells and IHCs may be essential for maintaining hair cell viability. We propose that after cisplatin damage, activation of PI3K signaling increases survival of supporting cells. Through several potential mechanisms including secretion of extracellular molecules or cell-cell signaling, the increased number of supporting cells promotes survival of nearby hair cells. The study implicates supporting cells as a cellular target for preventing hair cell loss.

AUTHOR CONTRIBUTIONS

AJ and KYK designed, performed the experiments and wrote the manuscript. Y-LMY helped with cell counts.

ACKNOWLEDGMENTS

We would also like to acknowledge Theresa Choi for her expertise and help in flow cytometry.

REFERENCES

Backman, S. A., Stambolic, V., Suzuki, A., Haight, J., Elia, A., Pretorius, J., et al. (2001). Deletion of Pten in mouse brain causes seizures, ataxia and defects in soma size resembling Lhermitte-Duclos disease. *Nat. Genet.* 29, 396–403. doi: 10.1038/ng782

Belyanskaya, L. L., Hopkins-Donaldson, S., Kurtz, S., Simões-Wüst, A. P., Yousefi, S., Simon, H. U., et al. (2005). Cisplatin activates Akt in small cell lung cancer cells and attenuates apoptosis by survivin upregulation. *Int. J. Cancer* 117, 755–763. doi: 10.1002/ijc.21242

Bird, J. E., Daudet, N., Warchol, M. E., and Gale, J. E. (2010). Supporting cells eliminate dying sensory hair cells to maintain epithelial integrity in the avian inner ear. *J. Neurosci.* 30, 12545–12556. doi: 10.1523/JNEUROSCI.3042-10.2010

Brand, Y., Levano, S., Radojevic, V., Naldi, A. M., Setz, C., Ryan, A. F., et al. (2015). All Akt isoforms (Akt1, Akt2, Akt3) are involved in normal hearing, but only Akt2 and Akt3 are involved in auditory hair cell survival in the mammalian inner ear. *PLoS One* 10:e0121599. doi: 10.1371/journal.pone.0121599

Brand, Y., Setz, C., Levano, S., Listyo, A., Chavez, E., Pak, K., et al. (2011). Simvastatin protects auditory hair cells from gentamicin-induced toxicity and activates Akt signaling *in vitro*. *BMC Neurosci.* 12:114. doi: 10.1186/1471-2202-12-114

Cantley, L. C., and Neel, B. G. (1999). New insights into tumor suppression: PTEN suppresses tumor formation by restraining the phosphoinositide 3-kinase/AKT pathway. *Proc. Natl. Acad. Sci. U S A* 96, 4240–4245. doi: 10.1073/pnas.96.8.4240

Chung, W.-H., Pak, K., Lin, B., Webster, N., and Ryan, A. (2006). A PI3K pathway mediates hair cell survival and opposes gentamicin toxicity in neonatal rat organ of corti. *J. Assoc. Res. Otolaryngol.* 7, 373–382. doi: 10.1007/s10162-006-0050-y

Dan, H. C., Sun, M., Kaneko, S., Feldman, R. I., Nicosia, S. V., Wang, H. G., et al. (2004). Akt phosphorylation and stabilization of X-linked inhibitor of apoptosis protein (XIAP). *J. Biol. Chem.* 279, 5405–5412. doi: 10.1074/jbc.M312044200

Datta, S. R., Brunet, A., and Greenberg, M. E. (1999). Cellular survival: a play in three Akts. *Genes Dev.* 13, 2905–2927. doi: 10.1101/gad.13.22.2905

Datta, S. R., Dudek, H., Tao, X., Masters, S., Fu, H., Gotoh, Y., et al. (1997). Akt phosphorylation of BAD couples survival signals to the cell-intrinsic death machinery. *Cell* 91, 231–241. doi: 10.1016/s0092-8674(00)80405-5

Doillon, C. J., Faure, R. L., Posner, B. I., and Savard, P. E. (1999). Peroxovanadium compounds as inhibitors of angiogenesis. *Angiogenesis* 3, 361–369. doi: 10.1023/A:1026577418765

Gómez-Casati, M. E., Murtie, J., Taylor, B., and Corfas, G. (2010). Cell-specific inducible gene recombination in postnatal inner ear supporting cells and glia. *J. Assoc. Res. Otolaryngol.* 11, 19–26. doi: 10.1007/s10162-009-0191-x

Haake, S. M., Dinh, C. T., Chen, S., Eshraghi, A. A., and Van De Water, T. R. (2009). Dexamethasone protects auditory hair cells against TNFα-initiated apoptosis via activation of PI3K/Akt and NFκB signaling. *Hear. Res.* 255, 22–32. doi: 10.1016/j.heares.2009.05.003

Hayakawa, J., Ohmichi, M., Kurachi, H., Kanda, Y., Hisamoto, K., Nishio, Y., et al. (2000). Inhibition of BAD phosphorylation either at serine 112 via extracellular signal-regulated protein kinase cascade or at serine 136 via Akt cascade sensitizes human ovarian cancer cells to cisplatin. *Cancer Res.* 60, 5988–5994.

Helmuth, J. A., Paul, G., and Sbalzarini, I. F. (2010). Beyond co-localization: inferring spatial interactions between sub-cellular structures from microscopy images. *BMC Bioinformatics* 11:372. doi: 10.1186/1471-2105-11-372

Jadali, A., and Kwan, K. Y. (2016). Activation of PI3K signaling prevents aminoglycoside-induced hair cell death in the murine cochlea. *Biol. Open* 5, 698–708. doi: 10.1242/bio.016758

Jadali, A., Zhichao, S., Alejandra, S. L., Alana, T.-R., and Kelvin, K. (2016). Initiating differentiation in immortalized multipotent otic progenitor cells. *J. Vis. Exp.* 107. doi: 10.3791/53692

Jiang, K., Pereira, E., Maxfield, M., Russell, B., Goudelock, D. M., and Sanchez, Y. (2003). Regulation of Chk1 includes chromatin association and 14-3-3 binding following phosphorylation on Ser-345. *J. Biol. Chem.* 278, 25207–25217. doi: 10.1074/jbc.M300070200

Jin, Z. H., Kurosu, T., Yamaguchi, M., Arai, A., and Miura, O. (2005). Hematopoietic cytokines enhance Chk1-dependent G2/M checkpoint activation by etoposide through the Akt/GSK3 pathway to inhibit apoptosis. *Oncogene* 24, 1973–1981. doi: 10.1038/sj.onc.1208408

Kurosu, T., Nagao, T., Wu, N., Oshikawa, G., and Miura, O. (2013). Inhibition of the PI3K/Akt/GSK3 pathway downstream of BCR/ABL, Jak2-V617F, or FLT3-ITD downregulates DNA damage-induced Chk1 activation as well as G2/M arrest and prominently enhances induction of apoptosis. *PLoS One* 8:e79478. doi: 10.1371/journal.pone.0079478

Kwan, K. Y., Shen, J., and Corey, D. P. (2015). C-MYC transcriptionally amplifies SOX2 target genes to regulate self-renewal in multipotent otic progenitor cells. *Stem Cell Reports* 4, 47–60. doi: 10.1016/j.stemcr.2014.11.001

Liu, Q., Guntuku, S., Cui, X. S., Matsuoka, S., Cortez, D., Tamai, K., et al. (2000). Chk1 is an essential kinase that is regulated by Atr and required for the G_2/M DNA damage checkpoint. *Genes Dev.* 14, 1448–1459.

Ljungberg, M. C., Sunnen, C. N., Lugo, J. N., Anderson, A. E., and D'Arcangelo, G. (2009). Rapamycin suppresses seizures and neuronal hypertrophy in a mouse model of cortical dysplasia. *Dis. Model. Mech.* 2, 389–398. doi: 10.1242/dmm.002386

Madisen, L., Zwingman, T. A., Sunkin, S. M., Oh, S. W., Zariwala, H. A., Gu, H., et al. (2010). A robust and high-throughput Cre reporting and characterization system for the whole mouse brain. *Nat. Neurosci.* 13, 133–140. doi: 10.1038/nn.2467

May, L. A., Kramarenko, I. I., Brandon, C. S., Voelkel-Johnson, C., Roy, S., Truong, K., et al. (2013). Inner ear supporting cells protect hair cells by secreting HSP70. *J. Clin. Invest.* 123, 3577–3587. doi: 10.1172/JCI68480

Mellado Lagarde, M. M., Wan, G., Zhang, L., Gigliello, A. R., McInnis, J. J., Zhang, Y., et al. (2014). Spontaneous regeneration of cochlear supporting cells after neonatal ablation ensures hearing in the adult mouse. *Proc. Natl. Acad. Sci. U S A* 111, 16919–16924. doi: 10.1073/pnas.1408064111

Monzack, E. L., and Cunningham, L. L. (2013). Lead roles for supporting actors: critical functions of inner ear supporting cells. *Hear. Res.* 303, 20–29. doi: 10.1016/j.heares.2013.01.008

Monzack, E. L., May, L. A., Roy, S., Gale, J. E., and Cunningham, L. L. (2015). Live imaging the phagocytic activity of inner ear supporting cells in response to hair cell death. *Cell Death Differ.* 22, 1995–2005. doi: 10.1038/cdd.2015.48

Niida, H., Katsuno, Y., Banerjee, B., Hande, M. P., and Nakanishi, M. (2007). Specific role of Chk1 phosphorylations in cell survival and checkpoint activation. *Mol. Cell. Biol.* 27, 2572–2581. doi: 10.1128/mcb.01611-06

Ramírez-Camacho, R., García-Berrocal, J. R., Buján, J., Martín-Marero, A., and Trinidad, A. (2004). Supporting cells as a target of cisplatin-induced inner ear damage: therapeutic implications. *Laryngoscope* 114, 533–537. doi: 10.1097/00005537-200403000-00027

Rybak, L. P., Mukherjea, D., Jajoo, S., and Ramkumar, V. (2009). Cisplatin ototoxicity and protection: clinical and experimental studies. *Tohoku J. Exp. Med.* 219, 177–186. doi: 10.1620/tjem.219.177

Schacht, J., Talaska, A. E., and Rybak, L. P. (2012). Cisplatin and aminoglycoside antibiotics: hearing loss and its prevention. *Anat. Rec. (Hoboken)* 295, 1837–1850. doi: 10.1002/ar.22578

Schmid, A. C., Byrne, R. D., Vilar, R., and Woscholski, R. (2004). Bisperoxovanadium compounds are potent PTEN inhibitors. *FEBS Lett.* 566, 35–38. doi: 10.1016/j.febslet.2004.03.102

Shimada, M., Niida, H., Zineldeen, D. H., Tagami, H., Tanaka, M., Saito, H., et al. (2008). Chk1 is a histone H3 threonine 11 kinase that regulates DNA damage-induced transcriptional repression. *Cell* 132, 221–232. doi: 10.1016/j.cell.2007.12.013

Siddik, Z. H. (2003). Cisplatin: mode of cytotoxic action and molecular basis of resistance. *Oncogene* 22, 7265–7279. doi: 10.1038/sj.onc.1206933

Sorensen, C. S., Hansen, L. T., Dziegielewski, J., Syljuasen, R. G., Lundin, C., Bartek, J., et al. (2005). The cell-cycle checkpoint kinase Chk1 is required for mammalian homologous recombination repair. *Nat. Cell Biol.* 7, 195–201. doi: 10.1038/ncb1212

Stankovic, K., Rio, C., Xia, A., Sugawara, M., Adams, J. C., Liberman, M. C., et al. (2004). Survival of adult spiral ganglion neurons requires erbB receptor signaling in the inner ear. *J. Neurosci.* 24, 8651–8661. doi: 10.1523/JNEUROSCI.0733-04.2004

Takai, H., Tominaga, K., Motoyama, N., Minamishima, Y. A., Nagahama, H., Tsukiyama, T., et al. (2000). Aberrant cell cycle checkpoint function and early embryonic death in $Chk1^{(-/-)}$ mice. *Genes Dev.* 14, 1439–1447.

van Ruijven, M. W., de Groot, J. C., Hendriksen, F., and Smoorenburg, G. F. (2005). Immunohistochemical detection of platinated DNA in the cochlea of cisplatin-treated guinea pigs. *Hear. Res.* 203, 112–121. doi: 10.1016/j.heares.2004.12.007

Vermes, I., Haanen, C., Steffens-Nakken, H., and Reutelingsperger, C. (1995). A novel assay for apoptosis. Flow cytometric detection of phosphatidylserine expression on early apoptotic cells using fluorescein labelled Annexin V. *J. Immunol. Methods* 184, 39–51. doi: 10.1016/0022-1759(95)00072-i

Vlahos, C. J., Matter, W. F., Hui, K. Y., and Brown, R. F. (1994). A specific inhibitor of phosphatidylinositol 3-kinase, 2- (4-morpholinyl)-8-phenyl-4H-1-benzopyran-4-one (LY294002). *J. Biol. Chem.* 269, 5241–5248.

Wan, G., Corfas, G., and Stone, J. S. (2013). Inner ear supporting cells: rethinking the silent majority. *Semin Cell Dev. Biol.* 24, 448–459. doi: 10.1016/j.semcdb.2013.03.009

Wang, D., and Lippard, S. J. (2005). Cellular processing of platinum anticancer drugs. *Nat. Rev. Drug Discov.* 4, 307–320. doi: 10.1038/nrd1691

Zhang, Y., and Hunter, T. (2014). Roles of Chk1 in cell biology and cancer therapy. *Int. J. Cancer* 134, 1013–1023. doi: 10.1002/ijc.28226

Zhao, H., and Piwnica-Worms, H. (2001). ATR-mediated checkpoint pathways regulate phosphorylation and activation of human Chk1. *Mol. Cell. Biol.* 21, 4129–4139. doi: 10.1128/mcb.21.13.4129-4139.2001

11

Protecting Mammalian Hair Cells from Aminoglycoside-Toxicity: Assessing Phenoxybenzamine's Potential

Paromita Majumder[1]*, *Paulette A. Moore*[1], *Guy P. Richardson*[2] *and Jonathan E. Gale*[1,3]*

[1] *UCL Ear Institute, University College London, London, UK,* [2] *Sussex Neuroscience, School of Life Sciences, University of Sussex, Falmer, UK,* [3] *Department of Cell and Developmental Biology, University College London, London, UK*

Edited by:
Peter S. Steyger,
Oregon Health & Science University,
USA

Reviewed by:
Allison B. Coffin,
Washington State University, USA
Federico Kalinec,
University of California, Los Angeles,
USA

***Correspondence:**
Paromita Majumder
paromita.majumder@gmail.com
Jonathan E. Gale
j.e.gale@ucl.ac.uk

Aminoglycosides (AGs) are widely used antibiotics because of their low cost and high efficacy against gram-negative bacterial infection. However, AGs are ototoxic, causing the death of sensory hair cells in the inner ear. Strategies aimed at developing or discovering agents that protect against aminoglycoside ototoxicity have focused on inhibiting apoptosis or more recently, on preventing antibiotic uptake by the hair cells. Recent screens for ototoprotective compounds using the larval zebrafish lateral line identified phenoxybenzamine as a potential protectant for aminoglycoside-induced hair cell death. Here we used live imaging of FM1-43 uptake as a proxy for aminoglycoside entry, combined with hair-cell death assays to evaluate whether phenoxybenzamine can protect mammalian cochlear hair cells from the deleterious effects of the aminoglycoside antibiotic neomycin. We show that phenoxybenzamine can block FM1-43 entry into mammalian hair cells in a reversible and dose-dependent manner, but pre-incubation is required for maximal inhibition of entry. We observed differential effects of phenoxybenzamine on FM1-43 uptake in the two different types of cochlear hair cell in mammals, the outer hair cells (OHCs) and inner hair cells (IHCs). The requirement for pre-incubation and reversibility suggests an intracellular rather than an extracellular site of action for phenoxybenzamine. We also tested the efficacy of phenoxybenzamine as an otoprotective agent. In mouse cochlear explants the hair cell death resulting from 24 h exposure to neomycin was steeply dose-dependent, with 50% cell death occurring at ~230 μM for both IHC and OHC. We used 250 μM neomycin in subsequent hair-cell death assays. At 100 μM with 1 h pre-incubation, phenoxybenzamine conferred significant protection to both IHCs and OHCs, however at higher concentrations phenoxybenzamine itself showed clear signs of ototoxicity and an additive toxic effect when combined with neomycin. These data do not support the use of phenoxybenzamine as a therapeutic agent in mammalian inner ear. Our findings do share parallels with the observations from the zebrafish lateral line model but they also highlight the necessity for validation in the mammalian system and the potential for differential effects on sensory hair cells from different species, in different systems and even between cells in the same organ.

Keywords: hair cells, cochlea, aminoglycosides, ototoxicity, FM 1-43, organotypic culture, mechanoelectrical transduction channels, inner ear

INTRODUCTION

Aminoglycosides (AGs) are widely used antibiotics because of their low cost and high efficacy against gram-negative bacterial infection. AGs are both nephrotoxic (Toubeau et al., 1986; Hock and Anderson, 1995) and ototoxic (Greenwood, 1959) affecting the vestibular and auditory organs (Matz et al., 2004). Among the AGs neomycin is highly toxic, particularly in the hearing organ, the cochlea (Forge and Schacht, 2000). In the cochlea, AGs first affect the high-frequency hair cells found at the basal end of the cochlea, subsequently extending to the lower-frequency regions at the apical end of cochlear spiral (Aran and Darrouzet, 1975; Stebbins et al., 1979; for review see Forge and Schacht, 2000).

In order to access the apical surface of hair cells AGs must first pass through the blood labyrinth barrier which is composed of a highly specialized capillary network in the stria vascularis (Shi, 2016). Studies with fluorescently-tagged gentamicin showed that it travels from the stria vascularis capillaries into marginal cells and then into the endolymph (Wang and Steyger, 2009; Wang et al., 2010) at which point it comes into contact with the apical surface of the hair cells. AGs can enter into hair cells via an endocytic route (Hashino and Shero, 1995) or via the mechanotransduction (MET) channels, located in the hair cell's stereociliary bundle (Gale et al., 2001; Marcotti et al., 2005; Dai et al., 2006; Wang and Steyger, 2009; Alharazneh et al., 2011) a route that is facilitated by the low calcium concentration of the endolymph (Marcotti et al., 2005).

When mammalian cochlear hair cells die there is no endogenous regenerative process that can replace them and thus hearing loss is permanent. Stem cell based therapies are being pursued and may well be available in the longer term. In the shorter term, however, it is important that we discover therapies that might protect hair cells from damage and death as a result of ototoxic medication, noise-induced hearing loss and aging.

New aminoglycoside antibiotics derived from the structural backbones of existing AGs are being produced to generate less ototoxicity whilst still being effective antibiotics (Matt et al., 2012; Duscha et al., 2014; Shulman et al., 2014; Huth et al., 2015). Until such antibiotics are available, a protective agent that could be applied along with any known ototoxin would be very advantageous. There have been a number of screens to identify compounds that might confer hair-cell protection during ototoxicity, including screens of FDA-approved drugs that could bypass some of the approval requirements (Ou et al., 2009). Many of these have used the zebrafish lateral line system as a screening model. One of the compounds that came through two separate screens using two different sets of FDA-approved compounds was phenoxybenzamine (also known as N-(2-chloroethyl)-N-(1-methyl-2-phenoxyethyl) benzylamine hydrochloride or dibenzyline) which was one of seven drugs which showed protection against aminoglycoside-induced hair-cell death potentially by blocking aminoglycoside uptake by hair cells (Ou et al., 2009; Vlasits et al., 2012). In zebrafish it was noted that pre-incubation of phenoxybenzamine was required to see efficacy in increasing hair-cell survival (Vlasits et al., 2012). Although phenoxybenzamine is a well characterized drug that is known to cross the blood brain barrier (Diop and Dausse, 1986) and so perhaps the blood labyrinth barrier, it has not been tested on mammalian cochlear hair cells.

Phenoxybenzamine is a well-known alpha-1-A and alpha-2-A adrenergic receptor antagonist (Thoenen et al., 1964). Among alpha 1-A and 2-A receptors, phenoxybenzamine has a slow onset and long lasting effect compared with other alpha adrenergic blockers and it is used to reduce the vasoconstriction caused by epinephrine (adrenaline) and norepinephrine. Phenoxybenzamine acts by covalently binding to the receptor resulting in the inhibition of ligand binding. It is used to reduce the hypertension caused by pheochromocytoma, for lower urinary tract problems (e.g., neurogenic bladder; Te, 2002), benign prostatic hyperplasia (Kumar and Dewan, 2000) and in complex regional pain syndrome (Inchiosa, 2013). Phenoxybenzamine is also known to block 5-HT2 serotonin receptors (Frazer and Hensley, 1999), in some cases acting as an irreversible blocker (Doggrell, 1995).

In this study we evaluated whether the protective effects of phenoxybenzamine that are observed in zebrafish hair cells (Ou et al., 2009; Vlasits et al., 2012) are also observed in mammalian inner hair cells (IHCs) and outer hair cells (OHCs). We first investigated the effects of phenoxybenzamine on the rapid FM1-43 entry into hair cells that occurs via the mechanoelectrical-transduction channels and mimics aminoglycoside entry (Gale et al., 2001). Second, we tested whether phenoxybenzamine could protect hair cells during neomycin ototoxicity.

MATERIALS AND METHODS

Materials

Phenoxybenzamine hydrochloride was obtained from Santa Cruz Biotechnology, Dallas, TX, USA and neomycin and ciprofloxacin from Sigma-Aldrich, UK. Leibovitz's L15 (L15), DMEM/F12, FM1-43FX and fetal bovine serum (FBS) were acquired from ThermoFisher scientific, UK and the cell and tissue adhesive Cell-Tak was supplied by BD Biosciences, UK. All other chemicals were obtained from Sigma-Aldrich, UK.

Postnatal Cochlea Isolation and Culture

In accordance with the United Kingdom Animals (Scientific Procedures) Act of 1986 (Schedule 1 procedures), cochleae were extracted from C57BL/6 wild-type mice at postnatal day 3–6 (P3-P6). The isolated cochleae were micro-dissected in Leibovitz L15 medium. The apical cochlear turn was discarded and the remaining 1.5 turns separated into "middle" and "basal" coils. The stria-vascularis was kept in place and Reissner's membrane was cut allowing the cochlear coils to be "fileted" open and then placed onto Cell-Tak® coated Matek (Ashland, MA, USA) dishes (Majumder et al., 2015). Explant cultures were incubated in DMEM/F12 supplemented with 1% FBS and ciprofloxacin (10 μg/ml) at 37°C in a 5% CO_2/95% air atmosphere overnight prior to experimentation.

Live FM1-43 Imaging and Analysis

All experiments were conducted at room temperature (20–22°C). FM1-43 (6 μM) was prepared from a 10 mM stock solution.

The control culture was loaded with 6 μM FM1-43 for 30 s and then immediately washed (five 10 s washes, followed by three slower, 2 min washes) in L15 or HBHBSS prior to imaging with a Zeiss 510NLO upright confocal microscope (excitation 488 nm, emission 500–550 nm) using a 40× (NA 0.8) water immersion objective. Confocal image stacks (~20 planes, 2 μm intervals) were acquired exactly 20 min after exposure to FM1-43. The confocal laser power and gain settings were identical for all live imaging experiments to enable data comparison. To evaluate whether phenoxybenzamine was more effective when pre-incubated, in a subset of experiments it was applied for 30 or 60 min prior to FM1-43 loading and the loading was performed in the continued presence of phenoxybenzamine (including the washout solution). To test for reversibility of the block, after 30 min of phenoxybenzamine incubation explants were washed for varying amounts of time before testing with FM1-43. Images were analyzed using ImageJ (NIH, USA). A running two frame average was applied to the *Z* planes and to maintain consistency ROIs were drawn two planes (i.e., ~4 μm) below the FM1-43 fluorescence signal from the hair-cell stereocilia. ROIs covered the extent of the cell body in that plane. Average intensities from the ROIs were recorded and the background fluorescence (measured in a non-cellular region) was subtracted. Measurements were taken from 30 OHCs and 10 IHCs per explant.

Ototoxic Hair Cell Death and Protection Assay

To determine a dose-response curve, middle and basal coil cochlear explants were exposed to 0, 10, 100, 200, 250, 400 or 1000 μM neomycin for 24 h. To determine whether phenoxybenzamine confers protection against neomycin ototoxicity, cochlear explants were pre-treated for 1 h in 0, 50, 100 or 200 μM phenoxybenzamine followed by 24 h co-treatment in phenoxybenzamine and 250 μM neomycin in DMEM/F12 media at 37°C in a 5% CO_2/95% air atmosphere. After all experiments, explants were fixed with 4% paraformaldehyde in 0.1 M phosphate buffered saline (PBS, pH 7.2) at room temperature for 30–45 min for immunostaining and later evaluation for pyknotic and surviving hair cells.

Immunohistochemistry, Image Acquisition and Analysis

After fixation the explants were rinsed three times with PBS and incubated in blocking solution (PBS, 10% secondary host antibody serum and 0.5% Triton X-100) for 2 h. Subsequently, the explants were incubated with a mouse monoclonal anti-myosin 7A antibody, deposited to the DSHB by Orten, D.J. (DSHB Hybridoma Product MYO7A 138-1, used at 1:250) or a rabbit polyclonal anti-myosin 7A (25–6790, Proteus BioScience, used at 1:1000) primary antibody in blocking solution overnight at 4°C. Samples were then washed in PBS and incubated for 2 h at room temperature with 4′,6′-diamidino-2-phenylindole (DAPI 1 μM), AlexaFluor647 phalloidin (33 nM) and goat anti-rabbit-Atto488 or goat anti-mouse-Atto488 secondary antibodies in blocking solution. The explants were rinsed three times with PBS and imaged using the multiphoton Zeiss 510 NLO upright confocal microscope. DAPI was imaged using the a two-photon Chameleon-XR Ti:Sapphire laser tuned to 720 nm (435–485 nm bandpass filter), Atto488 was imaged using the 488 nm (500–550 nm bandpass filter) and AlexaFluor647 phalloidin using the 633 nm (long pass filter 650 nm) laser lines. Images were acquired at 1.5 μm *Z* intervals using either Achroplan 40× (NA 0.8) or Achroplan 63× Vis-IR (NA 1.0) water immersion objectives.

Z stacks (25–30 planes, 1.5 μm intervals) were acquired from two different regions in each explant. Image stacks were visualized using ZEN Lite software (Carl Zeiss Ltd, Germany) to identify pyknotic and surviving hair cells. The hair cells were considered pyknotic when they presented with condensed and marginated chromatin in the nuclei (Li et al., 1995; Lahne and Gale, 2008). Here we have used the characteristic pattern of pyknosis that we observe with the DAPI and myosin 7A staining during the death of IHCs and OHCs (**Figure 1**).

Hair cells with normal nuclei were considered to be viable surviving hair cells. Counts from the two regions sampled were averaged so that each explant counted as one N sample. Images were independently evaluated by two individuals.

Statistics

For live imaging experiments, all the data are presented as the mean ± SEM and ANOVA was applied with *post hoc* Tukey-Kramer's with significance set at $p < 0.05$. For hair-cell survival and pyknosis, all the data are presented as the mean ± SEM and the statistical test used was Students's *t*-test with significance set as $p < 0.05$.

RESULTS

Phenoxybenzamine Blocks Rapid FM 1-43 Entry in Mammalian Hair Cells if Preincubated

To evaluate the nature of phenoxybenzamine's interaction with mammalian MET channels, we measured FM1-43 uptake by hair cells in cochlear explant cultures from postnatal day 3–6 mice. A brief (30 s) exposure to FM1-43 ensured that rapid entry through the MET channels was the primary uptake pathway as opposed to a slower endocytic mechanism. FM1-43 uptake was hair cell specific and irreversible with OHCs taking up approximately twice as much FM1-43 as IHCs as described previously (Gale et al., 2001). When 100 μM phenoxybenzamine was simply co-applied during FM-143 exposure there was no significant effect on FM1-43 uptake in either IHCs or OHCs. In contrast, when phenoxybenzamine was also pre-incubated for either 30 or 60 min, we found a significant reduction in FM1-43 uptake in OHCs, and a small reduction in uptake in IHCs that failed to reach significance (**Figures 2A,B**). Pre-incubation substantially reduced FM1-43 uptake to 28% of control levels in OHCs and 60% in IHCs respectively, significantly different to uptake both in the controls and in samples in which compounds were co-applied together (**Figure 2C**). The block of FM1-43 uptake was reversible upon washout although the recovery from block was not immediate. Comparing a 1 min washout with a 60 min

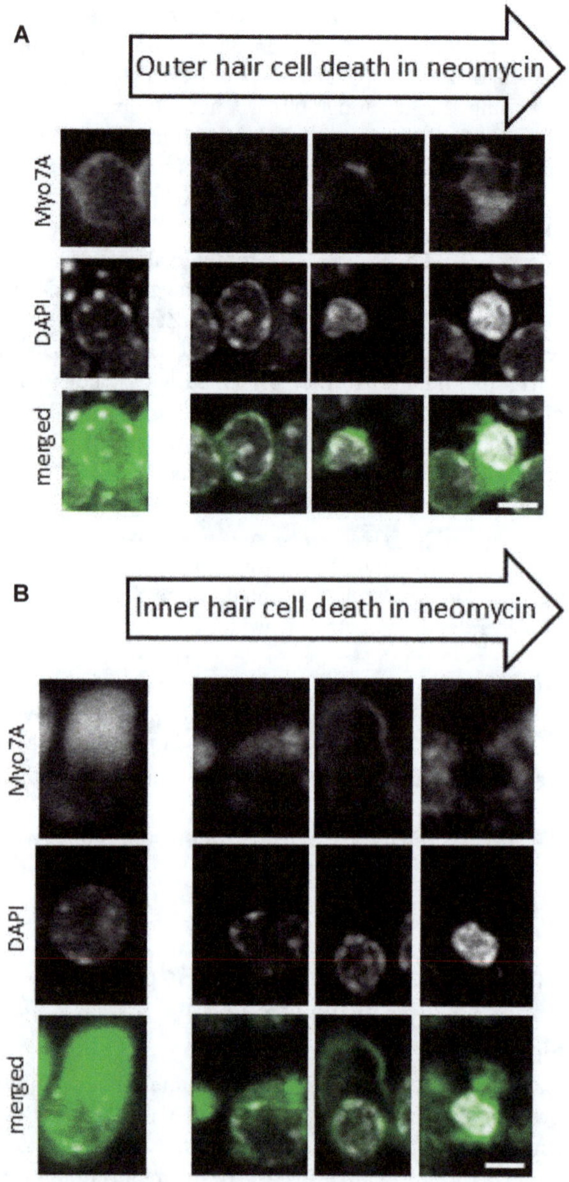

FIGURE 1 | Progression of neomycin-induced hair cell death. A sequence of images representing different stages of cell death that are observed after 24 h of neomycin exposure for both outer hair cells (OHCs) **(A)** and inner hair cells (IHCs) **(B)**. Anti-myosin 7A labeling (upper panel), 4′,6′-diamidino-2-phenylindole (DAPI) staining of nuclear chromatin (middle panel), Myo7A/DAPI merged image (lower panel). Since individual cells undergo cell death at different times each cell is at a different stage in the cell death process and the images have been compiled into a pseudo-time series as indicated by the arrows. Scale bar 5 μm.

washout we can see that the recovery was ~15% in OHCs after 1 min but was complete after 60 min (**Figure 3**). Recovery appeared to be faster but more variable in IHCs and on average we observed an overshoot in the recovery, but we note that the blocking effect of phenoxybenzamine was less robust in IHCs than in OHCs.

In order to determine whether the blockade of FM1-43 entry was dose-dependent, we varied the concentrations of phenoxybenzamine from 0 μM to 200 μM, pre-incubating for 30 min prior to FM1-43 application. The IC50 for the block of FM1-43 uptake by phenoxybenzamine differed slightly between OHC (logIC50 −4.185, 65 μM) and IHC (logIC50 −4.424, 38 μM) however, the Hill coefficient was strikingly different being 4 for OHC and 0.9 for IHC (**Figure 4**). One simple interpretation of these data is that there is a difference in the molecular nature of the MET channel in the two cochlear hair cell types. An alternative explanation is that the MET channel activity is reduced indirectly via a process that is affected by phenoxybenzamine and that is more prevalent in OHCs. We note that higher concentrations of phenoxybenzamine could not be tested due to problems with solubility that have been reported by others (Nisa et al., 2010).

Phenoxybenzamine Can Protect Hair Cells from Neomycin-Induced Ototoxicity

For the next experiments we set out to determine a concentration of neomycin that gave us ≥50% toxicity in our mouse cochlear explant culture model after 24 h of exposure. Cochlear explants were treated with neomycin at a range of concentrations from 0 μM to 1000 μM. At the end of the 24-h exposure explants were fixed and triple-labeled with DAPI, fluorescent phalloidin and antibodies to myosin 7A. *Z*-stack images were then collected using a confocal microscope (**Figure 5A**). Since hair cells are known to be able to survive without a hair bundle (Gale et al., 2002), we focused our analysis on the hair-cell soma and nuclear chromatin markers, as shown in **Figure 1**, to quantify the number of surviving hair cells, using the image stacks. A steep dose-dependence was observed for neomycin-induced hair cell death for both OHC and IHC (**Figure 5B**), with 50% cell death constants of 228 μM (log −3.642) and 232 μM (log −3.635) and different Hill coefficients of 4.7 and 1.9, respectively. Based on these experiments we decided to use 250 μM neomycin in subsequent experiments to test whether phenoxybenzamine could provide any protection in this 24 h ototoxicity model.

Given the requirement for drug pre-incubation, in test explants phenoxybenzamine (50, 100 or 200 μM) was applied for 1 h prior to the addition of neomycin in the presence of phenoxybenzamine. After 24 h explants were fixed, the same triple-labeling protocol was applied to all explants and image stacks collected and analyzed to quantify the number of surviving and pyknotic hair cells. At a concentration of 50 μM phenoxybenzamine did not offer significant protection against neomycin-induced ototoxicity (data not shown). In the presence of 100 μM phenoxybenzamine, however, the number of surviving OHC and IHC per 100 μm length of the cochlea was significantly higher, 27.9 ± 3.5 and 9.0 ± 1.0 respectively, compared to 17.6 ± 3.1 and 5.0 ± 1.4 with neomycin alone ($p < 0.05$). Using either the untreated control or phenoxybenzamine-treated alone explants to calculate the percent survival reveals that phenoxybenzamine increased OHC survival from 47% to 86% and IHC survival from 46% to 98% (**Figure 6**). Although phenoxybenzamine significantly reduced

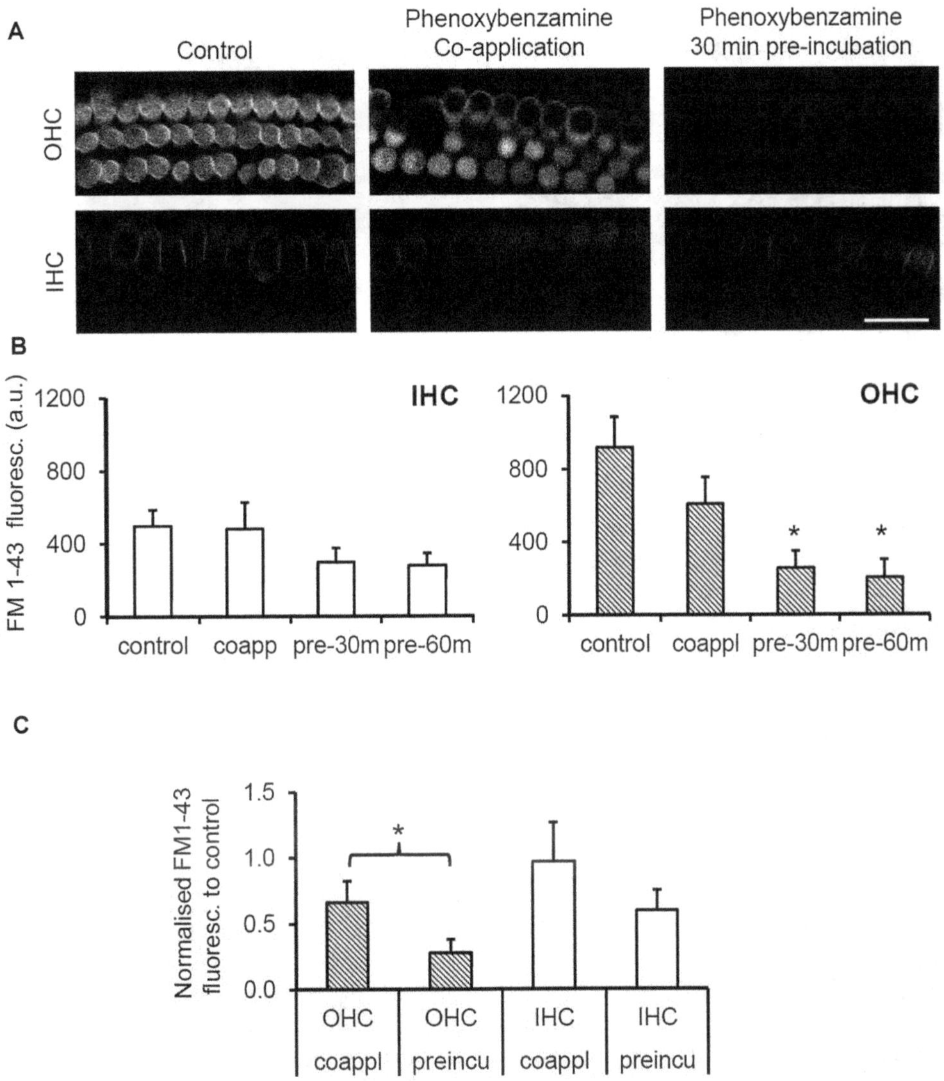

FIGURE 2 | Phenoxybenzamine (PB) significantly reduces rapid FM1-43 uptake in OHCs but not in inner cells. (A) Confocal images of FM1-43 uptake after brief exposure (30 s) in OHCs (upper panels) and IHCs (lower panel) under control conditions (left panel), either when co-applied with 100 μM PB (middle panel) or when explants were pre-incubated in PB for 30 min prior to FM1-43 application (right panel). **(B)** Quantification of FM1-43 fluorescence reveals that pre-incubation with phenoxybenzamine for 30 min or 60 min significantly reduces uptake in OHCs but not IHCs. Maximal inhibition of FM1-43 uptake is achieved in 30 min. **(C)** Pre-incubating with phenoxybenzamine is significantly more effective at blocking the rapid uptake of FM1-43. Expressed as a % of control, the uptake was reduced from 66% to 28% in OHCs and from 97% to 60% in IHCs. N numbers: control = 12; 100 μM PB-co-app = 6; 30 min pre-incubation = 9; 60 min pre-incubation = 6. Statistical test: ANOVA Tukey-Kramer's test, $^*p < 0.05$ in **(B)**; Student's t-test, $^*p < 0.05$ in **(C)**.

the number of neomycin-induced pyknotic OHC nuclei, we also observed a small but significant increase in pyknotic OHC and IHC nuclei when phenoxybenzamine was applied alone indicating the potential toxicity of the drug in the cochlea. The phenoxybenzamine-induced toxicity was more evident, particularly in OHCs at the highest concentration used (200 μM). In addition we observed that at 200 μM, rather than protecting hair cells against neomycin, phenoxybenzamine significantly enhanced the neomycin-induced toxicity in OHCs, whereas enhancement of toxicity was not observed in IHC (**Supplementary Figure S1**).

DISCUSSION

Phenoxybenzamine was one of a small number of compounds identified from two high-throughput drug screens for neomycin ototoxicity using zebrafish larvae (Ou et al., 2009; Vlasits et al., 2012). In zebrafish lateral line hair cells, the blockade of neomycin uptake into hair cells is thought to be the primary mode of action for the otoprotective effect of phenoxybenzamine (Ou et al., 2009). Here we used mammalian cochlear explant cultures from postnatal mice to evaluate the possible otoprotective effect of phenoxybenzamine. Testing

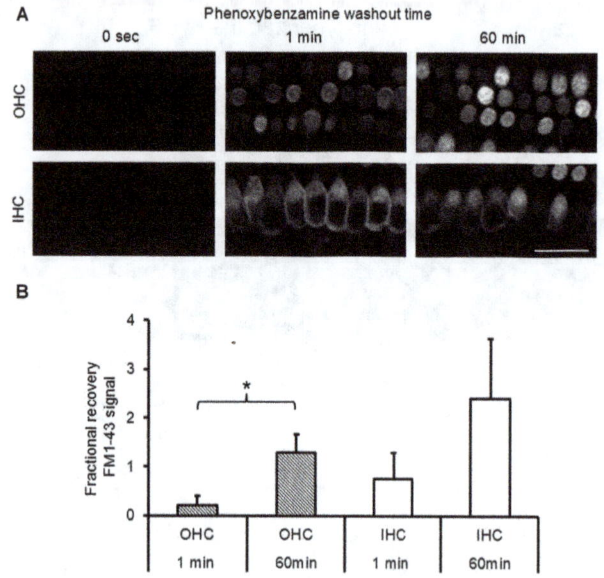

FIGURE 3 | Phenoxybenzamine block of FM1-43 entry is reversible. **(A)** After a 30 min pre-incubation in 100 μM phenoxybenzamine explants were washed for 1 min or 60 min in HBSS before being exposed to 6 μM FM1-43 for 30 s. Confocal images of the FM1-43 fluorescence signal in OHCs (upper panels) and IHCs (lower panel) when applied at 0 s, 1 min or 60 min after phenoxybenzamine washout. **(B)** The block by phenoxybenzamine is completely reversed 60 min after wash out. The fractional recovery of the FM1-43 signals was calculated from $F_{recov} = (F - F_{min})/(F_{max} - F_{min})$, where F_{min} is the signal from 30 min pre-incubation (n = 9) and F_{max} = control (no phenoxybenzamine) signal (n = 12) and F = 1 min (4) or 60 min (6). A F_{recov} value of 1 is equal to control (F_{max}). Student's t-test; $^*p < 0.05$.

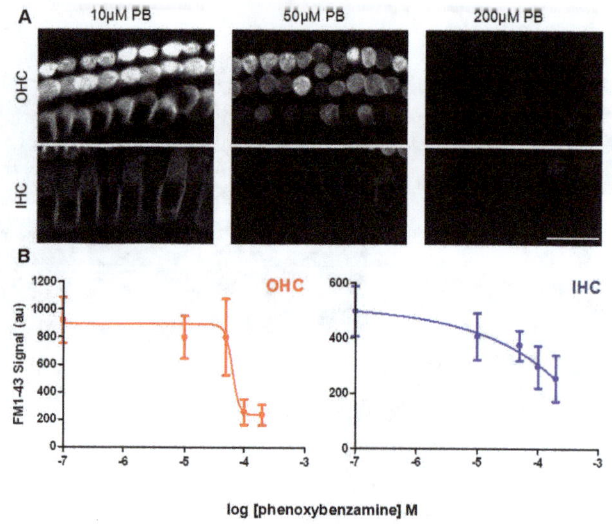

FIGURE 4 | Phenoxybenzamine block of FM1-43 entry is dose-dependent. **(A)** Confocal images of rapid FM-143 uptake assessed after 30 min of pre-incubation in 10, 50 or 200 μM phenoxybenzamine. Images at the focal planes of the OHC and IHC are shown. **(B)** Quantification of the rapid FM1-43 uptake in the presence of different concentrations of phenoxybenzamine reveal the reduction in FM1-43 uptake as a function of increasing phenoxybenzamine concentration in both OHC (red) and IHC (blue). The IC50 and Hill coefficient values from the curve fits are provided in the main text. N numbers: control (12); 10 μM PB (3); 50 μM PB (4); 100 μM (9); 200 μM (4). Scale bar: 20 μm.

compounds in the mammalian system is critical given the clear differences between the mammalian cochlea and the lateral line, not least because there are two distinctly different types of hair cell in the cochlea. We first characterized the effect of phenoxybenzamine on rapid FM1-43 uptake, which we use as mimic of neomycin entry since it permeates the mechanoelectrical transducer channels and has been shown to reduce the toxic effects of neomycin (Gale et al., 2001).

In zebrafish hair cells phenoxybenzamine blocks the uptake of both FM1-43 and gentamicin-Texas Red (Ou et al., 2009; Vlasits et al., 2012). We now show that phenoxybenzamine can block FM1-43 entry in both IHCs and OHCs in the mammalian cochlea. The IC50 for the blocking effect was quite similar between the two hair cell types (40–60 μM), however there was a ~4 fold difference in the Hill coefficient with the block in OHCs showing a steep dependence indicating cooperative binding, whereas in IHCs the coefficient was close to 1 suggesting non-cooperative binding of phenoxybenzamine. To better understand the mode of action, we compared pre-incubation of phenoxybenzamine with simple co-application and found that maximal inhibition was achieved by pre-incubation (**Figure 2**) as previously described in zebrafish (Vlasits et al., 2012). A 30 min pre-incubation was already maximal and no further block was observed when we extended the time of incubation to 60 min. Phenoxybenzamine is known to bind covalently to adrenergic receptors and serotonin receptors and in zebrafish the hair-cell survival effected by phenoxybenzamine persisted after phenoxybenzamine washout (Ou et al., 2009). In our live FM1-43 uptake assay, although the phenoxybenzamine effect remained for the first minute (at least in OHCs), the block was fully reversible after 60 min of washout. We observed differences in the effect of phenoxybenzamine on FM1-43 uptake in OHCs and IHCs. If the site of action of phenoxybenzamine in mammalian hair cells is within the mechanoelectrical transduction channel itself, this would suggest that there are significant differences in the structure of the channel between IHC and OHCs. Given the pre-incubation requirement, a simple explanation for this could that there is an intracellular binding site for phenoxybenzamine that is not present in IHCs. An alternative and perhaps more likely explanation is that there may be indirect effects of phenoxybenzamine on the mechanoelectrical transduction channels via regulatory molecules that are more prevalent in OHCs compared to IHCs.

We next examined whether the otoprotection seen in the lateral line with phenoxybenzamine is also observed in mammalian cochlear hair cells. The effects of AGs are both time and dose-dependent and we first set out to determine a neomycin-dose response curve for 24 h of exposure in our mouse cochlear explant model. We found a steep dose-dependence for neomycin-induced hair cell-death, particularly for OHCs (Hill coefficient of 4.7 compared to 1.9 in IHCs, **Figure 5**). The IC50 or

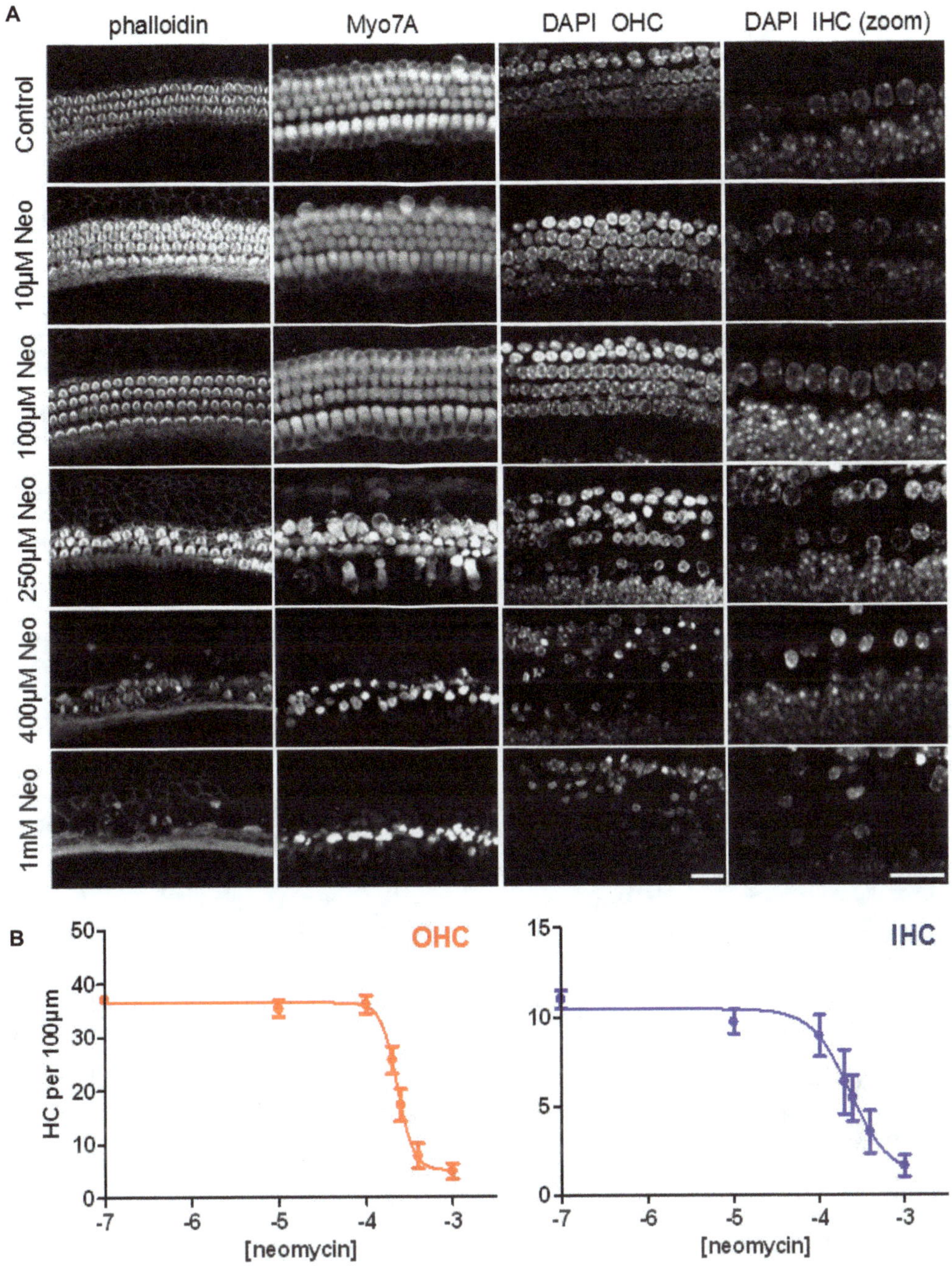

FIGURE 5 | Steep dose-dependent increase in hair-cell death after 24 h exposure to neomycin. (A) Confocal images of three different cellular markers: phalloidin, labeling F-actin; myosin7A (Myo7A), for the hair cell soma and DAPI which showing nuclear condensation and pyknosis in neomycin-treated examples. The right hand panels show a higher magnification (zoom) of the DAPI label in the IHC region. **(B)** Quantification of the numbers of surviving hair cells (expressed per 100 μm) reveals the steep dose-dependency of neomycin toxicity after 24 h of drug exposure. The 50% cell-death constants are similar between OHC (228 μM) and IHC (232 μM) but the Hill coefficients were quite different (4.7 and 1.9 respectively). N numbers: 0.1 μM (10); 10 μM (9); 100 μM (9); 200 μM (5); 250 μM (9); 400 μM (8); 1000 μM (10). Scale bar: 20 μm.

50% cell-death constant for neomycin was ~250 μM for both OHCs and IHCs and we used this concentration in subsequent assays in order to promote ~50% hair cell loss/survival, allowing either a protective effect or an enhancement of hair-cell death to be identified.

When used at a concentration of 100 μM phenoxybenzamine produced a significant protection of both OHC and IHCs, resulting in survival of both OHCs (86% survival) and IHCs (98% survival) relative to controls, i.e., phenoxybenzamine treatment alone. A small amount of toxicity was noted

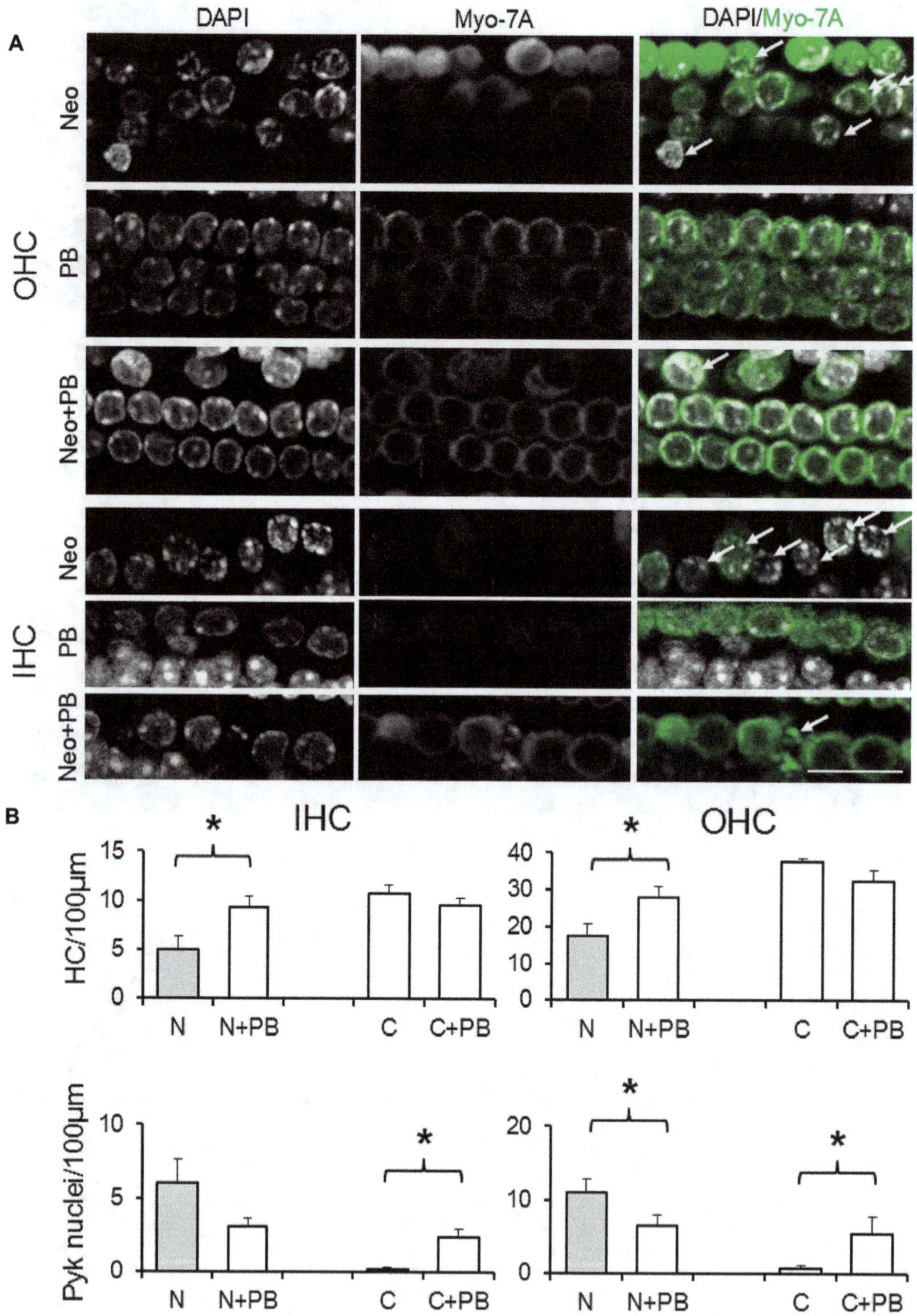

FIGURE 6 | Phenoxybenzamine confers protection against neomycin ototoxicity. (A) Representative confocal images showing the protective effect of the 100 μM phenoxybenzamine on the neomycin-induced hair cell death in both OHC and IHC. Images for phenoxybenzamine alone (PB), neomycin-alone for 250 μM for 24 h (Neo) or pre-incubation and continued presence of phenoxybenzamine during the neomycin exposure (Neo+PB). Images showing condensed chromation and pyknotic nuclei (DAPI staining, arrows) and the absence of the myosin7A labeling in missing/damaged hair cells. **(B)** Quantification of IHC and OHC survival (from myosin7A, upper graphs) and pyknotic hair cell nuclei (from DAPI images, lower graphs) in control C, 250 μM neomycin-treated (N), phenoxybenzamine alone (C+PB) or neomycin and phenoxybenzamine treated (N+PB) explants. N numbers: Neo (11); Neo+PB (8); PB alone (9); control (10). $^*p < 0.05$ (compared to control). Scale bar, 20 μm.

in the phenoxybenzamine-alone controls, based on the assessment of nuclear chromatin and pyknosis (**Figures 1, 6**). At a higher concentration, 200 μM phenoxybenzamine in combination with neomycin produced different effects on the two types of hair cell. The IHCs were still protected but there was an enhancement of toxicity in OHCs indicating an additive effect of phenoxybenzamine and neomycin. When phenoxybenzamine was applied alone at 200 μM for 24 h it resulted in a small amount of OHC death but did not affect IHCs. The stronger block of FM1-43 uptake in OHCs compared to IHCs that we have shown could explain the differential toxicity if we assume that activity of the MET channels is essential for cell survival. Another possible explanation for the phenoxybenzamine-induced toxicity observed in OHCs is that it results from the differential expression of known phenoxybenzamine targets. We checked cochlear gene expression on gEAR portal[1] and found that both serotonin receptors and adrenergic receptors are differentially expressed by OHCs and IHCs (Liu et al., 2014) providing some support for this as an alternative hypothesis for the observed toxicity. Importantly, however, phenoxybenzamine protects both IHCs and OHCs from neomycin-induced toxicity and the simplest explanation is that this is due to a reduction in neomycin uptake via the MET channels, consistent with our FM1-43 uptake assay (a mimic for the neomycin uptake).

The lack of a significant effect of phenoxybenzamine on FM1-43 uptake in IHCs compared to OHCs, but the presence of a protective effect from neomycin suggests a greater complexity here. The primary pathway for the aminoglycoside entry into hair cells is now considered to be via the MET channels located at the top of the stereocilia, consistent with AGs acting as open-channel blockers (Kroese et al., 1989; Ricci, 2002; Marcotti et al., 2005) as described for FM1-43 (Gale et al., 2001). However, the contribution of other ion channels to the uptake of AGs into hair cells has been less well characterized. Channels such as the transient receptor potential (TRP) class members such as TRPC3, TRPV4, TRPA1 and PRPML3 which are expressed in the cochlea have not been ruled out as possible entry pathways (Castiglioni and García-Añoveros, 2007; Cuajungco et al., 2007; Asai et al., 2010; Stepanyan et al., 2011; Quick et al., 2012). AGs block a variety of ion channels such as large-conductance Ca^{2+}-activated K^+ channels (Nomura et al., 1990), N-type and P/Q type Ca^{2+} channels (Pichler et al., 1996), ryanodine receptors (Mead and Williams, 2002a,b), P2X receptors (Lin et al., 1993) and nicotinic acetylcholine receptors (Blanchet et al., 2000). Similar to its effects on the MET channels, FM1-43 is also known to block TRPC3/TRPC6 channels (Quick et al., 2012). Phenoxybenzamine could be affecting any of the above channels, however, investigating these different ion channels is outside of the remit of this current work. In these present experiments a somewhat unexpected result was the consistent difference we observed between IHC and OHCs. Differences in the nature of the MET channels between these two cell types have been described (Beurg et al., 2006, 2009) and although the our results were generated from a different type of assay, they support the possibility of there being alternative channel isoforms expressed in the two cell types.

In recent years high-throughput screening in non-mammalian models has proven to be very useful in identify new compounds for preventing hair-cell death. The data presented here indicate the importance of follow up studies in mammalian hair-cell models. Our study did identify consistency between results from zebrafish lateral line screens and the mammalian cochlea: from the mode of action of phenoxybenzamine on FM1-43 uptake to the requirement for pre-incubation to achieve maximal inhibition. The particular sensitivity of OHCs to phenoxybenzamine is, however, something that would tend to preclude its clinical use. Nonetheless, the differential effects of phenoxybenzamine on IHC and OHCs could turn out to be of significance in our understanding of the molecular mechanisms regulating MET channels.

[1]http://umgear.org/index.html

AUTHOR CONTRIBUTIONS

All authors contributed to the initial conception and design of the work. PM undertook the majority of data analysis and drafted the manuscript. JEG contributed to data analysis and to the writing and revision of the manuscript. PAM collected data and undertook data analysis as part of an undergraduate project in Sussex and a Masters project at UCL. GR contributed to initial experimental design and manuscript revision.

ACKNOWLEDGMENTS

PM was supported by an Action On Hearing Loss Pauline Ashley award (PA12 to PM), by a Conselho Nacional de Desenvolvimento Cientifico e Tecnológico (CNPq) fellowship (249335/2013-1 to PM) and by an Action On Hearing Loss International Grant (G52 to JG). PAM was a BSc Neuroscience student at the University of Sussex and an MSc Neuroscience student at UCL. The authors would like to thank Professor Jonathan Ashmore for helpful discussions.

SUPPLEMENTARY MATERIAL

FIGURE S1 | Higher concentrations of phenoxybenzamine confer some protection against neomycin ototoxicity for IHCs but are toxic to OHCs. (A) Quantification of hair cell survival in the presence of 200 μM phenoxybenzamine (PB) alone or in the presence of neomycin for both IHCs and OHCs. N numbers: Neo (11); control (4); Neo+PB 50 μM (4); 50 μM PB alone (4); Neo+PB 200 μM (5); 200 μM PB alone (4). $^*P < 0.05$ and $^{**}P < 0.005$. **(B)** Representative confocal images showing F-actin (phalloidin), myosin 7a (Myo7a), for the hair cell soma and DAPI showing nuclear condensation and pyknosis in neomycin-treated examples.

REFERENCES

Alharazneh, A., Luk, L., Huth, M., Monfared, A., Steyger, P. S., Cheng, A. G., et al. (2011). Functional hair cell mechanotransducer channels are required for aminoglycoside ototoxicity. *PLoS One* 6:e22347. doi: 10.1371/journal.pone.0022347

Aran, J. M., and Darrouzet, J. (1975). Observation of click-evoked compound VIII nerve responses before, during and over seven months after kanamycin treatment in the guinea pig. *Acta Otolaryngol.* 79, 24–32. doi: 10.3109/00016487509124650

Asai, Y., Holt, J. R., and Géléoc, G. S. (2010). A quantitative analysis of the spatiotemporal pattern of transient receptor potential gene expression in the developing mouse cochlea. *J. Assoc. Res. Otolaryngol.* 11, 27–37. doi: 10.1007/s10162-009-0193-8

Beurg, M., Evans, M. G., Hackney, C. M., and Fettiplace, R. (2006). A large-conductance calcium-selective mechanotransducer channel in mammalian cochlear hair cells. *J. Neurosci.* 26, 10992–11000. doi: 10.1523/JNEUROSCI.2188-06.2006

Beurg, M., Fettiplace, R., Nam, J.-H., and Ricci, A. J. (2009). Localization of inner hair cell mechanotransducer channels using high-speed calcium imaging. *Nat. Neurosci.* 12, 553–558. doi: 10.1038/nn.2295

Blanchet, C., Eróstegui, C., Sugasawa, M., and Dulon, D. (2000). Gentamicin blocks ACh-evoked K^+ current in guinea-pig outer hair cells by impairing Ca^{2+} entry at the cholinergic receptor. *J. Physiol.* 525, 641–654. doi: 10.1111/j.1469-7793.2000.t01-1-00641.x

Castiglioni, A. J., and García-Añoveros, J. (2007). MechanoTRPs and TRPA1. *Curr. Top. Membr.* 59, 171–189. doi: 10.1016/S1063-5823(06)59008-8

Cuajungco, M. P., Grimm, C., and Heller, S. (2007). TRP channels as candidates for hearing and balance abnormalities in vertebrates. *Biochim. Biophys. Acta* 1772, 1022–1027. doi: 10.1016/j.bbadis.2007.01.002

Dai, C. F., Mangiardi, D., Cotanche, D. A., and Steyger, P. S. (2006). Uptake of fluorescent gentamicin by vertebrate sensory cells *in vivo*. *Hear. Res.* 213, 64–78. doi: 10.1016/j.heares.2005.11.011

Diop, L., and Dausse, J. P. (1986). Specific binding of 3H-nicergoline in rat brain: comparison with the selective alpha 1-antagonist 3H-prazosin. *J. Pharmacol.* 17, 65–74.

Doggrell, S. A. (1995). Increase in affinity and loss of 5-hydroxytryptamine 2a-receptor reserve for 5- hydroxytryptamine on the aorta of spontaneously hypertensive rats. *J. Auton. Pharmacol.* 15, 371–377. doi: 10.1111/j.1474-8673.1995.tb00403.x

Duscha, S., Boukari, H., Shcherbakov, D., Salian, S., Silva, S., Kendall, A., et al. (2014). Identification and evaluation of improved 4'-*O*-(alkyl) 4,5-disubstituted 2-deoxystreptamines as next-generation aminoglycoside antibiotics. *MBio* 5:e01827. doi: 10.1128/mBio.01827-14

Forge, A., and Schacht, J. (2000). Aminoglycoside antibiotics. *Audiol. Neurootol.* 5, 3–22. doi: 10.1159/000013861

Frazer, A., and Hensley, J. (1999). "Serotonin receptors," in *Basic Neurochemistry: Molecular, Cellular and Medical Aspects*, 6th Edn. eds G. J. Siegel, B. W. Agranoff and R. W. Albers (Philadelphia: Lippincott-Raven), 263–292.

Gale, J. E., Marcotti, W., Kennedy, H. J., Kros, C. J., and Richardson, G. P. (2001). FM1-43 dye behaves as a permeant blocker of the hair-cell mechanotransducer channel. *J. Neurosci.* 21, 7013–7025.

Gale, J. E., Meyers, J. R., Periasamy, A., and Corwin, J. T. (2002). Survival of bundleless hair cells and subsequent bundle replacement in the bullfrog's saccule. *J Neurobiol.* 50, 81–92. doi: 10.1002/neu.10002

Greenwood, G. J. (1959). Neomycin ototoxicity; report of a case. *AMA Arch. Otolaryngol.* 69, 390–397. doi: 10.1001/archotol.1959.00730030400002

Hashino, E., and Shero, M. (1995). Endocytosis of aminoglycoside antibiotics in sensory hair cells. *Brain Res.* 704, 135–140. doi: 10.1016/0006-8993(95)01198-6

Hock, R., and Anderson, R. J. (1995). Prevention of drug-induced nephrotoxicity in the intensive care unit. *J. Crit. Care* 10, 33–43. doi: 10.1016/0883-9441(95)90029-2

Huth, M. E., Han, K.-H., Sotoudeh, K., Hsieh, Y.-J., Effertz, T., Vu, A. A., et al. (2015). Designer aminoglycosides prevent cochlear hair cell loss and hearing loss. *J. Clin. Invest.* 125, 583–592. doi: 10.1172/JCI77424

Inchiosa, M. A. Jr. (2013). Phenoxybenzamine in complex regional pain syndrome: potential role and novel mechanisms. *Anesthesiol. Res. Pract.* 2013:978615. doi: 10.1155/2013/978615

Kroese, A. B., Das, A., and Hudspeth, A. J. (1989). Blockage of the transduction channels of hair cells in the bullfrog's sacculus by aminoglycoside antibiotics. *Hear. Res.* 37, 203–217. doi: 10.1016/0378-5955(89)90023-3

Kumar, V. L., and Dewan, S. (2000). Alpha adrenergic blockers in the treatment of benign hyperplasia of the prostate. *Int. Urol. Nephrol.* 32, 67–71. doi: 10.1023/A:1007108201320

Lahne, M., and Gale, J. E. (2008). Damage-induced activation of ERK1/2 in cochlear supporting cells is a hair cell death-promoting signal that depends on extracellular ATP and calcium. *J. Neurosci.* 28, 4918–4928. doi: 10.1523/JNEUROSCI.4914-07.2008

Li, L., Nevill, G., and Forge, A. (1995). Two modes of hair cell loss from the vestibular sensory epithelia of the guinea pig inner ear. *J. Comp. Neurol.* 355, 405–417. doi: 10.1002/cne.903550307

Lin, X., Hume, R. I., and Nuttall, A. L. (1993). Voltage-dependent block by neomycin of the ATP-induced whole cell current of guinea-pig outer hair cells. *J. Neurophysiol.* 70, 1593–1605.

Liu, H., Pecka, J. L., Zhang, Q., Soukup, G. A., Beisel, K. W., and He, D. Z. Z. (2014). Characterization of transcriptomes of cochlear inner and outer hair cells. *J. Neurosci.* 34, 11085–11095. doi: 10.1523/JNEUROSCI.1690-14.2014

Majumder, P., Duchen, M. R., and Gale, J. E. (2015). Cellular glutathione content in the organ of Corti and its role during ototoxicity. *Front. Cell. Neurosci.* 9:143. doi: 10.3389/fncel.2015.00143

Marcotti, W., van Netten, S. M., and Kros, C. J. (2005). The aminoglycoside antibiotic dihydrostreptomycin rapidly enters mouse outer hair cells through the mechano -electrical transducer channels. *J. Physiol.* 567, 505–521. doi: 10.1113/jphysiol.2005.085951

Matt, T., Ng, C. L., Lang, K., Sha, S.-H., Akbergenov, R., Shcherbakov, D., et al. (2012). Dissociation of antibacterial activity and aminoglycoside ototoxicity in the 4-monosubstituted 2-deoxystreptamine apramycin. *Proc. Natl. Acad. Sci. U S A* 109, 10984–10989. doi: 10.1073/pnas.1204073109

Matz, G., Rybak, L., Roland, P. S., Hannley, M., Friedman, R., Manolidis, S., et al. (2004). Ototoxicity of ototopical antibiotic drops in humans. *Otolaryngol. Head Neck Surg.* 130, S79–S82. doi: 10.1016/j.otohns.2003.12.007

Mead, F., and Williams, A. J. (2002a). Block of the ryanodine receptor channel by neomycin is relieved at high holding potentials. *Biophys. J.* 82, 1953–1963. doi: 10.1016/s0006-3495(02)75544-6

Mead, F., and Williams, A. J. (2002b). Ryanodine-induced structural alterations in the RyR channel suggested by neomycin block. *Biophys. J.* 82, 1964–1974. doi: 10.1016/s0006-3495(02)75545-8

Nisa, N., Blokpoel, M. C., Robertson, B. D., Tyndall, J. D. A., Lun, S., Bishai, W. R., et al. (2010). Targeting the chromosome partitioning protein ParA in tuberculosis drug discovery. *J. Antimicrob. Chemother.* 65, 2347–2358. doi: 10.1093/jac/dkq311

Nomura, K., Maruse, K., Watanabe, K., and Sokabe, M. (1990). Aminoglycoside blockade of Ca^{2+}-activated K^+ channel from rat brain synaptosomal membranes incorporated into planar bilayers. *J. Membr. Biol.* 115, 241–251. doi: 10.1007/bf01868639

Ou, H. C., Cunningham, L. L., Francis, S. P., Brandon, C. S., Simon, J. A., Raible, D. W., et al. (2009). Identification of FDA-approved drugs and bioactives that protect hair cells in the zebrafish (*Danio rerio*) lateral line and mouse (*Mus musculus*) utricle. *J. Assoc. Res. Otolaryngol.* 10, 191–203. doi: 10.1007/s10162-009-0158-y

Pichler, M., Wang, Z., Grabner-Weiss, C., Reimer, D., Hering, S., Grabner, M., et al. (1996). Block of P/Q-type calcium channels by therapeutic concentrations of aminoglycoside antibiotics. *Biochemistry* 35, 14659–14664. doi: 10.1021/bi961657t

Quick, K., Zhao, J., Eijkelkamp, N., Linley, J. E., Rugiero, F., Cox, J. J., et al. (2012). TRPC3 and TRPC6 are essential for normal mechanotransduction in subsets of sensory neurons and cochlear hair cells. *Open Biol.* 2:120068. doi: 10.1098/rsob.120068

Ricci, A. (2002). Differences in mechano-transducer channel kinetics underlie tonotopic distribution of fast adaptation in auditory hair cells. *J. Neurophysiol.* 87, 1738–1748. doi: 10.1152/jn.00574.2001

Shi, X. (2016). Pathophysiology of the cochlear intrastrial fluid-blood barrier (review). *Hear. Res.* 338, 52–63. doi: 10.1016/j.heares.2016.01.010

Shulman, E., Belakhov, V., Wei, G., Kendall, A., Meyron-Holtz, E. G., Ben-Shachar, D., et al. (2014). Designer aminoglycosides that selectively inhibit cytoplasmic rather than mitochondrial ribosomes show decreased ototoxicity: a strategy for the treatment of genetic diseases. *J. Biol. Chem.* 289, 2318–2330. doi: 10.1074/jbc.M113.533588

Stebbins, W. C., Hawkins, J. E. Jr., Johnson, L. G., and Moody, D. B. (1979). Hearing thresholds with outer and inner hair cell loss. *Am. J. Otolaryngol.* 1, 15–27. doi: 10.1016/s0196-0709(79)80004-6

Stepanyan, R. S., Indzhykulian, A. A., Vélez-Ortega, A. C., Boger, E. T., Steyger, P. S., Friedman, T. B., et al. (2011). TRPA1-mediated accumulation of aminoglycosides in mouse cochlear outer hair cells. *J. Assoc. Res. Otolaryngol.* 12, 729–740. doi: 10.1007/s10162-011-0288-x

Te, A. E. (2002). A modern rationale for the use of phenoxybenzamine in urinary tract disorders and other conditions. *Clin. Ther.* 24, 851–861; discussion 837. doi: 10.1016/s0149-2918(02)80003-0

Thoenen, H., Hürlimann, A., and Haefely, W. (1964). Dual site of action of phenoxybenzamine in the cat's spleen: blockade of α-adrenergic receptors and inhibition of re-uptake of neurally released norepinephrine. *Experientia* 20, 272–273. doi: 10.1007/bf02151802

Toubeau, G., Laurent, G., Carlier, M. B., Abid, S., Maldague, P., Heuson-Stiennon, J. A., et al. (1986). Tissue repair in rat kidney cortex after short treatment with aminoglycosides at low doses. A comparative biochemical and morphometric study. *Lab. Invest.* 54, 385–393.

Vlasits, A. L., Simon, J. A., Raible, D. W., Rubel, E. W., and Owens, K. N. (2012). Screen of FDA-approved drug library reveals compounds that protect hair cells from aminoglycosides and cisplatin. *Hear. Res.* 294, 153–165. doi: 10.1016/j.heares.2012.08.002

Wang, Q., Kachelmeier, A., and Steyger, P. S. (2010). Competitive antagonism of fluorescent gentamicin uptake in the cochlea. *Hear. Res.* 268, 250–259. doi: 10.1016/j.heares.2010.06.008

Wang, Q., and Steyger, P. S. (2009). Trafficking of systemic fluorescent gentamicin into the cochlea and hair cells. *J. Assoc. Res. Otolaryngol.* 10, 205–219. doi: 10.1007/s10162-009-0160-4

12

Cyclodextrins and Iatrogenic Hearing Loss: New Drugs with Significant Risk

Mark A. Crumling[1], *Kelly A. King*[2]* *and R. Keith Duncan*[1]*

[1]*Department of Otolaryngology-Head & Neck Surgery, Kresge Hearing Research Institute, University of Michigan, Ann Arbor, MI, United States,* [2]*Audiology Unit, Otolaryngology Branch, National Institute on Deafness and Other Communication Disorders, National Institutes of Health, Bethesda, MD, United States*

Edited by:
Peter S. Steyger,
Oregon Health & Science University,
United States

Reviewed by:
Fred Pereira,
Baylor College of Medicine,
United States
Federico Kalinec,
University of California, Los Angeles,
United States

***Correspondence:**
Kelly A. King
kingke@nidcd.nih.gov
R. Keith Duncan
rkduncan@umich.edu

Cyclodextrins are a family of cyclic oligosaccharides with widespread usage in medicine, industry and basic sciences owing to their ability to solubilize and stabilize guest compounds. In medicine, cyclodextrins primarily act as a complexing vehicle and consequently serve as powerful drug delivery agents. Recently, uncomplexed cyclodextrins have emerged as potent therapeutic compounds in their own right, based on their ability to sequester and mobilize cellular lipids. In particular, 2-hydroxypropyl-β-cyclodextrin (HPβCD) has garnered attention because of its cholesterol chelating properties, which appear to treat a rare neurodegenerative disorder and to promote atherosclerosis regression related to stroke and heart disease. Despite the potential health benefits, use of HPβCD has been linked to significant hearing loss in several species, including humans. Evidence in mice supports a rapid onset of hearing loss that is dose-dependent. Ototoxicity can occur following central or peripheral drug delivery, with either route resulting in the preferential loss of cochlear outer hair cells (OHCs) within hours of dosing. Inner hair cells and spiral ganglion cells are spared at doses that cause ~85% OHC loss; additionally, no other major organ systems appear adversely affected. Evidence from a first-to-human phase 1 clinical trial mirrors animal studies to a large extent, indicating rapid onset and involvement of OHCs. All patients in the trial experienced some permanent hearing loss, although a temporary loss of function can be observed acutely following drug delivery. The long-term impact of HPβCD use as a maintenance drug, and the mechanism(s) of ototoxicity, are unknown. β-cyclodextrins preferentially target membrane cholesterol, but other lipid species and proteins may be directly or indirectly involved. Moreover, as cholesterol is ubiquitous in cell membranes, it remains unclear why OHCs are preferentially susceptible to HPβCD. It is possible that HPβCD acts upon several targets—for example, ion channels, tight junctions (TJ), membrane integrity, and bioenergetics—that collectively increase the sensitivity of OHCs over other cell types.

Keywords: ototoxicity, cochlea, outer hair cell, Niemann-Pick disease type C, cholesterol, cyclodextrin, deafness

INTRODUCTION

Ototoxicity in the form of iatrogenic hearing loss arising from various pharmacological treatments has been well-described for more than 1000 years (Schacht and Hawkins, 2006). In these cases, drug treatments, often administered for life-threatening diseases, bring to bear a dilemma balancing the risk to hearing with the desire to remedy disease. Recently, a new class of ototoxic compounds was identified—cyclodextrins (Ward et al., 2010; Crumling et al., 2012; Davidson et al., 2016). Though these compounds have many roles in industrial and medicinal applications as solvents and stabilizers, the risk to hearing only became apparent when highly concentrated doses of cyclodextrin were being evaluated as a treatment for the devastating neurological disorder, Niemann-Pick Disease Type C (NPC). In this review article, we summarize the nature of these compounds, the evidence of cyclodextrin-induced hearing loss in human patients and animal models, and speculate about potential mechanisms that may underlie this ototoxicity.

Cyclodextrin Types and Structure

Cyclodextrins are ring-shaped oligosaccharides formed in nature by the digestion of cellulose by bacteria. They are composed of varying numbers of glucose units held together by α-1, 4 glycosidic bonds. The naturally occurring varieties contain at least six glucose units, with the most common having six, seven, or eight (so called, α-, β-, and γ- cyclodextrins, respectively). Cyclodextrins with more than eight glucose members are less common in nature and less well characterized, and compounds with five glucose units are only synthetic. Bountiful research has been poured into α-, β-, and γ- cyclodextrins and their properties are well characterized. The ring these molecules form (**Figure 1A**) is often depicted as a cup-shaped toroid (**Figure 1B**). The outside of the cup is hydrophilic, and the inside is more hydrophobic. Thus, these chemicals are water soluble with the ability to contain hydrophobic guest molecules within them, singly or as dimers (**Figure 1B**; López et al., 2011, 2013). The resulting increase in solubility and stability of the guest compounds is the predominant basis for the vast medical, industrial and scientific uses of cyclodextrins. Much effort has been expended on improving and tailoring this characteristic by chemical substitution of the hydrogen in the hydroxyl groups, which form the mouths of the toroidal openings, extending from the glucose units. Some common substitutions at these sites are methyl, hydroxylpropyl and sulfobutylether groups. Adding these groups occurs with different efficiencies and results in different sets of impurities along with the intended reaction product. It is chemically difficult to achieve substitution of all possible sites, so a reaction process results in a "degree of substitution", often expressed as the average number of substituted groups present per molecule or per glucose unit. Different processes produce varied degrees of substitution, and this can have advantages, since both the nature of the substituent group and the degree of substitution influence the performance of the cyclodextrin in ways that can be useful.

Uses of Cyclodextrins

The ability of cyclodextrins to hold guest compounds has been harnessed in many ways. The food industry has capitalized on this property to entrap various ingredients, masking or preserving flavors in food products. As food additives, the natural α-, β-, and γ- cyclodextrins have the Generally Recognized as Safe (GRAS) label by the U.S. Food and Drug Administration (FDA; Notices 000155, 000074, 000046, respectively), subject to certain percent composition limits. The α- and β-cyclodextrins do not cross the intestinal barrier in significant amounts and are fermented by gut bacteria or excreted whole; γ-cyclodextrins are metabolized by mammalian α-amylases into linear oligosaccharides. Consequently, cyclodextrins in food or otherwise consumed orally do not usually enter the

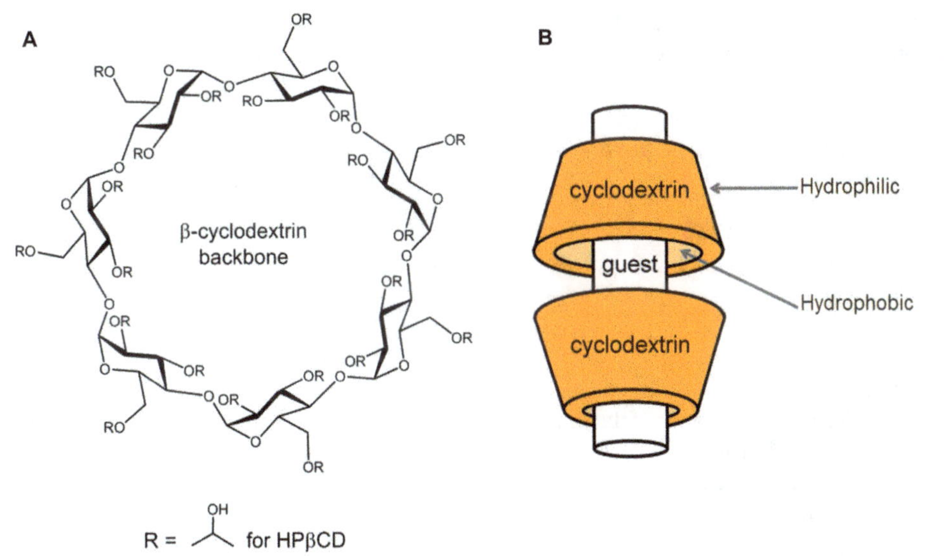

FIGURE 1 | Basic structure of a β-cyclodextrin and mode of complexation with guest compounds. **(A)** The chemical structure of a β-cyclodextrin backbone is illustrated, depicting the seven glucose units and sites of chemical substitution (R). In the native cyclodextrin, a hydrogen occupies each R site. As an example, in the case of 2-hydroxypropyl-β-cyclodextrin (HPβCD), the R sites are occupied to varying numbers by 2-hydroxypropyl groups, as shown. **(B)** Guest compounds can incorporate into the hydrophobic interior of the toroidal cyclodextrin molecule, where they are protected from water. The drawing is modeled after the interaction of HPβCD with cholesterol, where HPβCD dimers can encapsulate one cholesterol molecule (López et al., 2011, 2013).

circulation in significant amounts (Frijlink et al., 1990), and thus are generally safe.

Pharmaceutical applications primarily involve the use of cyclodextrins to increase the stability and solubility of drug compounds, but the ability to form inclusion complexes has also been exploited in scavenging applications where injected cyclodextrins can bind to active compounds and end their action on target systems. As constituents of drug formulations, several modified and unmodified cyclodextrins are in the FDA's Inactive Ingredient Database, suggesting that they are relatively inert up to certain dosages. Safety is greatly increased by hydroxypropyl and sulfobutylether substitution, which has allowed so-modified cyclodextrins to be administered parenterally at high doses to experimental animals with little morbidity and mortality and few obvious side effects (Gould and Scott, 2005). High dosing due to the relative safety of the substituted versions has opened the door to cyclodextrins being used for their own drug effects, rather than just for the actions of guest compounds.

New medical applications have arisen from the insight that uncomplexed cyclodextrins—those with an empty central cavity—can extract and shuttle membrane lipids. Therapeutic applications include treatments for atherosclerosis, Alzheimer's disease, Parkinson's disease, infectious disease, and lipid storage disorders (Dass and Jessup, 2000; Graham et al., 2003; Yao et al., 2012; Ottinger et al., 2014; Oliveri and Vecchio, 2016; Zimmer et al., 2016). A recent report generated considerable excitement, showing that 2-hydroxypropyl-β-cyclodextrin (HPβCD) reversed atherosclerosis and limited the formation of new sclerotic plaques in mice, even when the mice were fed a cholesterol-rich diet (Zimmer et al., 2016). The affordability and (reported) safety of HPβCD makes it attractive compared to other treatments for cardiovascular disease, especially for patients who are sensitive to statins or cannot maintain a low-fat, low-cholesterol diet. Similar dosing has been used successfully to treat a mouse model of Alzheimer's disease (Yao et al., 2012), further increasing the clinical interest in HPβCD. However, the true surge in attention given HPβCD has been driven by its ability to normalize lipid homeostasis and prolong survival in animal models of NPC.

Cyclodextrins in Treatment of Niemann-Pick Disease Type C

NPC is a rare (1:120,000–1:150,000) autosomal recessive disorder of lipid metabolism characterized by endolysosomal accumulation of unesterified cholesterol (Vanier and Millat, 2003; Vanier, 2010). It is part of a family of metabolic storage disorders, and the hallmark phenotype includes hepatic dysfunction and progressive neurodegeneration. It is panethnic, primarily affects children, and is fatal in all cases.

Biallelic mutations in one of two genes (*NPC1* and *NPC2*) result in NPC, although the two complementation groups appear biochemically indistinguishable and the majority of cases (approximately 95%) occur from DNA-variants in *NPC1* (Carstea et al., 1997; Naureckiene et al., 2000; Ikonen and Hölttä-Vuori, 2004), which, to date, is associated with hundreds of pathogenic mutations. NPC proteins reside in late endosomes/lysosomes, and their exact functions remain unclear (Vanier, 2010); affected cells fail to mobilize cholesterol across cell membranes resulting in excessive and ultimately pathological storage of exogenous, unesterified cholesterol and other lipid moieties in cells and tissues throughout the body (Liscum and Faust, 1987; Liscum et al., 1989). The effect is preferentially severe in neurons and lipid-dense regions of the central nervous system.

The NPC phenotype is complex and heterogeneous. Classical onset occurs in childhood, although presentation can range from the perinatal period to adulthood (Vanier and Millat, 2003), and there is often a diagnostic delay. Early clinical markers tend to involve the hepatic system, however, diagnosis is usually tied to onset of neurological symptoms, such as cerebellar ataxia, dysarthria and cognitive impairment. Vertical supranuclear gaze palsy is considered nearly pathognomic, particularly when coupled with gelastic cataplexy (loss of muscle tone that can be triggered by laughing). Although variable, most patients die in adolescence, 10–15 years after onset of neurological disease (Ory et al., 2017).

Pharmaceutical statins used to treat hypercholesterolemia and dietary cholesterol restriction have not proven effective at preventing or slowing neurological progression in NPC (Patterson et al., 1993; Somers et al., 2001). Miglustat (Zavesca), a small iminosugar that crosses the blood-brain barrier and inhibits an early enzyme in the glycosphingolipid pathway (Patterson et al., 2007), is used for the treatment of Gaucher disease, another disorder of lysosomal storage. Miglustat is an approved therapy for neurological symptoms of NPC in at least 45 countries (Patterson and Walkley, 2017); however its ability to delay neurological progression is modest, and it does not mobilize intracellular cholesterol in NPC. It is currently not approved in the United States for the treatment of NPC, although many patients pursue off-label usage if cost or insurance coverage is not prohibitive.

Recognition of a cyclodextrin derivative as a potential therapeutic intervention for NPC was first reported by Camargo et al. (2001), although the described effect on neurological symptoms was slight and, at the time, cyclodextrin was not considered to be a viable therapy for patients. Renewed attention came when, serendipitously, parallel work from the Dietschy and Walkley labs using HPβCD as an excipient to administer the drug allopregnanolone in a mouse model for NPC showed that HPβCD alone was effective at treating the disease (Davidson et al., 2009; Liu et al., 2009). This confirmed and expanded earlier evidence that HPβCD is efficacious at mobilizing cholesterol in cells (Kilsdonk et al., 1995; Liu et al., 2003). The combination of these discoveries launched an extensive exploration of HPβCD as a potential disease-altering therapy for NPC.

To date, in both feline and mouse models, HPβCD has increased lifespan and ameliorated the neurodegenerative phenotype. In $Npc1^{-/-}$ mice, intraperitoneal administration of HPβCD improved liver function, delayed onset and slowed progression of neurological disease while significantly increasing lifespan (Camargo et al., 2001; Davidson et al., 2009). Cats with a single spontaneous missense mutation in *NPC1* develop a phenotype similar to that observed in humans with classical juvenile onset (Lowenthal et al., 1990), and direct intracisternal administration of HPβCD into presymptomatic NPC1 cats prevented onset of cerebellar dysfunction for over a year. In symptomatic animals it slowed neurodegeneration while increasing lifespan. Subcutaneous HPβCD administration was effective at treating peripheral hepatic disease, but required higher doses to treat neurological disease, resulting in pulmonary toxicities (Vite et al., 2015).

It is not clear how HPβCD mechanistically alters the course of NPC disease progression, yet biomarkers show reduced neuronal storage and extended Purkinje cell survival in treated animals. Preclinical studies have confirmed the route of administration impacts efficacy and toxicity, likely related, in part, to HPβCD not crossing the blood-brain barrier at appreciable levels (Pontikis et al., 2013). When HPβCD is delivered directly to the CNS in $NPC1^{-/-}$ cats, the effect on survival duration is more than three times as much as when the drug is administered systemically (Vite et al., 2015).

Compelling preclinical data and a unique and innovative partnership established between the scientific and family stakeholder communities (Walkley et al., 2016) have accelerated the move of HPβCD into human phase 1/2a clinical trials, exploring both intravenous (IV) and intrathecal drug delivery using two different preparations (Trappsol Cyclo and VTS-270, respectively). The published results of these early phase studies, focused largely on safety and dosing, show high promise and indicate therapeutic efficacy at treating NPC1 disease in patients (Ory et al., 2017). An ongoing phase 2b/3 clinical trial is nearing completion, and in early 2016 the FDA granted a Breakthrough Therapy designation for a HPβCD preparation (VTS-270), which had previously been given Orphan Drug status. The combination of these designations by the FDA acknowledges the high therapeutic potential to address an unmet need in a rare disease population, and may serve to fast-track HPβCD approval as a therapy for NPC. Preclinical and now, first-in-human data demonstrate it is generally well tolerated, with a single salient toxicity observed thus far across species and now in humans: hearing loss. Despite its ototoxic properties, approval of HPβCD as a therapy for NPC seems likely, and exploration into its use to treat other, more common diseases such as atherosclerosis, is underway (Coisne et al., 2016; Zimmer et al., 2016). Establishing the ototoxic profile and causative mechanisms is critical if HPβCD ototoxicity is to be mitigated or prevented.

HPβCD OTOTOXICITY

Animal Models

Although the toxicology of cyclodextrins has been studied for decades, only in the last several years has their effect on hearing been appreciated. Prior to the discovery of ototoxicity, cyclodextrins, particularly HPβCD, had been administered parentally at doses that were high enough to be ototoxic (reviewed in Frömming and Szejtli, 1994; Gould and Scott, 2005). However, it appears that such doses were given infrequently, and audiological testing was not a priority. Behavioral effects of hearing loss also seem to have gone unnoticed. Only when research on the use of HPβCD to treat NPC in preclinical models prompted routine testing in animals at multi-thousand mg/kg parenteral doses, did the ototoxicity of HPβCD come to light.

HPβCD Ototoxicity in Cats

The first hint of HPβCD ototoxicity came from NPC research in cats (Ward et al., 2010). Human patients with *NPC1* mutations can have disease-related hearing loss (Pikus, 1991; King et al., 2014), and because of this, the auditory system of NPC cats was being monitored by auditory brainstem response (ABR) recording in experiments on HPβCD as a therapy. NPC cats turned out not to share the auditory phenotype with humans. However, hearing abnormalities were found in animals treated with HPβCD. Elevated ABR thresholds were noted after receiving a single subcutaneous injection of HPβCD at 8000 mg/kg (Ward et al., 2010). Comparable results were found after a single intrathecal injection of 4000 mg/kg brain weight. The elevated thresholds remained unchanged for up to 12 weeks after these single injections. These experiments indicated that single doses capable of altering NPC symptoms were harmful to the auditory system. When subcutaneous injections were given to normal cats weekly at 4000 mg/kg, ABR thresholds were significantly elevated by 4 weeks after the first injection, though single injections at this dose caused no significant threshold shift. This deviation from the behavior with a single subcutaneous injection means that there was a buildup of cyclodextrin or there was an accumulation of effect produced by the cyclodextrin on the auditory system, turning an innocuous dose into one that causes hearing loss. Interestingly, two cats treated at 4000 mg/kg brain weight intrathecally every 2 weeks for 13 weeks showed no response to short-duration, predominantly high frequency, broadband clicks in the ABR testing at the highest level available (125 dB SPL). In a subsequent study (Vite et al., 2015), several groups of NPC cats received HPβCD intracisternally at different concentrations and dosing frequencies. Successful disease treatment was always associated with ototoxicity. The threshold shifts were ~30–50 dB for 30–120 mg HPβCD given intracisternally at 14-day intervals.

HPβCD Ototoxicity in Mice

From the evaluation of hearing in cats, the permanence of HPβCD induced hearing loss was uncertain and the site of injury was unclear. Moreover, the generalization of the ototoxicity to other mammalian species was unknown. Reports now confirm generalization to mouse (Crumling et al., 2012; Cronin et al., 2015; Patterson et al., 2016). Mice injected with a single subcutaneous dose of 8000 mg/kg HPβCD had ABR thresholds at 4, 16 and 32 kHz that were ~60 dB above those of control animals (Crumling et al., 2012). These elevated thresholds were accompanied by elimination of distortion product otoacoustic emission (DPOAE) responses, indicating outer hair cell (OHC) dysfunction to a degree suggesting that most, if not all, of the ABR deficits were due to OHC pathophysiology. Inspection of organ of Corti whole-mount preparations revealed that the presence of inner hair cells was the same as vehicle-injected controls, but there was a total loss of OHCs over the basal-most ~85% of the sensory epithelium, indicating that the hearing loss produced by HPβCD is permanent under these conditions and confirming the predominant involvement of OHCs.

Surprisingly, while most mice injected at 8000 mg/kg displayed widespread damage to the organ of Corti and physiological losses, the histology and audiometry of some animals were unaffected by the dosing, appearing to be normal (Crumling et al., 2012). There was no middle ground in the ototoxicity, with the effect of HPβCD appearing to be an all-or-none phenomenon. At intermediate doses, the average threshold shifts were reduced but no individual animal displayed intermediate threshold shifts. Instead, the proportion of animals with normal or ~60-dB-elevated ABR thresholds changed to produce an intermediate mean response compared to higher doses (Patterson et al., 2016). This result is similar to that in animals co-treated with an aminoglycoside and a loop diuretic. This combination can produce rapid loss of hair cells, even at doses where the individual drugs do not cause an organ of Corti lesion. In this situation, the loop diuretic allows the aminoglycoside to cross the blood-labyrinth barrier in higher amounts than it achieves when administered alone, with a critical result being high endolymph concentration, allowing the aminoglycoside to enter hair cells via permeation through mechanotransduction channels. In mice, high-dose combinations of kanamycin and bumetanide or furosemide have been seen to eliminate all OHCs in about 80% of animals, while the remaining animals were unaffected by the combination or only had scattered OHC loss (Oesterle et al., 2008; Taylor et al., 2008). Later experiments with kanamycin and a more moderate IV furosemide dose (Jansen et al., 2013; Żak et al., 2016) produced a similar dichotomy. To explain corresponding outcomes in cyclodextrin ototoxicity, we envision a two-stage process, where HPβCD would facilitate its own entry into the cochlea only at a high concentration, perhaps achieved by build-up at blood-labyrinth capillary junctions. Once the concentration threshold is crossed, the flood of HPβCD would inevitably achieve an intracochlear concentration that is deadly to all OHCs that experience it. In this way, small differences in the ability of HPβCD to cross into the cochlea could have big effects on intracochlear concentration and the survival of OHCs.

A threshold for extreme HPβCD entry into the cochlea could be a mechanism of the all or no response to single doses, but that does not mean that no HPβCD enters the cochlea at sub-lethal levels. Similar to cats, a single, low subcutaneous dose in mice can leave no overt lasting physiological or histological defects in the cochlea, but with repeated dosing, detectable deficits can result. In an experiment in mice (Crumling et al., 2012), 4000 mg/kg HPβCD did not produce a threshold shift at 4 kHz, 7–10 days after a single dose. However, with weekly administration at this dose, ABR thresholds at 4 kHz began to elevate about 5 weeks after the start of the HPβCD course. Despite the dosing remaining constant, at about 8 weeks the elevation started to reverse reaching pre-drug threshold levels several weeks later, even while continuing the weekly drug injections. This is reminiscent of the phenomenon in noise-induced hearing loss referred to as "toughening" or "conditioning" (Clark et al., 1987; Sinex et al., 1987; Canlon et al., 1988). It may represent low HPβCD levels inducing homeostatic mechanisms at the hair cell or cochlear level that counteract some facet of HPβCD action, thereby allowing the acoustic sensitivity of the cochlea to return to normal while the animal is still receiving HPβCD.

Since treatment of NPC with HPβCD will inevitably require a combination of systemic and central routes of administration—to treat peripheral and central manifestations of the disease—it was important to determine whether otherwise benign systemic and central doses would act synergistically to cause ototoxic effects (Cronin et al., 2015). Penetration of the brain with HPβCD can be increased compared to systemic delivery by administering the compound into cerebrospinal fluid, as has been done in cats (intrathecal and intracisternal injection; Ward et al., 2010; Vite et al., 2015). This strategy increases benefit for the NPC brain, but fails to treat the disease outside the CNS, where systemic dosing is needed. In mice, HPβCD delivered at 500 mg/kg brain weight into cerebrospinal fluid intracerebroventricularly (ICV), left 4 and 16 kHz ABR thresholds statistically unaffected at 1 week after injection. Likewise, these frequencies were unaffected by a subcutaneous injection at 3000 mg/kg. When the two were combined, however, thresholds increased by 40–50 dB and included widespread OHC loss. Thus, seemingly innocuous doses can become devastating to the ear if administered by different routes close in time. This is further evidence that HPβCD is in the cochlea even when hair cells do not die. A mixture of affected and unaffected animals could still be seen with ICV dosing in this series of experiments, suggesting that the all-or-none mechanism is shared by subcutaneous and ICV delivery routes.

Ototoxicity of Other Cyclodextrins in Mice

The beneficial effect of HPβCD in NPC (and likewise, the ototoxicity) is thought to arise largely from its cholesterol-binding ability. While HPβCD is good at carrying cholesterol, it is not unique among cyclodextrins in this regard. Various α-, β-, and γ-cyclodextrins have been tested in NPC mice for their ability to normalize disease characteristics and screened for ototoxicity in normal mice (Davidson et al., 2016). The two best cyclodextrins at reversing disease abnormalities were HPβCD and 2-hydroxypropyl-γ-cyclodextrin (HPγCD). After one subcutaneous injection at 8000 mg/kg, all animals tested with HPβCD had ABR threshold shifts of about 60 dB. Interestingly, most animals given an equimolar dose of HPγCD had threshold shifts of about 40 dB, but the ABR thresholds of some animals were unaffected. The production of affected and unaffected animals was similar to that seen with single doses of HPβCD, and this segregation persisted after weekly injections that were carried out until the age of 28 weeks. Thus, with a stable dose level of HPγCD, there did not seem to be an expansion of a cochlear lesion with repeated dosing. These results provide evidence that the all-or-none nature of cyclodextrin-ototoxicity reflects biological interanimal variability and not methodological variance related to the injection. The elevated thresholds of HPβCD treated animals remained stable throughout the course of injections, indicating no recovery at this dose but also no additional injury. Because the ototoxicity of HPγCD under comparable circumstances, with equimolar dosing, was less than with HPβCD, it is attractive to think that HPγCD is a better alternative for treatment of NPC. However, its efficacy in disease treatment was correspondingly less than that of HPβCD.

Human Ototoxicity

Use of HPβCD to treat human NPC disease was first described in peer-reviewed literature for two children by Matsuo et al. (2013, 2014), who reported no measurable change in hearing via ABR after 2 years of both IV and ICV dosing. No auditory data were shown, and no description of test parameters was provided. Maarup et al. (2015) described outcomes in a 12-year-old boy with NPC1 who was given 27 treatments total, roughly every 2 weeks, of 200 mg intrathecal HPβCD over the course of 1.5 years. Pure-tone audiometry was performed prior to the initial exposure and then again before each dose. A progressive increase in threshold at 8 kHz was reported bilaterally, that was greater in the right ear than the left, which was considered ongoing at the time of publication. No impact was observed at lower test frequencies, and the ABR was reported as stable. A summary of the case-study literature to date on compassionate use of HPβCD, which is primarily a collation of abstracts, is presented by Megías-Vericat et al. (2017); detailed accounts of hearing and ototoxicity are not provided.

Recently, results of the only cohort study to date on the use of HPβCD in patients with NPC were published (Ory et al., 2017). This was an open-label, non-randomized, phase 1/2a dose escalation study assessing safety and efficacy of intrathecal administration of HPβCD. Detailed audiology is reported on 14 patients aged 4–24 years at enrollment with genetically confirmed *NPC1* mutations and neurological manifestations, who were followed for 18 months at the National Institutes of Health Clinical Center, Bethesda, MD, USA (Institutional review board-approved protocol 13-CH-0016). Patients were sequentially assigned, in cohorts of three, to receive starting doses ranging from 50 mg to 900 mg intrathecal HPβCD. Doses were administered monthly and advanced, based on tolerance and safety data from individuals and from higher dose cohorts, up to 1200 mg. Comprehensive audiometry, including pure-tone behavioral assessment (0.25–20 kHz) and measurement of DPOAEs, occurred prior to HPβCD exposure (baseline) and then monthly, before each infusion. Some patients were seen for additional testing during acute phases post exposure. A suprathreshold neurodiagnostic ABR was collected at baseline and then every 6 months. Two patients were unable to provide reliable behavioral responses to pure-tone stimuli due to advanced disease status, and their hearing was monitored via DPOAE and ultimately tone burst (0.5–4 kHz) ABR threshold.

All patients in the trial eventually experienced permanent changes in hearing (Ory et al., 2017). Although hearing loss is a manifestation of NPC disease (Pikus, 1991; King et al., 2014), the hearing loss observed in this trial was time-locked to HPβCD exposure. Notably, pre-existing hearing loss in this population complicates the ototoxic profile of HPβCD. At the 18-month time point, change in hearing was more strongly correlated with hearing at baseline than with mean or median total HPβCD dosages; those patients with better hearing at the outset exhibited greater decline in hearing than those with more pre-existing hearing loss. This analysis was limited to a high frequency pure-tone average (4/6/8 kHz).

All patients had some degree of disease-related pre-existing hearing loss, but only half were considered candidates for hearing aids at the time of enrollment. Following 18 months of monthly HPβCD exposure, all patients were audiometrically considered candidates for hearing aids to support communication, and self-reported outcomes by patients and families choosing to use hearing aids were positive. The ototoxic effect typically began in the highest test frequencies and progressively moved to lower test frequencies; 2–8 kHz were most affected (analysis of ultra-high frequency hearing, above 8 kHz, was not reported). The type of loss was sensorineural and the combination of DPOAE and neurodiagnostic ABR data support a site of lesion that is predominantly OHC (King et al., 2015). Variable susceptibility across patients was observed, suggesting one or more factors potentiate the ototoxic properties of the drug. Two siblings showed particular sensitivity to the ototoxic potential of HPβCD exposure, limiting their total dosage, which suggests genetic involvement.

The onset of the hearing loss in humans appears to be rapid, which aligns with preclinical reports (Cronin et al., 2015; Lichtenhan et al., 2017). Some patients reported auditory symptoms (e.g., tinnitus, aural fullness) within hours of the infusion, and loss of OAE and changes in pure-tone thresholds were documented hours after administration. An unanticipated observation was a temporary component to the hearing loss in some cases. Serial monitoring of a subset of patients receiving doses of 600 mg and higher revealed cases in which OAEs were lost and pure-tone thresholds were elevated, followed by a partial or full recovery within a 3–5 week timeframe, prior to subsequent dosing (King et al., 2015, 2016). A similar temporary depression of auditory function has been reported in mice receiving repeated HPβCD exposure (Crumling et al., 2012). The mechanism(s) behind this remains unclear. Objective changes in auditory function often correlated with subjective reports from patients, who noted recovery in their auditory symptoms in the week or two following their infusion. Importantly, not all patients experienced temporary changes in hearing; some patients had no acute change in hearing following a given dose, and others had acute and permanent change. One patient, the youngest and smallest in the cohort, experienced significant and permanent decline in hearing following the initial exposure to 900 mg HPβCD (King et al., 2016).

Data presented by Ory et al. (2017) represent the first cohort of patients systematically evaluated for intrathecal HPβCD safety and efficacy, including comprehensive audiology. The results are promising, as treated patients showed evidence for slowed disease progression. The ototoxicity after 18 months of dosing was considered an expected and acceptable adverse event, when placed in the context of a devastating disease. Treatment of NPC with HPβCD, however, will be a maintenance therapy and it remains unclear what the ototoxic profile will be after years of exposure. ABR threshold data to broadband click stimuli from cats treated intrathecally at therapeutic levels showed profound hearing loss (Vite et al., 2015); although this short-duration click does not effectively probe lower frequency regions of the cochlea, it is possible that chronic exposure may cause widespread cochlear damage. It is also unclear what affect age has on the risk for ototoxicity, but it can be predicted that, should HPβCD be approved as a therapy for NPC, very young patients, newly diagnosed through advances in whole exome sequencing, may be candidates for treatment. The risk for functionally significant hearing loss before development of speech and language should be weighed carefully with potential benefits of early-life treatment of the disease.

CYCLODEXTRIN TOXICOLOGY

Given their widespread use as chemical excipients in drug formulations, as food additives, and as chemical stabilizers in a plethora of industrial products, the toxicological profile of cyclodextrins has been extensively studied and most varieties exhibit low toxicity at low concentrations. Even so, there can be considerable deleterious toxicological effects including death depending on formulation, concentration, and route of delivery. **Table 1** shows the LD_{50} data for rats given oral or IV administrations of unmodified cyclodextrins (reviewed by Del Valle, 2004). The greater safety profile for oral delivery likely reflects metabolism by bacteria in upper and lower intestinal tracts and reduced drug absorption compared to IV delivery. Toxicity from IV administration is largely a result of kidney damage, where filtration causes the formation of microcrystals composed of cyclodextrin and possibly deposits of cholesterol, resulting in nephrosis (Frank et al., 1976). Renal damage can occur with modified cyclodextrins as well, depending on concentration, since excretion in urine is the major means of drug elimination. Nephrotoxicity is of particular importance given the link between kidney and inner ear pathology from a variety of ototoxins.

The derivation of modified cyclodextrins has been and continues to be an exciting area of medicinal chemistry research, where substitutions of reactive moieties for various functional groups can range from simple modifications that increase solubility and safety (e.g., methylated, hydroxypropylated and sulfobutylated cyclodextrins) to supramolecular scaffolds and nanoparticles used in drug delivery (Stella and Rajewski, 1997; Varan et al., 2017). Derivatives of β-cyclodextrins, and specifically HPβCD, are widely studied and safety profiles have been extensively reviewed (for example see Gould and Scott, 2005). In an acute study in monkey, a single IV dose of 10,000 mg/kg HPβCD produced no mortality or observed toxicological effects, except hematuria in several animals (Brewster et al., 1990). In a study by AstraZeneca, continuous IV infusion in rat for 7 days reaching an effective dose of 2400 mg/kg/day of HPβCD lowered serum cholesterol and caused minor injury to the kidney (Gould and Scott, 2005). Mild histopathology, with no or limited physiological effects, from this and other short-term studies was generally reversible after cessation of drug treatment. Similarly, examination of several organ systems, including kidney, after 8000 mg/kg subcutaneous HPβCD in mice revealed only minor histopathological effects 3 days post-injection (e.g., edema, vacuolization), even while demonstrating hearing loss and severe OHC loss in those same animals (Cronin et al., 2015). What then underlies HPβCD-induced ototoxicity, and specifically OHC death, for doses that are seemingly benign to other organs and systems?

TABLE 1 | Toxicology of naturally occurring cyclodextrins in the rat (compiled from Del Valle, 2004).

Cyclodextrin type	Oral LD_{50}	IV LD_{50}
α-cyclodextrin	>10,000 mg/kg	500–750 mg/kg
β-cyclodextrin	>5000 mg/kg	450–790 mg/kg
γ-cyclodextrin	≫8000 mg/kg	4000 mg/kg

Can Indirect Mechanisms Lead to Ototoxicity?

In considering the potential cause(s) of HPβCD-induced ototoxicity, we must first address whether HPβCD ototoxicity is due to the cyclodextrin itself or some indirect effect of HPβCD treatment. These indirect effects could arise, for example, from impurities in the drug formulation or transport of toxic guest compounds "hitching a ride" to the ear during drug delivery. The main by-products of HPβCD synthesis are unreacted β-cyclodextrin and propylene glycol. The amount of impurities increases with the degree of substitution, as greater amounts of NaOH and propylene oxide are required for the reaction (Malanga et al., 2016). A variety of commercial HPβCD products have been examined and proven ototoxic, including formulations from Sigma-Aldrich (C0926, H107; Ward et al., 2010; Crumling et al., 2012; Cronin et al., 2015), Roche (Kleptose HPB; Davidson et al., 2016), and a highly characterized and purified form of Kleptose HPB used in the phase 2/3 clinical trials (VTS-270; Davidson et al., 2016; Ory et al., 2017; Yergey et al., 2017). Moreover, recent reports show little effect of degree of substitution on cell toxicity (Malanga et al., 2016). Since propylene glycol is a presumed ototoxin, it is possible that this contaminant is responsible for the ototoxicity after HPβCD treatment. The toxicity of propylene glycol has been reported for highly concentrated drug applications to the round window or via infusions into the middle ear (Vernon et al., 1978; Morizono et al., 1980), but the sensory epithelium appears well-preserved, with damage primarily occurring in the middle ear and ossification developing in scala tympani and scala vestibuli. Therefore, otopathology due to propylene glycol is quite distinct from that due to HPβCD treatment. Furthermore, the concentrations of this impurity are likely below normal dose limits. Propylene glycol is a common solvent for pharmaceuticals and dose limits for IV administration are on the order of 69 g per day for humans (Lim et al., 2014). Pharmacopoeial specifications (EP/USP) for HPβCD formulations limit propylene glycol contamination to a maximum of 2.5%. Highly purified, commercial formulations of HPβCD such as Kleptose HPB contain less than 0.2% propylene glycol (Machielse and Darling, 2017). If this formulation was given to an average human at 8000 mg/kg, the propylene glycol contamination would be less than 1 g, far below the dose limit for humans. Yet, Kleptose HPB (aka VTS-270) is ototoxic in mice and humans (Davidson et al., 2016; Ory et al., 2017). Therefore, HPβCD ototoxicity does not appear to be related to impurities in drug formulation.

Another possibility for indirect ototoxicity is that HPβCD complexes with endogenous compounds prior to entering the inner ear, carrying potentially damaging substances into the cochlea. When HPβCD is injected systemically, it passes through various tissue and vascular compartments, enabling exchange with myriad sterols, phospholipids and proteins. Cholesterol—the most likely endogenous guest compound—is extracted from plasma membranes by cyclodextrin with two distinct kinetic rates on the order of 10 s and 10 min, likely reflecting exchange from different membrane compartments (Rouquette-Jazdanian et al., 2006). Once in the bloodstream, extraction of cholesterol by cyclodextrins from lipoprotein complexes is expected to occur on similar timescales because the exchange of cholesterol between lipoproteins occurs with a $t_{1/2}$ of 4–45 min (Lund-Katz et al., 1982). Even so, although HPβCD is excreted intact in urine (Stella and He, 2008), the amount of cholesterol in the urine was unchanged in mice—wildtype and NPC mutants—after a single subcutaneous dose of 4000 mg/kg HPβCD (Taylor et al., 2012). It is likely that guest compounds, including cholesterol, are mobilized between local cellular and tissue compartments rather than redistributed from one region to another (i.e., from distal compartments to the inner ear). Therefore, it is unlikely that transport of extracochlear, endogenous, toxic guest compounds is responsible for HPβCD-induced ototoxicity.

Cyclodextrin Cytotoxicity May Involve Membrane Perturbation and Caspase-Dependent Cell Death

Similar to the *in vivo* toxicology of cyclodextrins, *in vitro* cytotoxicity arising from cyclodextrin exposure depends on formulation and concentration. Cell viability after cyclodextrin treatment has been reported for a variety of cultured lines of epithelial cells, including Calu-3 cells (human airway, Matilainen et al., 2008) and Caco-2 cells (human colorectal adenocarcinoma, Kiss et al., 2010). In both examples, HPβCD was less toxic than other forms, showing good viability (80% or better) when used at concentrations of 200 mM for up to 4 h, whereas methylated forms of β-cyclodextrin caused substantial cell death at 10–50 mM. The difference in cytotoxicity among the various derivatives was tightly associated with two factors: (1) their degree of cholesterol solubilization; and (2) the number and position of methyl groups on methylated derivatives (Kiss et al., 2010). Non-methylated β-cyclodextrins, like HPβCD and sulfobutylether-β-cyclodextrin, show lower cholesterol affinity but also lower cytotoxicity (Kiss et al., 2010; Wang et al., 2011).

Reported mechanisms of cytotoxicity generally involve cholesterol depletion from the plasma membrane or intracellular compartments, but the link between cholesterol depletion and cell death remains unclear. Membrane damage, quantified by the release of cytoplasmic enzymes, is a common observation (Boulmedarat et al., 2005; Wang et al., 2011; Hinzey et al., 2012), presumably due to cholesterol extraction and membrane perturbation. Both apoptotic and necrotic cell death pathways appear to be involved, but the balance of these effects is dependent on the type of cyclodextrin as well as the cell type being examined (Wang et al., 2011; Onodera et al., 2013). In some instances, cyclodextrin-induced apoptosis follows activation of executioner caspase-3 as well as a loss of mitochondrial transmembrane potential and cytochrome release (CytC) (Onodera et al., 2013), but it remains unclear whether this occurs through drug effects on the plasma membrane leading to activation of apoptosis inducible factors or direct effects of cyclodextrin on intracellular organelles. In all cases, these effects are associated with methylated β-cyclodextrins. HPβCD concentrations may have to exceed 200 mM to cause similar effects in these cell lines. Why then do OHCs appear to be sensitive to HPβCD concentrations as low as 10 mM (Takahashi et al., 2016)?

Potential Mechanisms of HPβCD Ototoxicity

Based on the actions of β-cyclodextrins in other systems, these compounds could target at least four aspects of OHC physiology, as depicted in **Figure 2**. These targets include intracellular organelles that govern a variety of cell stress pathways, membrane resident proteins, and cell-cell junctions that regulate ion flux between fluid compartments surrounding the OHCs. Oxidative stress is a major effector of hair cell death in acquired forms of hearing loss (for review see Dinh et al., 2015; Jiang et al., 2017). Cyclodextrin-induced cytotoxicity in other systems raises the possibility that mitochondrial dysfunction and oxidative stress form a common link with this new ototoxin as well. Several reports suggest that cyclodextrins can enter cells through endocytosis (Rosenbaum et al., 2010; Fenyvesi et al., 2014), deplete cholesterol in mitochondrial membranes, and alter mitochondrial bioenergetics (Ziolkowski et al., 2010; **Figure 2C**). Cyclodextrins can also disrupt ganglioside-rich domains at the mitochondria-associated endoplasmic reticulum (ER) membranes, linking cyclodextrin treatment to several stress pathways that are also common to other forms of hearing loss (Sano et al., 2009). Though ubiquitous in cell membranes, cholesterol is heterogeneously distributed in mammalian cells; the plasma membrane accounts for 60%–90% of cellular cholesterol and the ER about 1% (Das et al., 2014). Cholesterol homeostasis, one of the mostly tightly controlled processes in mammalian cells, is intimately related to synthesis in the ER and transport between other organelles and the plasma membrane. It is possible that high concentrations of cyclodextrin perturb this balance and overwhelm homeostatic processes to negatively impact vesicular transport between organelles and a large array of cellular processes. It is important to note that most studies linking cholesterol distribution/content and cell function utilize methylated cyclodextrins, so it remains to be seen whether these observations can be extended to HPβCD. Also, if oxidative stress and perturbation of general cell function are the major effectors of HPβCD ototoxicity, it is difficult to explain the rapid nature of the injury and the specificity of OHC death without nephrotoxicity. Further examination of cell death pathways initiated by inner ear exposure to HPβCD is required.

Unique features of OHCs may help explain their sensitivity to HPβCD. Here, it is important to consider the non-homogeneous

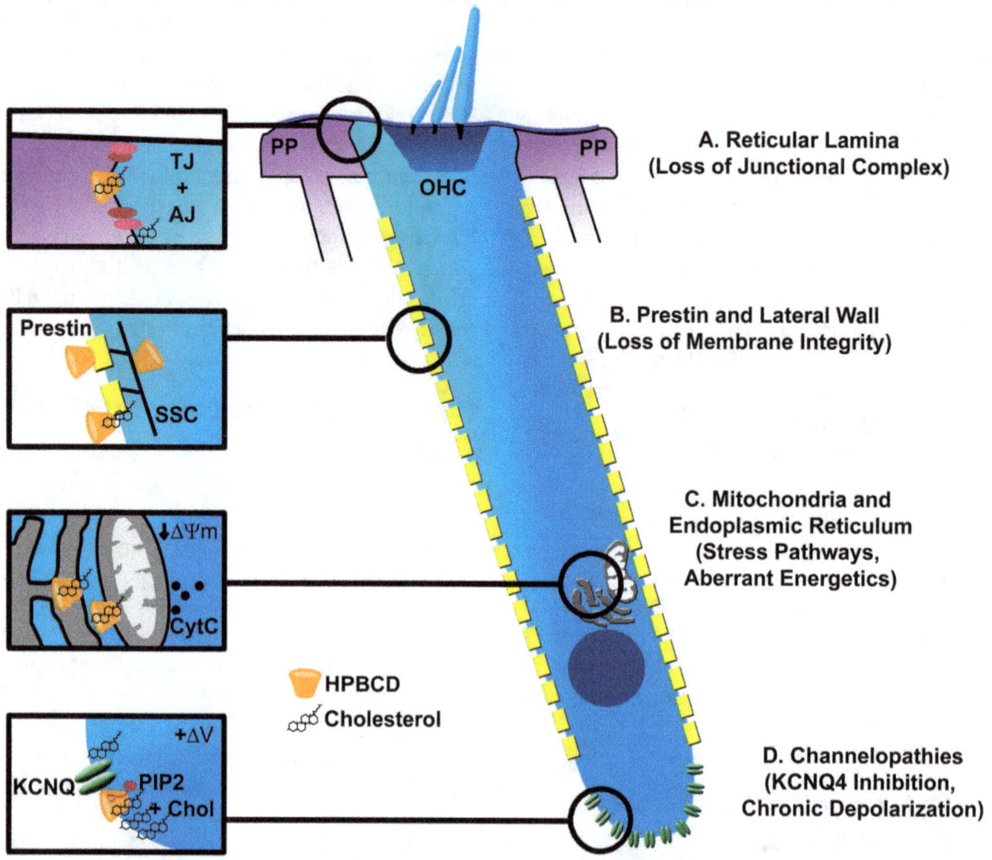

FIGURE 2 | Possible sites of pathologic interaction of cyclodextrins with outer hair cells (OHCs). **(A)** Cyclodextrins disrupt cell-cell junctional complexes (TJ, tight junctions; AJ, adherens junctions), which could breach the reticular lamina of the organ of Corti, allowing the high-potassium endolymph to bathe OHCs, leading to their excitotoxic death by prolonged depolarization. **(B)** The trilaminate structure of the OHC lateral wall is composed of prestin-rich plasma membrane connected to subsurface cisterane (SSC) by a cortical lattice. Removal of membrane cholesterol by cyclodextrins alters OHC membrane fluidity, stiffness and prestin-based motility. Since cholesterol level in the lateral wall appears low, it is unclear if cyclodextrin modifies these properties by interacting with plasma membrane lipids, membrane resident proteins like prestin, or the SSC. Nonetheless, loss of membrane integrity may be one mechanism of cyclodextrin-induced ototoxicity. **(C)** Since cyclodextrins can be endocytosed, they can potentially affect the membranes of intracellular organelles. Mitochondria and the endoplasmic reticulum (ER) represent common targets of other ototoxins. Specifically, cyclodextrins have been shown to reduce the mitochondrial membrane potential ($\Delta\Psi$m) and cause cytochrome release (CytC). Altered function in either organelle could contribute to OHC demise. **(D)** Cholesterol is non-uniformly distributed in the OHC plasma membrane, being enriched at the apical and basal poles of the cell. High concentrations at the base overlap with the expression of KCNQ4-type potassium channels, which also require the phospholipid PIP2 for proper function. Disruption of a channel-PIP2-cholesterol complex by cyclodextrin could cause loss of KCNQ4 current, chronic depolarization and ultimately excitotoxic death.

distribution of cholesterol in the OHC membrane. Cholesterol markers, filipin and theonellamide, intensely label apical and basal OHC regions with little or no staining along the lateral wall (Nguyen and Brownell, 1998; Takahashi et al., 2016). Interestingly, regions of low and high cholesterol mirror the non-homogeneous distribution of key OHC membrane-resident proteins, prestin and KCNQ4, respectively (Mustapha et al., 2009). One of the more obvious features unique to OHCs is related to their function in cochlear amplification via the abundant membrane motor protein prestin and the complex trilaminate structure of the OHC lateral wall (**Figure 2B**). Indeed, prestin function is exquisitely sensitive to cyclodextrin treatment, such that the voltage-sensitivity of prestin is shifted to more depolarized or hyperpolarized potentials depending on whether cholesterol is depleted or enriched in the OHC membrane (Rajagopalan et al., 2007; Takahashi et al., 2016). Moreover, cholesterol depletion, under certain conditions, alters the fluidity of the OHC lateral membrane (Organ and Raphael, 2009; Yamashita et al., 2015), and recent data suggest involvement of the trilaminate structure of the lateral wall, possibly including the intricate subsurface cistern and its cytoskeletal connections to the plasma membrane (Yamashita et al., 2015). These data suggest potential impacts on membrane integrity, but the exact site of action remains unclear. Interestingly, OHCs from prestin knockout mice are partially protected from HPβCD ototoxicity (Takahashi et al., 2016), suggesting a link between HPβCD and prestin/membrane function in ototoxicity. However, the mechanism of protection in the knockout mice remains unclear. The preservation of OHCs in the knockout animals could reflect the large-scale redistribution of cholesterol throughout the OHC membrane, which would undoubtedly change how HPβCD interacts with the OHCs. Moreover, only a portion of the mutant OHCs were protected from HPβCD, though prestin was absent from both resistant and susceptible OHCs alike. More study is required. It would be interesting to determine whether knock-in of mutated, dysfunctional prestin preserves the normal distribution of lipids in the OHC lateral wall and then renders sensitivity or resistance to HPβCD. It will also be important to determine the pharmacokinetics of HPβCD accumulation in the inner ear fluid spaces to determine whether drug concentration in perilymph reaches levels required to catastrophically damage the OHC membrane (~10 mM).

Other membrane resident proteins, such as ion channels, could be affected by cyclodextrin as well. In chick hair cells, methyl-β-cyclodextrin depleted membrane cholesterol, disrupted membrane microdomains, and altered major ion channel conductances (Purcell et al., 2011). All major ion channel classes are sensitive to perturbations in membrane cholesterol (Levitan et al., 2010), but the effects are heterogeneous and highly context dependent. Membrane perturbation can alter channel density, electrical activity and localization in specific membrane compartments (Levitan et al., 2010; Purcell et al., 2011; Mercer et al., 2012). It is important to emphasize that cholesterol can inhibit or activate the same channel type in different tissues. The potassium channel, KCNQ4, is the dominant potassium conductance in OHCs. Mutations in KCNQ4 are associated with DFNA2, a nonsyndromic progressive form of sensorineural hearing loss characterized by loss of OHCs (Nie, 2008). Expression of KCNQ4 at the basal pole of the OHC overlaps in distribution with cholesterol and other lipids (Santi et al., 1994; Nguyen and Brownell, 1998; **Figure 2D**). Additionally, KCNQ channel activation is modulated by cholesterol (Chun et al., 2010), possibly through the coordinated perturbation of PIP2, which is required for KCNQ channel gating (Suh and Hille, 2008). A complete understanding of HPβCD effects on OHC physiology is required to fully appreciate the potential mechanisms underlying ototoxicity from this drug.

Finally, it should be noted that HPβCD effects on other structures within the inner ear could indirectly affect OHC health or modulate their susceptibility to direct influence of the drug. One possibility is altered ion homeostasis within the cochlear duct. Direct application of HPβCD into the guinea pig cochlea does not seem to impact endocochlear potential (Lichtenhan et al., 2017) and histopathological effects on the mouse lateral wall appear absent (Crumling et al., 2012; Cronin et al., 2015). However, in many epithelial systems, cyclodextrins effectively disrupt tight-junction barriers (Francis et al., 1999; Lynch et al., 2007), leading to one of their major uses in drug delivery (epidermal patches). Human mutations associated with the integrity of a partition between cochlear fluid compartments—the reticular lamina—are associated with deafness, largely due to OHC loss (Ben-Yosef et al., 2003; Kamitani et al., 2015). Presumably, disruption of the reticular lamina would cause potassium flux into the fluid surrounding the basal pole of the OHCs, resulting in chronic depolarization and possibly cell death (Zenner, 1986; Zenner et al., 1994; **Figure 2A**).

Each of the potential mechanisms discussed above underscores the unique susceptibility of OHCs to various insults. HPβCD entry into the cochlear duct could induce one or more events that lead to the selective injury of OHCs. More investigation is warranted to determine whether any of these potential mechanisms are at play. Only then can proper interventions be developed.

SUMMARY AND FUTURE DIRECTIONS

Cyclodextrin use is expanding in medicine, far beyond use as pharmacological excipients. In NPC, HPβCD is the only viable treatment option currently under consideration. In other lipid-related diseases where alternative treatment options exist, HPβCD still potentially offers greater affordability, increased safety, and uniquely attractive properties. To harness the power of this versatile drug, it is imperative to address iatrogenic hearing loss as the major factor limiting further use.

Basic pharmacokinetic and pharmacodynamic studies are needed to understand the relationship between dose, route of administration, accumulation in the ear, transient and permanent hearing loss, and long-term otopathology. These studies could be accomplished by pairing drug injection, auditory tests and pathology with mass spectrometry, which could be used to detect HPβCD in tissue or fluid samples (Jiang et al., 2014), or with radiolabeled HPβCD, which could be used to probe uptake in cellular compartments (Pontikis et al., 2013). These studies could resolve how peak drug concentration and accumulated exposure relate to pathology, and they could define appropriate drug concentrations and exposure durations in *in vitro* models of OHC response to cyclodextrin. Of primary importance to current clinical trials is a greater understanding of the risk from long-term exposure to repeated doses. With long-term use and with combined systemic and central drug administration, otopathology may extend beyond OHC loss to eventually include damage to other cochlear structures including inner hair cells and auditory neurons. Moreover, future studies should examine whether there is risk to hearing from cyclodextrin-based drug formulations, where dissociation of guest compounds might free the excipient to accumulate in the ear and cause injury. Once we know more about the concentrations of HPβCD that reach and reside in the ear over time, we can more fully examine the physiological response of the cochlea during and following peak exposures and build suitable *in vitro* models for examining OHC physiology in response to clinically relevant concentrations of HPβCD.

Along with studies linking pharmacokinetics to injury, we need greater mechanistic insight into the means of HPβCD uptake into the cochlea, the molecular changes that result from HPβCD exposure in the cochlea, and the cell-death pathways that are involved in OHC loss. In this review article, we hypothesized that HPβCD transiently disrupts the blood-labyrinth barrier, facilitating entry into the cochlear duct. Effects on this barrier should be examined further, pathways that are involved in OHC loss. In this review article, we hypothesized that HPβCD transiently disrupts the blood-labyrinth barrier, facilitating entry into the cochlear duct. Effects on this barrier should be examined further, including examination of changes to endocochlear potential, the morphology of vascular beds, and paracellular extravasation of the drug into the cochlea. The studies with radiolabeled HPβCD could also be informative here to determine whether there is cellular uptake and whether the drug is targeted to specific cellular compartments. Basic morphological studies are needed to derive the primary mechanisms of cell death (e.g., apoptosis, necrosis, or a combination of these) and could reveal key structural changes (e.g., loss of membrane integrity, apoptotic or necrotic nuclei) or molecular changes (e.g., caspase-dependent/independent apoptosis) that lead to OHC demise.

Figure 2 illustrates several potential targets that could link cyclodextrin effects to cholesterol perturbation, cellular dysfunction and ultimately cell death. One of these targets includes the junctional complexes between sensory and non-sensory cells that separate fluid compartments in the cochlea. Morphological studies could help resolve whether these junctional complexes along the reticular lamina are disrupted after HPβCD administration. Other potential targets include membrane processes essential for OHC function, like prestin-mediated motility, lateral wall stiffness and fluidity, and ion channel function. It remains unclear whether systemic administration of HPβCD alters OHC physiology. With a greater understanding of HPβCD pharmacokinetics, OHC function could be examined *in vitro* using drug applications that mirror *in vivo* drug concentrations; alternatively, OHC function could be assessed *in vitro* at specified points after systemic drug injection. Finally, from the evidence that cyclodextrins can negatively impact mitochondrial function and the link between mitochondrial dysfunction, oxidative stress and hearing loss from other ototoxins, future studies should examine potential relationships between HPβCD treatment and OHC oxidative stress.

Preventative approaches, namely adjuvants that might prevent HPβCD ototoxicity, must be pursued in parallel with mechanistic studies since there is now overwhelming evidence that human patient hearing is at risk. Moreover, the potential expansion of NPC clinical trials to young presymptomatic patients raises the specter of causing hearing loss during critical phases of cognitive development in otherwise phenotypically normal patients. Such preventative measures might focus on antioxidants that are currently in clinical trial for other forms of acquired hearing loss (e.g., NCT02903355, NCT01727492), compounds that would modulate OHC excitability and membrane function, and compounds that might modulate uptake and egress of HPβCD into and from the cochlear duct. The results from both mechanistic and therapeutic studies will undoubtedly shape our understanding of cochlear physiology and OHC structure-function specifically. A conundrum has been raised in this review article: HPβCD operates primarily through cholesterol manipulation and cholesterol is a ubiquitous component of cell membranes, yet OHCs show exceptional sensitivity to HPβCD exposure, more so than apparently any other cell in the body. Certainly, we stand to gain major insights into OHC physiology and OHC membrane function by further pursuing the mechanisms of cyclodextrin ototoxicity.

AUTHOR CONTRIBUTIONS

MAC, KAK and RKD contributed to conception and design, review and interpretation of literature and drafting and revising the manuscript.

ACKNOWLEDGMENTS

The authors thank Lisa Cunningham and Michael Hoa for their careful review of the manuscript and Taylor Sodano for assistance with chemical structure depiction.

REFERENCES

Ben-Yosef, T., Belyantseva, I. A., Saunders, T. L., Hughes, E. D., Kawamoto, K., Van Itallie, C. M., et al. (2003). Claudin 14 knockout mice, a model for autosomal recessive deafness DFNB29, are deaf due to cochlear hair cell degeneration. *Hum. Mol. Genet.* 12, 2049–2061. doi: 10.1093/hmg/ddg210

Boulmedarat, L., Bochot, A., Lesieur, S., and Fattal, E. (2005). Evaluation of buccal methyl-β-cyclodextrin toxicity on human oral epithelial cell culture model. *J. Pharm. Sci.* 94, 1300–1309. doi: 10.1002/jps.20350

Brewster, M. E., Estes, K. S., and Bodor, N. (1990). An intravenous toxicity study of 2-hydroxypropyl-β-cyclodextrin, a useful drug solubilizer, in rats and monkeys. *Int. J. Pharm.* 59, 231–243. doi: 10.1016/0378-5173(90)90114-j

Camargo, F., Erickson, R. P., Garver, W. S., Hossain, G. S., Carbone, P. N., Heidenreich, R. A., et al. (2001). Cyclodextrins in the treatment of a mouse model of Niemann-Pick C disease. *Life Sci.* 70, 131–142. doi: 10.1016/s0024-3205(01)01384-4

Canlon, B., Borg, E., and Flock, A. (1988). Protection against noise trauma by pre-exposure to a low level acoustic stimulus. *Hear. Res.* 34, 197–200. doi: 10.1016/0378-5955(88)90107-4

Carstea, E. D., Morris, J. A., Coleman, K. G., Loftus, S. K., Zhang, D., Cummings, C., et al. (1997). Niemann-Pick C1 disease gene: homology to mediators of cholesterol homeostasis. *Science* 277, 228–231. doi: 10.1126/science.277.5323.228

Chun, Y. S., Shin, S., Kim, Y., Cho, H., Park, M. K., Kim, T. W., et al. (2010). Cholesterol modulates ion channels via down-regulation of phosphatidylinositol 4,5-bisphosphate. *J. Neurochem.* 112, 1286–1294. doi: 10.1111/j.1471-4159.2009.06545.x

Clark, W. W., Bohne, B. A., and Boettcher, F. A. (1987). Effect of periodic rest on hearing loss and cochlear damage following exposure to noise. *J. Acoust. Soc. Am.* 82, 1253–1264. doi: 10.1121/1.395261

Coisne, C., Tilloy, S., Monflier, E., Wils, D., Fenart, L., and Gosselet, F. (2016). Cyclodextrins as emerging therapeutic tools in the treatment of cholesterol-associated vascular and neurodegenerative diseases. *Molecules* 21:E1748. doi: 10.3390/molecules21121748

Cronin, S., Lin, A., Thompson, K., Hoenerhoff, M., and Duncan, R. K. (2015). Hearing loss and otopathology following systemic and intracerebroventricular delivery of 2-hydroxypropyl-β-cyclodextrin. *J. Assoc. Res. Otolaryngol.* 16, 599–611. doi: 10.1007/s10162-015-0528-6

Crumling, M. A., Liu, L., Thomas, P. V., Benson, J., Kanicki, A., Kabara, L., et al. (2012). Hearing loss and hair cell death in mice given the cholesterol-chelating agent hydroxypropyl-β-cyclodextrin. *PLoS One* 7:e53280. doi: 10.1371/journal.pone.0053280

Das, A., Brown, M. S., Anderson, D. D., Goldstein, J. L., and Radhakrishnan, A. (2014). Three pools of plasma membrane cholesterol and their relation to cholesterol homeostasis. *Elife* 3:e02882. doi: 10.7554/eLife.02882

Dass, C. R., and Jessup, W. (2000). Apolipoprotein A-I, cyclodextrins and liposomes as potential drugs for the reversal of atherosclerosis. A review. *J. Pharm. Pharmacol.* 52, 731–761. doi: 10.1211/0022357001774606

Davidson, C. D., Ali, N. F., Micsenyi, M. C., Stephney, G., Renault, S., Dobrenis, K., et al. (2009). Chronic cyclodextrin treatment of murine Niemann-Pick C disease ameliorates neuronal cholesterol and glycosphingolipid storage and disease progression. *PLoS One* 4:e6951. doi: 10.1371/journal.pone.0006951

Davidson, C. D., Fishman, Y. I., Puskas, I., Szemán, J., Sohajda, T., McCauliff, L. A., et al. (2016). Efficacy and ototoxicity of different cyclodextrins in Niemann-Pick C disease. *Ann. Clin. Transl. Neurol.* 3, 366–380. doi: 10.1002/acn3.306

Del Valle, E. M. M. (2004). Cyclodextrins and their uses: a review. *Process Biochem.* 39, 1033–1046. doi: 10.1016/s0032-9592(03)00258-9

Dinh, C. T., Goncalves, S., Bas, E., Van De Water, T. R., and Zine, A. (2015). Molecular regulation of auditory hair cell death and approaches to protect sensory receptor cells and/or stimulate repair following acoustic trauma. *Front. Cell. Neurosci.* 9:96. doi: 10.3389/fncel.2015.00096

Fenyvesi, F., Réti-Nagy, K., Bacsó, Z., Gutay-Tóth, Z., Malanga, M., Fenyvesi, É., et al. (2014). Fluorescently labeled methyl-β-cyclodextrin enters intestinal epithelial Caco-2 cells by fluid-phase endocytosis. *PLoS One* 9:e84856. doi: 10.1371/journal.pone.0084856

Francis, S. A., Kelly, J. M., McCormack, J., Rogers, R. A., Lai, J., Schneeberger, E. E., et al. (1999). Rapid reduction of MDCK cell cholesterol by methyl-β-cyclodextrin alters steady state transepithelial electrical resistance. *Eur. J. Cell Biol.* 78, 473–484. doi: 10.1016/s0171-9335(99)80074-0

Frank, D. W., Gray, J. E., and Weaver, R. N. (1976). Cyclodextrin nephrosis in the rat. *Am. J. Pathol.* 83, 367–382.

Frijlink, H. W., Visser, J., Hefting, N. R., Oosting, R., Meijer, D. K., and Lerk, C. F. (1990). The pharmacokinetics of β-cyclodextrin and hydroxypropyl-β-cyclodextrin in the rat. *Pharm. Res.* 7, 1248–1252. doi: 10.1023/A:1015929720063

Frömming, K.-H., and Szejtli, J. Z. (1994). *Cyclodextrins in Pharmacy.* Dordrecht, Boston: Kluwer Academic Publishers.

Gould, S., and Scott, R. C. (2005). 2-Hydroxypropyl-β-cyclodextrin (HP-β-CD): a toxicology review. *Food Chem. Toxicol.* 43, 1451–1459. doi: 10.1016/j.fct.2005.03.007

Graham, D. R., Chertova, E., Hilburn, J. M., Arthur, L. O., and Hildreth, J. E. (2003). Cholesterol depletion of human immunodeficiency virus type 1 and simian immunodeficiency virus with β-cyclodextrin inactivates and permeabilizes the virions: evidence for virion-associated lipid rafts. *J. Virol.* 77, 8237–8248. doi: 10.1128/jvi.77.15.8237-8248.2003

Hinzey, A. H., Kline, M. A., Kotha, S. R., Sliman, S. M., Butler, E. S., Shelton, A. B., et al. (2012). Choice of cyclodextrin for cellular cholesterol depletion for vascular endothelial cell lipid raft studies: cell membrane alterations, cytoskeletal reorganization and cytotoxicity. *Indian J. Biochem. Biophys.* 49, 329–341.

Ikonen, E., and Hölttä-Vuori, M. (2004). Cellular pathology of Niemann-Pick type C disease. *Semin Cell Dev. Biol.* 15, 445–454. doi: 10.1016/j.semcdb.2004.03.001

Jansen, T. T., Bremer, H. G., Topsakal, V., Hendriksen, F. G., Klis, S. F., and Grolman, W. (2013). Deafness induction in mice. *Otol. Neurotol.* 34, 1496–1502. doi: 10.1097/MAO.0b013e318291c610

Jiang, M., Karasawa, T., and Steyger, P. S. (2017). Aminoglycoside-induced cochleotoxicity: a review. *Front. Cell. Neurosci.* 11:308. doi: 10.3389/fncel.2017.00308

Jiang, H., Sidhu, R., Fujiwara, H., De Meulder, M., de Vries, R., Gong, Y., et al. (2014). Development and validation of sensitive LC-MS/MS assays for quantification of HP-β-CD in human plasma and CSF. *J. Lipid Res.* 55, 1537–1548. doi: 10.1194/jlr.D050278

Kamitani, T., Sakaguchi, H., Tamura, A., Miyashita, T., Yamazaki, Y., Tokumasu, R., et al. (2015). Deletion of tricellulin causes progressive hearing loss associated with degeneration of cochlear hair cells. *Sci. Rep.* 5:18402. doi: 10.1038/srep18402

Kilsdonk, E. P., Yancey, P. G., Stoudt, G. W., Bangerter, F. W., Johnson, W. J., Phillips, M. C., et al. (1995). Cellular cholesterol efflux mediated by cyclodextrins. *J. Biol. Chem.* 270, 17250–17256. doi: 10.1074/jbc.270.29.17250

King, K. A., Gordon-Salant, S., Yanjanin, N., Zalewski, C., Houser, A., Porter, F. D., et al. (2014). Auditory phenotype of Niemann-Pick disease, type C1. *Ear Hear.* 35, 110–117. doi: 10.1097/AUD.0b013e3182a362b8

King, K., Zalewski, C., Farhat, N., Keener, L. A., Bianconi, S., Hoa, M., et al. (2015). "HPβCD therapy in humans with NPC1 disease: audiological outcomes," in *Association for Research in Otolaryngology 38th Annual Midwinter Meeting*, (Baltimore, MD).

King, K. A., Zalewski, C., Farhart, N., Keener, L. A., Bianconi, S., Hoa, M., et al. (2016). "The ototoxic profile of HPβCD in children with NPC1: 18-month outcomes of the phase 1 clinical trial," in *American Academy of Audiology Annual Meeting*, (Phoenix, AZ).

Kiss, T., Fenyvesi, F., Bácskay, I., Váradi, J., Fenyvesi, E., Iványi, R., et al. (2010). Evaluation of the cytotoxicity of β-cyclodextrin derivatives: evidence for the role of cholesterol extraction. *Eur. J. Pharm. Sci.* 40, 376–380. doi: 10.1016/j.ejps.2010.04.014

Levitan, I., Fang, Y., Rosenhouse-Dantsker, A., and Romanenko, V. (2010). Cholesterol and ion channels. *Subcell. Biochem.* 51, 509–549. doi: 10.1007/978-90-481-8622-8_19

Lichtenhan, J. T., Hirose, K., Buchman, C. A., Duncan, R. K., and Salt, A. N. (2017). Direct administration of 2-Hydroxypropyl-β-Cyclodextrin into guinea pig cochleae: effects on physiological and histological measurements. *PLoS One* 12:e0175236. doi: 10.1371/journal.pone.0175236

Lim, T. Y., Poole, R. L., and Pageler, N. M. (2014). Propylene glycol toxicity in children. *J. Pediatr. Pharmacol. Ther.* 19, 277–282. doi: 10.5863/1551-6776-19.4.277

Liscum, L., and Faust, J. R. (1987). Low density lipoprotein (LDL)-mediated suppression of cholesterol synthesis and LDL uptake is defective in Niemann-Pick type C fibroblasts. *J. Biol. Chem.* 262, 17002–17008.

Liscum, L., Ruggiero, R. M., and Faust, J. R. (1989). The intracellular transport of low density lipoprotein-derived cholesterol is defective in Niemann-Pick type C fibroblasts. *J. Cell Biol.* 108, 1625–1636. doi: 10.1083/jcb.108.5.1625

Liu, S. M., Cogny, A., Kockx, M., Dean, R. T., Gaus, K., Jessup, W., et al. (2003). Cyclodextrins differentially mobilize free and esterified cholesterol from primary human foam cell macrophages. *J. Lipid Res.* 44, 1156–1166. doi: 10.1194/jlr.m200464-jlr200

Liu, B., Turley, S. D., Burns, D. K., Miller, A. M., Repa, J. J., and Dietschy, J. M. (2009). Reversal of defective lysosomal transport in NPC disease ameliorates liver dysfunction and neurodegeneration in the *Npc1*$^{-/-}$ mouse. *Proc. Natl. Acad. Sci. U S A* 106, 2377–2382. doi: 10.1073/pnas.0810895106

López, C. A., de Vries, A. H., and Marrink, S. J. (2011). Molecular mechanism of cyclodextrin mediated cholesterol extraction. *PLoS Comput. Biol.* 7:e1002020. doi: 10.1371/journal.pcbi.1002020

López, C. A., de Vries, A. H., and Marrink, S. J. (2013). Computational microscopy of cyclodextrin mediated cholesterol extraction from lipid model membranes. *Sci. Rep.* 3:2071. doi: 10.1038/srep02071

Lowenthal, A. C., Cummings, J. F., Wenger, D. A., Thrall, M. A., Wood, P. A., and de Lahunta, A. (1990). Feline sphingolipidosis resembling Niemann-Pick disease type C. *Acta Neuropathol.* 81, 189–197. doi: 10.1007/bf00334507

Lund-Katz, S., Hammerschlag, B., and Phillips, M. C. (1982). Kinetics and mechanism of free cholesterol exchange between human serum high- and low-density lipoproteins. *Biochemistry* 21, 2964–2969. doi: 10.1021/bi00541a025

Lynch, R. D., Francis, S. A., McCarthy, K. M., Casas, E., Thiele, C., and Schneeberger, E. E. (2007). Cholesterol depletion alters detergent-specific solubility profiles of selected tight junction proteins and the phosphorylation of occludin. *Exp. Cell Res.* 313, 2597–2610. doi: 10.1016/j.yexcr.2007.05.009

Maarup, T. J., Chen, A. H., Porter, F. D., Farhat, N. Y., Ory, D. S., Sidhu, R., et al. (2015). Intrathecal 2-hydroxypropyl-β-cyclodextrin in a single patient with Niemann-Pick C1. *Mol. Genet. Metab.* 116, 75–79. doi: 10.1016/j.ymgme.2015.07.001

Machielse, B. N., and Darling, A. (2017). *Hydroxypropyl β-Cyclodextrin Compositions and Methods.* United States Patent Application 9675634.

Malanga, M., Szemán, J., Fenyvesi, É., Puskás, I., Csabai, K., Gyémánt, G., et al. (2016). "Back to the future": a new look at hydroxypropyl β-cyclodextrins. *J. Pharm. Sci.* 105, 2921–2931. doi: 10.1016/j.xphs.2016.04.034

Matilainen, L., Toropainen, T., Vihola, H., Hirvonen, J., Järvinen, T., Jarho, P., et al. (2008). *In vitro* toxicity and permeation of cyclodextrins in Calu-3 cells. *J. Control. Release* 126, 10–16. doi: 10.1016/j.jconrel.2007.11.003

Matsuo, M., Shraishi, K., Wada, K., Ishitsuka, Y., Doi, H., Maeda, M., et al. (2014). Effects of intracerebroventricular administration of 2-hydroxypropyl-β-cyclodextrin in a patient with Niemann-Pick Type C disease. *Mol. Genet. Metab. Rep.* 1, 391–400. doi: 10.1016/j.ymgmr.2014.08.004

Matsuo, M., Togawa, M., Hirabaru, K., Mochinaga, S., Narita, A., Adachi, M., et al. (2013). Effects of cyclodextrin in two patients with Niemann-Pick Type C disease. *Mol. Genet. Metab.* 108, 76–81. doi: 10.1016/j.ymgme.2012.11.005

Megías-Vericat, J. E., García-Robles, A., Company-Albir, M. J., Fernández-Megía, M. J., Pérez-Miralles, F. C., López-Briz, E., et al. (2017). Early experience with compassionate use of 2 hydroxypropyl-β-cyclodextrin for Niemann-Pick type C disease: review of initial published cases. *Neurol. Sci.* 38, 727–743. doi: 10.1007/s10072-017-2833-9

Mercer, A. J., Szalewski, R. J., Jackman, S. L., Van Hook, M. J., and Thoreson, W. B. (2012). Regulation of presynaptic strength by controlling Ca^{2+} channel mobility: effects of cholesterol depletion on release at the cone ribbon synapse. *J. Neurophysiol.* 107, 3468–3478. doi: 10.1152/jn.00779.2011

Morizono, T., Paparella, M. M., and Juhn, S. K. (1980). Ototoxicity of propylene glycol in experimental animals. *Am. J. Otolaryngol.* 1, 393–399. doi: 10.1016/s0196-0709(80)80020-2

Mustapha, M., Fang, Q., Gong, T. W., Dolan, D. F., Raphael, Y., Camper, S. A., et al. (2009). Deafness and permanently reduced potassium channel gene expression and function in hypothyroid Pit1dw mutants. *J. Neurosci.* 29, 1212–1223. doi: 10.1523/JNEUROSCI.4957-08.2009

Naureckiene, S., Sleat, D. E., Lackland, H., Fensom, A., Vanier, M. T., Wattiaux, R., et al. (2000). Identification of HE1 as the second gene of Niemann-Pick C disease. *Science* 290, 2298–2301. doi: 10.1126/science.290.5500.2298

Nguyen, T. V., and Brownell, W. E. (1998). Contribution of membrane cholesterol to outer hair cell lateral wall stiffness. *Otolaryngol. Head Neck Surg.* 119, 14–20. doi: 10.1016/s0194-5998(98)70167-6

Nie, L. (2008). KCNQ4 mutations associated with nonsyndromic progressive sensorineural hearing loss. *Curr. Opin. Otolaryngol. Head Neck Surg.* 16, 441–444. doi: 10.1097/MOO.0b013e32830f4aa3

Oesterle, E. C., Campbell, S., Taylor, R. R., Forge, A., and Hume, C. R. (2008). Sox2 and JAGGED1 expression in normal and drug-damaged adult mouse inner ear. *J. Assoc. Res. Otolaryngol.* 9, 65–89. doi: 10.1007/s10162-007-0106-7

Oliveri, V., and Vecchio, G. (2016). Cyclodextrins as protective agents of protein aggregation: an overview. *Chem. Asian. J.* 11, 1648–1657. doi: 10.1002/asia.201600259

Onodera, R., Motoyama, K., Okamatsu, A., Higashi, T., Kariya, R., Okada, S., et al. (2013). Involvement of cholesterol depletion from lipid rafts in apoptosis induced by methyl-β-cyclodextrin. *Int. J. Pharm.* 452, 116–123. doi: 10.1016/j.ijpharm.2013.04.071

Organ, L. E., and Raphael, R. M. (2009). Lipid lateral mobility in cochlear outer hair cells: regional differences and regulation by cholesterol. *J. Assoc. Res. Otolaryngol.* 10, 383–396. doi: 10.1007/s10162-009-0171-1

Ory, D. S., Ottinger, E. A., Farhat, N. Y., King, K. A., Jiang, X., Weissfeld, L., et al. (2017). Intrathecal 2-hydroxypropyl-β-cyclodextrin decreases neurological disease progression in Niemann-Pick disease, type C1: a non-randomised, open-label, phase 1–2 trial. *Lancet* 390, 1758–1768. doi: 10.1016/s0140-6736(17)31465-4

Ottinger, E. A., Kao, M. L., Carrillo-Carrasco, N., Yanjanin, N., Shankar, R. K., Janssen, M., et al. (2014). Collaborative development of 2-hydroxypropyl-β-cyclodextrin for the treatment of Niemann-Pick type C1 disease. *Curr. Top. Med. Chem.* 14, 330–339. doi: 10.2174/1568026613666131127160118

Patterson, I., Halsey, K., Liu, L., Schrepfer, T., and Duncan, R. (2016). "Ion channel modulation limits cyclodextrin-induced ototoxicity," in *Association for Research in Otolaryngology 39th Annual Midwinter Meeting,* (San Diego, CA).

Patterson, M. C., Di Bisceglie, A. M., Higgins, J. J., Abel, R. B., Schiffmann, R., Parker, C. C., et al. (1993). The effect of cholesterol-lowering agents on hepatic and plasma cholesterol in Niemann-Pick disease type C. *Neurology* 43, 61–64. doi: 10.1212/wnl.43.1_part_1.61

Patterson, M. C., Vecchio, D., Prady, H., Abel, L., and Wraith, J. E. (2007). Miglustat for treatment of Niemann-Pick C disease: a randomised controlled study. *Lancet Neurol.* 6, 765–772. doi: 10.1016/s1474-4422(07)70194-1

Patterson, M. C., and Walkley, S. U. (2017). Niemann-Pick disease, type C and Roscoe Brady. *Mol. Genet. Metab.* 120, 34–37. doi: 10.1016/j.ymgme.2016.11.008

Pikus, A. (1991). Audiologic profile in Niemann-Pick C. *Ann. N Y Acad. Sci.* 630, 313–314. doi: 10.1111/j.1749-6632.1991.tb19618.x

Pontikis, C. C., Davidson, C. D., Walkley, S. U., Platt, F. M., and Begley, D. J. (2013). Cyclodextrin alleviates neuronal storage of cholesterol in Niemann-Pick C disease without evidence of detectable blood-brain barrier permeability. *J. Inherit. Metab. Dis.* 36, 491–498. doi: 10.1007/s10545-012-9583-x

Purcell, E. K., Liu, L., Thomas, P. V., and Duncan, R. K. (2011). Cholesterol influences voltage-gated calcium channels and BK-type potassium channels in auditory hair cells. *PLoS One* 6:e26289. doi: 10.1371/journal.pone.0026289

Rajagopalan, L., Greeson, J. N., Xia, A., Liu, H., Sturm, A., Raphael, R. M., et al. (2007). Tuning of the outer hair cell motor by membrane cholesterol. *J. Biol. Chem.* 282, 36659–36670. doi: 10.1074/jbc.m705078200

Rosenbaum, A. I., Zhang, G., Warren, J. D., and Maxfield, F. R. (2010). Endocytosis of β-cyclodextrins is responsible for cholesterol reduction in Niemann-Pick type C mutant cells. *Proc. Natl. Acad. Sci. U S A* 107, 5477–5482. doi: 10.1073/pnas.0914309107

Rouquette-Jazdanian, A. K., Pelassy, C., Breittmayer, J. P., and Aussel, C. (2006). Revaluation of the role of cholesterol in stabilizing rafts implicated in T cell receptor signaling. *Cell. Signal.* 18, 105–122. doi: 10.1016/j.cellsig.2005.03.024

Sano, R., Annunziata, I., Patterson, A., Moshiach, S., Gomero, E., Opferman, J., et al. (2009). GM1-ganglioside accumulation at the mitochondria-associated ER membranes links ER stress to Ca^{2+}-dependent mitochondrial apoptosis. *Mol. Cell* 36, 500–511. doi: 10.1016/j.molcel.2009.10.021

Santi, P. A., Mancini, P., and Barnes, C. (1994). Identification and localization of the GM1 ganglioside in the cochlea using thin-layer chromatography and cholera toxin. *J. Histochem. Cytochem.* 42, 705–716. doi: 10.1177/42.6.8189033

Schacht, J., and Hawkins, J. E. (2006). Sketches of otohistory. Part 11: ototoxicity: drug-induced hearing loss. *Audiol. Neurootol.* 11, 1–6. doi: 10.1159/000088850

Sinex, D. G., Clark, W. W., and Bohne, B. A. (1987). Effects of periodic rest on physiological measures of auditory sensitivity following exposure to noise. *J. Acoust. Soc. Am.* 82, 1265–1273. doi: 10.1121/1.395829

Somers, K. L., Brown, D. E., Fulton, R., Schultheiss, P. C., Hamar, D., Smith, M. O., et al. (2001). Effects of dietary cholesterol restriction in a feline model of Niemann-Pick type C disease. *J. Inherit. Metab. Dis.* 24, 427–436. doi: 10.1023/A:1010588112003

Stella, V. J., and He, Q. (2008). Cyclodextrins. *Toxicol. Pathol.* 36, 30–42. doi: 10.1177/0192623307310945

Stella, V. J., and Rajewski, R. A. (1997). Cyclodextrins: their future in drug formulation and delivery. *Pharm. Res.* 14, 556–567. doi: 10.1023/A:1012136608249

Suh, B. C., and Hille, B. (2008). PIP2 is a necessary cofactor for ion channel function: how and why? *Annu. Rev. Biophys.* 37, 175–195. doi: 10.1146/annurev.biophys.37.032807.125859

Takahashi, S., Homma, K., Zhou, Y., Nishimura, S., Duan, C., Chen, J., et al. (2016). Susceptibility of outer hair cells to cholesterol chelator 2-hydroxypropyl-β-cyclodextrine is prestin-dependent. *Sci. Rep.* 6:21973. doi: 10.1038/srep21973

Taylor, A. M., Liu, B., Mari, Y., Liu, B., and Repa, J. J. (2012). Cyclodextrin mediates rapid changes in lipid balance in *Npc1*$^{-/-}$ mice without carrying cholesterol through the bloodstream. *J. Lipid Res.* 53, 2331–2342. doi: 10.1194/jlr.m028241

Taylor, R. R., Nevill, G., and Forge, A. (2008). Rapid hair cell loss: a mouse model for cochlear lesions. *J. Assoc. Res. Otolaryngol.* 9, 44–64. doi: 10.1007/s10162-007-0105-8

Vanier, M. T. (2010). Niemann-Pick disease type C. *Orphanet J. Rare Dis.* 5:16. doi: 10.1186/1750-1172-5-16

Vanier, M. T., and Millat, G. (2003). Niemann-pick disease type C. *Clin. Genet.* 64, 269–281. doi: 10.1034/j.1399-0004.2003.00147.x

Varan, G., Varan, C., Erdogar, N., Hincal, A. A., and Bilensoy, E. (2017). Amphiphilic cyclodextrin nanoparticles. *Int. J. Pharm.* 531, 457–469. doi: 10.1016/j.ijpharm.2017.06.010

Vernon, J., Brummett, R., and Walsh, T. (1978). The ototoxic potential of propylene glycol in guinea pigs. *Arch. Otolaryngol.* 104, 726–729. doi: 10.1001/archotol.1978.00790120052008

Vite, C. H., Bagel, J. H., Swain, G. P., Prociuk, M., Sikora, T. U., Stein, V. M., et al. (2015). Intracisternal cyclodextrin prevents cerebellar dysfunction and Purkinje cell death in feline Niemann-Pick type C1 disease. *Sci. Transl. Med.* 7:276ra26.

Walkley, S. U., Davidson, C. D., Jacoby, J., Marella, P. D., Ottinger, E. A., Austin, C. P., et al. (2016). Fostering collaborative research for rare genetic disease: the example of niemann-pick type C disease. *Orphanet J. Rare Dis.* 11:161. doi: 10.1186/s13023-016-0540-x

Wang, H., Xie, X., Zhang, F., Zhou, Q., Tao, Q., Zou, Y., et al. (2011). Evaluation of cholesterol depletion as a marker of nephrotoxicity *in vitro* for novel β-cyclodextrin derivatives. *Food Chem. Toxicol.* 49, 1387–1393. doi: 10.1016/j.fct.2011.03.026

Ward, S., O'Donnell, P., Fernandez, S., and Vite, C. H. (2010). 2-hydroxypropyl-β-cyclodextrin raises hearing threshold in normal cats and in cats with Niemann-Pick type C disease. *Pediatr. Res.* 68, 52–56. doi: 10.1203/pdr.0b013e3181df4623

Yamashita, T., Hakizimana, P., Wu, S., Hassan, A., Jacob, S., Temirov, J., et al. (2015). Outer hair cell lateral wall structure constrains the mobility of plasma membrane proteins. *PLoS Genet.* 11:e1005500. doi: 10.1371/journal.pgen.1005500

Yao, J., Ho, D., Calingasan, N. Y., Pipalia, N. H., Lin, M. T., and Beal, M. F. (2012). Neuroprotection by cyclodextrin in cell and mouse models of Alzheimer disease. *J. Exp. Med.* 209, 2501–2513. doi: 10.1084/jem.20121239

Yergey, A. L., Blank, P. S., Cologna, S. M., Backlund, P. S., Porter, F. D., and Darling, A. J. (2017). Characterization of hydroxypropyl-β-cyclodextrins used in the treatment of Niemann-Pick Disease type C1. *PLoS One* 12:e0175478. doi: 10.1371/journal.pone.0175478

Żak, M., van der Linden, C. A., Bezdjian, A., Hendriksen, F. G., Klis, S. F., and Grolman, W. (2016). Scar formation in mice deafened with kanamycin and furosemide. *Microsc. Res. Tech.* 79, 766–772. doi: 10.1002/jemt.22695

Zenner, H. P. (1986). K^{+}-induced motility and depolarization of cochlear hair cells. Direct evidence for a new pathophysiological mechanism in Ménière's disease. *Arch. Otorhinolaryngol.* 243, 108–111. doi: 10.1007/bf00453760

Zenner, H. P., Reuter, G., Zimmermann, U., Gitter, A. H., Fermin, C., and LePage, E. L. (1994). Transitory endolymph leakage induced hearing loss and tinnitus: depolarization, biphasic shortening and loss of electromotility of outer hair cells. *Eur. Arch. Otorhinolaryngol.* 251, 143–153. doi: 10.1007/bf00181826

Zimmer, S., Grebe, A., Bakke, S. S., Bode, N., Halvorsen, B., Ulas, T., et al. (2016). Cyclodextrin promotes atherosclerosis regression via macrophage reprogramming. *Sci. Transl. Med.* 8:333ra50. doi: 10.1126/scitranslmed.aad6100

Ziolkowski, W., Szkatula, M., Nurczyk, A., Wakabayashi, T., Kaczor, J. J., Olek, R. A., et al. (2010). Methyl-β-cyclodextrin induces mitochondrial cholesterol depletion and alters the mitochondrial structure and bioenergetics. *FEBS Lett.* 584, 4606–4610. doi: 10.1016/j.febslet.2010.10.023

13

d-Tubocurarine and Berbamine: Alkaloids that are Permeant Blockers of the Hair Cell's Mechano-Electrical Transducer Channel and Protect from Aminoglycoside Toxicity

Nerissa K. Kirkwood[1], *Molly O'Reilly*[1], *Marco Derudas*[2], *Emma J. Kenyon*[1], *Rosemary Huckvale*[2], *Sietse M. van Netten*[3], *Simon E. Ward*[2], *Guy P. Richardson*[1] and *Corné J. Kros*[1*]

[1] Sussex Neuroscience, School of Life Sciences, University of Sussex, Brighton, United Kingdom, [2] Sussex Drug Discovery Centre, School of Life Sciences, University of Sussex, Brighton, United Kingdom, [3] Institute of Artificial Intelligence and Cognitive Engineering, University of Groningen, Groningen, Netherlands

Edited by:
Peter S. Steyger,
Oregon Health & Science University,
United States

Reviewed by:
Jung-Bum Shin,
University of Virginia, United States
Gregory I. Frolenkov,
University of Kentucky, United States

***Correspondence:**
Corné J. Kros
c.j.kros@sussex.ac.uk

Aminoglycoside antibiotics are widely used for the treatment of life-threatening bacterial infections, but cause permanent hearing loss in a substantial proportion of treated patients. The sensory hair cells of the inner ear are damaged following entry of these antibiotics via the mechano-electrical transducer (MET) channels located at the tips of the hair cell's stereocilia. d-Tubocurarine (dTC) is a MET channel blocker that reduces the loading of gentamicin-Texas Red (GTTR) into rat cochlear hair cells and protects them from gentamicin treatment. Berbamine is a structurally related alkaloid that reduces GTTR labeling of zebrafish lateral-line hair cells and protects them from aminoglycoside-induced cell death. Both compounds are thought to reduce aminoglycoside entry into hair cells through the MET channels. Here we show that dTC ($\geq$6.25 μM) or berbamine ($\geq$1.55 μM) protect zebrafish hair cells *in vivo* from neomycin (6.25 μM, 1 h). Protection of zebrafish hair cells against gentamicin (10 μM, 6 h) was provided by $\geq$25 μM dTC or $\geq$12.5 μM berbamine. Hair cells in mouse cochlear cultures are protected from longer-term exposure to gentamicin (5 μM, 48 h) by 20 μM berbamine or 25 μM dTC. Berbamine is, however, highly toxic to mouse cochlear hair cells at higher concentrations ($\geq$30 μM) whilst dTC is not. The absence of toxicity in the zebrafish assays prompts caution in extrapolating results from zebrafish neuromasts to mammalian cochlear hair cells. MET current recordings from mouse outer hair cells (OHCs) show that both compounds are permeant open-channel blockers, rapidly and reversibly blocking the MET channel with half-blocking concentrations of 2.2 μM (dTC) and 2.8 μM (berbamine) in the presence of 1.3 mM Ca^{2+} at −104 mV. Berbamine, but not dTC, also blocks the hair cell's basolateral K^+ current, $I_{K,neo}$, and modeling studies indicate that berbamine permeates the MET channel more readily than dTC. These studies reveal key properties of MET-channel blockers required for the future design of successful otoprotectants.

Keywords: hair cell, mechanotransduction, hearing loss, ototoxicity, aminoglycosides, d-tubocurarine, berbamine

INTRODUCTION

Aminoglycoside antibiotics are prescribed worldwide as an effective treatment for serious and life-threatening conditions including tuberculosis, sepsis, neonatal infections, and those associated with cystic fibrosis (Rizzi and Hirose, 2007; Durante-Mangoni et al., 2009). The potency of these drugs against such infections ensures their continued use despite the knowledge that they are both nephro- and ototoxic (Forge and Schacht, 2000). Whilst kidney damage is reversible, a degree of permanent hearing loss is found in around 20–30% of patients treated with these antibiotics (Rizzi and Hirose, 2007; Schacht et al., 2012). The hearing loss is the result of damage caused to the sensory hair cells in the inner ear, an organ in which the aminoglycosides are found to selectively accumulate, with the basal, high-frequency outer hair cells (OHCs) being those that are predominantly affected (Forge and Schacht, 2000; Nakashima et al., 2000).

The main route of aminoglycoside entry into the hair cells is via their mechano-electrical transducer (MET) channels, large non-selective cation channels located at the tips of the hair cells' stereocilia (Marcotti et al., 2005; Alharazneh et al., 2011; Vu et al., 2013). Evidence for the molecular identity of the MET channel is increasingly suggesting that the transmembrane channel-like (TMC) family proteins, TMC1, and TMC2, are prime candidates (Kawashima et al., 2011, 2015; Pan et al., 2013; Kurima et al., 2015; Corey and Holt, 2016; Fettiplace, 2016). Once inside the cells the aminoglycosides disrupt various pathways and organelles, resulting in the activation of multiple signaling cascades including those involving the caspases (Forge and Li, 2000; Matsui et al., 2002, 2004; Owens et al., 2007). In the absence of alternative antibiotics of similar efficacy, identifying methods to protect the hair cells from this damage is crucial. Although one approach is to interrupt the intracellular pathways this may prove complex as, for example, the two closely-related aminoglycosides neomycin and gentamicin have been found to activate distinct cell-death pathways in zebrafish lateral line hair cells (Owens et al., 2009; Coffin et al., 2013a,b). Arguably, a more effective and universal method would be to administer compounds that block the MET channels and prevent aminoglycoside entry into the cells.

d-Tubocurarine (dTC), historically known as the main active component of the arrow poison, curare, is a naturally occurring alkaloid obtained from the bark of the South American plant *Chondrodendron tomentosum* (Perotti, 1977). It is a nicotinic antagonist that has been shown to block the acetylcholine receptor response in mature guinea-pig OHCs (Housley and Ashmore, 1991; Eróstegui et al., 1994) as well as the MET channels in neonatal mouse cochlear OHCs (Glowatzki et al., 1997). A study into the pore of the MET channels in turtle auditory hair cells reported that curare acts as a non-permeant blocker of these channels (Farris et al., 2004), making this an interesting molecule to investigate for potential otoprotective properties. The co-application of 1 mM curare was shown to significantly reduce the loading of 3 μM Texas Red conjugated gentamicin (GTTR) into rat cochlear inner hair cells (IHCs) and OHCs (Alharazneh et al., 2011) suggesting a competitive block of the pore, and the presence of 1 mM curare during the exposure of rat cochlear cultures to 0.1 mM gentamicin prevented hair-cell death from occurring during a subsequent 48-h antibiotic-free period (Alharazneh et al., 2011).

Looking for other potential MET channel blockers, we identified berbamine as having a very similar chemical structure to dTC. Berbamine is a naturally occurring alkaloid that is present in a number of plant species within the *Berberidaceae* family (Rahmatullah et al., 2014). It has been used in Eastern medicine for centuries to treat inflammation and related conditions such as rheumatoid arthritis and is still of interest to date for its potential anti-cancer properties (Ji et al., 2009; Meng et al., 2013; Rahmatullah et al., 2014; Zhao et al., 2016). Studies on zebrafish lateral line hair cells have revealed that 25 μM berbamine can protect these cells from the damage caused by 50–400 μM of either neomycin or gentamicin (Kruger et al., 2016). Furthermore, these authors found that berbamine blocked the loading of both GTTR and FM1-43, a styryl dye that acts as a permeant blocker of the hair cells' MET channels (Gale et al., 2001), leading Kruger et al. (2016) to conclude that berbamine is providing protection by competitively blocking the MET channels.

The zebrafish lateral line system is a useful and effective model for initial screening, with the hair cells being both structurally and functionally similar to mammalian inner ear hair cells and externally located, making them easily accessible for pharmacological studies. A degree of caution is however required as to date only three of the compounds that have been identified to protect lateral line hair cells have also been shown to protect mammalian inner ear hair cells (PROTO1, tacrine, and phenoxybenzamine; Owens et al., 2008; Ou et al., 2009; Majumder et al., 2017). We therefore sought to ascertain if berbamine would protect mammalian hair cells from the toxic side effects of aminoglycoside antibiotics and, likewise, if dTC would protect zebrafish lateral line hair cells. Furthermore, we fully characterized how dTC blocks the MET channel in mammalian OHCs and whether berbamine, like dTC, acts in a similar fashion or otherwise. Comparisons between the two structurally related molecules will assist in understanding the features/characteristics of a compound that are required to provide optimum otoprotection.

MATERIALS AND METHODS

Zebrafish Husbandry and Embryo Generation

Zebrafish embryos were obtained from sibling crosses of adult AB fish. Embryos were staged following standard protocols (Kimmel et al., 1995; Westerfield, 2000) and raised at 28.5°C in E3 medium (1 mM NaCl, 0.17 mM KCl, 0.33 mM $MgSO_4$, 0.33 mM $CaCl_2$).

Zebrafish Protection Assay

AB larvae (4 days post fertilization, dpf) were pre-incubated with 3 μM of Yo-Pro-1 (Molecular Probes Y3603) for 30 min to label the hair cells, washed and pipetted into 96-well plates (three larvae per well). Larvae were co-incubated with serial dilutions of test compound (dTC or berbamine) ranging from 200 to 1.55 μM with 6.25 μM neomycin sulfate (Sigma N1876) for 1 h, or with 10 μM gentamicin sulfate (Sigma G3632) for 6 h. Plates were screened on a Zeiss IM35 inverted microscope with a 16X objective. Trunk neuromasts 3–9 were viewed for qualitative assessment of damage. Images of trunk neuromast 4 of all three larvae in each well were taken on a Nikon D5000 at 40X magnification and individual cells within the neuromast counted for quantitative analysis. Experiments were repeated at least four times.

Mouse Cochlear Culture Preparation

Cochlear cultures were prepared from wild-type CD-1 mice as previously described by Russell and Richardson (1987). In brief, postnatal day 2 (P2) pups of either sex were killed by cervical dislocation following Home Office guidelines. Decapitated heads were surface sterilized by three 1-min washes in 80% ethanol. Sagittal incisions were made down the midline of the head and cochleae were removed. Subsequent dissections were performed in Hanks' Balanced Salt Solution (HBSS; Thermo Shandon 14025050) buffered with 10 mM Hepes (Sigma H0887) (HBHBSS). Cochleae were removed from the bony labyrinth and explanted onto collagen-coated (Corning 354236) coverslips in cochlear culture medium (93% DMEM-F12, 7% fetal bovine serum and 10 $\mu g.ml^{-1}$ ampicillin). The coverslips complete with cochleae were then sealed in Maximow slide assemblies and the cultures were left to grow and adhere to the collagen in a 37°C incubator before use.

Mouse Cochlear Culture Protection Assay

Following 24 h incubation coverslips with adherent cochleae were removed from the Maximow slide assemblies, placed in 35 mm petri dishes (Greiner Bio-One 627161) and incubated for 48 h in the presence of 1 ml of cochlear culture medium that had been diluted with DMEM-F12 to reduce the serum concentration to 1.4%, together with 5 μM gentamicin (Sigma G3632) and varying concentrations of berbamine or dTC. Following 48-h incubation, cultures were washed in phosphate buffered saline (PBS), fixed in 3.7% formaldehyde (Sigma F1635) in 0.1 M sodium phosphate buffer pH 7.4, and stained with TRITC-phalloidin (Sigma P1951). Cultures were mounted on glass slides with Vectashield (Vector Laboratories H-1000) and imaged using a Zeiss Axioplan2 microscope. Images were obtained from the middle of the basal coil at a position ~20% along the length of the cochlea, measured from the basal tip. For quantification, the OHCs in these images were counted and averaged across a number of experiments. Image width was 220 μm and was aligned along the length of the cochlea.

Mouse Cochlear Culture Electrophysiology

Recordings were made from OHCs in organotypic cultures that had been maintained for 1–3 days *in vitro*. The organotypic cultures were transferred to the microscope chamber on their collagen-coated coverslips and the chamber was continuously perfused with an extracellular solution containing (in mM): 135 NaCl, 5.8 KCl, 1.3 $CaCl_2$, 0.9 $MgCl_2$, 0.7 NaH_2PO_4, 5.6 D-glucose, 10 HEPES-NaOH, 2 sodium pyruvate. MEM amino acids solution (50X) and MEM vitamins solution (100X) were added to a final concentration of 1X from concentrates (Fisher Scientific). The pH was adjusted to 7.48 with 1 molar NaOH (osmolality ~308 mOsmol kg^{-1}). The organs of Corti were observed with an upright microscope (Olympus) with Nomarski differential interference contrast optics (40X water-immersion objective). Whole-cell patch-clamp recordings were obtained from basal-coil OHCs at room temperature (20–23°C) using an Optopatch (Cairn Research) patch-clamp amplifier. For MET current recordings patch pipettes (2.5–3.0 MΩ) contained the following (in mM): 137 CsCl, 2.5 $MgCl_2$, 1 EGTA-CsOH, 2.5 Na_2ATP, 10 sodium phosphocreatine, 5 HEPES-CsOH; pH adjusted to 7.3 with CsOH (osmolality ~295 mOsmol kg^{-1}). For recording basolateral potassium currents patch pipettes contained (in mM): 131 KCl, 3 $MgCl_2$, 5 Na_2ATP, 1 EGTA-KOH, 5 HEPES, 10 sodium phosphocreatine, pH adjusted to 7.28 with KOH (osmolality ~295 mOsmol kg^{-1}). Patch pipettes were coated with surf wax (Mr. Zogs SexWax) to minimize the fast capacitance transient across the wall of the patch pipette. MET currents were elicited by stimulating the OHC hair bundles using a fluid jet from a pipette (tip diameter 8–10 μm) driven by a piezoelectric disc (Kros et al., 1992; Marcotti et al., 2005). Mechanical stimuli (filtered at 1.0 kHz, 8-pole Bessel) were applied as 45 Hz sinusoids or, to quantify kinetics of block, voltage steps, with driver voltage amplitudes of ±40 V, sufficient to elicit large, saturating MET currents. Currents were acquired using pClamp (Molecular Devices) software and stored on a computer for off-line analysis. To look at extracellular block the compounds were locally superfused onto the OHCs at concentrations ranging from 300 nM to 100 μM in a solution containing (in mM): 145 NaCl, 5.8 KCl, 1.3 $CaCl_2$, 0.9 $MgCl_2$, 0.7 NaH_2PO_4, 5.6 glucose, 10 HEPES-NaOH, 2 sodium pyruvate. The pH was adjusted to 7.48 with NaOH (osmolality ~305 mOsmol kg^{-1}). This solution, without any compound, was superfused as a control solution before and after the application of each compound. A modest negative pressure applied to the tip of the fluid jet pipette resulted in the compound-containing solution being sucked into the pipette during superfusion. This prevented mixing and dilution of the compound with bath solution during fluid jet stimulation. To look at intracellular block the compounds were included in the patch-pipette solution at concentrations ranging from 100 μM to 1 mM. MET currents obtained at the beginning of each recording were used as controls, by which time the compounds would not yet have diffused into the cells.

MET current size was determined by measuring the difference between the minimum current during the inhibitory phase of the sinewave and the current ~6 ms after the onset of the excitatory phase of the sinewave, a time point at which the current would have reached near steady state. The current sizes were averaged for each 22 ms phase of the sinewave, omitting the first cycle. Basolateral currents were determined by measuring the steady-state current toward the end of the voltage-step. Series resistance compensation was applied (50–80%) and the average residual series resistance was calculated to be 1.73 ± 0.10 MΩ ($n = 78$). The average maximum MET current size was 1.54 ± 0.08 nA ($n = 66$), and the average maximum basolateral current was 2.09 ± 0.11 nA ($n = 12$). This would result in a maximum voltage drop across the residual series resistance of 2.7 and 3.6

mV respectively, considered sufficiently small to not require any correction to quoted voltage values. All voltages reported include a −4 mV correction for the liquid junction potential between extra- and intra-cellular solutions.

Two-Barrier One Binding-Site Model of Permeant Block of the MET Channel

The model used is a modification of that used for describing permeation and block by dihydrostreptomycin (DHS; Marcotti et al., 2005), to allow for values of the Hill coefficient (a measure of the degree of cooperativity of the binding process of blocker molecules to the binding site) that are greater or less than unity (van Netten and Kros, 2007). Assuming that the fraction of unblocked transducer channels is indicated by *C*, the fraction of blocked channels by *CB*, the extra- and intracellular blocker by B_o and B_i, the Hill coefficient by n_H, and using the forward (k_1, k_2) and reverse (k_{-1}, k_{-2}) rate constants, the reaction equation is given by:

$$C + n_H B_0 \underset{k_{-1}}{\overset{k_1}{\Leftrightarrow}} CB_{n_H} \underset{k_{-2}}{\overset{k_2}{\Leftrightarrow}} C + n_H B_i. \quad (1)$$

Introducing the time variable *t*, the dynamics of the two fractions are denoted by $C(t)$ and $CB(t) = 1 - C(t)$. The rate of change of $C(t)$ is dependent on the four rate constants k_1, k_{-1}, k_2, k_{-2} of the transitions across the barriers and the intra- and extracellular blocker concentrations, $[B_i]$ and $[B_o]$. We assume that the intracellular compound concentration B_i is small and it is therefore set to zero ($[B_i = 0]$).

The voltage across the MET channel is assumed to vary with a fixed gradient so that it linearly changes the free energy across the membrane, effectively tilting the overall free energy profile in proportion to the membrane potential *V*. The maxima of the free energy related to the barriers are defined as E_1 and E_2 and the minimum free energy related to the binding site as E_b, with respect to $V = 0$. We further assume that the two barriers are located at both sides of the membrane so that their fractional positions across the membrane are $\delta_1 = 0$ (outside), and $\delta_2 = 1$ (inside). This is a simplification of, but otherwise similar to, that used in a previous study of block by DHS, where the barriers were positioned just inside the field (Marcotti et al., 2005).

Block of GTTR Loading in Mouse Cochlear Cultures

Cochlear cultures on the collagen-coated coverslips were transferred from the Maximow slide assemblies into a viewing chamber in which they were incubated for 5 min in HBHBSS together with 1% DMSO and 100 μM of compound (dTC or berbamine) or 1% DMSO vehicle alone. GTTR was then added to a final concentration of 0.2 μM and left for 10 min. The cultures were washed three times and imaged using a 60X dipping lens on a Zeiss Axioplan2 microscope. Fluorescence intensity values were obtained from ten cells for each condition from images captured at a time point 27 min from the start of the experiment. Experiments for each condition were repeated three times (30 cells total) and the intensity values averaged. Images were obtained from a region that was ~800 μm from the basal tip of the cochlea.

Compound Analysis

Structures of dTC and berbamine were prepared, energy minimized (using MMFF94x forcefield) and flexibly aligned using Molecular Operating Environment (MOE) 2015.10. pKa was calculated using MarvinSketch 16.8.15.0, ChemAxon (https://www.chemaxon.com).

Statistical Analysis

Values of half-blocking concentration (K_D) and Hill coefficient (n_H) determined from fitting dose-response curves were tested for significant differences using 95% confidence intervals (CI). This is equivalent to $p < 0.05$ being the criterion for statistical significance. Multiple comparisons were made using 1-way ANOVA with Dunnett (cell counts) or Tukey (GTTR fluorescence) post tests. Compounds were considered fully protective if the cell counts differed significantly from the cell counts in the presence of aminoglycoside antibiotic (neomycin or gentamicin) alone, but not from the cell counts in the control medium. Compounds were considered partially protective if cell counts differed significantly from both aminoglycoside and control media. Means are quoted and shown in Figures ± SEM. Level of statistical significance is shown in Figures as follows: $^{*}p < 0.05$; $^{**}p < 0.01$; $^{***}p < 0.001$.

Study Approval

Animals were raised following Home Office guidelines. All experiments were performed in accordance with the Home Office Animals (Scientific Procedures) Act 1986 and approved by the University of Sussex Animal Welfare and Ethical Review Board.

RESULTS

d-Tubocurarine and Berbamine Protect Zebrafish Lateral Line Hair Cells from Aminoglycoside Damage

In order to assess the protective capabilities of dTC and berbamine against aminoglycoside damage, a protection assay was performed using hair cells in the lateral line organs of zebrafish larvae at 4 dpf. This time point ensures the reliable loading of Yo-Pro 1 (Santos et al., 2006; Kindt et al., 2012). dTC was found to fully protect against damage induced by 6.25 μM neomycin in zebrafish larvae at concentrations ≥12.5 μM, with partial protection at 6.25 μM (**Figures 1A–F, 2A**). Full protection against damage induced by 10 μM gentamicin was only observed at concentrations ≥50 μM dTC, with partial protection at 25 μM (**Figures 1G–L, 2B**). Berbamine protected at somewhat lower concentrations compared to dTC. It fully protected against neomycin-induced neuromast damage in zebrafish larvae at concentrations ≥12.5 μM, with partial protection even down to 1.55 μM, the lowest concentration tested (**Figures 1M–R, 2C**). Berbamine offered full protection against gentamicin damage at 25 μM and above, with partial protection at 12.5 μM (**Figures 1S–X, 2D**). No signs of toxicity due to either compound were observed at the highest concentration tested (200 μM).

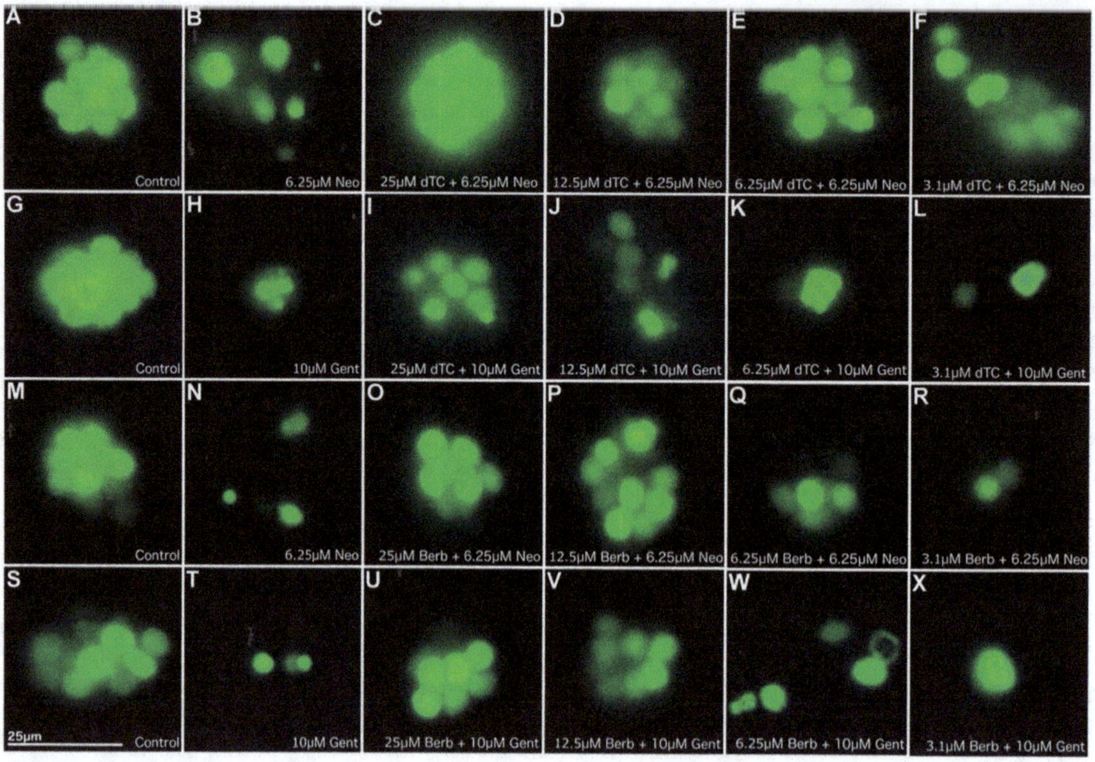

FIGURE 1 | d-Tubocurarine and berbamine protect lateral line hair cells in zebrafish from gentamicin and neomycin induced damage. Zebrafish were treated with: **(A,G,M,S)** E3 alone **(B)** 6.25 μM neomycin, or **(C–F)** 25, 12.5, 6.25, or 3.1 μM of dTC plus 6.25 μM neomycin, **(H)** 10 μM gentamicin, **(I–L)** 25, 12.5, 6.25, or 3.1 μM of dTC plus 10 μM gentamicin, **(N)** 6.25 μM neomycin, **(O–R)** 25, 12.5, 6.25, or 3.1 μM of berbamine plus 6.25 μM neomycin, **(T)** 10 μM gentamicin, **(U–X)** 25, 12.5, 6.25, or 3.1 μM of berbamine plus 10 μM gentamicin. Neuromasts were pre-stained with 3 μM Yo-Pro1. $n > 3$ independent experiments with at least 3 fish per well. Images were obtained with a 40X objective. Scale bar = 25 μm.

d-Tubocurarine and Berbamine Protect Mouse Cochlear Hair Cells from Aminoglycoside Damage, but Berbamine Is Toxic at Higher Concentrations

dTC and berbamine were subsequently tested in mouse cochlear cultures to see if they would protect mammalian cochlear hair cells from the damage induced by exposure to 5 μM gentamicin for 48 h (**Figures 3A–D**). Such treatment results in the nearly complete loss of OHCs from the basal 35% of the cochlea, but has little effect if any on the survival of IHCs. dTC and berbamine were found to be protective at minimum concentrations of 25 μM and 20 μM, respectively, as quantified in **Figures 4A,B**, which show counts of OHCs in a 220 μm wide segment of the basal coil of the cochlea. As a further criterion to assess the suitability of a compound for use as an otoprotectant we examined the hair-bundle morphology. No hair-bundle damage was observed during exposure to either compound.

To determine if either compound had any adverse effects on hair cells in the absence of gentamicin, they were tested alone at a higher concentration of 50 μM. Berbamine was found to be generally cytotoxic and killed both the IHCs and OHCs as well as other cell types in the entire organ of Corti, whereas dTC had no adverse effects on hair cells or hair-bundle morphology at this concentration (**Figures 3E, 4A**). Berbamine was tested alone at the lower concentrations of 20 and 30 μM and found to be equally toxic at 30 μM as it was at 50 μM (no IHCs or OHCs could be identified) but not at 20 μM, the concentration at which it showed protection against 5 uM gentamicin (**Figures 3F, 4B**). When 30 μM berbamine was tested together with 5 μM gentamicin, the same cytotoxic effect was observed as with 30 μM berbamine alone. While berbamine can thus protect from gentamicin toxicity, albeit over a narrow concentration range, we saw no evidence that gentamicin could protect from berbamine cytotoxicity.

d-Tubocurarine and Berbamine Block MET Channel Currents in Mouse Cochlear Hair Cells

To determine whether the protection observed for both compounds may be the result of a direct interaction with the hair cells' MET channels, thereby reducing or preventing aminoglycoside entry, we examined the effect of dTC and berbamine on the MET currents in basal-coil OHCs, the cells that are predominantly affected by aminoglycoside ototoxicity. Although dTC has previously been described as a MET channel blocker (Glowatzki et al., 1997; Farris et al., 2004), no such

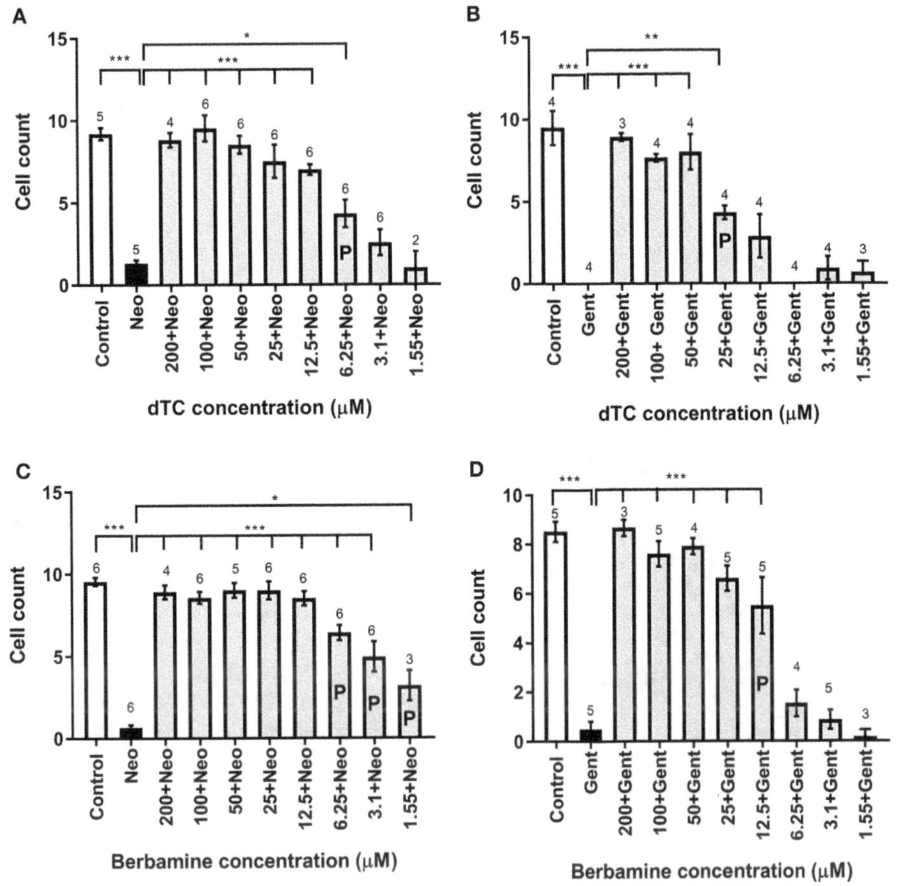

FIGURE 2 | Cell count analysis for lateral line hair cell protection against gentamicin and neomycin by d-tubocurarine and berbamine. **(A–D)** A range of concentrations (1.55–200 μM) of either dTC or berbamine with either neomycin or gentamicin are compared to neomycin or gentamicin alone. Number of hair cells were counted in trunk neuromast 4. **(A)** dTC against neomycin, **(B)** dTC against gentamicin, **(C)** berbamine against neomycin and **(D)** berbamine against gentamicin. Cells counts that are significantly different from aminoglycoside alone are indicated above the bars, with the number of stars representing the level of significance. The letter **P** in the bars indicates concentrations that were deemed partially protective, because cell counts were also significantly different from the control (A: ***; **B**: ***; **C**: ***; **D**: **). Numbers above the bars indicate experimental replicates, with cell numbers in three neuromasts counted and averaged for each replicate. *$p < 0.05$; **$p < 0.01$; ***$p < 0.001$.

study has been carried out with berbamine. MET currents were recorded at membrane potentials ranging from −164 to +96 mV before, during and after superfusion with dTC or berbamine at concentrations ranging from 300 nM to 100 μM (dTC), or 1 to 30 μM (berbamine). During exposure to either dTC or berbamine, a reduction in the current sizes was seen when the cells were stepped to hyperpolarized potentials. This reduction was less pronounced at depolarized potentials, with the level of the reduction being dependent upon the concentration of the compound. Examples of MET current block by dTC and berbamine at a concentration of 3 μM are shown in **Figures 5A,B**. Note that currents before and after application of the compounds appear as rectified versions of the sinewave stimulus. During superfusion of the compounds the currents look similar at positive potentials, but at negative potentials the MET currents can be seen to decline rapidly on each cycle after an initial inward current peak. This is suggestive of an open-channel blocking mechanism, where the blocker can only interact with the open channel. The block of the channel and subsequent washout were both rapid, with the currents making a full recovery upon re-exposure to the control superfusion solution, indicating that the block by both dTC and berbamine is completely reversible (**Figures 5A,B**).

Average normalized current-voltage curves show the extracellular block by dTC and berbamine at a range of concentrations (**Figures 6A,B**). These curves clearly demonstrate both the increase in the block with increasing compound concentration and the voltage dependence of the block, with minimal block at the depolarized potentials and stronger block at the hyperpolarized potentials.

To examine whether either compound has an effect on the MET currents when applied from the intracellular side of the channel, dTC and berbamine were included in the intracellular patch pipette solution at varying concentrations to enable their entry into the cells. Transducer currents were recorded in the same way as for the extracellular experiments, but omitting

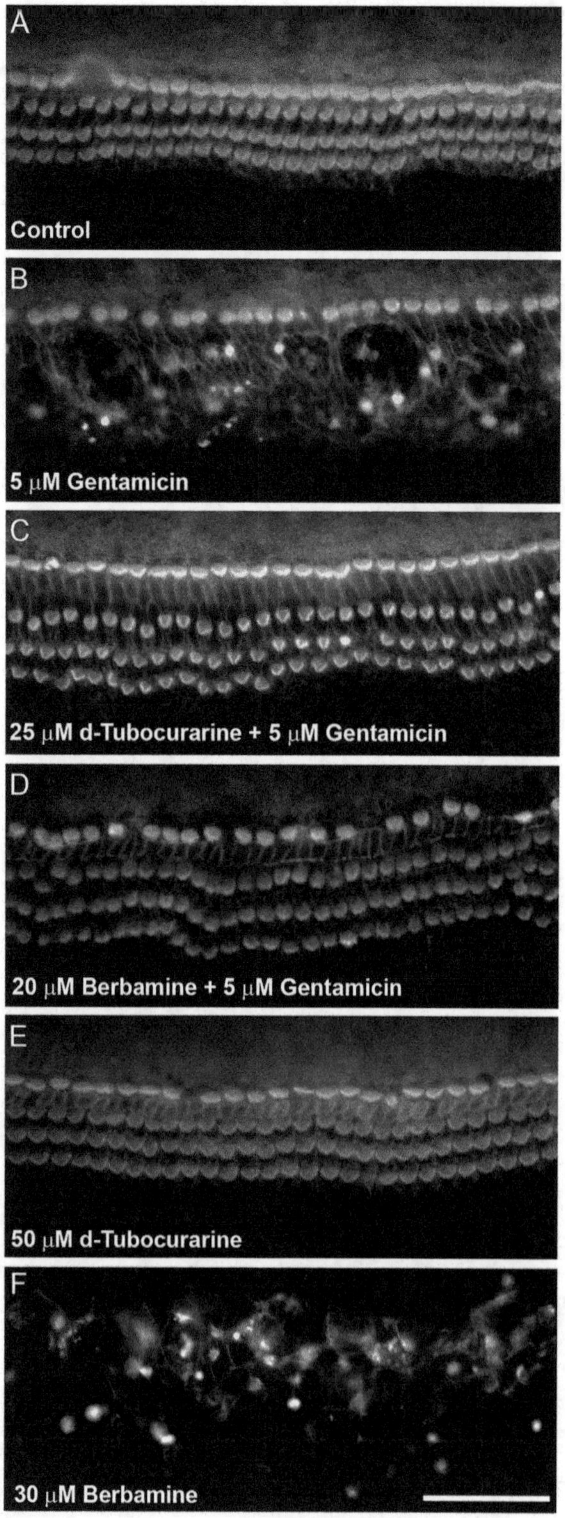

FIGURE 3 | d-Tubocurarine and berbamine protect cochlear OHCs from gentamicin damage. Protection assay using cultures prepared from CD-1 mice at postnatal day 2 (P2). Cultures were stained with TRITC-phalloidin at the end of the experiment allowing visualization of the actin-rich stereocilia. **(A)** Control culture incubated for 48 h in the presence of medium alone. The sensory hair *(Continued)*

FIGURE 3 | Continued
cell loss shown in **(B)** caused by 48 h incubation with 5 μM gentamicin can be prevented by co-incubation with 25 μM dTC **(C)** or 20 μM berbamine **(D)**. Cells incubated in 50 μM dTC in the absence of gentamicin were not damaged **(E)**, whereas 30 μM berbamine resulted in widespread loss of IHCs, OHCs and other cell types **(F)**. Scale bar = 50 μm.

any local superfusion of the cells. Intracellular berbamine at concentrations of 100 and 300 μM was found to have no effect on the size of the MET currents (data not shown). A higher concentration of 1 mM resulted in the rapid loss of the cells and the inability to maintain whole-cell recordings in every cell tested. Conversely, intracellular dTC, at concentrations ranging from 100 μM to 1 mM, was found to reduce the current size when cells were depolarized but not when they were hyperpolarized, indicating a block of the channel from the intracellular side. Average normalized current-voltage curves showing this intracellular block are shown (**Figure 6C**). Again, these curves clearly demonstrate the voltage dependence of the block and the increase in block with increasing compound concentration.

Dose-response curves for the extracellular block of the MET channels by dTC and berbamine were generated (**Figures 7A,B**). These curves were derived from the currents measured at −104 mV, near the membrane potential at which the block was seen to be the strongest, and fitted with the equation:

$$\frac{I}{I_C} = \frac{1}{1 + \left(\frac{[B]}{K_D}\right)^{n_H}} \tag{2}$$

where I_C is the control current in the absence of the compound, $[B]$ is the concentration of the blocking compound, K_D is the half-blocking concentration and n_H is the Hill coefficient. From these curves, the K_D for dTC was found to be 2.2 μM (95% CI 1.7 μM to 2.7 μM), a value very similar to the previously reported value for neonatal mouse OHC MET channel block of 2.3 μM (Glowatzki et al., 1997). The K_D for berbamine was found to be 2.8 μM (95% CI 2.4–3.2 μM), similar to the styryl dye FM1-43 (2.4 μM at −104 mV: Gale et al., 2001) and not significantly different from dTC. Both dTC and berbamine have a higher affinity for the MET channel than DHS, which has a reported K_D of 10 μM (Marcotti et al., 2005). The Hill coefficients calculated from the dose-response curve fits were 1.02 for berbamine and 0.80 for dTC, the latter a value that is significantly smaller than one ($p < 0.05$). These values suggest that, in the case of berbamine, a single molecule interacts with and blocks the channel whereas for dTC two molecules are involved, showing negative cooperativity (Wyman and Gill, 1990).

A dose-response curve for the intracellular block of the MET channels by dTC was generated, derived from the currents measured at +96 mV and fitted with Equation (2) (not shown). From this curve dTC was found to block the intracellular side of the channel with a K_D of 880 μM (95% CI 700–1,070 μM) and a Hill coefficient of 0.92, values similar to those found for the intracellular block of the MET channel by DHS (Marcotti

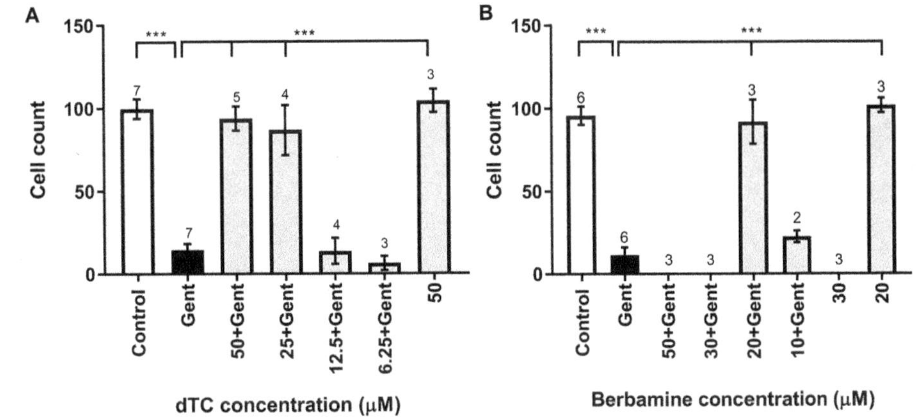

FIGURE 4 | Quantification of survival of OHCs exposed to gentamicin and otoprotective compounds. **(A,B)** Bar charts showing average numbers of OHCs remaining after 48 h in medium alone (control), in medium containing 5 μM gentamicin, in 5 μM gentamicin plus different concentrations of compounds, and in medium containing the compound alone. Number of OHCs were counted in a 220 μm wide field. Significant protection occurs at dTC concentrations of 25 μM and above **(A)** and for 20 μM berbamine **(B)**. While 50 μM dTC alone does not cause OHC damage, OHCs are obliterated at ≥30 μM berbamine, with or without gentamicin. Numbers above the bars indicate experimental replicates. ***$p < 0.001$.

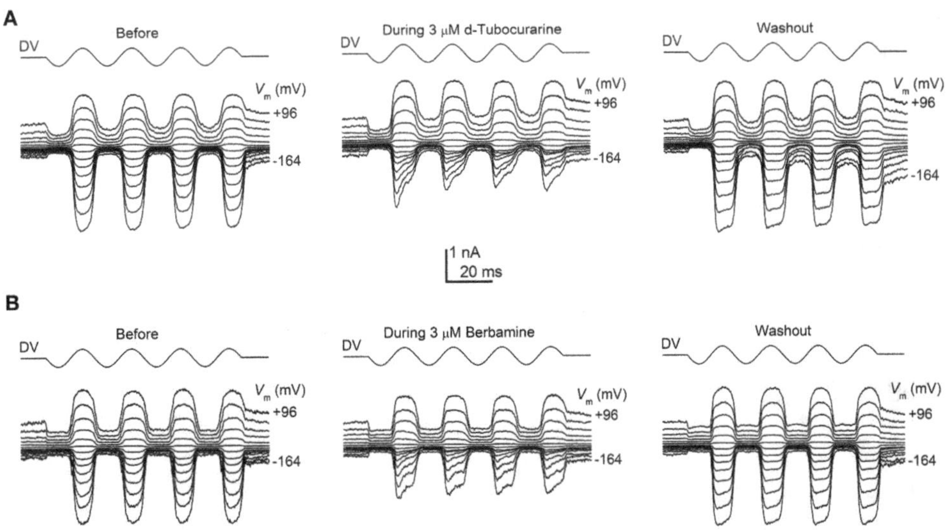

FIGURE 5 | Extracellular d-tubocurarine and berbamine block the OHC MET channel. **(A,B)** MET currents recorded from P2+2 OHCs before, during and after superfusion with a solution containing 3 μM dTC **(A)** or 3 μM berbamine **(B)**. Both compounds can be seen to predominantly block the MET currents at hyperpolarized potentials with the block fully reversible as seen from the washouts. Membrane potentials were stepped between −164 mV and +96 mV and MET currents were recorded in response to a sinewave delivered by a fluid jet (45 Hz sinusoid, ±40 V driver voltage, DV) shown above each trace. The capacitances of the cells were 6.9 pF **(A)** and 7.8 pF **(B)**.

et al., 2005; Corns et al., 2016). These values show that the affinity of dTC for the MET channel is greatly reduced when blocking from the intracellular side as opposed to the extracellular side.

Fractional block curves for both dTC and berbamine at all concentrations tested were plotted (**Figures 8A,B**). The data were fitted with a two-barrier, one binding-site (2B1BS) model similar to that previously used to describe the block of the MET currents by DHS (Marcotti et al., 2005) but adapted to allow for Hill coefficients different from one (van Netten and Kros, 2007; see Section Materials and Methods). For plotting the fractional block, the half-blocking concentration K_D in Equation (2) above becomes voltage-dependent as follows:

$$K_D = \left[K_1(V)\right]^{\frac{1}{nH}} \text{ with}$$
$$K_1(V) = \exp\left(\frac{E_b}{kT} + \frac{\delta_b V}{V_s}\right) \cdot \left(1 + \exp\left(-\frac{\Delta E}{kT} - \frac{V}{V_s}\right)\right), \quad (3)$$

where $\Delta E = E_2 - E_1$, the slope factor: $V_s = \frac{kT}{ze_0}$, is the ratio of thermal energy (kT, i.e., Boltzmann's constant multiplied by absolute temperature) and effective charge of the blocker molecule (ze_0, i.e., valence multiplied by elementary charge) and

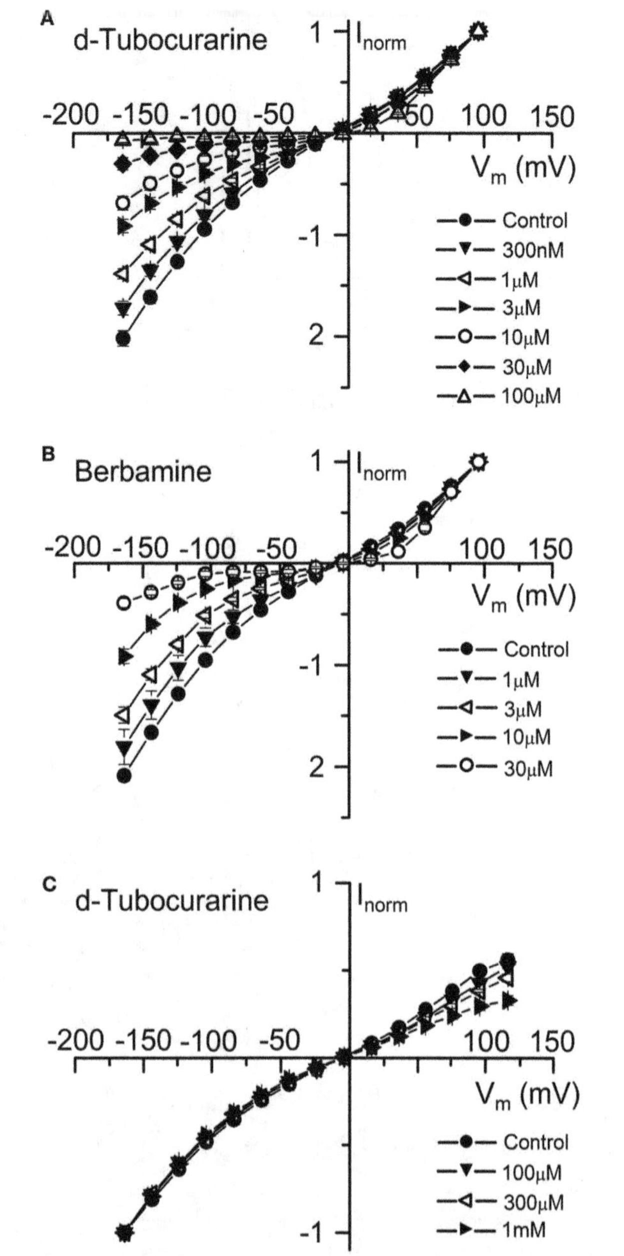

FIGURE 6 | Normalized current-voltage curves reveal the voltage-dependence of d-tubocurarine and berbamine MET channel block. **(A,B)** Average normalized current-voltage curves for the peak MET currents recorded before and during extracellular superfusion with 300 nM to 100 μM dTC **(A)**, or 1 to 30 μM extracellular berbamine **(B)**. Currents were normalized to the peak current measured at +96 mV. For the two compounds, block increases with both increasing hyperpolarization and compound concentration. Inclusion of 0.1 to 1 mM dTC in the patch-pipette resulted in a block of the MET currents from the intracellular side at depolarized potentials **(C)**. Currents in **(C)** were normalized to the peak current measured at −164 mV. Numbers of cells and peak current **(A)** Control: 43, 0.92 ± 0.05 nA; 300 nM: 5, 1.01 ± 0.14 nA; 1 μM: 6, 1.00 ± 0.09 nA; 3 μM: 9, 0.89 ± 0.10 nA; 10 μM: 5, 0.75 ± 0.09 nA; 30 μM: 13, 0.78 ± 0.10 nA; 100 μM: 5, 0.32 ± 0.03 nA **(B)** Control: 37, 0.65 ± 0.07 nA; 1 μM: 6, 0.76 ± 0.19 nA; 3 μM: 14, 0.51 ± 0.10 nA; 10 μM: 8, 0.54 ± 0.11 nA; 30 μM: 9, 0.38 ± 0.11 nA **(C)** Control: 10, −1.86 ± 0.13 nA; 100 μM: 3, −1.84 ± 0.31 nA; 300 μM: 2, −1.95 ± 0.12 nA; 1 mM: 5, −1.40 ± 0.13 nA.

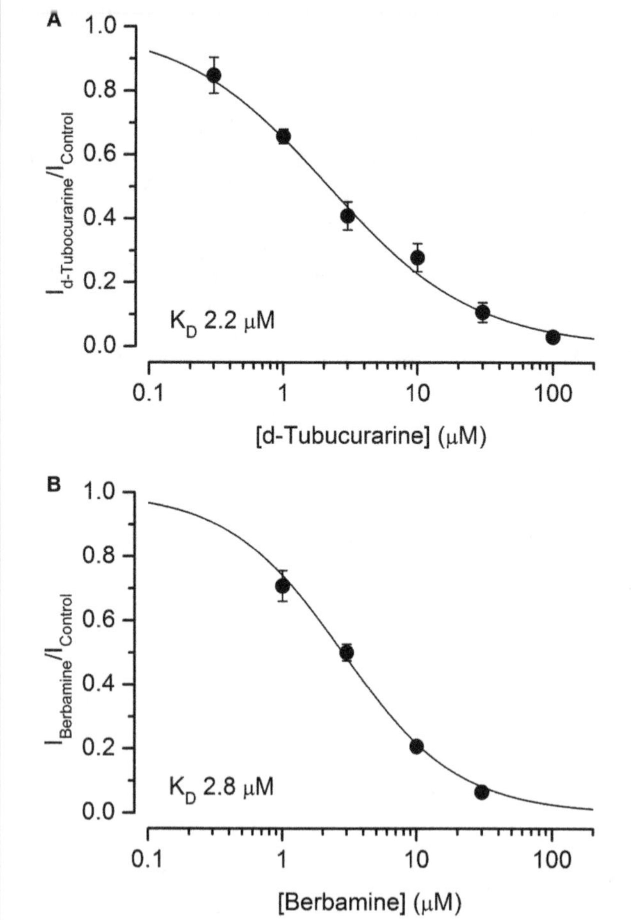

FIGURE 7 | d-Tubocurarine and berbamine block MET channels with similar half-blocking concentrations. **(A,B)** Dose-response curves of MET channel block by dTC **(A)** and berbamine **(B)** derived from currents recorded at −104 mV and fit with Equation (2). dTC: K_D 2.2 μM, Hill coefficient 0.80; berbamine: K_D 2.8 μM, Hill coefficient 1.02. From 5 to 14 cells were used for each data set.

δ_b is the relative electrical distance of the binding site along the membrane.

The data and fitted curves show that block is voltage-dependent for both compounds, with block being released strongly at positive potentials but also, to a lesser extent, at extreme negative potentials—the latter indicative of permeant block in which the compounds enter the cell with a sufficiently strong electrical driving force. This release at hyperpolarized potentials was more pronounced for berbamine than for dTC. The membrane potential of maximum block was −118 mV for dTC and −94 mV for berbamine.

Large step stimuli were applied to the cells before and during superfusion of the compounds to confirm whether or not the channel is required to open before block can occur, i.e., whether the compounds act as open-channel blockers, as suggested by the MET currents recorded in response to sinusoidal stimuli (**Figures 5A,B**), and to quantify the time course of the block. Currents were recorded in response to a large force step

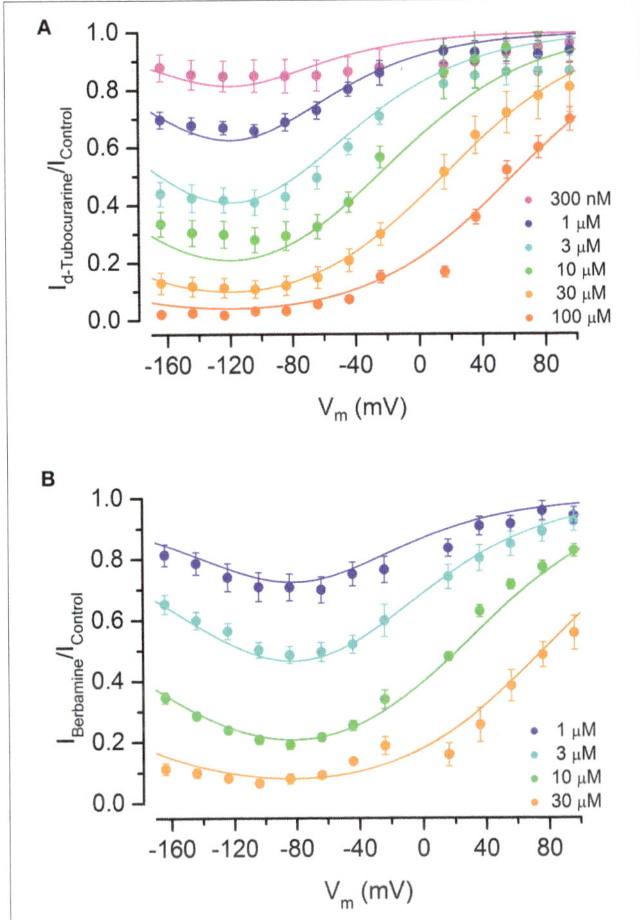

FIGURE 8 | Fractional block of the MET currents by d-tubocurarine and berbamine shows that both are permeant blockers. **(A,B)** Fraction of the MET current remaining during dTC **(A)** or berbamine **(B)** superfusion relative to the control current at the same membrane potential. Concentrations ranged from 300 nM to 100 μM (dTC) or 1 to 30 μM (berbamine). Data are fitted with a two-barrier, one binding-site model (see Section Materials and Methods). A release of the block at extreme hyperpolarized potentials indicates that both compounds can enter the cells. Maximum current block is seen at −118 mV (dTC) and −94 mV (berbamine). Fitted parameters were for dTC ΔE 4.96 kT; E_b −8.67 kT; z 1.09; δ_b 0.52, and for berbamine ΔE 2.68 kT; E_b −12.0 kT; z 0.94; δ_b 0.57. Number of cells **(A)** 300 nM: 5, 1 μM: 6, 3 μM: 9, 10 μM: 5, 30 μM: 13, 100 μM: 5 **(B)** 1 μM: 6, 3 μM: 14, 10 μM: 8, 30 μM: 9.

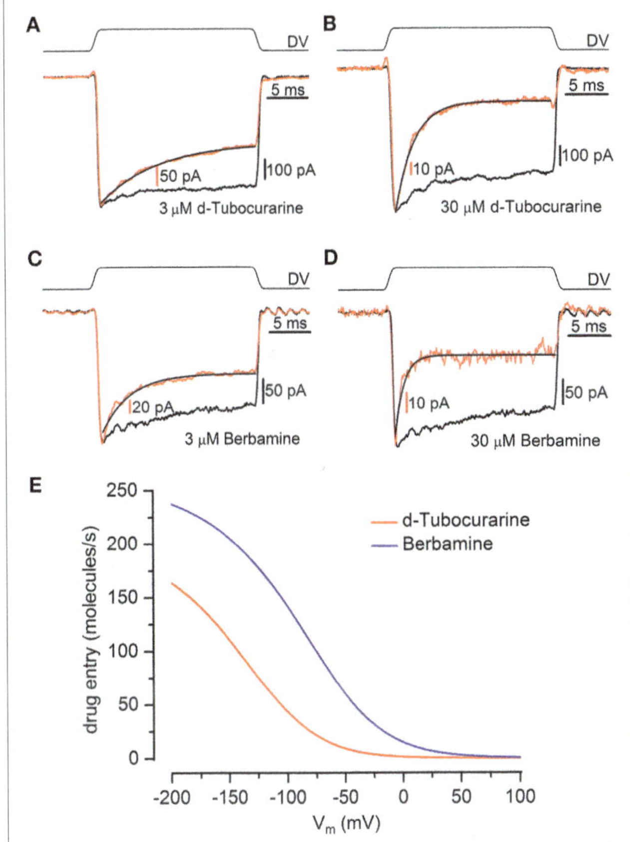

FIGURE 9 | Kinetics of MET channel block reveal d-tubocurarine and berbamine act as open channel blockers. **(A–D)** Transducer currents were recorded from OHCs in response to a mechanical step delivered by a fluid-jet (±40 V driver voltage, DV), shown above each trace [**(A,B)** P2+2; **(C,D)** P2+3]. From a holding potential of −84 mV, cells were exposed to an initial saturating inhibitory stimulus, resulting in the closure of the MET channels, followed by a saturating excitatory step eliciting rapidly activating inward currents. Currents (averaged from 10 repetitions) before (black trace) and during (red trace) superfusion of 3 μM dTC **(A)**, 30 μM dTC **(B)**, 3 μM berbamine **(C)**, and 30 μM berbamine **(D)** were scaled and superimposed. Maximum transducer currents were; **(A)** −679 pA before and −369 pA during 3 μM dTC application, **(B)** −742 pA before and −137 pA during 30 μM dTC application, **(C)** −271 pA before and −211 pA during 3 μM berbamine application and **(D)** −271 pA before and −67 pA during 30 μM berbamine application. Both dTC and berbamine can be seen to act as open channel blockers from the decline in current size observed following the excitatory step. The currents during compound superfusion were fitted with single exponentials **(A)** τ = 6.9 ms **(B)** τ = 2.1 ms **(C)** τ = 3.2 ms **(D)** τ = 0.83 ms. **(E)** Entry rates into the OHC of extracellular dTC and berbamine as a function of membrane potential. At all membrane potentials berbamine enters the cell more rapidly than dTC. Rates calculated for 1 μM compound, 80 channels, p_{open} 0.1.

before and during superfusion with different concentrations of each compound (3–30 μM; examples of recordings are shown in **Figures 9A–D**). In the absence of the blockers the force steps result in large, saturating MET currents showing minimal adaptation. Upon superfusion of either dTC or berbamine the currents activate with the same rapid time course, followed by an exponential decline in the currents, with the speed of the decline increasing with increasing concentration. This decline in the current following channel opening indicates that both compounds act as open-channel blockers and can only access their binding site once the channel is open. The time constants measured from the MET current decline allow for a calculation of the rate constants for entry into the channel from the extracellular side (k_1; see Marcotti et al., 2005; van Netten and Kros, 2007). Mean values of the time constants were, for dTC, 6.7 ± 0.6 ms (n = 7 OHCs) for 3 μM and 2.1 ± 0.2 ms (n = 6) for 30 μM. For berbamine at 3 μM the time constant was 4.7 ± 0.4 ms (n = 10), at 10 μM 2.45 ± 0.15 (n = 5) and at 30 μM 0.97 ± 0.22 ms (n = 3). From these values, the entry rates into the hair cells can be calculated. At all potentials berbamine enters more avidly than dTC (**Figure 9E**).

Effect of the Compounds on the Basolateral Potassium Currents in Mouse Outer Hair Cells

dTC is a known nicotinic antagonist that has also been shown to block various potassium channels including the apamin-sensitive potassium current in neurones (Goh and Pennefather, 1987), cloned small conductance calcium-activated potassium (SK) channels (Ishii et al., 1997) and a calcium-dependent potassium current in rat tumoral pituitary cells (Vacher et al., 1998). During the first postnatal week OHCs express a slow outward K^+ current ($I_{K,neo}$) activated at potentials positive to −50 mV (Marcotti and Kros, 1999). We therefore investigated whether dTC or berbamine could suppress this current and confer additional protection through causing a shift in resting membrane potential, with any depolarization of the cell potentially resulting in a reduced driving force for the positively charged aminoglycosides to enter the cells. Currents were elicited by applying a series of hyperpolarising and depolarizing voltage steps from the holding potential of −84 mV and currents recorded before and during exposure to 30 μM of each compound. Berbamine was found to substantially reduce $I_{K,neo}$ whereas dTC had no effect at this concentration (**Figure 10A**). Average normalized current-voltage curves for all cells recorded from are shown (**Figure 10B**).

Notably, neither compound elicited a reduction in the resting membrane potential when it was perfused onto OHCs under current clamp at a concentration of 30 μM (**Figure 10C**). In fact the reverse was observed, with similar increases in resting membrane potential during both dTC and berbamine superfusion. This hyperpolarization, which would lead to an increase in the electrical force driving the aminoglycosides to enter the hair cells, eliminates changes in resting membrane potential as a potential protective mechanism for both dTC and berbamine.

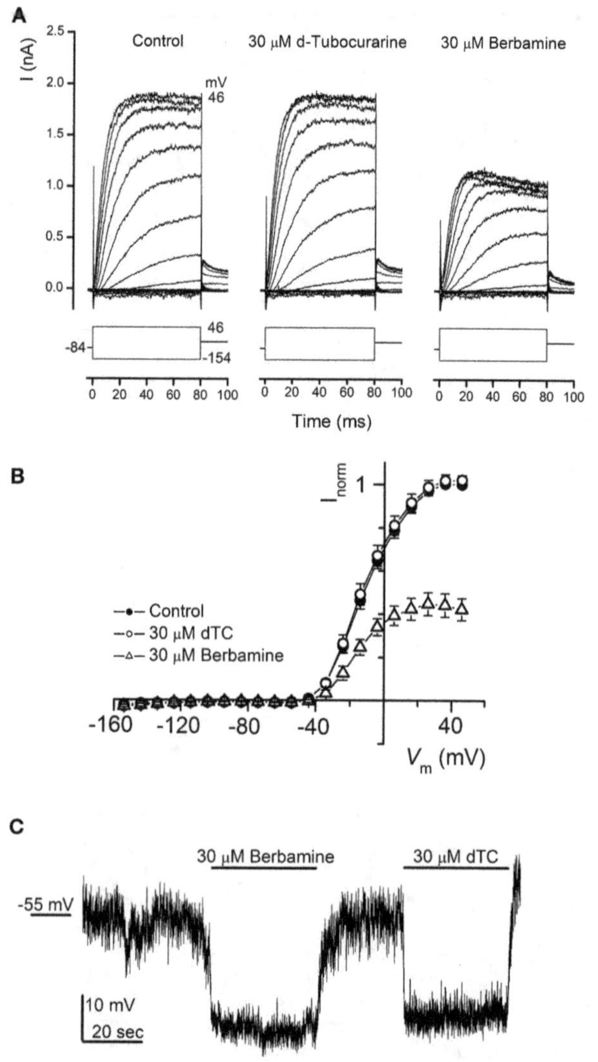

FIGURE 10 | Basolateral potassium currents are blocked by berbamine but not by d-tubocurarine. **(A)** Currents from an OHC recorded before and during exposure to 30 μM dTC or berbamine reveal a decrease in current size during berbamine, but not dTC superfusion. Currents were recorded in response to 10 mV hyperpolarizing and depolarizing voltage steps from a holding potential of −84 mV. Schematic representations of the voltage step protocols are shown below each trace. The leakage currents have been subtracted but the membrane potentials have not been adjusted for the residual series resistance (3.0 MΩ). The capacitance of the cell was 6.7 pF. **(B)** Average normalized steady-state I-V curves for all cells before (closed symbols; $n = 12$) and during exposure to 30 μM dTC (open circles; $n = 9$) or 30 μM berbamine (open triangles; $n = 8$). **(C)** Monitoring membrane potential changes under current clamp revealed that exposure to both 30 μM berbamine and 30 μM dTC resulted in a hyperpolarization of the cell of more than 10 mV from the resting potential of −55 mV.

d-Tubocurarine and Berbamine Reduce GTTR Loading into Cochlear Hair Cells

In order to test whether either compound could block or reduce the accumulation of gentamicin into the OHCs, mouse cochlear cultures were exposed to a low concentration (0.2 μM) of GTTR in the presence of a large molar excess (100 μM) of each compound for a short period of time to enable a quantification of the gentamicin uptake (Steyger et al., 2003). For a negative control, cultures were incubated in 0.2 μM GTTR and 1% DMSO alone. Following a 5 min pre-incubation with dTC, berbamine or DMSO alone and a subsequent 10 min co-incubation with 0.2 μM GTTR, a significant decrease in GTTR loading was seen in OHCs that were exposed to GTTR in the presence of either dTC or berbamine compared to the DMSO vehicle controls (**Figures 11A–D**). The reduction in GTTR labeling observed with the two compounds was similar and not significantly different.

DISCUSSION

The results of this study show that berbamine protects hair cells in mouse cochlear cultures from gentamicin toxicity, and that dTC can protect zebrafish lateral line hair cells from the toxic side effects of both neomycin and gentamicin. Furthermore, we confirm previous observations showing that dTC can protect mammalian hair cells from gentamicin (Alharazneh et al., 2011) and that berbamine can protect zebrafish hair cells from aminoglycoside toxicity (Kruger et al., 2016). The two alkaloids dTC and berbamine are therefore versatile otoprotectants that work in both fish and mammals.

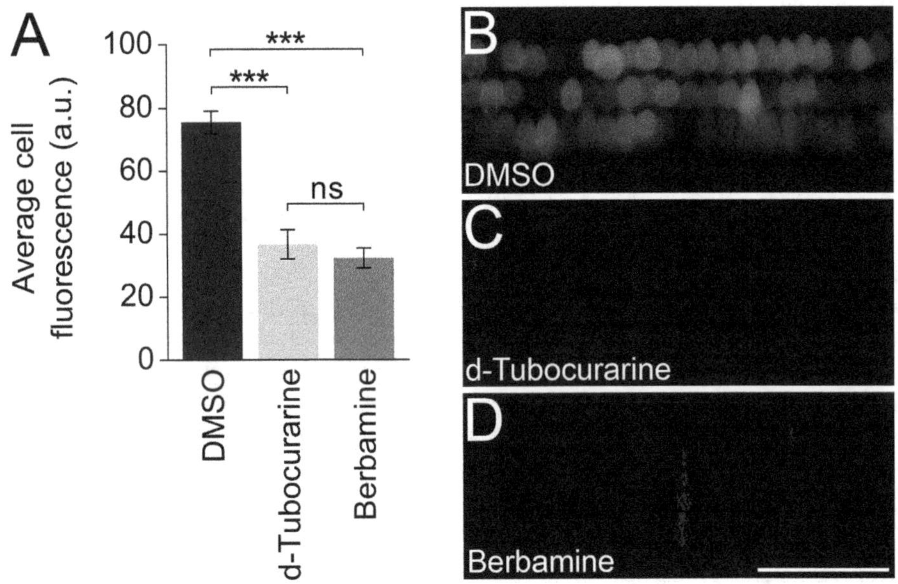

FIGURE 11 | d-Tubocurarine and berbamine reduce the loading of GTTR. **(A)** dTC and berbamine significantly reduced the fluorescent intensity of 0.2 μM GTTR compared to DMSO controls (***$p < 0.001$). No significant difference was seen between the reduction by dTC and berbamine. Fluorescent intensity was measured in arbitrary units (a.u.). Error bars are ±SEM. **(B–D)** Representative images taken following 10 min GTTR exposure in DMSO, dTC and berbamine. Scale bar = 50 μm.

Following on from this we set out to determine whether berbamine and dTC share the same mechanism of protection in mammals. The MET channels are the main entry site for the aminoglycosides into the hair cells (Marcotti et al., 2005) and a block of these channels has been suggested as the mechanism of protection for both berbamine in zebrafish lateral line hair cells (Kruger et al., 2016) and curare in rat OHCs (Alharazneh et al., 2011). Furthermore, previous studies have shown also that dTC is a MET channel blocker (Glowatzki et al., 1997; Farris et al., 2004). Our results clearly demonstrate that both compounds act as permeant blockers of the MET channel, rapidly and reversibly blocking the channels with similar half-blocking concentrations. Maximum block is seen at −118 mV for dTC and −94 mV for berbamine, with the block reducing at more hyperpolarized potentials, indicating both compounds can enter into the cells, albeit at a greatly reduced rate compared to the aminoglycoside DHS (Marcotti et al., 2005). For example, with the conditions chosen for **Figure 9E** (1 μM compound, 80 MET channels, p_{open} 0.1), the entry rates into the OHCs are 110 molecules/s for dTC and 205 molecules/s for berbamine, at a membrane potential of −150 mV. Taking the parameters for DHS permeation in the presence of 1.3 mM extracellular Ca^{2+} from Marcotti et al. (2005), the entry rate of 1 μM DHS into the cells would be some 1,130 molecules/s, an order of magnitude faster. For higher concentrations the entry rates started to saturate, so rates for dTC and berbamine can never approach those for DHS (e.g., for 100 μM rates were 319 molecules/s for dTC, 1107 molecules/s for berbamine and 11,460 molecules/s for DHS).

Whilst a previous study has reported that dTC is non-permeant and remains in the channel pore (Farris et al., 2004), this finding was based on studies in turtle auditory hair cells in which the cells were not hyperpolarized much beyond the potential at which we observe maximum block. The release of the block was therefore not observed. In our study cells were hyperpolarized to -164 mV, a potential at which a release of the block was clearly evident. This is a physiologically relevant membrane potential as the electrical driving force across the MET channels in the mammalian cochlea *in vivo* is generated by a positive endocochlear potential of +80 to +100 mV (Bosher and Warren, 1971) and a negative hair-cell resting potential of some −40 to −60 mV (Johnson et al., 2011). In turtle hair cells, Farris et al. reported K_D values for dTC block of 6.3 μM for the steady-state current and 16 μM for the peak current, values ~3-8 times higher than our (near steady-state) finding of 2.2 μM. They also calculated a Hill coefficient of 2 suggesting the cooperative binding of 2 dTC molecules in the channel pore as opposed to the negative cooperativity suggested by our finding of a Hill coefficient of 0.8. These observations imply marked differences between the turtle and mouse MET channels, highlighting the need for caution in interpreting results across species.

Both dTC and berbamine significantly reduce the loading of GTTR into the OHCs. This observation, together with the knowledge that they are both MET channel blockers with a reasonably high affinity for the channel pore, strongly suggests that protection is conferred via a competitive block of the channels. Both compounds can, however, enter the cells so it is possible that there are alternative and/or additional intracellular targets. This seems unlikely though as dTC and berbamine provide protection against both neomycin and gentamicin in zebrafish, a species in which these aminoglycosides activate distinct cell death pathways (Owens et al., 2009; Coffin et al.,

2013a,b) and may have different targets (Owens et al., 2008; Vlastis et al., 2012). Although berbamine and dTC are both permeant, open-channel blockers of the hair cell's MET channel that reduce GTTR loading into hair cells and protect against aminoglycoside toxicity, berbamine was found to be toxic to mammalian hair cells and other cell types in the developing organ of Corti at concentrations ≥30 μM. It also blocks the hair cell's basolateral K^+ current $I_{K,neo}$. As mentioned above, berbamine is more permeant than dTC, and the energy profiles (**Figure 12**) indicate substantial differences between their interactions with the MET channel, with dTC having higher entry and exit barriers. The latter feature would hinder its entry into the hair cells.

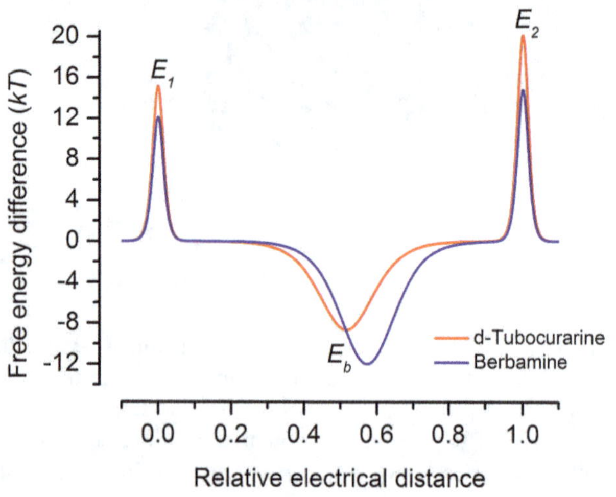

FIGURE 12 | Energy profiles for MET channel permeation and block by extracellular d-tubocurarine and berbamine. Energy profiles calculated from fits to the fractional-block curves and kinetics of MET current block are shown. Values for the free energies of the binding site E_b and barriers E1 and E_2 are shown in the absence of a voltage across the membrane (V_m = 0 mV). The voltage-independent extracellular barrier E_1, at an electrical distance of zero, has a free energy of 15.16 kT for dTC and 12.14 kT for berbamine. E_b is −8.67 kT for dTC and −12.0 kT for berbamine. The binding sites, δ_b, are located at an electrical distance from the extracellular side of 0.52 for dTC and 0.57 for berbamine. The intracellular barrier E_2, positioned at an electrical distance of one, is 20.13 kT for dTC and 14.82 kT for berbamine.

dTC is an alkaloid formed of two isoquinoline moieties linked via hydroxyl-benzyl groups to form an 18 atom macrocycle. It bears one fixed positive charge (quaternary nitrogen) and a pH dependent positive charge (tertiary nitrogen, calculated pKa ~8.0). Ionization simulation shows that at physiological pH ~80% of the molecule will bear two positive charges. The distance between the two positive charges of dTC (**Figure 13A**), with the stereochemistry of the carbon atoms next to the quaternary and the tertiary nitrogens being R and S respectively, is 8.89 Å. Whilst berbamine is an 18 atom macrocycle alkaloid that is structurally related to dTC and bears the same two isoquinoline moieties the latter are, however, linked differently. In comparison to dTC, berbamine does not bear any fixed positive charge but has instead two pH dependent ones, with the calculated pKa for the two tertiary nitrogens being ~7.4 and 8.2. Prediction of ionization status at physiological pH suggests that 50% of the molecules will bear two positive charges and ~40% only one positive charge. The distance between the two positive charges for berbamine, with the stereochemistry of the carbon atoms next to the two nitrogens being R and S (**Figure 13B**), is 10.18 Å, slightly higher than that in dTC. Flexible alignment of the two structures (**Figure 13C**) shows a good overall superimposition of the molecules; however, the isoquinoline moiety bearing the quaternary nitrogen of dTC and one of the two tertiary nitrogens of berbamine do not superimpose properly with the two nitrogens being 1.2 Å apart from each other.

Some of the differences between the structures of dTC and berbamine outlined above may explain why their properties and interactions with the MET channel are different. For example, the higher entry and exit energy barriers for dTC could tentatively be explained by the fact that a higher percentage of dTC molecules will bear two positive charges compared to berbamine molecules at physiological pH, thereby hindering the passage of dTC across the positive charges present at the mouth and exit of the channel (van Netten and Kros, 2007). Alternatively, the distance between the positive charges may critically determine the strength of interactions with the MET channel protein. As discussed earlier, dTC and berbamine are both less permeant than the aminoglycoside DHS (Marcotti et al., 2005), entering the cells at a substantially slower rate, by an order of magnitude. This may, in part, be explained by the fact that dTC and berbamine both

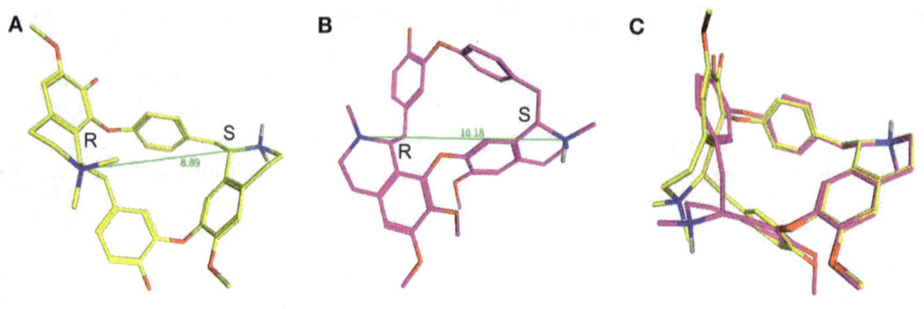

FIGURE 13 | d-Tubocurarine and berbamine share similar chemical structures. **(A,B)** Energy-minimized structures showing the distance between the positive charges for dTC (8.89 Å; yellow) and berbamine (10.18 Å; magenta) respectively. **(C)** A flexible alignment with the structures not minimized reveals dTC and berbamine share striking structural similarities.

have a more rigid structure, are less flexible compared to DHS, and may therefore be unable to adapt their conformation within the channel.

In the search for potential otoprotective compounds we have identified dTC as a promising lead compound for further investigation. dTC is a reasonably high-affinity MET channel blocker ($K_D = 2.2$ μM) that rapidly and reversibly blocks the channel. It has advantages over berbamine which include reduced permeability and a lack of toxicity up to 50 μM. By comparison berbamine had only a narrow range of protective concentrations in the cochlea, as it was found to be toxic at concentrations above 30 μM. Moreover, berbamine damaged OHCs when applied intracellularly at 1 mM. As berbamine was not toxic to neuromast hair cells, and protected these cells at lower concentrations than dTC, results from the zebrafish assay alone would have favored berbamine over dTC as a potential otoprotective compound. This points to the necessity to follow-up results from zebrafish screening with a mammalian otoprotection assay. One future approach would be to modify dTC in order to increase its affinity for the MET channel and eliminate its ability to enter the cells. In parallel one would need to reduce its action as a nicotinic antagonist to avoid blocking the middle ear reflex and the action of the olivocochlear bundle following trans-tympanic application.

AUTHOR CONTRIBUTIONS

Participated in research design: NK, MD, EK, RH, SvN, SW, GR, CK. Conducted experiments: NK, MO, EK, GR. Performed data analysis: NK, MO, MD, EK, RH, CK. Wrote or contributed to the writing of the manuscript: NK, MO, MD, EK, SvN, GR, CK.

REFERENCES

Alharazneh, A., Luk, L., Huth, M., Monfared, A., Steyger, P. S., Cheng, A. G., et al. (2011). Functional hair cell mechanotransducer channels are required for aminoglycoside ototoxicity. *PLoS ONE* 6:e22347. doi: 10.1371/journal.pone.0022347

Bosher, S. K., and Warren, R. L. (1971). A study of the electrochemistry and osmotic relationships of the cochlear fluids in the neonatal rat at the time of the development of the endocochlear potential. *J. Physiol.* 212, 739–761. doi: 10.1113/jphysiol.1971.sp009354

Coffin, A. B., Rubel, E. W., and Raible, D. W. (2013a). Bax, Bcl2 and p53 differentially regulate neomycin- and gentamicin-induced hair cell death in the zebrafish lateral line. *J. Assoc. Res. Otolaryngol.* 14, 645–659. doi: 10.1007/s10162-013-0404-1

Coffin, A. B., Williamson, K. L., Mamiya, A., Raible, D. W., and Rubel, E. W. (2013b). Profiling drug-induced cell death pathways in the zebrafish lateral line. *Apoptosis* 18, 393–408. doi: 10.1007/s10495-013-0816-8

Corey, D. P., and Holt, J. R. (2016). Are TMCs the mechanotransduction channels of vertebrate hair cells? *J. Neurosci.* 36, 10921–10926. doi: 10.1523/JNEUROSCI.1148-16.2016

Corns, L. F., Johnson, S. L., Kros, C. J., and Marcotti, W. (2016). Tmc1 point mutation affects Ca2+ sensitivity and block by dihydrostreptomycin of the mechanoelectrical transducer current of mouse outer hair cells. *J. Neurosci.* 36, 336–349. doi: 10.1523/JNEUROSCI.2439-15.2016

Durante-Mangoni, E., Grammatikos, A., Utili, R., and Falagas, M. E. (2009). Do we still need the aminoglycosides? *Int. J. Antimicrob. Agents* 33, 201–205. doi: 10.1016/j.ijantimicag.2008.09.001

Eróstegui, C., Norris, C. H., and Bobbin, R. P. (1994). *In vitro* pharmacologic characterisation of a cholinergic receptor on outer hair cells. *Hear. Res.* 74, 135–147. doi: 10.1016/0378-5955(94)90182-1

Farris, H. E., LeBlanc, C. L., Goswami, J., and Ricci, A. J. (2004). Probing the pore of the auditory hair cell mechanotransducer channel in turtle. *J. Physiol.* 558, 769–792. doi: 10.1113/jphysiol.2004.061267

Fettiplace, R. (2016). Is TMC1 the hair cell mechanotransducer channel? *Biophys. J.* 111, 3–9. doi: 10.1016/j.bpj.2016.05.032

Forge, A., and Li, L. (2000). Apoptotic death of hair cells in mammalian vestibular sensory epithelia. *Hear. Res.* 139, 97–115. doi: 10.1016/S0378-5955(99)00177-X

Forge, A., and Schacht, J. (2000). Aminoglycoside antibiotics. *Audiol. Neurootol.* 5, 3–22. doi: 10.1159/000013861

Gale, J. E., Marcotti, W., Kennedy, H. J., Kros, C. J., and Richardson, G. P. (2001). FM1-43 dye behaves as a permeant blocker of the hair-cell mechanotransducer channel. *J. Neurosci.* 21, 7013–7025.

Glowatzki, E., Ruppersberg, J. P., Zenner, H.-P., and Rüsch, A. (1997). Mechanically and ATP-induced currents of mouse outer hair cells are independent and differentially blocked by d-tubocurarine. *Neuropharmacology* 36, 1269–1275. doi: 10.1016/S0028-3908(97)00108-1

Goh, J. W., and Pennefather, P. S. (1987). Pharmacological and physiological properties of the after-hyperpolarization current of bull frog ganglion neurones. *J. Physiol.* 394, 315–330. doi: 10.1113/jphysiol.1987.sp016872

Housley, G. D., and Ashmore, J. F. (1991). Direct measurement of the action of acetylcholine on isolated outer hair cells of the guinea pig cochlea. *Proc. R. Soc. Lond. B* 244, 161–167. doi: 10.1098/rspb.1991.0065

Ishii, T. M., Maylie, J., and Adelman, J. P. (1997). Determinants of apamin and d-tubocurarine block in SK potassium channels. *J. Biol. Chem.* 272, 23195–23200. doi: 10.1074/jbc.272.37.23195

Ji, H., Li, X., and Zhang, H. (2009). Natural products and drug discovery. Can thousands of years of ancient medical knowledge lead us to new and powerful drug combinations in the fight against cancer and dementia? *EMBO Rep.* 10, 194–200. doi: 10.1038/embor.2009.12

Johnson, S. L., Beurg, M., Marcotti, W., and Fettiplace, R. (2011). Prestin-driven cochlear amplification is not limited by the outer hair cell membrane time constant. *Neuron* 70, 1143–1154. doi: 10.1016/j.neuron.2011.04.024

Kawashima, Y., Géléoc, G. S. G., Kurima, K., Labay, V., Lelli, A., Asai, Y., et al. (2011). Mechanotransduction in mouse inner ear hair cells requires transmembrane channel-like genes. *J. Clin. Invest.* 121, 4796–4809. doi: 10.1172/JCI60405

Kawashima, Y., Kurima, K., Pan, B., Griffith, A. J., and Holt, J. R. (2015). Transmembrane channel-like (TMC) genes are required for auditory and vestibular mechanosensation. *Pfulgers Arch.* 467, 85–94. doi: 10.1007/s00424-014-1582-3

Kimmel, C. B., Ballard, W. W., Kimmel, S. R., Ullmann, B., and Schilling, T. F. (1995). Stages of embryonic development of the zebrafish. *Dev. Dyn.* 203, 253–310. doi: 10.1002/aja.1002030302

Kindt, K. S., Finch, G., and Nicolson, T. (2012). Kinocilia mediate mechanosensitivity in developing zebrafish hair cells. *Dev. Cell* 23, 329–341. doi: 10.1016/j.devcel.2012.05.022

Kros, C. J., Rüsch, A., and Richardson, G. P. (1992). Mechano-electrical transducer currents in hair cells of the cultured neonatal mouse cochlea. *Proc. Biol. Sci.* 249, 185–193. doi: 10.1098/rspb.1992.0102

Kruger, M., Boney, R., Ordoobadi, A. J., Sommers, T. F., Trapani, J. G., and Coffin, A. B. (2016). Natural bizbenzoquinoline derivatives protect zebrafish lateral line sensory hair cells from aminoglycoside toxicity. *Front. Cell. Neurosci.* 10:83. doi: 10.3389/fncel.2016.00083

Kurima, K., Ebrahim, S., Pan, B., Sedlacek, M., Sengupta, P., Millis, B. A., et al. (2015). TMC 1 and TMC2 localize at the site of mechanotransduction in mammalian inner ear hair cell stereocilia. *Cell Rep.* 12, 1606–1617. doi: 10.1016/j.celrep.2015.07.058

Majumder, P., Moore, P. A., Richardson, G. P., and Gale, J. E. (2017). Protecting mammalian hair cells from aminoglycoside-toxicity: assessing phenoxybenzamine's potential. *Front. Cell. Neurosci.* 11:94. doi: 10.3389/fncel.2017.00094

Marcotti, W., and Kros, C. J. (1999). Developmental expression of the potassium current IK,n contributes to maturation of mouse outer hair cells. *J. Physiol.* 520, 653–660. doi: 10.1111/j.1469-7793.1999.00653.x

Marcotti, W., van Netten, S. M., and Kros, C. J. (2005). The aminoglycoside antibiotic dihydrostreptomycin rapidly enters mouse outer hair cells through the mechano-electrical transducer channels. *J. Physiol.* 567, 505–521. doi: 10.1113/jphysiol.2005.085951

Matsui, J. I., Gale, J. E., and Warchol, M. E. (2004). Critical signaling events during the aminoglycoside-induced death of sensory hair cells *in vitro*. *J. Neurobiol.* 61, 250–266. doi: 10.1002/neu.20054

Matsui, J. I., Ogilvie, J. M., and Warchol, M. E. (2002). Inhibition of capases prevents ototoxic and ongoing hair cell death. *J. Neurosci.* 22, 1218–1227.

Meng, Z., Li, T., Ma, X., Wang, X., Van Ness, C., Gan, Y., et al. (2013). Berbamine inhibits the growth of liver cancer cells and cancer-initiating cells by targeting Ca2+/calmodulin-dependent protein kinase II. *Mol. Cancer Ther.* 12, 2067–2077. doi: 10.1158/1535-7163.MCT-13-0314

Nakashima, T., Teranishi, M., Hibi, T., Kobayashi, M., and Umemura, M. (2000). Vestibular and cochlear toxicity of aminoglycosides – a review. *Acta Otolaryngol.* 120, 904–911. doi: 10.1080/00016480050218627

Ou, H. C., Cunningham, L. L., Francis, S. P., Brandon, C. S., Simon, J. A., Raible, D. W., et al. (2009). Identification of FDA-approved drugs and bioactives that protect hair cells in the zebrafish (*Danio rerio*) lateral line and mouse (*Mus musculus*) utricle. *J. Assoc. Res. Otolaryngol.* 10, 191–203. doi: 10.1007/s10162-009-0158-y

Owens, K. N., Coffin, A. B., Hong, L. S., Bennett, K. O., Rubel, E. W., and Raible, D. W. (2009). Response of mechanosensory hair cells of the zebrafish lateral line to aminoglycosides reveals distinct cell death pathways. *Hear. Res.* 253, 32–41. doi: 10.1016/j.heares.2009.03.001

Owens, K. N., Cunningham, D. E., MacDonald, G., Rubel, E. W., Raible, D. W., and Pujol, R. (2007). Ultrastructural analysis of aminoglycoside-induced hair cell death in the zebrafish lateral line reveals an early mitochondrial response. *J. Comp. Neurol.* 502, 522–543. doi: 10.1002/cne.21345

Owens, K. N., Santos, F., Roberts, B., Linbo, T., Coffin, A. B., Knisely, A. J., et al. (2008). Identification of genetic and chemical modulators of zebrafish mechanosensory hair cell death. *PLoS Genet.* 4:e1000020. doi: 10.1371/journal.pgen.1000020

Pan, B., Géléoc, G. S., Asai, Y., Horwitz, G. C., Kurima, K., Ishikawa, K., et al. (2013). TMC1 and TMC2 are components of the mechanotransduction channel in hair cells of the mammalian inner ear. *Neuron* 79, 504–515. doi: 10.1016/j.neuron.2013.06.019

Perotti, G. S. (1977). A review of d-tubocurarine in clinical usage. *AANA J.* 45, 182–186.

Rahmatullah, M., Jahan, R., Bashar, A., Al-Nahain, A., Majumder, S., Islam, T., et al. (2014). A review of berbamine – potential anticancer drug. *WJPPS* 3, 95–110.

Rizzi, M. D., and Hirose, K. (2007). Aminoglycoside ototoxicity. *Curr. Opin. Otolaryngol. Head Neck Surg.* 15, 352–357. doi: 10.1097/MOO.0b013e3282ef772d

Russell, I. J., and Richardson, G. P. (1987). The morphology and physiology of hair cells in organotypic cultures of the mouse cochlea. *Hear. Res.* 31, 9–24. doi: 10.1016/0378-5955(87)90210-3

Santos, F., MacDonald, G., Rubel, E. W., and Raible, D. W. (2006). Lateral line hair cell maturation is a determinant of aminoglycoside susceptibility in zebrafish (*Danio rerio*). *Hear. Res.* 213, 25–33. doi: 10.1016/j.heares.2005.12.009

Schacht, J., Talaska, A., and Rybak, L. (2012). Cisplatin and aminoglycoside antibiotics: hearing loss and its prevention. *Ant. Rec.* 295, 1837–1850. doi: 10.1002/ar.22578

Steyger, P. S., Peters, S. L., Rehling, J., and Hordichok, A. (2003). Uptake of gentamicin by bullfrog saccular hair cells *in vitro*. *J. Assoc. Res. Otolaryngol.* 4, 565–578. doi: 10.1007/s10162-003-4002-5

Vacher, P., Vacher, A. –M., and Mollard, P. (1998). Tubocurarine blocks a calcium-dependent potassium current in rat tumoral pituitary cells. *Mol. Cell. Endocrinol.* 139, 131–142. doi: 10.1016/S0303-7207(98)00066-5

van Netten, S. M., and Kros, C. J. (2007). Insights into the pore of the hair cell transducer channel from experiments with permeant blockers. *Curr. Top. Membr.* 59, 375–398. doi: 10.1016/S1063-5823(06)59013-1

Vlastis, A. L., Simon, J. A., Raible, D. W., Rubel, E. W., and Owens, K. N. (2012). Screen of FDA-approved drug library reveals compounds that protect hair cells from aminoglycosides and cisplatin. *Hear. Res.* 294, 153–165. doi: 10.1016/j.heares.2012.08.002

Vu, A. A., Nadaraja, G. S., Huth, M. E., Luk, L., Kim, J., Chai, R., et al. (2013). Integrity and regeneration of mechanotransduction machinery regulate aminoglycoside entry and sensory cell death. *PLoS ONE* 8:e54794. doi: 10.1371/journal.pone.0054794

Westerfield, M. (2000). *The Zebrafish Book: A Guide for the Laboratory Use of Zebrafish (Danio (Brachydanio) rerio)*. Eugene, OR: University of Oregon.

Wyman, J., and Gill, S. J. (1990). *Binding and Linkage: Functional Chemistry of Biological Marcromolecules*. Mill Valley, CA: University Science Books.

Zhao, Y., Lv, J. J., Chen, J., Jin, X. B., Wang, M. W., Su, Z. H., et al. (2016). Berbamine inhibited the growth of prostate cancer cells *in vivo* and *in vitro* via triggering intrinsic pathway of apoptosis. *Prostate Cancer Prostatic Dis.* 19, 358–366. doi: 10.1038/pcan.2016.29

14

The Contribution of Immune Infiltrates to Ototoxicity and Cochlear Hair Cell Loss

*Megan B. Wood and Jian Zuo **

Department of Developmental Neurobiology, St. Jude Children's Research Hospital, Memphis, TN, USA

Edited by:
Michael E. Smith,
Western Kentucky University, USA

Reviewed by:
Allison B. Coffin,
Washington State University, USA
Mark E. Warchol,
Washington University School of Medicine, USA

***Correspondence:**
Jian Zuo
jian.zuo@stjude.org

Cells of the immune system have been shown to infiltrate the cochlea after acoustic trauma or ototoxic drug treatment; however, the contribution of the immune system to hair cell loss in the inner ear is incompletely understood. Most studies have concentrated on the immediate innate response to hair cell damage using CD45 as a broad marker for all immune cells. More recent studies have used RNA sequencing, GeneChip arrays and quantitative PCR to analyze gene expression in the entire cochlea after auditory trauma, leading to a better understanding of the chemokines and cytokines that attract immune cells to the cochlea. Immune suppression by blocking cytokines or immune receptors has been proven to suppress hair cell damage. However, it is now understood that not all immune cells are detrimental to the cochlea. CX3CR1+ resident macrophages protect hair cells from damage mediated by infiltrating immune cells. Systemically, the immune response is associated with both protection and pathology, and it has been implicated in the regeneration of certain tissues after injury. This review focuses on the studies of immune cells in various models of hearing loss and highlights the steps that can be taken to elucidate the connection between the immune response and hearing loss. The interplay between the immune system and tissues that were previously thought to be immune privileged, such as the cochlea, is an emerging research field, to which additional studies of the immune component of the cochlear response to injury will make an important contribution.

Keywords: ototoxicity, CX3CR1+ macrophage, TLR4, noise-induced hearing loss, sterile inflammation

INTRODUCTION

In the cochlea, the loss of sensory hair cells in the organ of Corti or the connecting spiral ganglion neurons due to exposure to ototoxic drugs or excessive noise results in hearing loss. There is increasing evidence that the loss of one or both of these cell types is exacerbated by inflammation of the cochlea. The direct action of infiltrating immune cell types and their cytokines, as well as reactive oxygen species (ROS) and cytokines generated by resident cochlear cells, leads to irreparable damage to hair cells and neurons (Bánfi et al., 2004; Lang et al., 2016). Understanding the cell types and cellular products that lead to this cell death will provide valuable targets for combatting sensorineural hearing loss. Although Fredelius and Rask-Andersen (1990) first reported the infiltration of immune cells into the noise-damaged cochlea nearly 30 years ago, the phenomenon has attracted renewed interest in the last 10–15 years. The following review discusses the recent advances in our understanding of the role of the cells of the immune system in hearing loss due to noise and ototoxic drug treatment. It is hoped that our examination of the existing literature will serve as a basis for developing new ideas in this exciting area of research that may ultimately lead to new ways of preventing or treating hearing loss resulting from the aforementioned causes.

BASIC PATHWAYS IN STERILE INFLAMMATION

Inflammation in the ear caused by exposure to ototoxic drugs or excessive noise is unique in that the resulting immune response at the epithelial surface is not a response to a pathogen. Accordingly, it is termed sterile inflammation (Ma et al., 2000; Rock et al., 2010). In the past, it was thought that the immune system was unable to infiltrate into several sites of the body. Such "immune privileged" sites included the brain, the inner ear, the eye and the joint capsules among others. However, the multiple observations of immune responses in these sites have fundamentally changed our understanding, such that the immune system is now thought to be able to respond in all tissues, albeit with varying degrees of efficiency (Galea et al., 2007; Taylor, 2016). Furthermore, many of the tissues formerly considered to be "immune-privileged" have their own specific resident immune cell populations, with the microglia of the brain being the best characterized in this regard (Immig et al., 2015). When damage occurs in these tissues in the absence of a pathogen, cellular byproducts of the damage, termed damage-associated molecular patterns (DAMPs), stimulate pattern recognition receptors (PRRs; Tang et al., 2012). This PRR activation rapidly leads to the activation of resident macrophages, the release of pro-inflammatory cytokines, and ROS production, causing apoptosis of damaged cells and immune cell infiltration (Hume et al., 2001; Park et al., 2004; Tsung et al., 2007). Early inflammation caused by DAMP-PRR signaling is an evolutionarily conserved mechanism for controlling the spread of pathogens or necrotic tissue. In the absence of a pathogen, immune cells are recruited to sites of inflammation to clear debris and facilitate wound healing. Cells of the innate immune system are the first to respond to inflammation. Bone marrow-derived macrophages and neutrophils attempt to kill any damaged cells by nonspecific means, such as by releasing ROS, and they also phagocytose dead and dying cells. This activity mirrors the role of macrophages and neutrophils at the site of an infection, where they kill infected cells to stop the spread of the pathogen. The second wave of cells that infiltrates an area of active inflammation consists of T cells of the adaptive immune system. In the case of inflammation caused by a pathogen, T cells specifically kill cells infected with the pathogen, which they are able to recognize via interaction with a unique T-cell receptor (TCR). T cells also secrete cytokines to modify the activation states of innate cells that are present (Stein et al., 1992). In a sterile inflammatory site, T cells may recognize self-antigens as a result of the cell debris arising from damage and inflammation (Brodeur et al., 2015). T-regulatory cells also infiltrate the site to dampen inflammation and facilitate wound healing (Gazzinelli et al., 1992; Fontenot et al., 2003). In this way, the adaptive immune response first refines then curbs inflammation to bring about an effective resolution. Because inflammatory signaling after noise exposure or ototoxic insult happens quickly in the cochlea and appears to play a role in hair cell death, most research to date has concentrated on preventing the earliest stages of inflammation. However, the immune system is also involved in the resolving inflammation and in wound healing (Nahrendorf et al., 2007; Xu et al., 2014; Lindemans et al., 2015; Psachoulia et al., 2016). It is unclear whether the pro-regenerative resolution of inflammation mediated by the immune response does not occur in the inner ear or whether the cells of the cochlea do not respond to this resolution phase because they are unable to regenerate in response to immune signals.

GENE EXPRESSION IN THE EAR AFTER NOISE DAMAGE

New developments in detecting and sequencing mRNA have enabled the examination of gene transcription after noise damage. This is an important step toward understanding how the cochlea as a whole responds to damage. One of the first studies of transcription after noise damage compared the effect of noise on the lateral wall and organ of Corti in mouse strains that were susceptible or resistant to noise damage (Gratton et al., 2011). An important finding of this study was that C57BL/6 mice, which are susceptible to noise-induced hearing loss, express more genes related to an immune response after noise damage than do mice of resistant strains (Gratton et al., 2011). More recently, a group used RNA sequencing to compare the gene expression in the sensory epithelia of mice and rats 1 day after acoustic injury (Yang et al., 2016). Again, this study highlighted the upregulation of immune-response genes after noise damage, showing that this type of gene expression is conserved across mammalian species. Tan et al. (2016) took this approach a step further by investigating at immune-response gene and protein expression at multiple time points up to 14 days after noise damage. The expression of genes encoding TNF-α, IL-1β and Icaml increased as early as 6 h after injury with Icam-1 protein remaining elevated at 14 days after noise damage (Tan et al., 2016). Taken together, the results of these studies show that genes encoding cytokines, chemokines and innate immune responses to noise damage are expressed in the cochlea as early as 6 h after damage occurs. Moreover, there was considerable overlap among the genes whose expression was detected in these various studies.

Even though each of the studies described above used different strains of mice, namely CBA/CaJ, 129, C57BL/6, or B6.CAST, it appears that several genes involved in the inflammatory response are expressed following noise damage (Gratton et al., 2011; Tan et al., 2016; Yang et al., 2016). Fos, Socs3, Gpb2 and Icaml are all associated with the response to noise damage. Socs3 is especially interesting in this regard as it is expressed to dampen JAK/STAT-dependent cytokine signaling by marking signaling components for degradation (Bode et al., 1999; Babon et al., 2008). Regulation of cytokine signaling after damage may control the attraction of new immune cells and the activation of resident immune cells. Icam1 is expressed after NF-κB activation caused by TNF-α and enables recruited immune cells to follow other signals into the cochlea by facilitating the extravasation of the cells from the bloodstream through interaction with lymphocyte function-associated antigen 1 (LFA-1; Wilcox et al., 1990; Wertheimer et al., 1992; Ledebur and Parks, 1995; Suzuki and Harris, 1995). Fos and Gbp2 are both upregulated under conditions of cellular stress and can be expressed in response to interferons (Li et al., 2002; Wei et al., 2008). Although it is important to know that immune response genes can be detected in the cochlear tissue after noise damage, it is much more likely that only a subset of cell types upregulate these genes. Identifying these cell types will enable specific targeting of their contribution to hair cell loss.

CELL TYPES THAT INFILTRATE THE COCHLEA

The first marker used to identify immune cells infiltrating the cochlea after noise damage was CD45, also known as leukocyte common antigen (Kurtin and Pinkus, 1985; Tornabene et al., 2006). Hirose et al. (2005) used the combination of CD45 expression and morphology to characterize most of the infiltrating cells as monocytes or macrophages. Additional markers were subsequently explored, so that today the profile of infiltrating immune cells after noise damage currently includes CD45+, F4/80+, Iba-1+ CD11b+ and CX3CR1+ macrophages (Tornabene et al., 2006; Okano et al., 2008; Tan et al., 2008; Sato et al., 2010; Shi, 2010; Yang et al., 2015). Although these markers are important for identifying macrophage populations, the likelihood of all the infiltrating macrophages and resident macrophages having the same signature is low. The increased sensitivity of cell sorters and flow cytometers will enable a more complete characterization of the expression of these markers on infiltrating cells. The identification of the specific cell types that infiltrate the cochlea is still ongoing, but the timeline of the arrival of these cells after acoustic or ototoxic trauma has been more extensively studied.

Few truly comparable studies have examined the combination of cytokine expression, Icam1 expression, and immune cell infiltration with reference to the same parameters of hair cell damage (e.g., hair cell ablation, aminoglycoside/cisplatin ototoxicity and noise damage). This makes it difficult to draw conclusions about the overall immune response after hair cell or cochlear trauma. Nevertheless, it is worth critically synthesizing the information from these disparate studies to inform the future direction of the field. The immune response to each type of damage needs to be characterized, as noise damage affects more cell types than hair cell- specific ablation or aminoglycoside ototoxicity. The best information about the immune response that can be gleaned at present is a rough timeline of events after hair cell death. TNF-α, IL-1β and IL-6 are expressed before as early as 6 h and up to 1 day after damage (Fujioka et al., 2006; Wakabayashi et al., 2010; Tan et al., 2016). Chemokines such as CCL2, CCL4 and CXCL12 are expressed as early as 6 h after damage (Tornabene et al., 2006; Tan et al., 2008, 2016; Dai et al., 2010). Chemokine expression beginning at 24 h after noise seems to be due to ROS, as iNOS-deficient mice do not secrete CXCL12 from the lateral wall after injury to the blood-labyrinth barrier (Dai et al., 2010). By 3–4 days after damage, the numbers of CX3CR1+ and CD45+ cells in the cochlea reach a peak, with increased cell counts being observed until day 7 (Hirose et al., 2005; Kaur et al., 2015). Interestingly, a second peak of expression of TNF-α, IL-1β and IL-6 occurs after cell infiltration, starting at day 3–4 after damage (Oh et al., 2011; Tan et al., 2016). The cytokine expression that occurs as early as 6 h after noise damage could be a result of activation of resident CX3CR1+ macrophages and fibrocytes that are present at the initiation of damage, whereas the secondary peak in cytokine expression could be due to infiltrating immune cells; however, this has not been definitively shown (**Figure 1**; Okano et al., 2008; Oh et al., 2011; Kaur et al., 2015; Tan et al., 2016). In rats, IL-6 was expressed by type III and type IV fibrocytes of the lateral wall, but not Iba-1 positive macrophages, 6 h after noise damage (Fujioka et al., 2006). Fujioka et al. (2006) also showed that spiral ganglion neurons expressed IL-6 12 h after noise damage. In mice, the receptor for IL-6 and its signal transducer, gp130, are expressed in hair cells in the organ of Corti and the spiral ganglion neurons, meaning that these cells can respond to IL-6 released after noise damage (Wakabayashi et al., 2010). Furthermore, TNF-α, IL-1β and IL-6 staining after lipopolysaccharide (LPS) injection shows expression throughout the cochlea (Oh et al., 2011). The overall effect of these cytokines is to induce the activation of spiral ganglion neurons, lateral wall fibrocytes and immune cells and thereby increase inflammation through the secretion of more of the same cytokines such as TNF-α, IL-1β and IL-6 as well as chemokines such as CCL2 and CXCL12 (So et al., 2007; Dai et al., 2010). However, the specific expression of cytokines and chemokines by immune cells have not been explored. Many of these genes are direct targets of canonical NF-κB, a transcription factor that is upregulated after damage induced by noise or ototoxic drug (Masuda et al., 2005; So et al., 2007). One way in which these cytokines increase immune cell infiltration is by inducing Icam1 expression in the spiral ligament (Tan et al., 2016). Icam1 interacts with receptors on the surface of the immune cell to enable its extravasation into the cochlea (Wilcox et al., 1990; Suzuki and Harris, 1995). Future studies should concentrate on the cell types present and the cytokines expressed immediately after damage, as well as at a 3–4 days and 7–10 days or later after damage, in order to understand the waxing and waning of the whole immune response to damage in the cochlea.

EVIDENCE FOR RESIDENT MACROPHAGES

When GFP-labeled bone marrow was used to reconstitute a lethally irradiated mouse, GFP+ bone marrow cells populate the cochlea in the absence of damage to the tissue (Okano et al., 2008). Approximately 80% of these cells were identified as macrophages, based on their morphology and staining for F4/80,

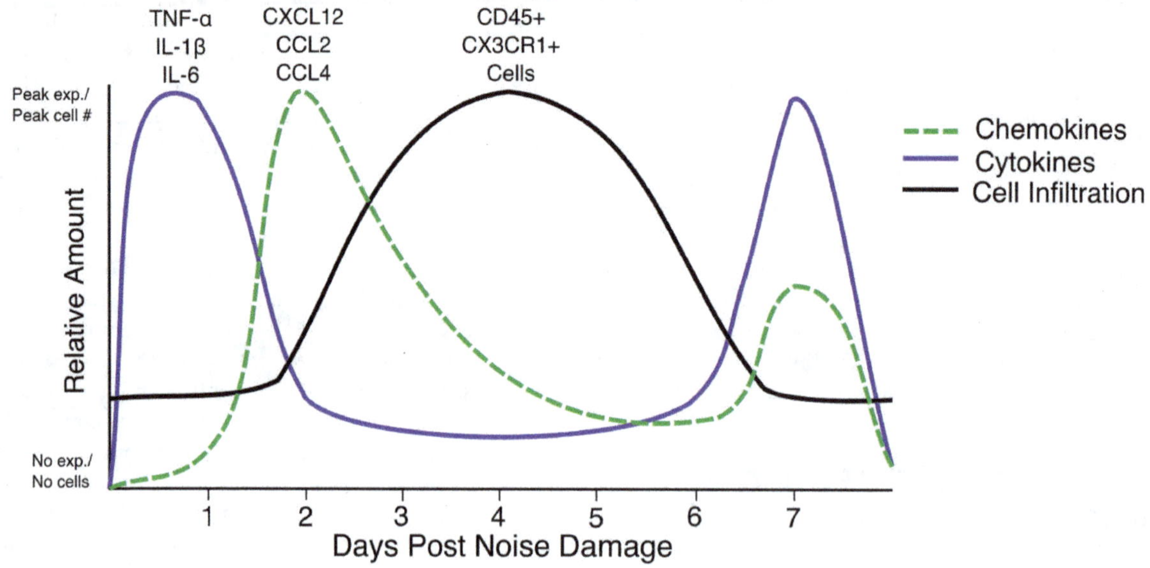

FIGURE 1 | Timeline of cytokine expression, chemokine expression and cell infiltration in the inner ear after noise damage. The relative amounts of each cytokine (blue line), chemokine (green dashed line) and cell infiltration (black line) in the first 7 days after noise damage are summarized in the above graph. Note that the cytokine and chemokine expression begins at zero expression as such expression has not been reported in the steady state. The line representing CD45+ and CX3CR1+ cells does not begin at zero as CX3CR1+ and CD45+ cells are present in the cochlea in the steady state. Peak exp.: peak expression. No exp.: No expression.

Iba-1, CD11b and CD68 (Okano et al., 2008; Sun et al., 2014). Resident macrophages are also positive for CX3CR1, which allows for chemoattraction to CX3CL1 expressed in the organ of Corti and the spiral ganglion; however, the specific chemotaxis of resident macrophages to these sources of CX3CL1 has not been proven (Sato et al., 2008, 2010; Kaur et al., 2015). In the CX3CR1gfp/gfp mouse model, fractalkine signaling is disrupted by GFP knock-in that also labels CX3CR1-expressing cells. Kanamycin treatment in this model results in an increased number of infiltrating CD45+ cells in the cochlea (Sato et al., 2010). Furthermore, transplanting CX3CR1gfp/gfp bone marrow into a wild-type mouse results in a similar phenotype of increased infiltration of CD45+ cells, suggesting that disruption of CX3CR1 signaling on immune cells is detrimental to hair cell survival after aminoglycoside exposure (Sato et al., 2010). When no CX3CR1 is expressed in mice that have a specific loss of all their hair cells, spiral ganglion cell death is increased (Kaur et al., 2015). Taken together, these results indicate that resident CX3CR1+ macrophages may have a valuable role in reducing immune cell infiltration and cell death after aminoglycoside treatment or in response to a specific hair cell lesion. Thus, further characterization of this protective function of CX3CR1+ macrophages will be valuable for understanding the positive role of immune cells in regulating the inflammatory response after cochlear damage.

TLR4 ACTIVATION

Toll-like receptor 4 (TLR4) is a PRR that recognizes multiple ligands, the best characterized of which is Gram-negative bacterial LPS (Liaunardy-Jopeace and Gay, 2014). TLR4 is one of the multiple PRRs that can be activated during sterile inflammation. The downstream effects of TLR4 are ROS production and canonical NF-κB activation (Park et al., 2004; Fan et al., 2007). Several studies have implicated TLR4 activation as one of the pathways leading to inflammation in the cochlea after noise damage or ototoxicity caused by aminoglycoside or cisplatin treatment. Although the exact ligand that activated TLR4 in each of these cases is unknown, each of these types of damage increases the expression of TLR4 in the cochlea within hours (Oh et al., 2011; Hirose et al., 2014; Vethanayagam et al., 2016). In turn, TLR4 activation leads to NF-κB activation and production of TNF-α, IL-1β and IL-6 (Oh et al., 2011). Interestingly, systemic LPS given to mimic a bacterial infection or sepsis amplifies the amount of inflammation in all three types of damage and increases the severity of hearing loss (Oh et al., 2011; Hirose et al., 2014; Vethanayagam et al., 2016). Cochleae deficient in TLR4 exhibit less inflammation, and especially less TNF-α expression, which in turn results in less hearing loss (Oh et al., 2011; Vethanayagam et al., 2016). These studies have furthered our understanding of the negative effects of innate inflammation in the inner ear while raising the possibility that systemic inflammation affects the inflammatory response of the inner ear.

IMMUNE MODULATION

Many mouse models and reagents are available for investigating the modulation of the immune response. Several studies have used these models and techniques in an effort to identify specific cytokines and signaling pathways that are stimulated as a result of cochlear trauma. In the first such study, the FDA-approved anti-TNF-α antibody etanercept was used in conjunction with cisplatin treatment to reduce inflammation in the cochlea (So et al., 2007). Blocking TNF-α release after cisplatin treatment reduced the amount of the canonical NF-κB constituent p65 and the amount of apoptosis throughout the cochlea, even though the outer hair cells were still damaged (So et al., 2007). In a second study, a neutralizing antibody to the IL-6R was used to block the effects of IL-6 released after noise damage (Wakabayashi et al., 2010). This resulted in significantly less infiltration of CD45+ Iba-1+ double-positive cells at day 3 after noise-induced damage, along with less cell death in the spiral ganglion. Furthermore, this study showed that a systemically administered antibody could cross the blood-labyrinth barrier after acoustic trauma, thereby opening the way to studying FDA-approved biologics for treating cochlear damage (Wakabayashi et al., 2010). In a third study, minocycline was used to reduce macrophage activation in order to prevent hair cell damage by CX3CR1+ macrophages (Sun et al., 2014). When minocycline was administered along with neomycin, mice had less microglia-like cell infiltration, less hair cell death, and a reduced threshold shift, which suggests the blockade of macrophage-induced inflammation is important for attenuating the effects of neomycin on hearing (Sun et al., 2014). Although these results appear to indicate that the immune system can be modulated to protect the cochlea from aminoglycoside ototoxicity, follow-up studies in adult mice are needed to verify that this is indeed the case. The most recent study of immune modulation in the cochlea (Vethanayagam et al., 2016) built upon the observation that systemic LPS worsened ototoxic hair cell loss; this study fully examined the role of TLR4 in cochlear inflammation by using TLR4 knockout mice. Compared to wild-type controls, TLR4 knockout mice retained more hair cells and had a lower ABR threshold after noise damage, as well as reduced levels of IL-6 in the organ of Corti (Vethanayagam et al., 2016). Although the TLR4 knockout mice ultimately had less hearing damage, they still exhibited infiltration of macrophages; however, these macrophages did not upregulate MHCII, which would have allowed them to present antigen to the CD4+ T cells of the adaptive immune system (Gloddek et al., 2002; Vethanayagam et al., 2016). Taken together, the results of these studies suggest that the early stimulation of innate receptors and inflammatory cytokines plays a role in hair cell death after damage, although these factors are not solely responsible for all the inflammation that occurs in the cochlea.

SUMMARY

Thus far, the investigations of the role of the immune system in the inner ear have focused on the early players in inflammation: TLR4 activation, pro-inflammatory cytokine and chemokine release and infiltrating cells of the innate immune system. All three of these major pathways are common to acoustic injury and to ototoxicity caused by both aminoglycosides or cisplatin. This has led researchers in the field to identify ways of systemically modulating the immune system to reduce inflammatory destruction of the inner ear. However, CX3CR1+ resident macrophages appear to regulate the influx of CD45+ cells after hair cell damage. The exact regulatory actions of these cells must be examined to discover ways to dampen damaging inflammation. Also, the role of adaptive immunity in the inner ear is yet to be explored. Infiltrating T cells could prolong inflammation by initiating a self-antigen-specific response (Brodeur et al., 2015). However, in other epithelial systems, adaptive immunity supports tissue regeneration by IL-22 signaling, by dampening the inflammatory response through the release of IL-10, and by polarizing macrophages to an anti-inflammatory phenotype (Gazzinelli et al., 1992; Lindemans et al., 2015; Siqueira Mietto et al., 2015).

Although the mechanisms that act in other tissues may not be applicable to the inner ear, further study is required in three areas in order to learn more about the full extent of the immune response in the inner ear after noise or ototoxic drug damage. First, it is imperative to identify all the cell types that enter the cochlea. Second, once the cell types have been identified, their specific functions must be explored to understand how their secreted products and cell interactions shape the inflammatory response in the inner ear. Finally, each of the PRR families should be investigated to obtain a better understanding of which DAMPs cause the initiation of the inflammatory response in the ear after damage. The results of these studies should reveal new targets for preventative therapies in the case of ototoxic drugs and new treatments for noise-induced hearing loss, and they should expand our fundamental knowledge of the immune response to sterile insults.

AUTHOR CONTRIBUTIONS

MBW assembled the literature and wrote the manuscript. JZ saw the need for a review of the material and provided input at every stage of the writing process.

ACKNOWLEDGMENTS

Dr. Hongbo Chi gave critical feedback to the editing of this manuscript in his area of expertise, immunology. We appreciate the work of Dr. Keith Laycock who edited the manuscript.

REFERENCES

Babon, J. J., Sabo, J. K., Soetopo, A., Yao, S., Bailey, M. F., Zhang, J. G., et al. (2008). The SOCS box domain of SOCS3: structure and interaction with the elonginBC-cullin5 ubiquitin ligase. *J. Mol. Biol.* 381, 928–940. doi: 10.1016/j.jmb.2008.06.038

Bánfi, B., Malgrange, B., Knisz, J., Steger, K., Dubois-Dauphin, M., and Krause, K. H. (2004). NOX3, a superoxide-generating NADPH oxidase of the inner ear. *J. Biol. Chem.* 279, 46065–46072. doi: 10.1074/jbc.M403046200

Bode, J. G., Nimmesgern, A., Schmitz, J., Schaper, F., Schmitt, M., Frisch, W., et al. (1999). LPS and TNFα induce SOCS3 mRNA and inhibit IL-6-induced activation of STAT3 in macrophages. *FEBS Lett.* 463, 365–370. doi: 10.1016/s0014-5793(99)01662-2

Brodeur, T. Y., Robidoux, T. E., Weinstein, J. S., Craft, J., Swain, S. L., and Marshak-Rothstein, A. (2015). IL-21 promotes pulmonary fibrosis through the induction of pro-fibrotic $CD8^+$ T cells. *J. Immunol.* 195, 5251–5260. doi: 10.4049/jimmunol.1500777

Dai, M., Yang, Y., Omelchenko, I., Nuttall, A. L., Kachelmeier, A., Xiu, R., et al. (2010). Bone marrow cell recruitment mediated by inducible nitric oxide synthase/stromal cell-derived factor-1α signaling repairs the acoustically damaged cochlear blood-labyrinth barrier. *Am. J. Pathol.* 177, 3089–3099. doi: 10.2353/ajpath.2010.100340

Fan, J., Li, Y., Levy, R. M., Fan, J. J., Hackam, D. J., Vodovotz, Y., et al. (2007). Hemorrhagic shock induces NAD(P)H oxidase activation in neutrophils: role of HMGB1-TLR4 signaling. *J. Immunol.* 178, 6573–6580. doi: 10.4049/jimmunol.178.10.6573

Fontenot, J. D., Gavin, M. A., and Rudensky, A. Y. (2003). Foxp3 programs the development and function of $CD4^+CD25^+$ regulatory T cells. *Nat. Immunol.* 4, 330–336. doi: 10.1038/ni904

Fredelius, L., and Rask-Andersen, H. (1990). The role of macrophages in the disposal of degeneration products within the organ of Corti after acoustic overstimulation. *Acta Otolaryngol.* 109, 76–82. doi: 10.3109/00016489009107417

Fujioka, M., Kanzaki, S., Okano, H., Masuda, M., Ogawa, K., and Okano, H. (2006). Proinflammatory cytokines expression in noise-induced damaged cochlea. *J. Neurosci. Res.* 83, 575–583. doi: 10.1002/jnr.20764

Galea, I., Bechmann, I., and Perry, V. H. (2007). What is immune privilege (not)? *Trends Immunol.* 28, 12–18. doi: 10.1016/j.it.2006.11.004

Gazzinelli, R. T., Oswald, I. P., James, S. L., and Sher, A. (1992). IL-10 inhibits parasite killing and nitrogen oxide production by IFN-gamma-activated macrophages. *J. Immunol.* 148, 1792–1796.

Gloddek, B., Bodmer, D., Brors, D., Keithley, E. M., and Ryan, A. F. (2002). Induction of MHC class II antigens on cells of the inner ear. *Audiol. Neurootol.* 7, 317–323. doi: 10.1159/000066158

Gratton, M., Eleftheriadou, A., Garcia, J., Verduzco, E., Martin, G. K., Lonsbury-Martin, B. L., et al. (2011). Noise-induced changes in gene expression in the cochleae of mice differing in their susceptibility to noise damage. *Hear. Res.* 277, 211–226. doi: 10.1016/j.heares.2010.12.014

Hirose, K., Discolo, C. M., Keasler, J. R., and Ransohoff, R. (2005). Mononuclear phagocytes migrate into the murine cochlea after acoustic trauma. *J. Comp. Neurol.* 489, 180–194. doi: 10.1002/cne.20619

Hirose, K., Li, S.-Z., Ohlemiller, K. K., and Ransohoff, R. M. (2014). Systemic lipopolysaccharide induces cochlear inflammation and exacerbates the synergistic ototoxicity of kanamycin and furosemide. *J. Assoc. Res. Otolaryngol.* 15, 555–570. doi: 10.1007/s10162-014-0458-8

Hume, D. A., Underhill, D. M., Sweet, M. J., Ozinsky, A. O., Liew, F. Y., and Aderem, A. (2001). Macrophages exposed continuously to lipopolysaccharide and other agonists that act via toll-like receptors exhibit a sustained and additive activation state. *BMC Immunol.* 2:11. doi: 10.1186/1471-2172-2-11

Immig, K., Gericke, M., Menzel, F., Merz, F., Krueger, M., Schiefenhövel, F., et al. (2015). CD11c-positive cells from brain, spleen, lung and liver exhibit site-specific immune phenotypes and plastically adapt to new environments. *Glia* 63, 611–625. doi: 10.1002/glia.22771

Kaur, T., Zamani, D., Tong, L., Rubel, E. W., Ohlemiller, K. K., Hirose, K., et al. (2015). Fractalkine signaling regulates macrophage recruitment into the cochlea and promotes the survival of spiral ganglion neurons after selective hair cell lesion. *J. Neurosci.* 35, 15050–15061. doi: 10.1523/JNEUROSCI.2325-15.2015

Kurtin, P. J., and Pinkus, G. S. (1985). Leukocyte common antigen—a diagnostic discriminant between hematopoietic and nonhematopoietic neoplasms in paraffin sections using monoclonal antibodies: correlation with immunologic studies and ultrastructural localization. *Hum. Pathol.* 16, 353–365. doi: 10.1016/s0046-8177(85)80229-x

Lang, H., Nishimoto, E., Xing, Y., Brown, L. N., Noble, K. V., Barth, J. L., et al. (2016). Contributions of mouse and human hematopoietic cells to remodeling of the adult auditory nerve after neuron loss. *Mol. Ther.* 24, 2000–2011. doi: 10.1038/mt.2016.174

Ledebur, H. C., and Parks, T. P. (1995). Transcriptional regulation of the intercellular adhesion molecule-1 gene by inflammatory cytokines in human endothelial cells. Essential roles of a variant NF-κB site and p65 homodimers. *J. Biol. Chem.* 270, 933–943. doi: 10.1074/jbc.270.2.933

Li, X., Massa, P. E., Hanidu, A., Peet, G. W., Aro, P., Savitt, A., et al. (2002). IKKα, IKKβ and NEMO/IKKγ are each required for the NF-κB-mediated inflammatory response program. *J. Biol. Chem.* 277, 45129–45140. doi: 10.1074/jbc.M205165200

Liaunardy-Jopeace, A., and Gay, N. J. (2014). Molecular and cellular regulation of toll-like receptor-4 activity induced by lipopolysaccharide ligands. *Front. Immunol.* 5:473. doi: 10.3389/fimmu.2014.00473

Lindemans, C. A., Calafiore, M., Mertelsmann, A. M., O'Connor, M. H., Dudakov, J. A., Jenq, R. R., et al. (2015). Interleukin-22 promotes intestinal stem cell-mediated epithelial regeneration. *Nature* 528, 560–564. doi: 10.1038/nature16460

Ma, C., Billings, P., Harris, J. P., and Keithley, E. M. (2000). Characterization of an experimentally induced inner ear immune response. *Laryngoscope* 110, 451–456. doi: 10.1097/00005537-200003000-00024

Masuda, M., Nagashima, R., Kanzaki, S., Fujioka, M., Ogita, K., and Ogawa, K. (2005). Nuclear factor-kappa B nuclear translocation in the cochlea of mice following acoustic overstimulation. *Brain Res.* 1068, 237–247. doi: 10.1016/j.brainres.2005.11.020

Nahrendorf, M., Swirski, F. K., Aikawa, E., Stangenberg, L., Wurdinger, T., Figueiredo, J. L., et al. (2007). The healing myocardium sequentially mobilizes two monocyte subsets with divergent and complementary functions. *J. Exp. Med.* 204, 3037–3047. doi: 10.1084/jem.20070885

Oh, G.-S., Kim, H.-J., Choi, J.-H., Shen, A., Kim, C.-H., Kim, S.-J., et al. (2011). Activation of lipopolysaccharide-TLR4 signaling accelerates the ototoxic potential of cisplatin in mice. *J. Immunol.* 186, 1140–1150. doi: 10.4049/jimmunol.1002183

Okano, T., Nakagawa, T., Kita, T., Kada, S., Yoshimoto, M., Nakahata, T., et al. (2008). Bone marrow-derived cells expressing Iba1 are constitutively present as resident tissue macrophages in the mouse cochlea. *J. Neurosci. Res.* 86, 1758–1767. doi: 10.1002/jnr.21625

Park, H. S., Jung, H. Y., Park, E. Y., Kim, J., Lee, W. J., and Bae, Y. S. (2004). Cutting edge: direct interaction of TLR4 with NAD(P)H oxidase 4 isozyme is essential for lipopolysaccharide-induced production of reactive oxygen species and activation of NF-κB. *J. Immunol.* 173, 3589–3593. doi: 10.4049/jimmunol.173.6.3589

Psachoulia, K., Chamberlain, K. A., Heo, D., Davis, S. E., Paskus, J. D., Nanescu, S. E., et al. (2016). IL4I1 augments CNS remyelination and axonal protection by modulating T cell driven inflammation. *Brain* 139, 3121–3136. doi: 10.1093/brain/aww254

Rock, K. L., Latz, E., Ontiveros, F., and Kono, H. (2010). The sterile inflammatory response. *Annu. Rev. Immunol.* 28, 321–342. doi: 10.1146/annurev-immunol-030409-101311

Sato, E., Shick, E. H., Ransohoff, R. M., and Hirose, K. (2008). Repopulation of cochlear macrophages in murine hematopoietic progenitor cell chimeras: the role of CX3CR1. *J. Comp. Neurol.* 506, 930–942. doi: 10.1002/cne.21583

Sato, E., Shick, E. H., Ransohoff, R. M., and Hirose, K. (2010). Expression of fractalkine receptor CX3CR1 on cochlear macrophages influences survival of hair cells following ototoxic injury. *J. Assoc. Res. Otolaryngol.* 11, 223–234. doi: 10.1007/s10162-009-0198-3

Shi, X. (2010). Resident macrophages in the cochlear blood-labyrinth barrier and their renewal via migration of bone-marrow-derived cells. *Cell Tissue Res.* 342, 21–30. doi: 10.1007/s00441-010-1040-2

Siqueira Mietto, B., Kroner, A., Girolami, E. I., Santos-Nogueira, E., Zhang, J., and David, S. (2015). Role of IL-10 in resolution of inflammation and functional recovery after peripheral nerve injury. *J. Neurosci.* 35, 16431–16442. doi: 10.1523/JNEUROSCI.2119-15.2015

So, H., Kim, H., Lee, J.-H., Park, C., Kim, Y., Kim, E., et al. (2007). Cisplatin cytotoxicity of auditory cells requires secretions of proinflammatory cytokines via activation of ERK and NF-κB. *J. Assoc. Res. Otolaryngol.* 8, 338–355. doi: 10.1007/s10162-007-0084-9

Stein, M., Keshav, S., Harris, N., and Gordon, S. (1992). Interleukin 4 potently enhances murine macrophage mannose receptor activity: a marker of alternative immunologic macrophage activation. *J. Exp. Med.* 176, 287–292. doi: 10.1084/jem.176.1.287

Sun, S., Yu, H., Yu, H., Honglin, M., Ni, W., Zhang, Y., et al. (2014). Inhibition of the activation and recruitment of microglia-like cells protects against neomycin-induced ototoxicity. *Mol. Neurobiol.* 51, 252–267. doi: 10.1007/s12035-014-8712-y

Suzuki, M., and Harris, J. P. (1995). Expression of intercellular adhesion molecule-1 during inner ear inflammation. *Ann. Otol. Rhinol. Laryngol.* 104, 69–75. doi: 10.1177/000348949510400111

Tan, B., Lee, M., and Ruan, R. (2008). Bone-marrow-derived cells that home to acoustic deafened cochlea preserved their hematopoietic identity. *J. Comp. Neurol.* 509, 167–179. doi: 10.1002/cne.21729

Tan, W. J. T., Thorne, P. R., and Vlajkovic, S. M. (2016). Characterisation of cochlear inflammation in mice following acute and chronic noise exposure. *Histochem. Cell Biol.* 146, 219–230. doi: 10.1007/s00418-016-1436-5

Tang, D., Kang, R., Coyne, C. B., Zeh, H. J., and Lotze, M. T. (2012). PAMPs and DAMPs: signal 0s that spur autophagy and immunity. *Immunol. Rev.* 249, 158–175. doi: 10.1111/j.1600-065X.2012.01146.x

Taylor, A. W. (2016). Ocular immune privilege and transplantation. *Front. Immunol.* 7:37. doi: 10.3389/fimmu.2016.00037

Tornabene, S. V., Sato, K., Pham, L., Billings, P., and Keithley, E. M. (2006). Immune cell recruitment following acoustic trauma. *Hear. Res.* 222, 115–124. doi: 10.1016/j.heares.2006.09.004

Tsung, A., Klune, J. R., Zhang, X., Jeyabalan, G., Cao, Z., Peng, X., et al. (2007). HMGB1 release induced by liver ischemia involves Toll-like receptor 4 dependent reactive oxygen species production and calcium-mediated signaling. *J. Exp. Med.* 204, 2913–2923. doi: 10.1084/jem.20070247

Vethanayagam, R. R., Yang, W., Dong, Y., and Hu, B. H. (2016). Toll-like receptor 4 modulates the cochlear immune response to acoustic injury. *Cell Death Dis.* 7:e2245. doi: 10.1038/cddis.2016.156

Wakabayashi, K., Fujioka, M., Kanzaki, S., Okano, H., Shibata, S., Yamashita, D., et al. (2010). Blockade of interleukin-6 signaling suppressed cochlear inflammatory response and improved hearing impairment in noise-damaged mice cochlea. *Neurosci. Res.* 66, 345–352. doi: 10.1016/j.neures.2009.12.008

Wei, L., Fan, M., Xu, L., Heinrich, K., Berry, M. W., Homayouni, R., et al. (2008). Bioinformatic analysis reveals cRel as a regulator of a subset of interferon-stimulated genes. *J. Interferon Cytokine Res.* 28, 541–551. doi: 10.1089/jir.2007.0136

Wertheimer, S. J., Myers, C. L., Wallace, R. W., and Parks, T. P. (1992). Intercellular adhesion molecule-1 gene expression in human endothelial cells. Differential regulation by tumor necrosis factor-α and phorbol myristate acetate. *J. Biol. Chem.* 267, 12030–12035.

Wilcox, C. E., Ward, A. M., Evans, A., Baker, D., Rothlein, R., and Turk, J. L. (1990). Endothelial cell expression of the intercellular adhesion molecule-1 (ICAM-1) in the central nervous system of guinea pigs during acute and chronic relapsing experimental allergic encephalomyelitis. *J. Neuroimmunol.* 30, 43–51. doi: 10.1016/0165-5728(90)90051-n

Xu, M. J., Feng, D., Wang, H., Guan, Y., Yan, X., and Gao, B. (2014). IL-22 ameliorates renal ischemia-reperfusion injury by targeting proximal tubule epithelium. *J. Am. Soc. Nephrol.* 25, 967–977. doi: 10.1681/ASN.2013060611

Yang, S., Cai, Q., Vethanayagam, R. R., Wang, J., Yang, W., and Hu, B. H. (2016). Immune defense is the primary function associated with the differentially expressed genes in the cochlea following acoustic trauma. *Hear. Res.* 333, 283–294. doi: 10.1016/j.heares.2015.10.010

Yang, W., Vethanayagam, R. R., Dong, Y., Cai, Q., and Hu, B. H. (2015). Activation of the antigen presentation function of mononuclear phagocyte populations associated with the basilar membrane of the cochlea after acoustic overstimulation. *Neuroscience* 303, 1–15. doi: 10.1016/j.neuroscience.2015.05.081

15

Aminoglycoside-Induced Cochleotoxicity

*Meiyan Jiang[1], Takatoshi Karasawa[1] and Peter S. Steyger[1,2]**

[1]Oregon Hearing Research Center, Oregon Health & Science University, Portland, OR, United States, [2]National Center for Rehabilitative Auditory Research, Portland VA Medical Center (VHA), Portland, OR, United States

Edited by:
Egidio D'Angelo,
University of Pavia, Italy

Reviewed by:
Jianxin Bao,
Northeast Ohio Medical University,
United States
Ivan Milenkovic,
Leipzig University, Germany

***Correspondence:**
Peter S. Steyger
steygerp@ohsu.edu

Aminoglycoside antibiotics are used as prophylaxis, or urgent treatment, for many life-threatening bacterial infections, including tuberculosis, sepsis, respiratory infections in cystic fibrosis, complex urinary tract infections and endocarditis. Although aminoglycosides are clinically-essential antibiotics, the mechanisms underlying their selective toxicity to the kidney and inner ear continue to be unraveled despite more than 70 years of investigation. The following mechanisms each contribute to aminoglycoside-induced toxicity after systemic administration: (1) drug trafficking across endothelial and epithelial barrier layers; (2) sensory cell uptake of these drugs; and (3) disruption of intracellular physiological pathways. Specific factors can increase the risk of drug-induced toxicity, including sustained exposure to higher levels of ambient sound, and selected therapeutic agents such as loop diuretics and glycopeptides. Serious bacterial infections (requiring life-saving aminoglycoside treatment) induce systemic inflammatory responses that also potentiate the degree of ototoxicity and permanent hearing loss. We discuss prospective clinical strategies to protect auditory and vestibular function from aminoglycoside ototoxicity, including reduced cochlear or sensory cell uptake of aminoglycosides, and otoprotection by ameliorating intracellular cytotoxicity.

Keywords: aminoglycosides, gentamicin, ototoxicity, cochleotoxicity, nephrotoxicity, inflammation, systemic administration

AMINOGLYCOSIDE ANTIBIOTICS

Aminoglycosides are among the most efficacious antibiotics used to treat serious Gram-negative infections by *Pseudomonas*, *Salmonella* and *Enterobacter* species (Forge and Schacht, 2000). The first identified aminoglycoside, streptomycin, was isolated from *Streptomyces griseus* in 1944 (Schatz et al., 1944), followed by neomycin from *Streptomyces fradiae* (Waksman and Lechevalier, 1949). In 1957 and 1963, kanamycin and gentamicin (**Figure 1**) were isolated from *Streptomyces kanamyceticus* (Umezawa et al., 1957) and the actinomycete *Micromonospora purpurea* (Weinstein et al., 1963) respectively, followed by tobramycin from *Streptomyces tenebrarius* (Wick and Welles, 1967) and amikacin, a semi-synthetic derivative of kanamycin A (Kawaguchi et al., 1972). Aminoglycosides with the–mycin suffix are derived from *Streptomyces* genera, while those from *Micromonospora* genera have the suffix–micin. Aminoglycosides can also treat selected Gram-positive infections like tuberculosis due to the intracellular *Mycobacterium tuberculosis* (Forge and Schacht, 2000). Clinically, aminoglycosides are often used in combination with β-lactams (like ampicillin) for combinatorial synergistic efficacy against a broad range of bacteria, especially when the causative microbe(s) is unknown (Dressel et al., 1999), and has been well-characterized for *Pseudomonas* and other Gram-negative bacteria (Niederman et al., 2001).

Nonetheless, these drugs can induce acute dose-dependent kidney failure (nephrotoxicity), and permanent hearing loss (cochleotoxicity; defined here as hearing loss in the conventional

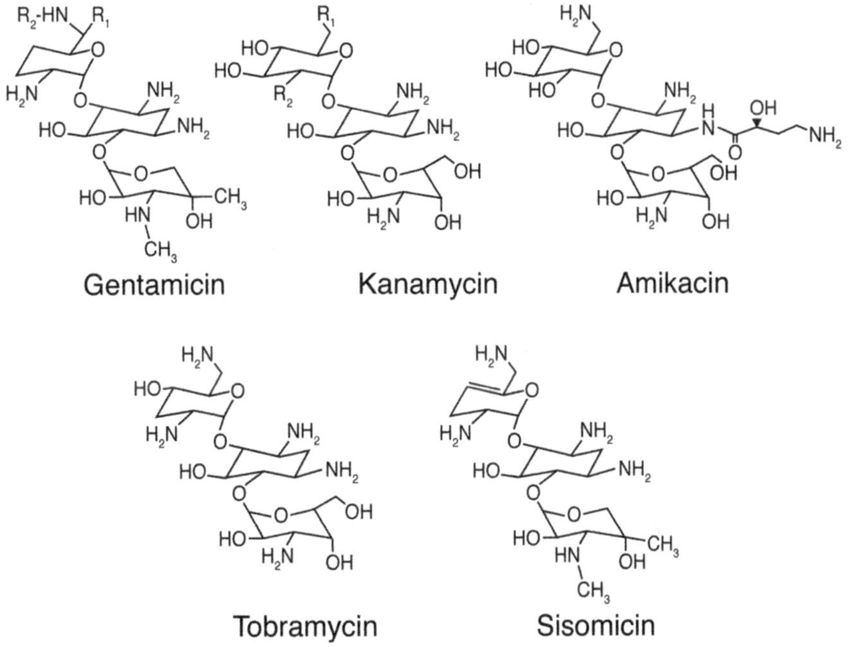

FIGURE 1 | Chemical structures of selected aminoglycoside antibiotics. For gentamicin C_1: $R_1 = R_2 = CH_3$; gentamicin C_2: $R_1 = CH_3$, $R_2 = H$; and gentamicin C_{1A}: $R_1 = R_2 = H$. For kanamycin A: $R_1 = NH_2$, $R_2 = OH$; kanamycin B: $R_1 = R_2 = NH_2$; and kanamycin C: $R_1 = OH$, $R_2 = NH_2$.

frequency range, i.e., <8 kHz) and/or balance disorders (vestibulotoxicity). Aminoglycoside-induced vestibulotoxicity and/or cochleotoxicity occurs in as many as 20% of patients who received these drugs intravenously for multiple days (Ariano et al., 2008; Al-Malky et al., 2015; Garinis et al., 2017a). Hearing loss delays speech acquisition, education and psychosocial development, reducing employability, income and tax revenues (Jones and White, 1990; Järvelin et al., 1997; Mehl and Thomson, 1998; Naramura et al., 1999; Tambs, 2004), with a socioeconomic burden >$1,393,000 in 2015 dollars over the life-time of each pre-lingually deafened child (Mohr et al., 2000). Similarly, for each adult that acquires hearing loss, the socioeconomic burden is >$350,000 in 2015 dollars over their remaining lifespan.

The bactericidal efficacy of aminoglycosides against a broad range of bacteria is directly related to peak concentration in the blood. Yet aminoglycosides have a narrow therapeutic index, and it is crucial to maintain or enhance their therapeutic efficacy while minimizing their side effects. The increasing prevalence of bacterial resistance to more commonly-used antibiotics, e.g., ampicillin, β-lactams (Puopolo and Eichenwald, 2010; Tsai et al., 2014) has resulted in the retention of aminoglycosides as a clinically necessary alternative treatment. Aminoglycosides also remain an attractive clinical antibiotic strategy due to their chemical stability at ambient temperature (particularly in sub-Sahara Africa), rapid bactericidal effect, lower incidence of resistance, and relative lower cost compared to newer, synthetic, more costly non-ototoxic medications.

Advances in molecular biology have enabled the bactericidal mechanisms of aminoglycosides, and subsequent emergence of bacterial resistance to these drugs, to be studied extensively (Shakil et al., 2008). Furthermore, the emerging bioactivities and potential applications of aminoglycosides continue to be extensively investigated. For example, the K20 derivative of kanamycin A with an octanesulfonyl chain is a broad-spectrum antifungal that targets fungal plasma membranes to protect agricultural crops (Shrestha et al., 2014). Selected aminoglycosides are being tested for their ability to read-through premature stop-codons in genetic mutations for the cystic fibrosis transmembrane conductance regulator (CFTR) and selected cancers (Du et al., 2006; Baradaran-Heravi et al., 2017).

Currently nine aminoglycosides are approved by the US Food and Drug Administration (FDA) for clinical use in the United States. Of these, gentamicin, tobramycin, and amikacin are the most common parental agents. Gentamicin is often preferred because of its low cost and reliable bactericidal activity. It is administered systemically in neonatal intensive care units (NICU), mostly for prophylaxis in preterm infants, and discontinued once sepsis is ruled out <72 h. If sepsis is confirmed, treatment may continue for another 10–15 days. Tobramycin is primarily used for treating *Pseudomonas aeruginosa*-induced respiratory infections in patients with cystic fibrosis. Amikacin is particularly effective against bacteria that are resistant to other aminoglycosides, since its chemical structure makes it less susceptible to inactivating enzymes. Gentamicin and tobramycin are considered more vestibulotoxic, while amikacin, neomycin and kanamycin are considered more cochleotoxic, though each drug affects both sensory systems to varying degrees.

Almost all cells take up aminoglycosides, and most cells are able to clear these drugs from their cytoplasm relatively quickly, by mechanisms as yet undetermined, except for inner ear hair cells and renal proximal tubule cells which retain these drugs for extended periods of time (Dai et al., 2006). It is thought that this retention of aminoglycosides, plus the higher metabolic rate of hair cells and proximal tubules cells, contributes to their susceptibility to these drugs. This review will focus on the trafficking and cellular uptake of systemically-administered aminoglycosides, and their subsequent intracellular cytotoxic mechanisms. We also review factors that potentiate ototoxicity, and approaches to ameliorate aminoglycoside-induced ototoxicity.

FUNCTIONAL ANATOMY OF THE COCHLEA AND KIDNEY

Cochlea

Within the temporal bone, the cochlea is a coiled, bony tube divided into three fluid-filled compartments by two tight junction-coupled cellular barriers located on Reissner's membrane and the basilar membrane (**Figure 2A**). The organ of Corti, residing on the basilar membrane, consists of sensory hair cells and adjacent supporting cells coupled together by apical tight junctions to form a reticular lamina. There are typically three rows of outer hair cells (OHCs), and a single row of inner hair cells (IHCs). The upper and lower fluid compartments, the scala vestibuli and scala tympani, respectively, are filled with perilymph similar to cerebrospinal fluid. These two compartments sandwich the inner compartment, the scala media, filled with endolymph. Uniquely, endolymph has high K^+ concentrations due to active trafficking via Na^+-K^+-ATPases, Na^+-K^+-Cl^- co-transporters and rectifying potassium channels ($K_{ir}4.1$) within the stria vascularis that generates an endocochlear potential (EP) as high as +100 mV. The stria vascularis is also a tight junction-coupled compartment and with the reticular lamina and Reissner's membrane encloses the scala media, ensuring electrochemical separation of endolymph and perilymph (**Figure 2A**).

Sound pressure waves entering the cochlea tonotopically vibrate the basilar membrane, deflecting the stereocilia projecting from the apices of hair cells into endolymph. These deflections gate the mechano-electrical transduction (MET) channels on the stereociliary membrane, enabling depolarizing transduction currents that trigger the release of the neurotransmitter glutamate, which in turn induces action potentials in the innervating afferent auditory neurons (Nordang et al., 2000; Oestreicher et al., 2002). Loss of the EP reduces cochlear sensitivity to sound.

Kidney Tubules (Nephron)

Drugs and toxins in the blood are excreted via ultra-filtration by the kidney. Renal arterial blood undergoes extravasation in kidney glomeruli, and the ultrafiltrate passes into the lumen of the proximal convoluted tubule (**Figure 2B**). Epithelial cells lining the proximal convoluted tubule are characterized by their extensive brush border of microvilli, maximizing the surface area available to incorporate ion channels, active transporters or exchangers and electrogenic symporters. The majority of essential nutrients, including 90% of glucose and amino acids, are resorbed from the ultrafiltrate in the proximal tubule. The tubule then descends into the medulla of the kidney and sharply reverses

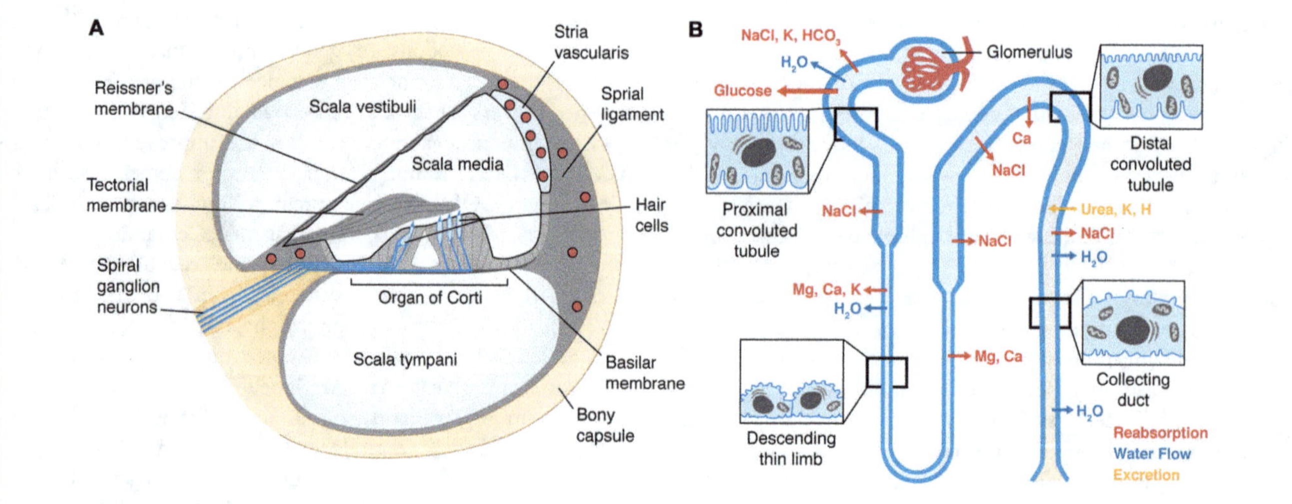

FIGURE 2 | (A) Cross-section of the cochlear duct, illustrating the perilymph-filled scala vestibuli and scala tympani, separated from the scala media by tight junctions between adjacent cells (black line) of Reissner's membrane and reticular lamina of the organ of Corti resting on the basilar membrane. Within the organ of Corti are four longitudinal rows of sensory hair cells (in sky blue), under the tectorial membrane. The hair cells are innervated by afferent and efferent fibers (blue lines). Within the lateral wall of the cochlea is the highly-vascularized stria vascularis (upper right); enclosing several capillary beds (red circles) lined by tight-junction-coupled endothelial cells (black lines enclosing red circles) that form the cochlear BLB. **(B)** A nephron (kidney tubule) showing the glomerulus encapsulating a single capillary bed that gathers the ultrafiltrate from blood. The proximal tubule has a brush border of microvilli that recovers the majority of essential nutrients and ions, and the distal tubule recaptures the remaining nutrients, and excretes specific ions. Sites of major ion movements are shown. Both schematic diagrams are not to relative scale.

direction to ascend back to the kidney cortex, and is collectively called the loop of Henle. In the descending limb, water is readily resorbed, increasing the osmolarity of the ultrafiltrate, which enables additional essential ions (Na^+, K^+ and Cl^-) to be resorbed in the ascending limb. As the tubule progresses into distal convoluted tubule, further cation reclamation (K^+, Ca^{2+}) occurs as H^+ is secreted into the remaining fluid, now recognized as urine that drains into the collecting duct and bladder prior to being voided.

Similarities and Differences between Cochlea and Kidney

There are many physiological similarities between the cochlea and kidney, principally the active transport of electrolytes or nutrients, and consequently, water follows to maintain iso-osmolarity. Gene expression analysis has identified at least 36 genes that are significantly expressed in both cochlea and kidney (Liu et al., 2004). More striking is the correlation of genetic syndromes that affect both cochlear and renal function (Izzedine et al., 2004). Both renal tubules and the stria vascularis are closely associated with basement membranes (of similar collagenous composition) that enclose blood vessels. Mutations in genes for collagen result in Alport's syndrome characterized by progressive glomerular kidney disease and high frequency hearing loss (Gratton et al., 2005). Bartter's syndrome results from a mutation in the gene for the protein barttin, a required subunit of voltage-gated chloride channels essential for salt and ion homeostasis in both the stria vascularis and renal ascending limb of Henle and distal tubule (Kramer et al., 2008). Hearing loss is associated in patients with lower estimated glomerular filtration rate and late chronic kidney disease (Seo et al., 2015).

Aminoglycosides are readily taken up by renal proximal tubule cells and cochlear cells (Dai et al., 2006), and more pertinently, they preferentially induce cytotoxicity in inner ear sensory hair cells and proximal tubule cells *in vivo* than for most other cell types (Humes, 1999). Other ototoxic compounds, like cisplatin and loop diuretics are also directly toxic to both organs (Humes, 1999). In addition, there is increased expression of Mpv17, a peroxisomal protein that metabolizes reactive oxygen species in renal glomeruli and the stria vascularis of the cochlea following aminoglycoside exposure (Meyer zum Gottesberge et al., 2002).

TRAFFICKING OF AMINOGLYCOSIDES *IN VIVO*

Intra-Cochlear Trafficking after Systemic Administration

In the 1980s, aminoglycosides were readily detected only in perilymph, but not endolymph, following intravenous infusion (Tran Ba Huy et al., 1986). Parental injection of gentamicin attenuated efferent inhibition of auditory neurons within 1–2 h, presumptively by blocking cholinergic activity at efferent synapses at the base of OHCs immersed in perilymph (Avan et al., 1996; Blanchet et al., 2000). The degree of the loss of inhibition may be predictive of subsequent permanent sensorineural hearing loss (Halsey et al., 2005).

In vitro, aminoglycosides are effective blockers of the MET channel on hair cell stereociliary membranes (Kroese et al., 1989) that, *in vivo*, are immersed in endolymph. Similar experiments then demonstrated that aminoglycosides rapidly permeate through MET channels into hair cells (Marcotti et al., 2005). Endolymph has a +80 mV potential, and when coupled with the cochlear hair cell receptor potential of −45 mV (IHCs) to −70 mV (OHCs), the potential across the apical membrane of hair cells of ∼125–150 mV (Pickles, 2012). Surprisingly, adjacent supporting cells can have resting potentials between −80 mV and −100 mV (Russell and Sellick, 1978, 1983). This potent electrophoretic force likely drives cations, including aminoglycosides, across membranes through open (non-selective) cation channels with the requisite physicochemical properties for aminoglycoside permeation.

To test whether aminoglycosides could enter hair cells from endolymph *in vivo*, perfusion of the scala tympani with artificial perilymph (to prevent aminoglycoside access to the basolateral membranes of hair cells) did not visibly affect hair cell uptake of intravenously-administered aminoglycosides. However, when aminoglycoside-laden artificial perilymph was perfused though the scala tympani, hair cell uptake of aminoglycosides over their basolateral membranes was markedly reduced compared to systemic delivery (Li and Steyger, 2011). These data strongly suggest that systemic aminoglycosides are predominantly and rapidly trafficked across the blood-labyrinth barrier into the stria vascularis, and cleared into endolymph prior to entering hair cells across their apical membranes. Aminoglycosides are taken up by most other cochlear cells, including fibrocytes in the lateral wall, spiral ganglion neurons, supporting cells in the organ of Corti (Imamura and Adams, 2003; Kitahara et al., 2005; Dai et al., 2006). Aminoglycosides are cleared from non-sensory cells, but can be retained by surviving hair cells for as long as 6 months (Imamura and Adams, 2003).

Cellular Changes Following Aminoglycoside Administration

After parental injection, basal OHCs preferentially take up aminoglycosides prior to hair cell death (Hiel et al., 1993). Multiple dosing with aminoglycosides can induce cell-specific changes in ion channel expression (see below) that may enhance drug uptake following subsequent aminoglycoside dosing, e.g., spiral ganglion cells (Kitahara et al., 2005). Aminoglycoside-induced hair cell death typically occurs in basal OHCs, and extends to IHCs and more apical OHCs with increasing cumulative dose (Forge and Schacht, 2000). The apices of dying hair cells are extruded as the surrounding supporting cell apices expand to seal the reticular lamina and prevent mixing of endolymph and perilymph, and retain optimal cochlear function in surviving hair cells. The expanded supporting cell apices, or scar, is characterized by the deposition of new junctional and cytoskeletal proteins at the site of the missing hair cell (Leonova and Raphael, 1997; Steyger et al., 1997). The hair cell bodies are typically phagocytosed by adjacent supporting cells and resident macrophages (Monzack et al., 2015).

Chronic kanamycin treatment leads to the selective loss of basal OHCs, presumptively isolating IHCs and their innervating afferent neurons which display a loss of auditory frequency selectivity and sensitivity (Dallos and Harris, 1978); however these basal IHCs also have damaged cytoskeletal networks (Hackney et al., 1990). Interestingly, significant elevations in auditory threshold occur in cochlear regions where OHCs appear morphologically intact following chronic aminoglycoside administration (Nicol et al., 1992; Koo et al., 2015). This may be due to cochlear synaptopathy, where aminoglycosides have disrupted the synapses between IHCs and their afferent neurons, as well as decreased neuronal density in the spiral ganglion of the cochlea (Oishi et al., 2015). Thus, cochlear synaptopathy may account for the greater degree of cochlear dysfunction relative to actual hair cell loss. Aminoglycosides can also induce vestibular synaptopathy, as described elsewhere in this Research Topic (Sultemeier and Hoffman, under review).

Nephrotoxicity

In the kidney, systemic administration of aminoglycosides can induce severe toxicity in the proximal tubule that preferentially takes up aminoglycosides compared to more distal tubular regions (Dai et al., 2006). Distal tubule cells are also functionally disrupted by aminoglycoside block of magnesium and other cation channels, leading to magnesium wasting and block of ion channel function (Kang et al., 2000). Overall, disruption of kidney function tends to be short-lived, as damaged and dying proximal tubule cells are replaced through cellular proliferation (Xie et al., 2001).

CELLULAR UPTAKE OF AMINOGLYCOSIDES

A major factor in susceptibility to aminoglycoside-induced toxicity is the cellular uptake of these drugs prior to inducing cell death.

Endocytosis

Aminoglycosides are endocytosed at the apical membranes of hair cells, i.e., from endolymph, and transported to lysosomes (Hashino et al., 1997; Hailey et al., 2017). Sufficient lysosomal sequestration of aminoglycosides was hypothesized to induce lysosomal lysis, releasing both aminoglycosides and catabolic hydrolases, to initiate cell death (Hashino et al., 1997; Kroemer and Jäättelä, 2005). However, blockade of endocytosis only marginally reduced hair cell uptake of aminoglycosides and did not prevent hair cell death (Alharazneh et al., 2011; Hailey et al., 2017). Aminoglycosides in the cytoplasm can be sequestered by endosomes prior to being trafficked to lysosomes, a novel form of autophagy (Hailey et al., 2017). Impeding the lysosomal trafficking of aminoglycoside-laden endosomes potentiated drug-induced hair cell death, suggesting that endosomal sequestration of aminoglycosides can partially protect hair cells (Hailey et al., 2017).

In the kidney, megalin, also known as the low density lipoprotein-related protein 2 (LRP2), associates with cubulin, a co-receptor, and when bound to aminoglycosides, the complex is endocytosed (Christensen and Nielsen, 2007). Megalin-deficient mice are profoundly deaf by 3 months of age (early-onset presbycusis) and have reduced renal uptake of aminoglycosides (Schmitz et al., 2002; Köonig et al., 2008). In the cochlea, megalin is expressed near the apical (endolymphatic) membrane of strial marginal cells, but is not expressed in cochlear hair cells (Köonig et al., 2008). This suggests that megalin-dependent endocytosis of aminoglycosides by marginal cells, i.e., clearance from endolymph, could provide partial otoprotection for hair cells.

Ion Channels

Aminoglycosides can permeate many ubiquitously-expressed non-selective cation channels with the requisite physicochemical properties to accommodate aminoglycosides. In addition to the inner ear and kidney, aminoglycosides are readily taken up by sensory neurons in the dorsal root and trigeminal ganglia, linguinal taste receptors, and sensory neurons of hair follicles (Dai et al., 2006). Each location expresses a variety of aminoglycoside-permeant ion channels, including non-selective Transient Receptor Potential (TRP) cation channels.

In the inner ear, aminoglycosides readily permeate the non-selective MET cation channel expressed on the stereociliary membranes of hair cells (Marcotti et al., 2005). Although the identity of MET channels (pore diameter ~1.25 nm) remain uncertain, their electrophysiological properties are well-characterized and major components, including transmembrane channel-like (TMC) 1 and TMC2 proteins, have been identified (Farris et al., 2006; Kawashima et al., 2011). Mutations in myosin VIIA, another component of the MET complex, dysregulate MET channel conductance, reducing drug uptake by hair cells (Kros et al., 2002). Extracellular cadherin-23 and protocadherin-15 proteins form the stereociliary tip-links that mechanically gate the MET channel, and mutation in these genes reduced aminoglycoside uptake, prolonging hair cell survival compared to wild-type hair cells (Vu et al., 2013). The conductance of MET channels is modulated by extracellular $[Ca^{2+}]$, and reduced by channel blockers like amiloride, curare or benzamil; each can reduce hair cell uptake of aminoglycosides and/or prolong hair cell survival (Marcotti et al., 2005; Coffin et al., 2009; Alharazneh et al., 2011; Hailey et al., 2017). Increasing the membrane potential difference between the extracellular fluid and the negatively-polarized cytoplasm increases cellular uptake of the cationic aminoglycosides in hair cells and renal cells (Marcotti et al., 2005; Myrdal and Steyger, 2005).

Several identified non-selective cation channels are candidates for aminoglycoside permeation, particularly TRP channels with pore diameters sufficient to admit the maximal cross-sectional diameter of aminoglycosides (0.8–0.9 nm). The TRP vanilloid receptor 1, TRPV1, was identified using a number of channel modulators (Myrdal and Steyger, 2005). TRPV1 is activated by heat (>43°C), and is also stimulated by capsaicin (or analogs) and protons (Caterina et al., 1997; Vellani et al., 2001). TRPV1 has a pore diameter of ~1 nm (Jara-Oseguera et al., 2008) that can be further dilated by agonists (Bautista and Julius, 2008). Capsaicin activation of cells heterologously expressing TRPV1 induces rapid cell death in streptomycin-containing culture media (Caterina et al., 1997), suggestive of aminoglycoside permeation and subsequent cytotoxicity. TRPV1 is expressed by hair cells and plays a critical role in cisplatin-induced toxicity (Zheng et al., 2003; Mukherjea et al., 2011).

TRPV4 channels are temperature-sensitive (25–34°C) cation channels that are also activated by osmotic swelling of cells, and chemically activated by 4α-phorbol 12,13-didecanoate (Liedtke et al., 2000; Vriens et al., 2004). TRPV4 has a large pore diameter (Shigematsu et al., 2010), is expressed on the apical surface of hair cells, and is aminoglycoside-permeant when overexpressed in kidney proximal tubule cell lines (Karasawa et al., 2008). Low [Ca^{2+}] increase the open probability of TRPV4 channels (Banke, 2011). Crucially, endolymph has low [Ca^{2+}] (Wangemann and Schacht, 1996), increasing the likelihood of aminoglycosides entering the cytoplasm of cells with membranous TRPV4 channels bathed by extracellular endolymph.

TRPA1 (TRP channel, subfamily A, member 1) channels are inflammatory, irritant and oxidative stress sensors (Kwan et al., 2006; Macpherson et al., 2007; Bessac et al., 2008), and appear to reside in the basolateral membrane of OHCs (Stepanyan et al., 2011). TRPA1 channels have a pore diameter of 1.1 nm and show agonist-induced dilation (to ~1.4 nm; Karashima et al., 2010), larger than the molecular diameter of aminoglycosides. The TRPA1 agonists, cinnamaldehyde and 4-hydroxynonenal (4-HNE), both increased OHC uptake of aminoglycosides, presumptively across their basolateral membranes *in vitro* (Stepanyan et al., 2011), suggesting that endogenous intracellular activation of basolateral TRPA1 channels due to oxidative stress, induced by noise (Henderson et al., 2006) or aminoglycoside exposure (Lesniak et al., 2005), could augment hair cell uptake of aminoglycosides from the scala tympani. The promiscuous permeation of several non-selective cation channels by aminoglycosides suggest that additional aminoglycoside-permeant channels will be identified (based on permeation by other cationic organic compounds). These include connexins (or gap junctions), pannexins (hemi-channels), canonical TRPC3 with a large inner chamber (~6 nm diameter) and P2X channels among others (Weber et al., 2004; Mio et al., 2007; Crumling et al., 2009; Torres et al., 2017).

Transporters

An electrogenic Na^+-ligand symporter, sodium glucose transporter 2 (SGLT2), resorbs 90% of lumenal glucose from renal ultra-filtrate in proximal tubules (Kanai et al., 1994). Inhibitors of SGLT2 inhibitors significantly block renal glucose reabsorption (Ghosh et al., 2012). SGLT2 has a large, hydrophilic and elastic vestibule, with an internal pore diameter of 3 nm, and an exit pore (into cytosol) of 1.5–2.5 nm, sufficient for aminoglycoside permeation. Aminoglycosides are complex sugars connected by glycosidic linkage (Neu and Gootz, 1996), and overexpression of SGLT2 in cell lines increased cellular uptake of aminoglycosides and exacerbated subsequent cytotoxicity (Jiang et al., 2014). Inhibition of SGLT2 by phlorizin reduced aminoglycoside-induced toxicity in proximal tubule cells *in vitro* and *in vivo*. However, phlorizin inhibition of SGLT2 *in vivo* did not reduce cochlear loading of aminoglycosides, potentially due to low cochlear expression levels of SGLT2, and/or by the phlorizin-induced elevation of serum aminoglycoside levels (Jiang et al., 2014). Since acute pharmacological inhibition or genomic loss of SGLT2 function did not affect auditory function (Jiang et al., 2014), this suggests that aminoglycoside (and glucose) trafficking across the blood-labyrinth barrier is accomplished by other molecular mechanisms, such as the facilitated glucose transporters (GLUTs; Ando et al., 2008). It is not yet known whether GLUTs are aminoglycoside-permeant and their pore dimensions remain to be determined, although it is known that the stria vascularis and organ of Corti both express GLUT5 (Belyantseva et al., 2000).

NOISE AND AMINOGLYCOSIDES

Loud sounds affect almost all cochlear cell types, including physically disrupting hair cell stereocilia, mitochondria, and the loss of synapses between hair cells and afferent neurons leading to transient and permanent hearing losses that accelerate the onset of presbycusis (Bohne et al., 2007; Kujawa and Liberman, 2015). Exposure to loud sounds synergistically potentiates the ototoxicity of aminoglycosides (Brown et al., 1978), presumptively by the summation of reactive oxygen species generated by each insult alone (Kopke et al., 1999). Loud sounds also break tip-links between stereocilia, closing the mechanically-gated MET channels (Husbands et al., 1999; Kurian et al., 2003). Sound levels that induce temporary threshold shifts (TTS) enhanced OHC uptake of aminoglycosides in mice, yet significantly reduced the number of tip links between OHC stereocilia (Li et al., 2015). This indicates that increased uptake of aminoglycosides by hair cells occurs by a mechanism distinct from MET channels. Loss of tip links would hyperpolarize hair cells, increasing the electrophoretic driving force from endolymph into hair cells, facilitating aminoglycoside permeation of other non-selective cation channels (Li et al., 2015).

The synergistic ototoxicity of loud sounds and aminoglycosides is not confined to simultaneous exposure. Loud sound exposure weeks prior to treatment with aminoglycosides can also potentiate aminoglycoside-induced hearing loss (Ryan and Bone, 1978). Low doses of aminoglycosides prior to loud sound exposure can *reduce* hearing loss compared to those exposed to loud sounds alone, a phenomenon called preconditioning (Fernandez et al., 2010), yet this is dependent on dosing regimen, age of treatment, anti-oxidant defenses and genetic background (Lautermann and Schacht, 1996; Kopke et al., 1999; Ohlemiller et al., 2011). Identifying the physiologic or genetic mechanisms behind these variations could establish who is at elevated risk of acquired hearing loss. These studies are clinically relevant as aminoglycosides are systemically administered in NICU, where sustained levels of higher ambient sound levels (Williams et al., 2007; Garinis et al., 2017b) could increase the risk of aminoglycoside-induced cochleotoxicity.

CO-THERAPEUTICS THAT POTENTIATE AMINOGLYCOSIDE-INDUCED OTOTOXICITY

Most prominent are the loop diuretics, administered to reduce high blood pressure and edema. In sufficient dosing it will cause temporary, or in some cases permanent, hearing loss. Loop diuretics block Na^+-K^+-Cl^- co-transporter trafficking of potassium into marginal cells, resulting in a loss of the EP (Higashiyama et al., 2003). This drug-induced loss of EP facilitates (by unknown mechanisms) greater entry of aminoglycosides into endolymph, and once the EP is restored, rapid and greater hair cell death (Rybak, 1982; Tran Ba Huy et al., 1983). This outcome is used experimentally to accelerate experimental timeframes in studies of cochlear repair and regeneration processes in mammals (Taylor et al., 2008).

Vancomycin, a glycopeptide antibiotic commonly-prescribed in the NICU (Rubin et al., 2002), can enhance aminoglycoside-induced ototoxicity in preclinical models (Brummett et al., 1990). Vancomycin alone induced acute nephrotoxicity in ~1–9% of neonates (Lestner et al., 2016), yet conflicting evidence for stand-alone vancomycin-induced ototoxicity in humans and preclinical models suggest that potential confounders and clinical settings (e.g., inflammation, see "Inflammation and Aminoglycosides" Section below) need to be considered in the analyses.

INFLAMMATION AND AMINOGLYCOSIDES

Until recently, the inner ear has been considered an immunologically-privileged site, as major components of the inflammatory response (e.g., immune cells, antibodies) are largely excluded by the blood-labyrinth barrier from inner ear tissues (Oh et al., 2012). This barrier is considered to reside at the endothelial cells of the non-fenestrated blood vessels traversing through the inner ear. However, recent pioneering studies show active inner ear participation in classical local and systemic inflammatory mechanisms, with unexpected and unintended consequences.

Middle ear infections increase the permeability of the round window to macromolecules, enabling pro-inflammatory signals and bacterial endotoxins in the middle ear to penetrate the round window into cochlear perilymph (Kawauchi et al., 1989; Ikeda et al., 1990). Spiral ligament fibrocytes lining the scala tympani respond to these immunogenic signals by releasing inflammatory chemokines that attract immune cells to migrate across the blood-labyrinth barrier into the cochlea, especially after hair cell death—another immunogenic signal (Oh et al., 2012; Kaur et al., 2015), and reviewed elsewhere in this Research Topic (Wood and Zuo, 2017). In addition, perivascular macrophages adjacent to cochlear blood vessels (Zhang et al., 2012), and supporting cells in the organ of Corti, exhibit glial-like (anti-inflammatory) phagocytosis of cellular debris following the death of nearby cells (Monzack et al., 2015). These data imply that inner ear tissues can mount a sterile inflammatory response similar to that observed after noise-induced cochlear cell death (Hirose et al., 2005; Fujioka et al., 2014).

In contrast, systemic inflammatory challenges experimentally do not generally modulate auditory function (Hirose et al., 2014b; Koo et al., 2015), with meningitis being a major exception. Nonetheless, systemic inflammation changes cochlear physiology, vasodilating cochlear blood vessels, although the tight junctions between endothelial cells of cochlear capillaries appear to be intact (Koo et al., 2015). Systemic inflammation also induces a 2–3 fold increase in the permeability of the blood-perilymph barrier (Hirose et al., 2014a), and increased cochlear levels of inflammatory markers (Koo et al., 2015). Systemic administration of immunogenic stimuli together with aminoglycosides triggered cochlear recruitment of mononuclear phagocytes into the spiral ligament over several days (Hirose et al., 2014b). Thus, cochlear tissues participate in the systemic inflammatory response induced by systemic immunogenic stimuli, as well as middle ear or intra-cochlear immunogenic stimuli from bacteria or cellular debris.

To date, most studies of aminoglycoside-induced ototoxicity have been conducted in healthy preclinical models, unlike the administration of aminoglycosides to those with severe infections (and consequent inflammation) in clinical settings. Preclinical models with systemic inflammation, induced by low doses of bacterial lipopolysaccharides displayed increased cochlear uptake of aminoglycosides, and enhanced levels of cochleotoxicity without altered serum drug levels (Koo et al., 2015). Inflammation also potentiates cisplatin-induced ototoxicity (Oh et al., 2011). The potential mechanisms by which systemic inflammation enhances aminoglycoside-induced ototoxicity is discussed elsewhere in this Research Topic (Jiang et al., under review). Much further work is required to unravel how inflammation affects: (i) cochlear physiology; and (ii) repair of cochlear lesions following noise exposure or ototoxicity, as discussed elsewhere in this Research Topic (Kalinec et al., 2017).

INTRACELLULAR MECHANISMS OF AMINOGLYCOSIDE COCHLEOTOXICITY

Although molecular mechanisms involving reactive oxygen species, c-Jun N-terminal kinase (JNK) and caspase signaling cascades have been described elsewhere in detail (Ylikoski et al., 2002; Matsui et al., 2004; Lesniak et al., 2005; Coffin et al., 2013), there are still gaps in understanding how aminoglycosides induce cytotoxicity. Below, we focus how mitochondria and endoplasmic reticula (ER) are also primary induction sites for aminoglycoside-induced cytotoxicity.

As antimicrobial agents, aminoglycosides target bacterial ribosomes and induce misreading during protein synthesis (Cox et al., 1964; Davies and Davis, 1968). A genetic study demonstrated that aminoglycoside susceptibility can be transmitted by matrilineal descent, suggesting mitochondrial inheritance (Hu et al., 1991). Analysis of mitochondrial ribosomes revealed that the A1555G polymorphism in 12S rRNA is associated with aminoglycoside-induced hearing loss (Prezant et al., 1993). Other mitochondrial 12S rRNA mutations, including C1494T and T1095C, also increase susceptibility to aminoglycoside ototoxicity (Zhao H. et al., 2004; Zhao L. et al., 2004). Mitochondrial mutations that lead to 12S rRNA binding with a higher affinity to aminoglycosides can cause misreading of the genetic code and mistranslated proteins is a primary mechanism of cytotoxicity (Hobbie et al., 2008; Qian and Guan, 2009). The variety of novel aminoglycoside-interacting proteins involved in mitochondrial respiration, in addition to other ribosomal or nuclear-targeting proteins with a basic-peptide motif, supports the hypothesis that mitochondrial function is a primary site of aminoglycoside-induced cytotoxicity (Kommareddi and Schacht, 2008). Additionally, mutations in *TRMU*, a nuclear modifier gene, can modulate the phenotypic manifestation of deafness-associated 12S rRNA mutations (Guan et al., 2006).

Aminoglycosides also induce ribotoxic stress by binding to cytosolic rRNA to inhibit protein synthesis in eukaryotes (Francis et al., 2013). Aminoglycosides have a higher binding affinity (K_d of 1.7 μM) for the 28S rRNA than for 12S rRNA, a concentration readily reached in hair cells at clinically-relevant concentrations (Marcotti et al., 2005; Francis et al., 2013). Through these mechanisms, aminoglycosides could further inhibit eukaryotic protein synthesis, and activate stress-induced apoptosis mechanisms.

Many cytosolic proteins also bind to aminoglycosides (Karasawa et al., 2010). Calreticulin, an ER chaperone protein (Horibe et al., 2004; Karasawa et al., 2011), assists in protein folding, quality control and degradation (Williams, 2006). Although calreticulin is ubiquitously expressed, it is highly expressed in cochlear marginal cells, and hair cell stereocilia (Karasawa et al., 2011). Calreticulin binds to Ca^{2+} and aminoglycosides at the same site (Karasawa et al., 2011). Aminoglycoside binding to calreticulin likely disrupts the chaperone activity, homeostatic calcium buffering or regulation of calreticulin activity in these cells that becomes cytotoxic (Bastianutto et al., 1995; Mesaeli et al., 1999). Aminoglycosides also dysregulate intracellular Ca^{2+} stores to facilitate toxic transfers of Ca^{2+} from the ER into mitochondria via inositol-1,4,5-triphosphate (IP_3) receptors (Esterberg et al., 2013). This, in turn, elevates mitochondrial Ca^{2+} that underlies elevated levels of both mitochondrial oxidation and cytoplasmic ROS prior to cell death (Esterberg et al., 2016).

Aminoglycosides can bind to another ER protein, CLIMP-63 (Karasawa et al., 2010), thought to anchor microtubules to the ER (Sandoz and van der Goot, 2015). CLIMP-63 is highly expressed in cultured HEI-OC1 cells derived from the murine organ of Corti. Aminoglycosides oligomerize CLIMP-63 that then bind to 14-3-3 proteins; knockdown of either CLIMP-63 or 14-3-3β suppressed aminoglycoside-induced apoptosis (Karasawa et al., 2010). 14-3-3 proteins are implicated in both pro- and anti-apoptosis mechanisms that involve p53, tumor suppressor gene, and binding of 14-3-3 proteins to MDMX, a negative regulator of p53, induces apoptosis (Okamoto et al., 2005). Thus, aminoglycoside binding to CLIMP-63 may promote p53-dependent apoptosis via 14-3-3 inhibition of MDMX.

POTENTIAL CLINICAL APPROACHES TO REDUCE AMINOGLYCOSIDE UPTAKE OR OTOTOXICITY

Over 5% of the world's population, ~360 million people, have hearing loss (WHO, 2012; Blackwell et al., 2014). Two major otoprotective strategies against aminoglycoside-induced hearing loss have been proposed. One is to reduce drug uptake by cells to prevent cytotoxicity; another is to interfere with mechanisms of aminoglycoside-induced cytotoxicity.

Reducing Cellular Uptake of Aminoglycosides

In the NICU, aminoglycosides, especially gentamicin, are often obligatory treatments to treat life-threatening sepsis (Cross et al., 2015). NICU environments have loud ambient sound levels (Williams et al., 2007; Garinis et al., 2017b), and a significantly increased incidence of hearing loss in NICU graduates (Yoon et al., 2003) that may be due to the synergistic effect of ambient sound levels increasing cochlear uptake of aminoglycosides (Li et al., 2015). Thus, efforts to reduce ambient sound levels in the NICU will be welcomed.

Inflammation caused by severe bacterial infections also increase cochlear uptake of aminoglycosides and subsequent ototoxicity (Koo et al., 2015). Administration of anti-inflammatory agents prior to or during aminoglycoside treatment may be effective as for etanercept, an antibody, that blocks the pro-inflammatory signaling receptor TNFα, in ameliorating noise-induced hearing loss (Arpornchayanon et al., 2013). Etanercept and perhaps other anti-inflammatory agents can reduce cochlear inflammation (Satoh et al., 2002), and could also reduce cochlear uptake of aminoglycosides, to better preserve auditory function, similar to glucocorticoids restoring auditory function by improving the ion homeostatic (mineralocorticoid) activity of the blood-labyrinth barrier (MacArthur et al., 2015).

The zebrafish lateral line is an excellent model to conduct high throughput screening of compounds that protect hair cells from ototoxicity (Harris et al., 2003). A recent screening of over 500 natural compounds identified four novel bisbenzylisoquinoline derivatives, berbamine, E6 berbamine, hernandezine, and isotetrandrine, as otoprotective agents that reduce hair cell uptake of aminoglycosides (Kruger et al., 2016; Kirkwood et al., 2017). Since these compounds block the aminoglycoside-permeant MET channels, these drugs are also expected be effective in reducing mammalian hair cell uptake of aminoglycosides *in vitro*, yet, verification is crucial (Majumder et al., 2017). It is also crucial to test *in vivo* following local or systemic administration to ensure these compounds can enter the compartmentalized endolymphatic fluids.

Reducing Aminoglycoside Cytotoxicity

Several anti-oxidants like *N*-acetylcysteine, D-methionine and edaravone reduce aminoglycoside-induced ototoxicity in preclinical models (Somdaş et al., 2015; Campbell et al., 2016; Turan et al., 2017), suggesting that drug-induced generation of reactive oxygen species leads to aminoglycoside-induced ototoxicity. Several anti-oxidants show otoprotection against both aminoglycosides and cisplatin, implying that induction of oxidative stress is a shared mechanism of cytotoxicity for these ototoxins (Lorito et al., 2011; Tate et al., 2017). If this is the case, then dosing regimens reducing cisplatin-induced ototoxicity may also translate to being otoprotective for aminoglycoside-induced ototoxicity. An *in vitro* screen to test for the otoprotective (or ototoxic) properties of antioxidants in the organ of Corti explants is described elsewhere in this Research Topic (Noack et al., 2017).

Another innovative strategy is to develop aminoglycosides like apramycin with minimal affinity for eukaryotic mitochondrial ribosomes while retaining strong activity against clinical pathogens (Matt et al., 2012). An alternative, pioneering method is to modify specific amine groups of sisomicin (a biosynthetic precursor of gentamicin), generating several designer aminoglycosides. One modified aminoglycoside, N1MS, displayed significantly reduced ototoxicity while retaining bactericidal efficacy in preclinical models (Huth et al., 2015).

Acetylation of histones, proteins required for chromatin regulation of gene transcription, is associated with gene transcription activation, and histone deacetylases (HDACs) regulate this process. Aminoglycosides also hypo-acetylate histones, reducing transcription factor binding to DNA, causing decreased levels of gene expression (Chen et al., 2009). Since HDACs remove histone acetylation, inhibitors of HDACs were found to provide otoprotection in cochlear explants (Chen et al., 2009), but not *in vivo* (Yang et al., 2017). In contrast, systemic HDAC inhibition using suberoylanilide hydroxamic acid (SAHA) resulted in almost complete protection against *combined* kanamycin and furosemide-induced ototoxicity, and this mechanism involved activating the NF-κB pathway (Layman et al., 2015), indicating that verification of candidate otoprotective agents requires testing in models that more closely resemble clinical situations, i.e., chronic dosing with aminoglycosides, preferably in the setting of inflammation (Koo et al., 2015). In the same vein, interfering with cell death signaling pathways also promoted acute hair cell survival and attenuated drug-induced hearing loss following chronic aminoglycoside dosing (Ylikoski et al., 2002).

Another promising approach involves activating heat shock proteins (HSPs), including HSP70, to promote hair cell survival against aminoglycoside ototoxicity (Taleb et al., 2008). Heat shock induces expression and secretion of HSP70 by supporting cells to effect otoprotection of hair cells (May et al., 2013). Intriguingly, exposure to sound sufficient to transiently stress the cochlea (without inducing permanent hearing loss, i.e., preconditioning) upregulated the expression of HSP70 (and HSP32) expression to significantly reduce aminoglycoside-induced hearing loss in preclinical models (Roy et al., 2013). Further discussion of the pro-survival and cell death factors influencing hair cell survival and hair cell death via autonomous and non-autonomous mechanisms are discussed elsewhere in this Research Topic (Francis and Cunningham, 2017).

CONCLUSION

Aminoglycoside antibiotics remain crucial pharmacotherapeutics for severe bacterial infections, despite their known side effects and the emergence of other (more labile) classes of broad-spectrum antibiotics. Aminoglycosides are also preferred due to their robust stability at ambient temperatures when used by itinerant healthcare providers in the field, and because of their bactericidal efficacy against bacteria resistant to other antibiotics. Increasing our understanding of aminoglycoside-induced (oto)toxicity requires greater insight into the mechanisms of cellular uptake kinetics, transcellular trafficking and intracellular disruption of physiological activities by aminoglycosides, especially in models that better mimic clinical settings such as exposure to higher levels of ambient sounds, co-therapeutics and/or inflammation that potentiate the degree of ototoxicity. Modifying dosing protocols, the structure of current aminoglycosides, and/or increased verification of candidate otoprotective agents could all enable aminoglycosides to be used more readily with reduced risks of lifelong ototoxicity in hospital.

AUTHOR CONTRIBUTIONS

This review was conceived, written and edited by each of the authors (MJ, TK and PSS).

ACKNOWLEDGMENTS

This work was supported by R01 awards (DC004555, DC12588) from the National Institute of Deafness and Other Communication Disorders. The illustrations were designed and drafted by Karen Thiebes, Simplified Science Publishing, LLC. The content is solely the responsibility of the authors and do not represent the official views of the NIH, Oregon Health and Science University or the VA Portland Health Care System.

REFERENCES

Alharazneh, A., Luk, L., Huth, M., Monfared, A., Steyger, P. S., Cheng, A. G., et al. (2011). Functional hair cell mechanotransducer channels are required for aminoglycoside ototoxicity. *PLoS One* 6:e22347. doi: 10.1371/journal.pone.0022347

Al-Malky, G., Dawson, S. J., Sirimanna, T., Bagkeris, E., and Suri, R. (2015). High-frequency audiometry reveals high prevalence of aminoglycoside ototoxicity in children with cystic fibrosis. *J. Cyst. Fibros.* 14, 248–254. doi: 10.1016/j.jcf.2014.07.009

Ando, M., Edamatsu, M., Fukuizumi, S., and Takeuchi, S. (2008). Cellular localization of facilitated glucose transporter 1 (GLUT-1) in the cochlear stria vascularis: its possible contribution to the transcellular glucose pathway. *Cell Tissue Res.* 331, 763–769. doi: 10.1007/s00441-007-0495-2

Ariano, R. E., Zelenitsky, S. A., and Kassum, D. A. (2008). Aminoglycoside-induced vestibular injury: maintaining a sense of balance. *Ann. Pharmacother.* 42, 1282–1289. doi: 10.1345/aph.1L001

Arpornchayanon, W., Canis, M., Ihler, F., Settevendemie, C., and Strieth, S. (2013). TNF-α inhibition using etanercept prevents noise-induced hearing loss by improvement of cochlear blood flow *in vivo*. *Int. J. Audiol.* 52, 545–552. doi: 10.3109/14992027.2013.790564

Avan, P., Erre, J. P., da Costa, D. L., Aran, J. M., and Popelar, J. (1996). The efferent-mediated suppression of otoacoustic emissions in awake guinea pigs and its reversible blockage by gentamicin. *Exp. Brain Res.* 109, 9–16. doi: 10.1007/bf00228621

Banke, T. G. (2011). The dilated TRPA1 channel pore state is blocked by amiloride and analogues. *Brain Res.* 1381, 21–30. doi: 10.1016/j.brainres.2011.01.021

Baradaran-Heravi, A., Niesser, J., Balgi, A. D., Choi, K., Zimmerman, C., South, A. P., et al. (2017). Gentamicin B1 is a minor gentamicin component with major nonsense mutation suppression activity. *Proc. Natl. Acad. Sci. U S A* 114, 3479–3484. doi: 10.1073/pnas.1620982114

Bastianutto, C., Clementi, E., Codazzi, F., Podini, P., De Giorgi, F., Rizzuto, R., et al. (1995). Overexpression of calreticulin increases the Ca^{2+} capacity of rapidly exchanging Ca^{2+} stores and reveals aspects of their lumenal microenvironment and function. *J. Cell Biol.* 130, 847–855. doi: 10.1083/jcb.130.4.847

Bautista, D., and Julius, D. (2008). Fire in the hole: pore dilation of the capsaicin receptor TRPV1. *Nat. Neurosci.* 11, 528–529. doi: 10.1038/nn0508-528

Belyantseva, I. A., Adler, H. J., Curi, R., Frolenkov, G. I., and Kachar, B. (2000). Expression and localization of prestin and the sugar transporter GLUT-5 during development of electromotility in cochlear outer hair cells. *J. Neurosci.* 20:RC116.

Bessac, B. F., Sivula, M., von Hehn, C. A., Escalera, J., Cohn, L., and Jordt, S. E. (2008). TRPA1 is a major oxidant sensor in murine airway sensory neurons. *J. Clin. Invest.* 118, 1899–1910. doi: 10.1172/JCI34192

Blackwell, D. L., Lucas, J. W., and Clarke, T. C. (2014). Summary health statistics for U.S. adults: national health interview survey, 2012. *Vital Health Stat.* 10, 1–161.

Blanchet, C., Erostegui, C., Sugasawa, M., and Dulon, D. (2000). Gentamicin blocks ACh-evoked K^{+} current in guinea-pig outer hair cells by impairing Ca^{2+} entry at the cholinergic receptor. *J. Physiol.* 525, 641–654. doi: 10.1111/j.1469-7793.2000.t01-1-00641.x

Bohne, B. A., Harding, G. W., and Lee, S. C. (2007). Death pathways in noise-damaged outer hair cells. *Hear. Res.* 223, 61–70. doi: 10.1016/j.heares.2006.10.004

Brown, J. J., Brummett, R. E., Meikle, M. B., and Vernon, J. (1978). Combined effects of noise and neomycin. Cochlear changes in the guinea pig. *Acta Otolaryngol.* 86, 394–400. doi: 10.3109/00016487809107518

Brummett, R. E., Fox, K. E., Jacobs, F., Kempton, J. B., Stokes, Z., and Richmond, A. B. (1990). Augmented gentamicin ototoxicity induced by vancomycin in guinea pigs. *Arch. Otolaryngol. Head Neck Surg.* 116, 61–64. doi: 10.1001/archotol.1990.01870010065019

Campbell, K. C., Martin, S. M., Meech, R. P., Hargrove, T. L., Verhulst, S. J., and Fox, D. J. (2016). D-methionine (D-met) significantly reduces kanamycin-induced ototoxicity in pigmented guinea pigs. *Int. J. Audiol.* 55, 273–278. doi: 10.3109/14992027.2016.1143980

Caterina, M. J., Schumacher, M. A., Tominaga, M., Rosen, T. A., Levine, J. D., and Julius, D. (1997). The capsaicin receptor: a heat-activated ion channel in the pain pathway. *Nature* 389, 816–824. doi: 10.1038/39807

Chen, F. Q., Schacht, J., and Sha, S. H. (2009). Aminoglycoside-induced histone deacetylation and hair cell death in the mouse cochlea. *J. Neurochem.* 108, 1226–1236. doi: 10.1111/j.1471-4159.2009.05871.x

Christensen, E. I., and Nielsen, R. (2007). Role of megalin and cubilin in renal physiology and pathophysiology. *Rev. Physiol. Biochem. Pharmacol.* 158, 1–22. doi: 10.1007/112_0604

Coffin, A. B., Reinhart, K. E., Owens, K. N., Raible, D. W., and Rubel, E. W. (2009). Extracellular divalent cations modulate aminoglycoside-induced hair cell death in the zebrafish lateral line. *Hear. Res.* 253, 42–51. doi: 10.1016/j.heares.2009.03.004

Coffin, A. B., Williamson, K. L., Mamiya, A., Raible, D. W., and Rubel, E. W. (2013). Profiling drug-induced cell death pathways in the zebrafish lateral line. *Apoptosis* 18, 393–408. doi: 10.1007/s10495-013-0816-8

Cox, E. C., White, J. R., and Flaks, J. G. (1964). Streptomycin action and the ribosome. *Proc. Natl. Acad. Sci. U S A* 51, 703–709. doi: 10.1073/pnas.51.4.703

Cross, C. P., Liao, S., Urdang, Z. D., Srikanth, P., Garinis, A. C., and Steyger, P. S. (2015). Effect of sepsis and systemic inflammatory response syndrome on neonatal hearing screening outcomes following gentamicin exposure. *Int. J. Pediatr. Otorhinolaryngol.* 79, 1915–1919. doi: 10.1016/j.ijporl.2015.09.004

Crumling, M. A., Tong, M., Aschenbach, K. L., Liu, L. Q., Pipitone, C. M., and Duncan, R. K. (2009). P2X antagonists inhibit styryl dye entry into hair cells. *Neuroscience* 161, 1144–1153. doi: 10.1016/j.neuroscience.2009.02.076

Dai, C. F., Mangiardi, D., Cotanche, D. A., and Steyger, P. S. (2006). Uptake of fluorescent gentamicin by vertebrate sensory cells *in vivo*. *Hear. Res.* 213, 64–78. doi: 10.1016/j.heares.2005.11.011

Dallos, P., and Harris, D. (1978). Properties of auditory nerve responses in absence of outer hair cells. *J. Neurophysiol.* 41, 365–383.

Davies, J., and Davis, B. D. (1968). Misreading of ribonucleic acid code words induced by aminoglycoside antibiotics. The effect of drug concentration. *J. Biol. Chem.* 243, 3312–3316.

Dressel, D. C., Tornatore-Reuscher, M. A., Boschman, C. R., Stosor, V., Zembower, T., Postelnick, M. J., et al. (1999). Synergistic effect of gentamicin plus ampicillin on enterococci with differing sensitivity to gentamicin: a phenotypic assessment of NCCLS guidelines. *Diagn. Microbiol. Infect. Dis.* 35, 219–225. doi: 10.1016/s0732-8893(99)00088-7

Du, M., Keeling, K. M., Fan, L., Liu, X., Kovaçs, T., Sorscher, E., et al. (2006). Clinical doses of amikacin provide more effective suppression of the human CFTR-G542X stop mutation than gentamicin in a transgenic CF mouse model. *J. Mol. Med. (Berl)* 84, 573–582. doi: 10.1007/s00109-006-0045-5

Esterberg, R., Hailey, D. W., Coffin, A. B., Raible, D. W., and Rubel, E. W. (2013). Disruption of intracellular calcium regulation is integral to aminoglycoside-induced hair cell death. *J. Neurosci.* 33, 7513–7525. doi: 10.1523/JNEUROSCI.4559-12.2013

Esterberg, R., Linbo, T., Pickett, S. B., Wu, P., Ou, H. C., Rubel, E. W., et al. (2016). Mitochondrial calcium uptake underlies ROS generation during aminoglycoside-induced hair cell death. *J. Clin. Invest.* 126, 3556–3566. doi: 10.1172/JCI84939

Farris, H. E., Wells, G. B., and Ricci, A. J. (2006). Steady-state adaptation of mechanotransduction modulates the resting potential of auditory hair cells, providing an assay for endolymph $[Ca^{2+}]$. *J. Neurosci.* 26, 12526–12536. doi: 10.1523/JNEUROSCI.3569-06.2006

Fernandez, E. A., Ohlemiller, K. K., Gagnon, P. M., and Clark, W. W. (2010). Protection against noise-induced hearing loss in young CBA/J mice by low-dose kanamycin. *J. Assoc. Res. Otolaryngol.* 11, 235–244. doi: 10.1007/s10162-009-0204-9

Forge, A., and Schacht, J. (2000). Aminoglycoside antibiotics. *Audiol. Neurootol.* 5, 3–22. doi: 10.1159/000013861

Francis, S. P., and Cunningham, L. L. (2017). Non-autonomous cellular responses to ototoxic drug-induced stress and death. *Front. Cell. Neurosci.* 11:252. doi: 10.3389/fncel.2017.00252

Francis, S. P., Katz, J., Fanning, K. D., Harris, K. A., Nicholas, B. D., Lacy, M., et al. (2013). A novel role of cytosolic protein synthesis inhibition in aminoglycoside ototoxicity. *J. Neurosci.* 33, 3079–3093. doi: 10.1523/JNEUROSCI.3430-12.2013

Fujioka, M., Okano, H., and Ogawa, K. (2014). Inflammatory and immune responses in the cochlea: potential therapeutic targets for sensorineural hearing loss. *Front. Pharmacol.* 5:287. doi: 10.3389/fphar.2014.00287

Garinis, A. C., Cross, C. P., Srikanth, P., Carroll, K., Feeney, M. P., Keefe, D. H., et al. (2017a). The cumulative effects of intravenous antibiotic treatments on hearing in patients with cystic fibrosis. *J. Cyst. Fibros.* 16, 401–409. doi: 10.1016/j.jcf.2017.01.006

Garinis, A. C., Liao, S., Cross, C. P., Galati, J., Middaugh, J. L., Mace, J. C., et al. (2017b). Effect of gentamicin and levels of ambient sound on hearing screening outcomes in the neonatal intensive care unit: a pilot study. *Int. J. Pediatr. Otorhinolaryngol.* 97, 42–50. doi: 10.1016/j.ijporl.2017.03.025

Ghosh, R. K., Ghosh, S. M., Chawla, S., and Jasdanwala, S. A. (2012). SGLT2 inhibitors: a new emerging therapeutic class in the treatment of type 2 diabetes mellitus. *J. Clin. Pharmacol.* 52, 457–463. doi: 10.1177/0091270011400604

Gratton, M. A., Rao, V. H., Meehan, D. T., Askew, C., and Cosgrove, D. (2005). Matrix metalloproteinase dysregulation in the stria vascularis of mice with

Alport syndrome: implications for capillary basement membrane pathology *Am. J. Pathol.* 166, 1465–1474. doi: 10.1016/s0002-9440(10)62363-2

Guan, M. X., Yan, Q., Li, X., Bykhovskaya, Y., Gallo-Teran, J., Hajek, P., et al. (2006). Mutation in TRMU related to transfer RNA modification modulates the phenotypic expression of the deafness-associated mitochondrial 12S ribosomal RNA mutations. *Am. J. Hum. Genet.* 79, 291–302. doi: 10.1086/506389

Hackney, C. M., Furness, D. N., and Steyger, P. S. (1990). "Structural abnormalities in inner hair cells following kanamycin-induced outer hair cell loss," in *Mechanics and Biophysics of Hearing. Lecture Notes in Biomathematics*, (Vol. 87) eds P. Dallos, C. D. Geisler, J. W. Matthews, M. Ruggero and C. R. Steele (New York, NY: Springer), 10–17.

Hailey, D. W., Esterberg, R., Linbo, T. H., Rubel, E. W., and Raible, D. W. (2017). Fluorescent aminoglycosides reveal intracellular trafficking routes in mechanosensory hair cells. *J. Clin. Invest.* 127, 472–486. doi: 10.1172/JCI85052

Halsey, K., Skjönsberg, A., Ulfendahl, M., and Dolan, D. F. (2005). Efferent-mediated adaptation of the DPOAE as a predictor of aminoglycoside toxicity. *Hear. Res.* 201, 99–108. doi: 10.1016/j.heares.2004.09.010

Harris, J. A., Cheng, A. G., Cunningham, L. L., MacDonald, G., Raible, D. W., and Rubel, E. W. (2003). Neomycin-induced hair cell death and rapid regeneration in the lateral line of zebrafish (Danio rerio). *J. Assoc. Res. Otolaryngol.* 4, 219–234. doi: 10.1007/s10162-002-3022-x

Hashino, E., Shero, M., and Salvi, R. J. (1997). Lysosomal targeting and accumulation of aminoglycoside antibiotics in sensory hair cells. *Brain Res.* 777, 75–85. doi: 10.1016/s0006-8993(97)00977-3

Henderson, D., Bielefeld, E. C., Harris, K. C., and Hu, B. H. (2006). The role of oxidative stress in noise-induced hearing loss. *Ear Hear.* 27, 1–19. doi: 10.1097/01.aud.0000191942.36672.f3

Hiel, H., Erre, J. P., Aurousseau, C., Bouali, R., Dulon, D., and Aran, J. M. (1993). Gentamicin uptake by cochlear hair cells precedes hearing impairment during chronic treatment. *Audiology* 32, 78–87. doi: 10.3109/00206099309072930

Higashiyama, K., Takeuchi, S., Azuma, H., Sawada, S., Yamakawa, K., Kakigi, A., et al. (2003). Bumetanide-induced enlargement of the intercellular space in the stria vascularis critically depends on Na^+ transport. *Hear. Res.* 186, 1–9. doi: 10.1016/s0378-5955(03)00226-0

Hirose, K., Discolo, C. M., Keasler, J. R., and Ransohoff, R. (2005). Mononuclear phagocytes migrate into the murine cochlea after acoustic trauma. *J. Comp. Neurol.* 489, 180–194. doi: 10.1002/cne.20619

Hirose, K., Hartsock, J. J., Johnson, S., Santi, P., and Salt, A. N. (2014a). Systemic lipopolysaccharide compromises the blood-labyrinth barrier and increases entry of serum fluorescein into the perilymph. *J. Assoc. Res. Otolaryngol.* 15, 707–719. doi: 10.1007/s10162-014-0476-6

Hirose, K., Li, S. Z., Ohlemiller, K. K., and Ransohoff, R. M. (2014b). Systemic lipopolysaccharide induces cochlear inflammation and exacerbates the synergistic ototoxicity of kanamycin and furosemide. *J. Assoc. Res. Otolaryngol.* 15, 555–570. doi: 10.1007/s10162-014-0458-8

Hobbie, S. N., Bruell, C. M., Akshay, S., Kalapala, S. K., Shcherbakov, D., and Böttger, E. C. (2008). Mitochondrial deafness alleles confer misreading of the genetic code. *Proc. Natl. Acad. Sci. U S A* 105, 3244–3249. doi: 10.1073/pnas.0707265105

Horibe, T., Matsui, H., Tanaka, M., Nagai, H., Yamaguchi, Y., Kato, K., et al. (2004). Gentamicin binds to the lectin site of calreticulin and inhibits its chaperone activity. *Biochem. Biophys. Res. Commun.* 323, 281–287. doi: 10.1016/j.bbrc.2004.08.099

Hu, D. N., Qui, W. Q., Wu, B. T., Fang, L. Z., Zhou, F., Gu, Y. P., et al. (1991). Genetic aspects of antibiotic induced deafness: mitochondrial inheritance. *J. Med. Genet.* 28, 79–83. doi: 10.1136/jmg.28.2.79

Humes, H. D. (1999). Insights into ototoxicity. Analogies to nephrotoxicity. *Ann. N Y Acad. Sci.* 884, 15–18. doi: 10.1111/j.1749-6632.1999.tb00278.x

Husbands, J. M., Steinberg, S. A., Kurian, R., and Saunders, J. C. (1999). Tip-link integrity on chick tall hair cell stereocilia following intense sound exposure. *Hear. Res.* 135, 135–145. doi: 10.1016/s0378-5955(99)00101-x

Huth, M. E., Han, K. H., Sotoudeh, K., Hsieh, Y. J., Effertz, T., Vu, A. A., et al. (2015). Designer aminoglycosides prevent cochlear hair cell loss and hearing loss. *J. Clin. Invest.* 125, 583–592. doi: 10.1172/JCI77424

Ikeda, K., Sakagami, M., Morizono, T., and Juhn, S. K. (1990). Permeability of the round window membrane to middle-sized molecules in purulent otitis media. *Arch. Otolaryngol. Head Neck Surg.* 116, 57–60. doi: 10.1001/archotol.1990.01870010061018

Imamura, S., and Adams, J. C. (2003). Distribution of gentamicin in the guinea pig inner ear after local or systemic application. *J. Assoc. Res. Otolaryngol.* 4, 176–195. doi: 10.1007/s10162-002-2036-8

Izzedine, H., Tankere, F., Launay-Vacher, V., and Deray, G. (2004). Ear and kidney syndromes: molecular versus clinical approach. *Kidney Int.* 65, 369–385. doi: 10.1111/j.1523-1755.2004.00390.x

Jara-Oseguera, A., Llorente, I., Rosenbaum, T., and Islas, L. D. (2008). Properties of the inner pore region of TRPV1 channels revealed by block with quaternary ammoniums. *J. Gen. Physiol.* 132, 547–562. doi: 10.1085/jgp.200810051

Järvelin, M. R., Mäki-Torkko, E., Sorri, M. J., and Rantakallio, P. T. (1997). Effect of hearing impairment on educational outcomes and employment up to the age of 25 years in northern Finland. *Br. J. Audiol.* 31, 165–175. doi: 10.3109/03005364000000019

Jiang, M., Wang, Q., Karasawa, T., Koo, J. W., Li, H., and Steyger, P. S. (2014). Sodium-glucose transporter-2 (SGLT2; SLC5A2) enhances cellular uptake of aminoglycosides. *PLoS One* 9:e108941. doi: 10.1371/journal.pone.0108941

Jones, E. M., and White, A. J. (1990). Mental health and acquired hearing impairment: a review. *Br. J. Audiol.* 24, 3–9. doi: 10.3109/03005369009077837

Kalinec, G., Lomberk, L., Urrutia, R., and Kalinec, F. (2017). Resolution of cochlear inflammation: novel target for preventing or ameliorating drug-, noise- and age-related hearing loss. *Front. Cell. Neurosci.* 11:192. doi: 10.3389/fncel.2017.00192

Kanai, Y., Lee, W. S., You, G., Brown, D., and Hediger, M. A. (1994). The human kidney low affinity Na^+/glucose cotransporter SGLT2. Delineation of the major renal reabsorptive mechanism for D-glucose. *J. Clin. Invest.* 93, 397–404. doi: 10.1172/jci116972

Kang, H. S., Kerstan, D., Dai, L., Ritchie, G., and Quamme, G. A. (2000). Aminoglycosides inhibit hormone-stimulated Mg^{2+} uptake in mouse distal convoluted tubule cells. *Can. J. Physiol. Pharmacol.* 78, 595–602. doi: 10.1139/y00-038

Karasawa, T., Wang, Q., David, L. L., and Steyger, P. S. (2010). CLIMP-63 is a gentamicin-binding protein that is involved in drug-induced cytotoxicity. *Cell Death Dis.* 1:e102. doi: 10.1038/cddis.2010.80

Karasawa, T., Wang, Q., David, L. L., and Steyger, P. S. (2011). Calreticulin binds to gentamicin and reduces drug-induced ototoxicity. *Toxicol. Sci.* 124, 378–387. doi: 10.1093/toxsci/kfr196

Karasawa, T., Wang, Q., Fu, Y., Cohen, D. M., and Steyger, P. S. (2008). TRPV4 enhances the cellular uptake of aminoglycoside antibiotics. *J. Cell Sci.* 121, 2871–2879. doi: 10.1242/jcs.023705

Karashima, Y., Prenen, J., Talavera, K., Janssens, A., Voets, T., and Nilius, B. (2010). Agonist-induced changes in Ca^{2+} permeation through the nociceptor cation channel TRPA1. *Biophys. J.* 98, 773–783. doi: 10.1016/j.bpj.2009.11.007

Kaur, T., Zamani, D., Tong, L., Rubel, E. W., Ohlemiller, K. K., Hirose, K., et al. (2015). Fractalkine signaling regulates macrophage recruitment into the cochlea and promotes the survival of spiral ganglion neurons after selective hair cell lesion. *J. Neurosci.* 35, 15050–15061. doi: 10.1523/JNEUROSCI.2325-15.2015

Kawaguchi, H., Naito, T., Nakagawa, S., and Fujisawa, K. I. (1972). BB-K 8, a new semisynthetic aminoglycoside antibiotic. *J. Antibiot.* 25, 695–708. doi: 10.7164/antibiotics.25.695

Kawashima, Y., Géléoc, G. S., Kurima, K., Labay, V., Lelli, A., Asai, Y., et al. (2011). Mechanotransduction in mouse inner ear hair cells requires transmembrane channel-like genes. *J. Clin. Invest.* 121, 4796–4809. doi: 10.1172/JCI60405

Kawauchi, H., Demaria, T. F., and Lim, D. J. (1989). Endotoxin permeability through the round window. *Acta Otolaryngol. Suppl.* 457, 100–115. doi: 10.3109/00016488809138892

Kirkwood, N. K., O'reilly, M., Derudas, M., Kenyon, E. J., Huckvale, R., Van Netten, S. M., et al. (2017). d-Tubocurarine and berbamine: alkaloids that are permeant blockers of the hair cell's mechano-electrical transducer channel and protect from aminoglycoside toxicity. *Front. Cell. Neurosci.* 11:262. doi: 10.3389/fncel.2017.00262

Kitahara, T., Li, H. S., and Balaban, C. D. (2005). Changes in transient receptor potential cation channel superfamily V (TRPV) mRNA expression in the mouse inner ear ganglia after kanamycin challenge. *Hear. Res.* 201, 132–144. doi: 10.1016/j.heares.2004.09.007

Kommareddi, P., and Schacht, J. (2008). Novel aminoglycoside-interacting proteins. *ARO Midwint. Meet. Abst.* 31:721.

Köonig, O., Rüttiger, L., Müller, M., Zimmermann, U., Erdmann, B., Kalbacher, H., et al. (2008). Estrogen and the inner ear: megalin knockout mice suffer progressive hearing loss. *FASEB J.* 22, 410–417. doi: 10.1096/fj.07-9171com

Koo, J. W., Quintanilla-Dieck, L., Jiang, M., Liu, J., Urdang, Z. D., Allensworth, J. J., et al. (2015). Endotoxemia-mediated inflammation potentiates aminoglycoside-induced ototoxicity. *Sci. Transl. Med.* 7:298ra118. doi: 10.1126/scitranslmed.aac5546

Kopke, R., Allen, K. A., Henderson, D., Hoffer, M., Frenz, D., and Van de Water, T. (1999). A radical demise. Toxins and trauma share common pathways in hair cell death. *Ann. N Y Acad. Sci.* 884, 171–191. doi: 10.1111/j.1749-6632.1999.tb08641.x

Kramer, B. K., Bergler, T., Stoelcker, B., and Waldegger, S. (2008). Mechanisms of Disease: the kidney-specific chloride channels ClCKA and ClCKB, the Barttin subunit, and their clinical relevance. *Nat. Clin. Pract. Nephrol.* 4, 38–46. doi: 10.1038/ncpneph0689

Kroemer, G., and Jäättelä, M. (2005). Lysosomes and autophagy in cell death control. *Nat. Rev. Cancer* 5, 886–897. doi: 10.1038/nrc1738

Kroese, A. B., Das, A., and Hudspeth, A. J. (1989). Blockage of the transduction channels of hair cells in the bullfrog's sacculus by aminoglycoside antibiotics. *Hear. Res.* 37, 203–217. doi: 10.1016/0378-5955(89)90023-3

Kros, C. J., Marcotti, W., van Netten, S. M., Self, T. J., Libby, R. T., Brown, S. D., et al. (2002). Reduced climbing and increased slipping adaptation in cochlear hair cells of mice with Myo7a mutations. *Nat. Neurosci.* 5, 41–47. doi: 10.1038/nn784

Kruger, M., Boney, R., Ordoobadi, A. J., Sommers, T. F., Trapani, J. G., and Coffin, A. B. (2016). Natural bizbenzoquinoline derivatives protect zebrafish lateral line sensory hair cells from aminoglycoside toxicity. *Front. Cell. Neurosci.* 10:83. doi: 10.3389/fncel.2016.00083

Kujawa, S. G., and Liberman, M. C. (2015). Synaptopathy in the noise-exposed and aging cochlea: primary neural degeneration in acquired sensorineural hearing loss. *Hear. Res.* 330, 191–199. doi: 10.1016/j.heares.2015.02.009

Kurian, R., Krupp, N. L., and Saunders, J. C. (2003). Tip link loss and recovery on chick short hair cells following intense exposure to sound. *Hear. Res.* 181, 40–50. doi: 10.1016/s0378-5955(03)00165-5

Kwan, K. Y., Allchorne, A. J., Vollrath, M. A., Christensen, A. P., Zhang, D. S., Woolf, C. J., et al. (2006). TRPA1 contributes to cold, mechanical, and chemical nociception but is not essential for hair-cell transduction. *Neuron* 50, 277–289. doi: 10.1016/j.neuron.2006.03.042

Lautermann, J., and Schacht, J. (1996). A sensitive animal model to assess acute and chronic ototoxic effects. *Arch. Otolaryngol. Head Neck Surg.* 122, 837–840. doi: 10.1001/archotol.1996.01890200027005

Layman, W. S., Williams, D. M., Dearman, J. A., Sauceda, M. A., and Zuo, J. (2015). Histone deacetylase inhibition protects hearing against acute ototoxicity by activating the Nf-kappaB pathway. *Cell Death Discov.* 1:15012. doi: 10.1038/cddiscovery.2015.12

Leonova, E. V., and Raphael, Y. (1997). Organization of cell junctions and cytoskeleton in the reticular lamina in normal and ototoxically damaged organ of Corti. *Hear. Res.* 113, 14–28. doi: 10.1016/s0378-5955(97)00130-5

Lesniak, W., Pecoraro, V. L., and Schacht, J. (2005). Ternary complexes of gentamicin with iron and lipid catalyze formation of reactive oxygen species. *Chem. Res. Toxicol.* 18, 357–364. doi: 10.1021/tx0496946

Lestner, J. M., Hill, L. F., Heath, P. T., and Sharland, M. (2016). Vancomycin toxicity in neonates: a review of the evidence. *Curr. Opin. Infect. Dis.* 29, 237–247. doi: 10.1097/QCO.0000000000000263

Li, H., Kachelmeier, A., Furness, D. N., and Steyger, P. S. (2015). Local mechanisms for loud sound-enhanced aminoglycoside entry into outer hair cells. *Front. Cell. Neurosci.* 9:130. doi: 10.3389/fncel.2015.00130

Li, H., and Steyger, P. S. (2011). Systemic aminoglycosides are trafficked via endolymph into cochlear hair cells. *Sci. Rep.* 1:159. doi: 10.1038/srep00159

Liedtke, W., Choe, Y., Marti-Renom, M. A., Bell, A. M., Denis, C. S., Sali, A., et al. (2000). Vanilloid receptor-related osmotically activated channel (VR-OAC), a candidate vertebrate osmoreceptor. *Cell* 103, 525–535. doi: 10.1016/s0092-8674(00)00143-4

Liu, X., Mohamed, J. A., and Ruan, R. (2004). Analysis of differential gene expression in the cochlea and kidney of mouse by cDNA microarrays. *Hear. Res.* 197, 35–43. doi: 10.1016/j.heares.2004.04.014

Lorito, G., Hatzopoulos, S., Laurell, G., Campbell, K. C., Petruccelli, J., Giordano, P., et al. (2011). Dose-dependent protection on cisplatin-induced ototoxicity—an electrophysiological study on the effect of three antioxidants in the Sprague-Dawley rat animal model. *Med. Sci. Monit.* 17, BR179–BR186. doi: 10.12659/msm.881894

MacArthur, C., Hausman, F., Kempton, B., and Trune, D. R. (2015). Intratympanic steroid treatments may improve hearing via ion homeostasis alterations and not immune suppression. *Otol. Neurotol.* 36, 1089–1095. doi: 10.1097/MAO.0000000000000725

Macpherson, L. J., Xiao, B., Kwan, K. Y., Petrus, M. J., Dubin, A. E., Hwang, S., et al. (2007). An ion channel essential for sensing chemical damage. *J. Neurosci.* 27, 11412–11415. doi: 10.1523/JNEUROSCI.3600-07.2007

Majumder, P., Moore, P. A., Richardson, G. P., and Gale, J. E. (2017). Protecting mammalian hair cells from aminoglycoside-toxicity: assessing Phenoxybenzamine's potential. *Front. Cell. Neurosci.* 11:94. doi: 10.3389/fncel.2017.00094

Marcotti, W., van Netten, S. M., and Kros, C. J. (2005). The aminoglycoside antibiotic dihydrostreptomycin rapidly enters mouse outer hair cells through the mechano-electrical transducer channels. *J. Physiol.* 567, 505–521. doi: 10.1113/jphysiol.2005.085951

Matsui, J. I., Gale, J. E., and Warchol, M. E. (2004). Critical signaling events during the aminoglycoside-induced death of sensory hair cells *in vitro*. *J. Neurobiol.* 61, 250–266. doi: 10.1002/neu.20054

Matt, T., Ng, C. L., Lang, K., Sha, S. H., Akbergenov, R., Shcherbakov, D., et al. (2012). Dissociation of antibacterial activity and aminoglycoside ototoxicity in the 4-monosubstituted 2-deoxystreptamine apramycin. *Proc. Natl. Acad. Sci. U S A* 109, 10984–10989. doi: 10.1073/pnas.1204073109

May, L. A., Kramarenko, I. I., Brandon, C. S., Voelkel-Johnson, C., Roy, S., Truong, K., et al. (2013). Inner ear supporting cells protect hair cells by secreting HSP70. *J. Clin. Invest.* 123, 3577–3587. doi: 10.1172/JCI68480

Mehl, A. L., and Thomson, V. (1998). Newborn hearing screening: the great omission. *Pediatrics* 101:E4. doi: 10.1542/peds.101.1.e4

Mesaeli, N., Nakamura, K., Zvaritch, E., Dickie, P., Dziak, E., Krause, K. H., et al. (1999). Calreticulin is essential for cardiac development. *J. Cell Biol.* 144, 857–868. doi: 10.1083/jcb.144.5.857

Meyer zum Gottesberge, A. M., Balz, V., and Felix, H. (2002). Mpv37 mouse strain—a model for the relationship between the kidney and the inner ear. *Adv. Otorhinolaryngol.* 59, 84–90. doi: 10.1159/000059244

Mio, K., Ogura, T., Kiyonaka, S., Hiroaki, Y., Tanimura, Y., Fujiyoshi, Y., et al. (2007). The TRPC3 channel has a large internal chamber surrounded by signal sensing antennas. *J. Mol. Biol.* 367, 373–383. doi: 10.1016/j.jmb.2006.12.043

Mohr, P. E., Feldman, J. J., Dunbar, J. L., McConkey-Robbins, A., Niparko, J. K., Rittenhouse, R. K., et al. (2000). The societal costs of severe to profound hearing loss in the United States. *Int. J. Technol. Assess. Health Care* 16, 1120–1135. doi: 10.1017/s0266462300103162

Monzack, E. L., May, L. A., Roy, S., Gale, J. E., and Cunningham, L. L. (2015). Live imaging the phagocytic activity of inner ear supporting cells in response to hair cell death. *Cell Death Differ.* 22, 1995–2005. doi: 10.1038/cdd.2015.48

Mukherjea, D., Jajoo, S., Sheehan, K., Kaur, T., Sheth, S., Bunch, J., et al. (2011). NOX3 NADPH oxidase couples transient receptor potential vanilloid 1 to signal transducer and activator of transcription 1-mediated inflammation and hearing loss. *Antioxid. Redox Signal.* 14, 999–1010. doi: 10.1089/ars.2010.3497

Myrdal, S. E., and Steyger, P. S. (2005). TRPV1 regulators mediate gentamicin penetration of cultured kidney cells. *Hear. Res.* 204, 170–182. doi: 10.1016/j.heares.2005.02.005

Naramura, H., Nakanishi, N., Tatara, K., Ishiyama, M., Shiraishi, H., and Yamamoto, A. (1999). Physical and mental correlates of hearing impairment in the elderly in Japan. *Audiology* 38, 24–29. doi: 10.3109/00206099909072999

Neu, H. C., and Gootz, T. D. (1996). "Antimicrobial chemotherapy," in *Medical Microbiology*, 4th Edn. ed. S. Baron (Galveston, TX: University of Texas Medical Branch at Galveston), 163–185.

Nicol, K. M., Hackney, C. M., Evans, E. F., and Pratt, S. R. (1992). Behavioural evidence for recovery of auditory function in guinea pigs following kanamycin administration. *Hear. Res.* 61, 117–131. doi: 10.1016/0378-5955(92)90042-l

Niederman, M. S., Mandell, L. A., Anzueto, A., Bass, J. B., Broughton, W. A., Campbell, G. D., et al. (2001). Guidelines for the management of adults with community-acquired pneumonia. Diagnosis, assessment of severity, antimicrobial therapy, and prevention. *Am. J. Respir. Crit. Care Med.* 163, 1730–1754. doi: 10.1164/ajrccm.163.7.at1010

Noack, V., Pak, K., Jalota, R., Kurabi, A., and Ryan, A. F. (2017). An antioxidant screen identifies candidates for improved protection of cochlear hair cells from gentamicin toxicity. *Front. Cell. Neurosci.* 11:242. doi: 10.3389/fncel.2017.00242

Nordang, L., Cestreicher, E., Arnold, W., and Anniko, M. (2000). Glutamate is the afferent neurotransmitter in the human cochlea. *Acta Otolaryngol.* 120, 359–362. doi: 10.1080/000164800750000568

Oestreicher, E., Wolfgang, A., and Felix, D. (2002). Neurotransmission of the cochlear inner hair cell synapse—implications for inner ear therapy. *Adv. Otorhinolaryngol.* 59, 131–139. doi: 10.1159/000059245

Oh, G. S., Kim, H. J., Choi, J. H., Shen, A., Kim, C. H., Kim, S. J., et al. (2011). Activation of lipopolysaccharide-TLR4 signaling accelerates the ototoxic potential of cisplatin in mice. *J. Immunol.* 186, 1140–1150. doi: 10.4049/jimmunol.1002183

Oh, S., Woo, J. I., Lim, D. J., and Moon, S. K. (2012). ERK2-dependent activation of c-Jun is required for nontypeable Haemophilus influenzae-induced CXCL2 upregulation in inner ear fibrocytes. *J. Immunol.* 188, 3496–3505. doi: 10.4049/jimmunol.1103182

Ohlemiller, K. K., Rybak Rice, M. E., Rosen, A. D., Montgomery, S. C., and Gagnon, P. M. (2011). Protection by low-dose kanamycin against noise-induced hearing loss in mice: dependence on dosing regimen and genetic background. *Hear. Res.* 280, 141–147. doi: 10.1016/j.heares.2011.05.007

Oishi, N., Duscha, S., Boukari, H., Meyer, M., Xie, J., Wei, G., et al. (2015). XBP1 mitigates aminoglycoside-induced endoplasmic reticulum stress and neuronal cell death. *Cell Death Dis.* 6:e1763. doi: 10.1038/cddis.2015.108

Okamoto, K., Kashima, K., Pereg, Y., Ishida, M., Yamazaki, S., Nota, A., et al. (2005). DNA damage-induced phosphorylation of MdmX at serine 367 activates p53 by targeting MdmX for Mdm2-dependent degradation. *Mol. Cell Biol.* 25, 9608–9620. doi: 10.1128/mcb.25.21.9608-9620.2005

Pickles, J. O. (2012). *An Introduction to the Physiology of Hearing.* Bingley, United Kingdom: Emerald Group Publishing Limited.

Prezant, T. R., Agapian, J. V., Bohlman, M. C., Bu, X., Oztas, S., Qiu, W. Q., et al. (1993). Mitochondrial ribosomal RNA mutation associated with both antibiotic-induced and non-syndromic deafness. *Nat. Genet.* 4, 289–294. doi: 10.1136/jmg.30.10.885

Puopolo, K. M., and Eichenwald, E. C. (2010). No change in the incidence of ampicillin-resistant, neonatal, early-onset sepsis over 18 years. *Pediatrics* 125, e1031–e1038. doi: 10.1542/peds.2009-1573

Qian, Y., and Guan, M. X. (2009). Interaction of aminoglycosides with human mitochondrial 12S rRNA carrying the deafness-associated mutation. *Antimicrob. Agents Chemother.* 53, 4612–4618. doi: 10.1128/AAC.00965-08

Roy, S., Ryals, M. M., Van den Bruele, A. B., Fitzgerald, T. S., and Cunningham, L. L. (2013). Sound preconditioning therapy inhibits ototoxic hearing loss in mice. *J. Clin. Invest.* 123, 4945–4949. doi: 10.1172/jci71353

Rubin, L. G., Sánchez, P. J., Siegel, J., Levine, G., Saiman, L., Jarvis, W. R., et al. (2002). Evaluation and treatment of neonates with suspected late-onset sepsis: a survey of neonatologists' practices. *Pediatrics* 110:e42. doi: 10.1542/peds.110.4.e42

Russell, I. J., and Sellick, P. M. (1978). Intracellular studies of hair cells in the mammalian cochlea. *J. Physiol.* 284, 261–290. doi: 10.1113/jphysiol.1978.sp012540

Russell, I. J., and Sellick, P. M. (1983). Low-frequency characteristics of intracellularly recorded receptor potentials in guinea-pig cochlear hair cells. *J. Physiol.* 338, 179–206. doi: 10.1113/jphysiol.1983.sp014668

Ryan, A. F., and Bone, R. C. (1978). Potentiation of kanamycin ototoxicity by a history of noise exposure. *Otolaryngology* 86, ORL-125–ORL-128. doi: 10.1177/019459987808600130

Rybak, L. P. (1982). Pathophysiology of furosemide ototoxicity. *J. Otolaryngol.* 11, 127–133.

Sandoz, P. A., and van der Goot, F. G. (2015). How many lives does CLIMP-63 have? *Biochem. Soc. Trans.* 43, 222–228. doi: 10.1042/BST20140272

Satoh, H., Firestein, G. S., Billings, P. B., Harris, J. P., and Keithley, E. M. (2002). Tumor necrosis factor-α, an initiator, and etanercept, an inhibitor of cochlear inflammation. *Laryngoscope* 112, 1627–1634. doi: 10.1097/00005537-200209000-00019

Schatz, A., Bugie, E., and Waksman, S. A. (1944). Streptomycin, a substance exhibiting antibiotic activity against gram-positive and gram-negative bacteria. *Proc. Soc. Exp. Biol. Med.* 55, 66–69. doi: 10.3181/00379727-55-14461

Schmitz, C., Hilpert, J., Jacobsen, C., Boensch, C., Christensen, E. I., Luft, F. C., et al. (2002). Megalin deficiency offers protection from renal aminoglycoside accumulation. *J. Biol. Chem.* 277, 618–622. doi: 10.1074/jbc.M109959200

Seo, Y. J., Ko, S. B., Ha, T. H., Gong, T. H., Bong, J. P., Park, D. J., et al. (2015). Association of hearing impairment with chronic kidney disease: a cross-sectional study of the Korean general population. *BMC Nephrol.* 16:154. doi: 10.1186/s12882-015-0151-0

Shakil, S., Khan, R., Zarrilli, R., and Khan, A. U. (2008). Aminoglycosides versus bacteria—a description of the action, resistance mechanism, and nosocomial battleground. *J. Biomed. Sci.* 15, 5–14. doi: 10.1007/s11373-007-9194-y

Shigematsu, H., Sokabe, T., Danev, R., Tominaga, M., and Nagayama, K. (2010). A 3.5-nm structure of rat TRPV4 cation channel revealed by Zernike phase-contrast cryoelectron microscopy. *J. Biol. Chem.* 285, 11210–11218. doi: 10.1074/jbc.M109.090712

Shrestha, S. K., Chang, C. W., Meissner, N., Oblad, J., Shrestha, J. P., Sorensen, K. N., et al. (2014). Antifungal amphiphilic aminoglycoside K20: bioactivities and mechanism of action. *Front. Microbiol.* 5:671. doi: 10.3389/fmicb.2014.00671

Somdaş, M. A., Korkmaz, F., Gürgen, S. G., Sagit, M., and Akçadag, A. (2015). N-acetylcysteine prevents gentamicin ototoxicity in a rat model. *J. Int. Adv. Otol.* 11, 12–18. doi: 10.5152/iao.2015.650

Stepanyan, R. S., Indzhykulian, A. A., Vélez-Ortega, A. C., Boger, E. T., Steyger, P. S., Friedman, T. B., et al. (2011). TRPA1-mediated accumulation of aminoglycosides in mouse cochlear outer hair cells. *J. Assoc. Res. Otolaryngol.* 12, 729–740. doi: 10.1007/s10162-011-0288-x

Steyger, P. S., Burton, M., Hawkins, J. R., Schuff, N. R., and Baird, R. A. (1997). Calbindin and parvalbumin are early markers of non-mitotically regenerating hair cells in the bullfrog vestibular otolith organs. *Int. J. Dev. Neurosci.* 15, 417–432. doi: 10.1016/s0736-5748(96)00101-3

Taleb, M., Brandon, C. S., Lee, F. S., Lomax, M. I., Dillmann, W. H., and Cunningham, L. L. (2008). Hsp70 inhibits aminoglycoside-induced hair cell death and is necessary for the protective effect of heat shock. *J. Assoc. Res. Otolaryngol.* 9, 277–289. doi: 10.1007/s10162-008-0122-2

Tambs, K. (2004). Moderate effects of hearing loss on mental health and subjective well-being: results from the Nord-Trondelag Hearing Loss Study. *Psychosom. Med.* 66, 776–782. doi: 10.1097/01.psy.0000133328.03596.fb

Tate, A. D., Antonelli, P. J., Hannabass, K. R., and Dirain, C. O. (2017). Mitochondria-targeted antioxidant mitoquinone reduces cisplatin-induced ototoxicity in guinea pigs. *Otolaryngol. Head Neck Surg.* 156, 543–548. doi: 10.1177/0194599816678381

Taylor, R. R., Nevill, G., and Forge, A. (2008). Rapid hair cell loss: a mouse model for cochlear lesions. *J. Assoc. Res. Otolaryngol.* 9, 44–64. doi: 10.1007/s10162-007-0105-8

Torres, J. L., Palomino, J., Moreno, R. D., and De Los Reyes, M. (2017). Pannexin channels increase propidium iodide permeability in frozen?thawed dog spermatozoa. *Reprod. Fertil. Dev.* doi: 10.1071/rd16267 [Epub ahead of print].

Tran Ba Huy, P., Bernard, P., and Schacht, J. (1986). Kinetics of gentamicin uptake and release in the rat. Comparison of inner ear tissues and fluids with other organs. *J. Clin. Invest.* 77, 1492–1500. doi: 10.1172/jci112463

Tran Ba Huy, P., Manuel, C., Meulemans, A., Sterkers, O., Wassef, M., and Amiel, C. (1983). Ethacrynic acid facilitates gentamicin entry into endolymph of the rat. *Hear. Res.* 11, 191–202. doi: 10.1016/0378-5955(83)90078-3

Tsai, M. H., Chu, S. M., Hsu, J. F., Lien, R., Huang, H. R., Chiang, M. C., et al. (2014). Risk factors and outcomes for multidrug-resistant Gram-negative bacteremia in the NICU. *Pediatrics* 133, e322–e329. doi: 10.1542/peds.2013-1248

Turan, M., Ciger, E., Arslanoglu, S., Börekci, H., and Önal, K. (2017). Could edaravone prevent gentamicin ototoxicity? An experimental study. *Hum. Exp. Toxicol.* 36, 123–127. doi: 10.1177/0960327116639360

Umezawa, H., Ueda, M., Maeda, K., Yagishita, K., Kondo, S., Okami, Y., et al. (1957). Production and isolation of a new antibiotic: kanamycin. *J. Antibiot. (Tokyo)* 10, 181–188.

Vellani, V., Mapplebeck, S., Moriondo, A., Davis, J. B., and McNaughton, P. A. (2001). Protein kinase C activation potentiates gating of the vanilloid receptor VR1 by capsaicin, protons, heat and anandamide. *J. Physiol.* 534, 813–825. doi: 10.1111/j.1469-7793.2001.00813.x

Vriens, J., Watanabe, H., Janssens, A., Droogmans, G., Voets, T., and Nilius, B. (2004). Cell swelling, heat, and chemical agonists use distinct pathways for the activation of the cation channel TRPV4. *Proc. Natl. Acad. Sci. U S A* 101, 396–401. doi: 10.1073/pnas.0303329101

Vu, A. A., Nadaraja, G. S., Huth, M. E., Luk, L., Kim, J., Chai, R., et al. (2013). Integrity and regeneration of mechanotransduction machinery regulate aminoglycoside entry and sensory cell death. *PLoS One* 8:e54794. doi: 10.1371/journal.pone.0054794

Waksman, S. A., and Lechevalier, H. A. (1949). Neomycin, a new antibiotic active against streptomycin-resistant bacteria, including tuberculosis organisms. *Science* 109, 305–307. doi: 10.1126/science.109.2830.305

Wangemann, P., and Schacht, J. (1996). "Homeostatic mechanisms in the cochlea," in *The Cochlea*, eds P. Dallos, A. N. Popper and R. R. Fay (New York, NY: Springer-Verlag), 130–185.

Weber, P. A., Chang, H. C., Spaeth, K. E., Nitsche, J. M., and Nicholson, B. J. (2004). The permeability of gap junction channels to probes of different size is dependent on connexin composition and permeant-pore affinities. *Biophys. J.* 87, 958–973. doi: 10.1529/biophysj.103.036350

Weinstein, M. J., Luedemann, G. M., Oden, E. M., and Wagman, G. H. (1963). Gentamicin, a new broad-spectrum antibiotic complex. *Antimicrob. Agents Chemother. (Bethesda)* 161, 1–7.

WHO. (2012). WHO global estimates on prevalence of hearing loss. Available online at: http://www.who.int/pbd/deafness/estimates

Wick, W. E., and Welles, J. S. (1967). Nebramycin, a new broad-spectrum antibiotic complex. IV. *In vitro* and *in vivo* laboratory evaluation. *Antimicrob. Agents Chemother. (Bethesda)* 7, 341–348.

Williams, D. B. (2006). Beyond lectins: the calnexin/calreticulin chaperone system of the endoplasmic reticulum. *J. Cell Sci.* 119, 615–623. doi: 10.1242/jcs.02856

Williams, A. L., van Drongelen, W., and Lasky, R. E. (2007). Noise in contemporary neonatal intensive care. *J. Acoust. Soc. Am.* 121, 2681–2690. doi: 10.1121/1.2717500

Wood, M. B., and Zuo, J. (2017). The contribution of immune infiltrates to ototoxicity and cochlear hair cell loss. *Front. Cell. Neurosci.* 11:106. doi: 10.3389/fncel.2017.00106

Xie, Y., Nishi, S., Iguchi, S., Imai, N., Sakatsume, M., Saito, A., et al. (2001). Expression of osteopontin in gentamicin-induced acute tubular necrosis and its recovery process. *Kidney Int.* 59, 959–974. doi: 10.1046/j.1523-1755.2001.059003959.x

Yang, C.-H., Liu, Z.-Q., Dong, D., Schacht, J., Arya, D., and Sha, S.-H. (2017). Histone deacetylase inhibitors are protective in acute but not in chronic models of ototoxicity. *Front. Cell. Neurosci.* 11:315. doi: 10.3389/fncel.2017.00315

Ylikoski, J., Xing-Qun, L., Virkkala, J., and Pirvola, U. (2002). Blockade of c-Jun N-terminal kinase pathway attenuates gentamicin-induced cochlear and vestibular hair cell death. *Hear. Res.* 163, 71–81. doi: 10.1016/s0378-5955(01)00380-x

Yoon, P. J., Price, M., Gallagher, K., Fleisher, B. E., and Messner, A. H. (2003). The need for long-term audiologic follow-up of neonatal intensive care unit (NICU) graduates. *Int. J. Pediatr. Otorhinolaryngol.* 67, 353–357. doi: 10.1016/s0165-5876(02)00400-7

Zhang, W., Dai, M., Fridberger, A., Hassan, A., Degagne, J., Neng, L., et al. (2012). Perivascular-resident macrophage-like melanocytes in the inner ear are essential for the integrity of the intrastrial fluid-blood barrier. *Proc. Natl. Acad. Sci. U S A* 109, 10388–10393. doi: 10.1073/pnas.1205210109

Zhao, H., Li, R., Wang, Q., Yan, Q., Deng, J. H., Han, D., et al. (2004). Maternally inherited aminoglycoside-induced and nonsyndromic deafness is associated with the novel C1494T mutation in the mitochondrial 12S rRNA gene in a large Chinese family. *Am. J. Hum. Genet.* 74, 139–152. doi: 10.1086/381133

Zhao, L., Young, W. Y., Li, R., Wang, Q., Qian, Y., and Guan, M. X. (2004). Clinical evaluation and sequence analysis of the complete mitochondrial genome of three Chinese patients with hearing impairment associated with the 12S rRNA T1095C mutation. *Biochem. Biophys. Res. Commun.* 325, 1503–1508. doi: 10.1016/j.bbrc.2004.10.199

Zheng, J., Dai, C., Steyger, P. S., Kim, Y., Vass, Z., Ren, T., et al. (2003). Vanilloid receptors in hearing: altered cochlear sensitivity by vanilloids and expression of TRPV1 in the organ of corti. *J. Neurophysiol.* 90, 444–455. doi: 10.1152/jn.00919.2002

16

Novel Peptide Vaccine GV1001 Rescues Hearing in Kanamycin/Furosemide-Treated Mice

*Shin Hye Kim [1], Gaon Jung [2], Sangjae Kim [3] and Ja-Won Koo [2,4]**

[1]Department of Otorhinolaryngology-Head and Neck Surgery, Korea University Medical Center, Korea University College of Medicine, Seoul, South Korea, [2]Department of Otorhinolaryngology-Head and Neck Surgery, Seoul National University Bundang Hospital, Seoul National University College of Medicine, Seongnam, South Korea, [3]GemVax & Kael Co., Ltd, Seongnam, South Korea, [4]Sensory Organ Research Institute, Seoul National University Medical Research Center, Seoul, South Korea

Edited by:
Peter S. Steyger,
Oregon Health & Science University,
United States

Reviewed by:
Bharath Ramaswamy,
University of Maryland, United States
Federico Kalinec,
University of California, Los Angeles,
United States

***Correspondence:**
Ja-Won Koo
jawonkoo@snubh.org

The cell-penetrating peptide GV1001 has been investigated as an anticancer agent and recently demonstrated anti-oxidant and anti-inflammatory effects. It has shown a protective effect on a kanamycin (KM)-induced ototoxicity mouse model. In the present study, we administered GV1001 at different time points after inducing hair cell damage, and examined if it rescues hair cell loss and restores hearing. A deaf mouse model was created by intraperitoneal injection of KM and furosemide. First, to test the early temporal change of hearing and extent of hair cell damage after KM and furosemide injection, hearing and outer hair cells (OHCs) morphology were evaluated on day 1, day 2 and day 3 after injection. In the second experiment, following KM and furosemide injection, GV1001, dexamethasone, or saline were given for three consecutive days at different time points: D0 group (days 0, 1, and 2), D1 group (days 1, 2, and 3), D3 group (days 3, 4, and 5) and D7 group (days 7, 8, and 9). The hearing thresholds were measured at 8, 16, and 32 kHz before ototoxic insult, and 7 days and 14 days after KM and furosemide injection. After 14 days, each turn of the cochlea was imaged to evaluate OHCs damage. GV1001-treated mice showed significantly less hearing loss and OHCs damage than the saline control group in the D0, D1 and D3 groups ($p < 0.0167$). However, there was no hearing restoration or intact hair cell in the D7 group. GV1001 protected against cochlear hair cell damage, and furthermore, delayed administration of GV1001 up to 3 days rescued hair cell damage and hearing loss in KM/furosemide-induced deaf mouse model.

Keywords: aminoglycoside, kanamycin, furosemide, ototoxicity, GV1001, peptide vaccine, deaf

INTRODUCTION

Aminoglycoside antibiotics are used in the treatment of gram-negative bacterial infections, multi-drug resistant tuberculosis, and other hospital acquired serious infections. Dose-limiting side effects include cochlear and/or vestibular toxicity and nephrotoxicity. Aminoglycosides result in hair cell death by either caspase-dependent or -independent mechanisms (Rybak and Ramkumar, 2007). Aminoglycoside induced hair cells impairment by first inducing disarray of stereocilia and inflammatory changes in inner ear structures (Nakagawa et al., 1998; Cunningham et al., 2002; Kitahara et al., 2005; Tabuchi et al., 2007), ultimately terminating in apoptotic cell death through the formation of reactive oxygen species (ROS) including free radicals (Forge and Fradis, 1985; Priuska and Schacht, 1995).

A novel peptide vaccine GV1001, which is a cell-penetrating peptide (16-amino-acid sequence) derived from the active site of human telomerase reverse transcriptase (hTERT), has been investigated as an anticancer agent. GV1001 has been used against advanced pancreatic cancer, melanoma, non-small cell lung cancer, advanced hepatocellular carcinoma, cutaneous T-cell lymphoma and B-cell chronic lymphocytic leukemia. As an anticancer agent, GV1001 binds multiple human leukocyte antigen (HLA) class II molecules and elicits combined CD4 and CD8 T-cell responses (Kyte et al., 2011).

Inflammatory reactions, oxidative stress and apoptotic cell death were reportedly prevented by GV1001 delivered to the kidney and various cancer and primary blood cell lines (Bernhardt et al., 2006; Brunsvig et al., 2006; Lee et al., 2013; Koo et al., 2014). Recently, GV1001 also demonstrated cellular proliferation, stem cell mobilization, anti-apoptotic, anti-aging and anti-oxidant effects (Martínez and Blasco, 2011; Park et al., 2014). GV1001 exerts anti-inflammatory effects by inhibiting leukocyte migration and the release of pro-inflammatory cytokines, such as interleukin-6 (IL-6) and monocyte chemoattractant protein-1 (MCP-1; Koo et al., 2014). GV1001 may be an effective anti-inflammatory peptide that downregulates the production of pro-inflammatory cytokines through the suppression of p38 mitogen-activated protein kinase (MAPK) and nuclear factor (NF)-κB following Enolase1 (ENO1) stimulation (Choi et al., 2015). GV1001 blocks β-amyloid toxicity by mimicking the extra-telomeric functions of hTERT, consequently showing anti-apoptotic and anti-oxidant effects in rat neural stem cells (Park et al., 2014). GV1001 exerts a protective effect in skin flap of rat against ischemia-reperfusion injury through anti-oxidant effects, reducing ROS and suppressing the inflammatory cascade (Lee et al., 2017).

Most therapeutic trials given at the same time or prior to administration of aminoglycoside have claimed effective in protecting aminoglycoside ototoxicity (Song and Schacht, 1996; Song et al., 1998; Sha and Schacht, 1999; Himeno et al., 2002; Wang et al., 2012; Campbell et al., 2016). GV1001 also has shown a protective effect on a kanamycin (KM)-induced ototoxicity mouse model in our previous study (manuscript under review). The anti-inflammatory, anti-oxidant and anti-apoptotic effects of GV1001 seem to be effective on KM-induced cochlear damage. However, experimental preclinical trials reporting rescue effect after cochlear damage are very rare.

Ototoxic hair cell injury in a mouse can be made either by multiple injections of KM or a single injection of KM with furosemide (Hirose et al., 2014). Though multiple injection of KM would be ideal to make an animal model of aminoglycoside ototoxicity, it usually takes around 2 weeks to induce ototoxicity (Jansen et al., 2013). Other shortcomings are chance of losing mice over the course of multiple injections and, variable and unclear onset of hearing loss if hearing is not tested frequently (Hirose and Sato, 2011). On the contrary, a deaf mouse model induced by single injection of KM and furosemide would not only be easier to conduct animal experiments, but the onset of hearing loss and hair cell damage is also immediate after injection of KM and furosemide as seen in this experiment.

In the present study, we administered GV1001 at different time points after inducing hair cell damage, and examined if it rescues hair cell loss and restores hearing in a KM/furosemide-induced ototoxicity mouse model.

MATERIALS AND METHODS

Deaf Mouse Model and Study Groups

A deaf mouse model (C57BL/6 mouse, 4–6 weeks of age, weight of 15–25 g) was created by intraperitoneal injection of KM (1000 mg/kg) followed by furosemide (100 mg/kg) within 30 min. The study protocols were approved by the Institutional Animal Care and Use Committee of Seoul National University Bundang Hospital (BA-1504-174-017). In Experiment 1, to assess the initial temporal change of hearing and the extent of hair cell damage in this deaf mouse model, total nine mice were divided into three groups: Day-1 (N = 3), Day-2 (N = 3) and Day-3 (N = 3). After injection of KM and furosemide on day 0, hearing loss and cochlear hair cell damage were evaluated on day 1, day 2 and day 3, respectively (Supplementary file S1).

In Experiment 2, to test the rescue effect of GV1001, total 120 mice were divided into the following three treatment groups: GV1001 (N = 40), dexamethasone (N = 40) and saline (N = 40). GV1001 (10 mg/kg; GemVax & Kael Co., Ltd, Seongnam, South Korea), dexamethasone (15 mg/kg), or saline was subcutaneously administered for three consecutive days after the injection of KM and furosemide. To compare the rescue effect of GV1001 on different time points, each group was divided into four subgroups according to the time points of GV1001, dexamethasone, and saline treatment: D0 group (days 0, 1 and 2), D1 group (days 1, 2 and 3), D3 group (days 3, 4 and 5), and D7 group (days 7, 8 and 9; Supplementary file S2).

Assessment of Hearing Loss

All of the mice underwent an auditory brainstem response (ABR) test (SmartEP; Intelligent Hearing Systems, Miami, FL, USA) under intraperitoneal injection of ketamine (100 mg/kg) and xylazine (10 mg/kg) after inhalation of isoflurane. During the ABR test, a heating pad was applied to maintain body temperature. Tone burst (envelope, Blackman; duration, 1562 μs; stimulation rate, 21.1/s) stimuli at 8, 16 and 32 kHz were delivered to the external auditory meatus through plastic earphones connected to an EC1 electrostatic speaker. Subdermal needle electrodes were applied behind the ipsilateral mastoid (reference electrode), behind the contralateral mastoid (active electrode), and on the vertex (ground electrode).

The evoked responses were amplified, and 1024 sweeps were averaged in real time. To acquire auditory thresholds, the sound intensity of the tone burst stimuli was lowered by 10 dB intervals from 90 dB SPL. The auditory threshold was defined as the lowest sound intensity at which the most robust and stable component was evoked around 4 ms (Wave III; Scimemi et al., 2014).

Tissue Preparation

Under anesthesia, venous blood was obtained before cardiac perfusion with PBS, followed by 4% paraformaldehyde (pH 7.4), and the cochlea and kidney were immersion-fixed (Koo et al., 2011). To prepare the cochlear whole-mount, the membranous labyrinth of the cochlea was dissected under a microscope and then fixed with 4% paraformaldehyde. Specimens were soaked in 0.3% Triton-X blocking solution for 1 h. Fixed tissues were labeled with Alexa 488-conjugated phalloidin for 1 h, washed, and then fixed with 4% paraformaldehyde. Specimens were mounted on slides with the anti-fade fluorescence mounting media VECTASHIELD® (Vector Laboratories, Burlington, ON, Canada), and examined using confocal microscopy (Carl Zeiss MicroImaging, Oberkochen, Germany) under uniform 63× magnification for all imaging analyses.

Each row of outer hair cells (OHCs) was evaluated for the presence or absence of hair cells. OHCs were considered missing if there was a gap in the normal hair cell array or if there were no apparent stereocilia or cuticular plates. The number of morphologically intact OHCs was counted manually and averaged in five different fields. The percentage of morphologically intact OHCs, defined as "intact OHCs rate", was calculated at each cochlear turn (apex/middle/base).

Assessment of Nephrotoxicity

The mice were anesthetized, and venous blood was collected to measure blood urea nitrogen (BUN) values prior to trans-cardiac perfusion with saline and 4% paraformaldehyde fixative (pH 7.4). The BUN values were measured using Stat Profile® Critical Care Xpress (Nova Biomedical, Waltham, MA, USA). The operating range for BUN was 6–102 mg/dL; the normal range of BUN in mice is 13–35 mg/dL (Stender et al., 2007).

Renal tubules were harvested and imaged by optical microscopy after hematoxylin and eosin (H&E) staining. The morphology was quantified as 0 (normal), 1 (areas of focal granulovacuolar epithelial cell degeneration and granular debris in the tubular lumens), 2 (tubular epithelial necrosis and desquamation seen easily but involving less than half of the cortical tubules), 3 (more than half of the proximal tubules showing desquamation and necrosis, and the involved tubules being found easily), and 4 (complete or almost complete tubular necrosis; Kapić et al., 2014). Ten consecutive fields were examined.

Statistical Analysis

Statistical analyses were performed using SPSS for Windows (ver. 21; SPSS Inc., Chicago, IL, USA) and STATA v. 14.0 for Windows software (Stata Corp., College Station, TX, USA). The Kruskal-Wallis H test with Bonferroni correction were performed to compare continuous variables among the three groups and four subgroups: p-values less than 0.0167 or 0.0083 when compare three or four groups, respectively, were considered statistically significant.

RESULTS

Early Temporal Change of Hearing and Cochlear Hair Cell after Kanamycin and Furosemide Injection

From the Experiment 1 designed to assess the initial temporal change of hearing and the extent of hair cell damage (**Figure 1A**), the hearing was markedly deteriorated even from the next day (Day-1 group) of KM and furosemide injection (**Figure 1B**). However, OHCs morphology of apical, middle and basal turns were intact in two out of three mice of the Day-1 group. Three

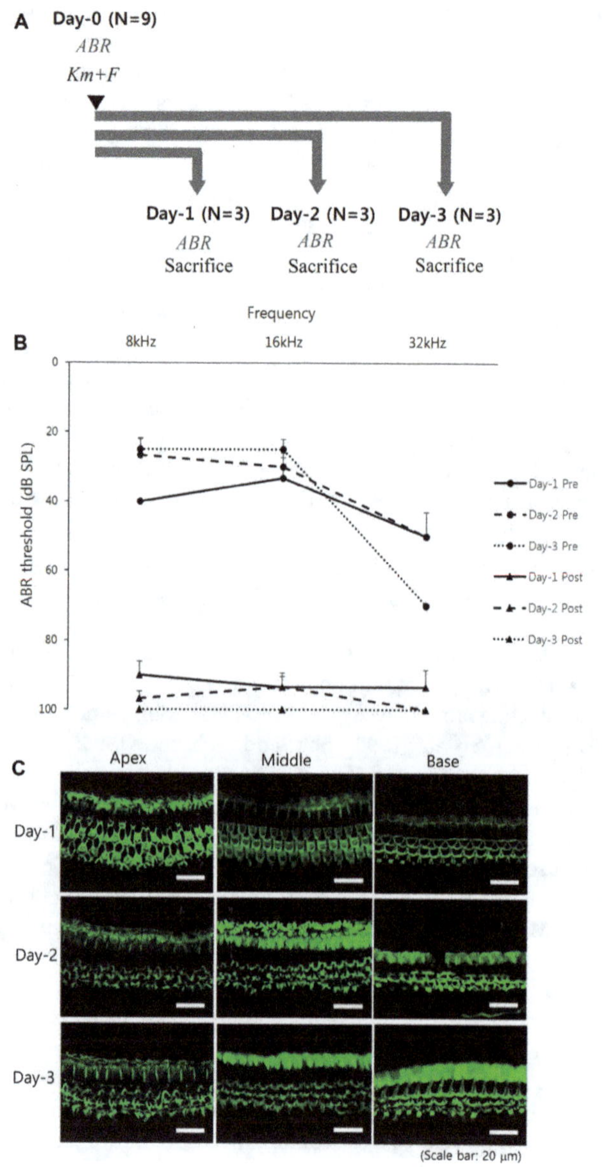

FIGURE 1 | Early temporal change of hearing and cochlear hair cell after kanamycin (KM) and furosemide injection (Experiment 1): **(A)** study design, **(B)** hearing thresholds over time, and **(C)** hair cell damage among the Day-1 (N = 3), Day-2 (N = 3), and Day-3 (N = 2) groups. Error bars in auditory brainstem response (ABR) indicate the standard error of the mean (SEM).

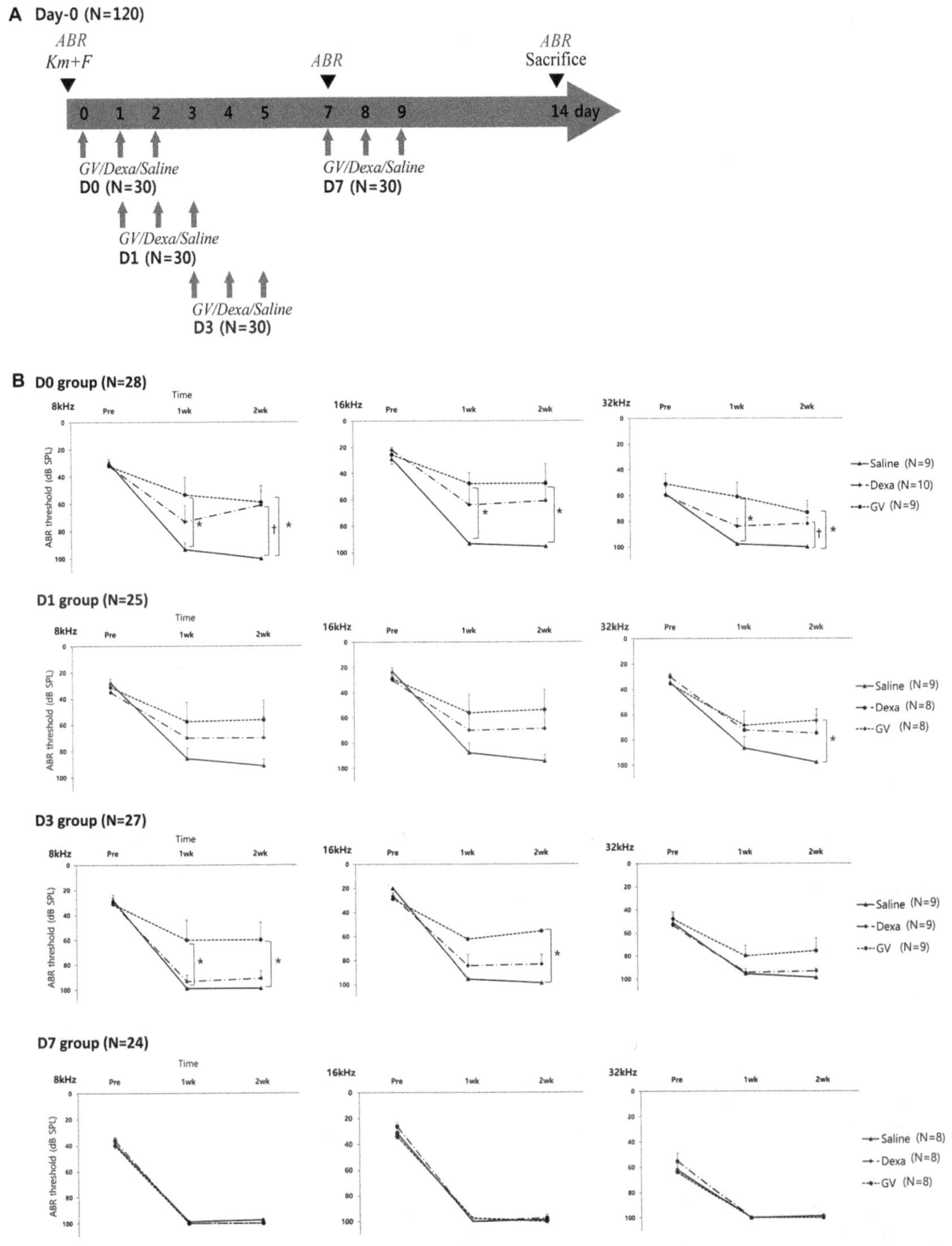

FIGURE 2 | Effect of GV1001, dexamethasone and saline treatment in KM/furosemide-induced ototoxicity mouse model (Experiment 2): **(A)** study design, **(B)** hearing thresholds over time among the saline, dexamethasone and GV1001 groups. According to the time points of GV1001, dexamethasone, and saline treatment, all mice were classified as D0 (N = 28), D1 (N = 25), D3 (N = 27) and D7 (N = 24) subgroups. Error bars in auditory brainstem response (ABR) indicate the SEM. Statistically significant differences ($p < 0.0167$) are marked between saline-GV1001 groups (*) and saline-dexamethasone groups (†).

rows of the OHCs were completely disorganized and missed in the remaining 1 mouse of the Day-1 group and all five mice of the Day-2 and Day-3 groups (1 mouse of the Day-3 group died, **Figure 1C**; Supplementary file S3).

Effect of GV1001 on Hearing Loss

In the Experiment 2 designed to test the rescue effect of GV1001 (**Figure 2A**), the hearing thresholds at 8, 16 and 32 kHz over 2 weeks were compared among the three groups

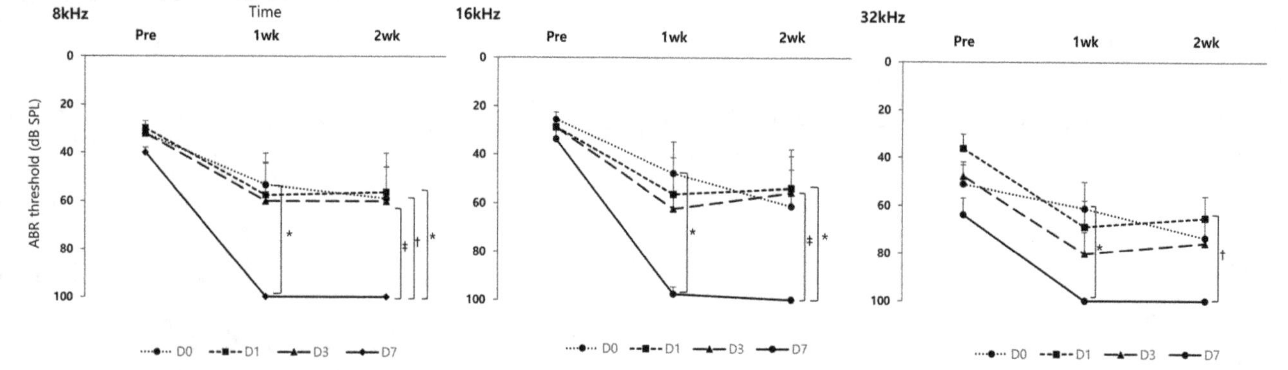

FIGURE 3 | Rescue effect of GV1001 on hearing loss according to the time points of GV1001 treatment: hearing thresholds over time among the D0 ($N = 9$), D1 ($N = 8$), D3 ($N = 9$) and D7 ($N = 8$) subgroups in the GV1001 group. Error bars indicate the SEM. Statistically significant difference ($p < 0.0083$) is marked between D0–D7 groups (*), D1–D7 groups (†), and D3–D7 groups (‡).

(GV1001, dexamethasone and saline) and four subgroups (D0, D1, D3 and D7; **Figure 2B**). After injection of KM and furosemide, the hearing thresholds increased in all three groups and all four subgroups. However, the hearing thresholds of the GV1001 group were relatively well preserved compared with those of the dexamethasone and saline groups with statistical significance ($p < 0.0167$).

Difference in the hearing thresholds between the GV1001 and saline control group was statistically significant at all six points in the D0 group: 8 kHz ($p = 0.007$), 16 kHz ($p = 0.006$), and 32 kHz ($p = 0.001$) at 1 week, and 8 kHz ($p = 0.013$), 16 kHz ($p = 0.008$), and 32 kHz ($p = 0.003$) at 2 weeks. In the D1 group, the significant difference between the GV1001 and saline control group showed at one points: 32 kHz ($p = 0.014$) at 2 weeks. In the D3 group, the significant difference between the GV1001 and saline control group showed at three points: 8 kHz ($p = 0.006$) at 1 week, and 8 kHz ($p = 0.005$) and 16 kHz ($p = 0.001$) at 2 weeks. On the other hand, a statistically significant difference to the saline control group, in the hearing thresholds of the dexamethasone group, was seen at two points in the only D0 group: 8 kHz ($p = 0.007$) and 32 kHz ($p = 0.012$) at 2 weeks. There was no statistically significant difference in the hearing thresholds between the GV1001 and dexamethasone group. In the D7 group, the hearing thresholds of all three groups were increased to nearly 100 dB SPL (complete hearing loss).

In the GV1001 group, when compared the hearing thresholds among the D0, D1, D3 and D7 groups, the hearing thresholds of the D0, D1 and D3 groups were found to be statistical significantly different vs. that of the D7 group ($p < 0.0083$; **Figure 3**). In comparison between D0 and D7 group, hearing thresholds at four points, 8 kHz ($p = 0.004$), 16 kHz ($p = 0.001$), and 32 kHz ($p = 0.001$) at 1 week, and 16 kHz ($p = 0.002$) at 2 weeks, were significantly different. In comparison between D1 and D7 group, hearing thresholds at three points, 32 kHz ($p = 0.003$) at baseline, and 8 kHz ($p = 0.004$) and 32 kHz ($p = 0.003$) at 2 weeks, showed statistically significant difference. Moreover, in comparison between D3 and D7 group, hearing thresholds at one points, 8 kHz ($p = 0.007$) at 2 weeks, showed statistically significant difference. However, we found no significant difference in the hearing thresholds at any treatment time points among the D0, D1 and D3 groups (Supplementary file S4).

Effect of GV1001 on Hair Cell Damage

Regarding the cochlear whole-mount results, almost all the OHCs in the saline group were lost or disorganized in all D0, D1, D3 and D7 groups (**Figure 4**). However, the count of morphologically intact hair cells were significantly higher in GV1001-treated mice than saline-treated mice in all D0, D1 and D3 groups, especially at the basal turns ($p < 0.0167$). In the D0 group (**Figure 4A**), the significant difference between the GV1001 and saline control group showed at all of the cochlear turns: apex ($p = 0.005$), middle ($p = 0.002$), and base ($p = 0.003$). In the D1 group (**Figure 4B**), the significant difference between the GV1001 and saline control group showed at the middle turn ($p = 0.005$) and basal turn ($p = 0.007$). In the D3 group (**Figure 4C**), the significant difference between the GV1001 and saline control group showed at the basal turn ($p = 0.008$). On the other hand, dexamethasone-treated mice showed a statistically significant intact OHCs morphology than the saline group at each cochlear turn only in the D0 group: apex ($p = 0.010$), middle ($p = 0.009$), and base ($p = 0.002$). However, the OHCs and hearing could not be rescued by dexamethasone or GV1001 when treated 7 days after injection of KM and furosemide (**Figure 4D**).

In the GV1001 group, when compared hair cell damage among the D0, D1, D3 and D7 groups, the number of intact hair cells of the D0 group was significantly higher than that of the D7 group ($p < 0.0083$): apex ($p = 0.005$), middle ($p = 0.003$), and base ($p = 0.005$; **Figure 5**), while the comparison between the D0 group with D1 group or D3 group did not show statistical significance (Supplementary file S4).

Effect of GV1001 on the Kidney

The BUN values of tested mice in the GV1001, dexamethasone, and saline groups ranged from 12 mg/dL to 33 (19.06 ± 4.77) mg/dL, and these values were within the normal range for BUN values in mice (8–33 mg/dL). Moreover, the renal tubules of all

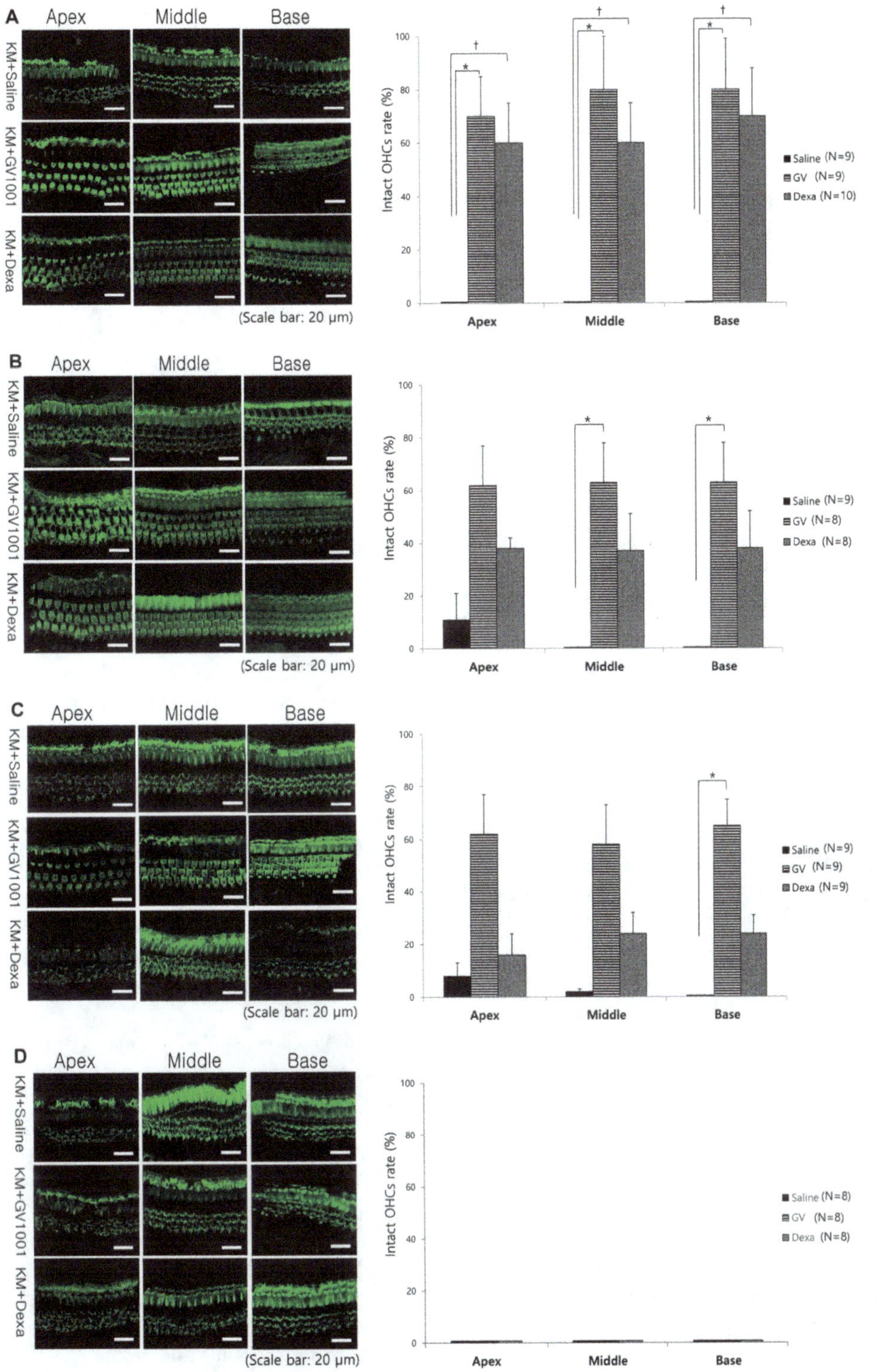

FIGURE 4 | Effect of GV1001, dexamethasone and saline treatment on cochlear hair cell damage: hair cell damage among the saline, dexamethasone and GV1001 groups in **(A)** D0 (N = 28), **(B)** D1 (N = 25), **(C)** D3 (N = 27) and **(D)** D7 (N = 24) subgroups. Error bars indicate the SEM. Statistical significant difference ($p < 0.0167$) is marked between saline-GV1001 groups (*) and saline-dexamethasone groups (†).

GV1001, dexamethasone, and saline treated mice showed normal morphology in the H&E staining. Thus, the administration of 10 mg/kg GV1001 was safe in mice and did not cause nephrotoxicity (Supplementary file S4).

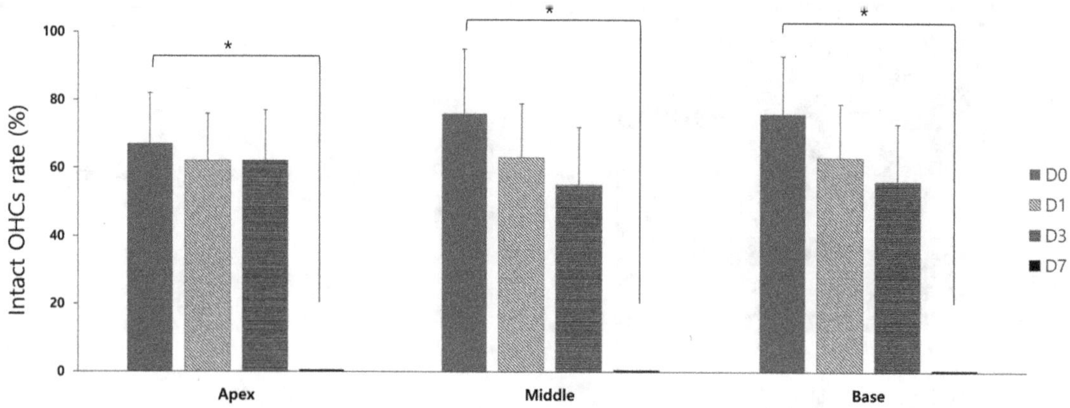

FIGURE 5 | Rescue effect of GV1001 on hair cell damage according to the time points of GV1001 treatment: hair cell damage among the D0 ($N = 9$), D1 ($N = 8$), D3 ($N = 9$) and D7 ($N = 8$) subgroups in the GV1001 group. Error bars indicate the SEM. Statistical significant difference ($p < 0.0083$) is marked between D0–D7 groups (*). OHCs, outer hair cells.

DISCUSSION

In the present study, cell penetrating peptide GV1001 was tested if it rescues hair cell loss and restores hearing after inducing hair cell damage using KM/furosemide-induced deaf mouse model. We also tested if there is a therapeutic window to reverse hair cell damage by investigating agents at different time points of D0, D1, D3 and D7. The KM/furosemide-induced ototoxicity mouse model was ideal for this experiment since substantial hearing loss was documented on the next day of KM and furosemide injection, and complete loss of OHCs was seen on the second day of injection. GV1001-treated mice showed significantly less hearing loss and less hair cell damage than the saline control group in the D0, D1 and D3 subgroups. Therefore, delayed administration of GV1001 up to 3 days could rescue hearing loss and hair cell damage, while hearing loss was irreversible if it was given 7 days after ototoxic insult in KM/furosemide-induced deaf mouse model.

The potential otoprotective effects of several antioxidants have been tested in animal models. Iron chelators such as desferoxamine and dihydroxybenzoate (in guinea pig, Song and Schacht, 1996; Song et al., 1998) as well as antioxidants such as lipoic acid (in mouse, Wang et al., 2012), α-tocopherol (in guinea pig, Fetoni et al., 2004), D-methionine (in guinea pig, Campbell et al., 2016), and salicylates (in guinea pig, Sha and Schacht, 1999) successfully reduced the aminoglycoside-induced ototoxicity. Moreover, intra-cochlear administration of dexamethasone attenuated aminoglycoside-induced ototoxicity in the guinea pig (Himeno et al., 2002). In this study, GV1001-administered mice showed less hearing loss, with reduced hair cell damage, vs. the dexamethasone- and saline-treated mice even after the onset of hearing loss. The anti-inflammatory, anti-oxidant and anti-apoptotic effects of GV1001 may explain why GV1001 rescues cochlear hair cells against KM/furosemide-induced ototoxicity.

Clinically, there are numerous therapeutic approaches to treat ototoxicity, including antioxidants, ROS scavengers, apoptosis inhibitors, neuroprotective compounds and anti-inflammatory drugs such as steroids (Atar and Avraham, 2005; Rybak and Whitworth, 2005; Maruyama et al., 2008; Tabuchi et al., 2010; Mukherjea et al., 2011; Mizutari et al., 2013). The treatment of N-acetylcysteine (NAC) significantly reduced the ototoxicity in hemodialysis patients with gentamicin-induced hearing loss (Feldman et al., 2007). Use of aspirin significantly reduced the incidence of hearing loss in patients receiving gentamicin and aspirin when compared to the incidence in placebo group (3% vs. 13%; Sha et al., 2006). Our previous study proved that GV1001 (0.1–100 mg/kg) itself did not have any detrimental effects on the inner ear or kidney. As shown in **Figures 2B, 4**, the saline-treated mice showed complete hearing loss and damaged cellular framework of OHCs. The normal range of BUN values of all 40 mice in the saline group indicated that the increased ototoxicity in the saline group was not potentiated by nephrotoxicity.

As well known, OHCs damage caused by aminoglycoside-induced ototoxicity is most prominent at the basal turn of the cochlea, and the hearing loss is more prominent in higher frequency range. This susceptibility of the basal turn of the cochlea is likely caused by a higher concentration of aminoglycoside at that structure than at the middle or apical turn, in a concentration-dependent manner (Dai et al., 2006; Dai and Steyger, 2008). Moreover, the susceptibility of the basal turn of the cochlea to ototoxic drugs can be explained by there being greater metabolic activity than at the apical turn of the cochlea (Sha et al., 2001). As shown in **Figure 4**, the OHCs damage caused by KM and furosemide and rescue effect of GV1001 were more prominent at the basal turn than the apical turn of the cochlea.

In this study, to assess the therapeutic effect of GV1001 against KM/furosemide-induced hair cell damage, we compared GV1001 (10 mg/kg) with dexamethasone (15 mg/kg) and saline by measuring the hearing thresholds and OHCs morphology. When compared with saline, the rescue effect of GV1001 was proven in all D0, D1 and D3 groups. As shown in **Figures 2B, 4**, the rescue effect of GV1001 seems to be superior to that of dexamethasone, but could not reach statistical significance in comparison of hearing thresholds and OHCs morphology between GV1001 and dexamethasone groups.

A previous study investigated the effect of different dexamethasone treatment times on OHCs survival following ototoxic insult with KM and furosemide. Mice pre-treated with dexamethasone (prior to 1 h of the insult) showed a statistically significant improvement in intact OHCs counts compared with the controls, but the mice subjected to dexamethasone post-treatment (at 1, 6, 12 and 72 h after the insult) showed highly variable OHCs counts (Fernandes and Lin, 2014). By contrast, in this study, GV1001 showed a rescue effect against OHCs damage even with delayed administration, i.e., at 3 days after the ototoxic insult.

The preventive effect of GV1001 pre-treatment against cochlear hearing loss and hair cell damage in a KM-induced deaf mouse model was verified in our previous study. As shown in **Figure 1**, all tested mice of the Day-1, Day-2 and Day-3 groups showed nearly complete hearing loss, but two out of three mice of the Day-1 group showed intact OHCs morphology. The cause of this discrepancy derived from phalloidin-stained at stereocilia of the OHCs. Two mice of the Day-1 group may have structurally intact OHCs morphology with loss of hearing function. The current study corroborated the rescue capacity of GV1001 against hair cell damage, as well as the ability to restore hearing even when administration was delayed by up to 3 days. Further study to investigate the underlying mechanisms of rescue effect of GV1001 will be needed.

In conclusion, we demonstrated that the cell-penetrating peptide GV1001 rescues hair cell damage and restores hearing in a KM/furosemide-induced deaf mouse model. Given that the rescue effect of GV1001 could be related to its anti-inflammatory, anti-oxidant, and anti-apoptotic activities, we predict that GV1001 could be useful not only in aminoglycoside-induced hearing loss, but also in acute cochlear hearing loss due to other causes. Because SNHL is caused by an imbalance in redox homeostasis and subsequent increase in ROS followed by the apoptotic pathway, GV1001 may have a potential clinical role in restoring hearing in cases of acute SNHL.

AUTHOR CONTRIBUTIONS

SHK analyzed data and wrote the manuscript. GJ performed the animal experiments and wrote the manuscript. SK provided technical assistance and wrote the manuscript. JWK designed the study and revised the manuscript. All authors read and approved the final manuscript.

REFERENCES

Atar, O., and Avraham, K. B. (2005). Therapeutics of hearing loss: expectations vs. reality. *Drug Discov. Today* 10, 1323–1330. doi: 10.1016/s1359-6446(05)03618-4

Bernhardt, S. L., Gjertsen, M. K., Trachsel, S., Møller, M., Eriksen, J. A., Meo, M., et al. (2006). Telomerase peptide vaccination of patients with non-resectable pancreatic cancer: a dose escalating phase I/II study. *Br. J. Cancer* 95, 1474–1482. doi: 10.1038/sj.bjc.6603437

Brunsvig, P. F., Aamdal, S., Gjertsen, M. K., Kvalheim, G., Markowski-Grimsrud, C. J., Sve, I., et al. (2006). Telomerase peptide vaccination: a phase I/II study in patients with non-small cell lung cancer. *Cancer Immunol. Immunother.* 55, 1553–1564. doi: 10.1007/s00262-006-0145-7

Campbell, K. C., Martin, S. M., Meech, R. P., Hargrove, T. L., Verhulst, S. J., and Fox, D. J. (2016). D-methionine (D-met) significantly reduces kanamycin-induced ototoxicity in pigmented guinea pigs. *Int. J. Audiol.* 55, 273–278. doi: 10.3109/14992027.2016.1143980

Choi, J., Kim, H., Kim, Y., Jang, M., Jeon, J., Hwang, Y., et al. (2015). The anti-inflammatory effect of GV1001 mediated by the downregulation of ENO1-induced pro-inflammatory cytokine production. *Immune Netw.* 15, 291–303. doi: 10.4110/in.2015.15.6.291

Cunningham, L. L., Cheng, A. G., and Rubel, E. W. (2002). Caspase activation in hair cells of the mouse utricle exposed to neomycin. *J. Neurosci.* 22, 8532–8540.

Dai, C. F., Mangiardi, D., Cotanche, D. A., and Steyger, P. S. (2006). Uptake of fluorescent gentamicin by vertebrate sensory cells *in vivo*. *Hear. Res.* 213, 64–78. doi: 10.1016/j.heares.2005.11.011

Dai, C. F., and Steyger, P. S. (2008). A systemic gentamicin pathway across the stria vascularis. *Hear. Res.* 235, 114–124. doi: 10.1016/j.heares.2007.10.010

Feldman, L., Efrati, S., Eviatar, E., Abramsohn, R., Yarovoy, I., Gersch, E., et al. (2007). Gentamicin-induced ototoxicity in hemodialysis patients is ameliorated by *N*-acetylcysteine. *Kidney Int.* 72, 359–363. doi: 10.1038/sj.ki.5002295

Fernandes, V. T., and Lin, V. Y. (2014). Development of an ototoxicity model in the adult CBA/CaJ mouse and determination of a golden window of corticosteroid intervention for otoprotection. *J. Otolaryngol. Head Neck Surg.* 43:12. doi: 10.1186/1916-0216-43-12

Fetoni, A. R., Sergi, B., Ferraresi, A., Paludetti, G., and Troiani, D. (2004). α-Tocopherol protective effects on gentamicin ototoxicity: an experimental study. *Int. J. Audiol.* 43, 166–171. doi: 10.1080/14992020400050023

Forge, A., and Fradis, M. (1985). Structural abnormalities in the stria vascularis following chronic gentamicin treatment. *Hear. Res.* 20, 233–244. doi: 10.1016/0378-5955(85)90028-0

Himeno, C., Komeda, M., Izumikawa, M., Takemura, K., Yagi, M., Weiping, Y., et al. (2002). Intra-cochlear administration of dexamethasone attenuates aminoglycoside ototoxicity in the guinea pig. *Hear. Res.* 167, 61–70. doi: 10.1016/s0378-5955(02)00345-3

Hirose, K., Li, S. Z., Ohlemiller, K. K., and Ransohoff, R. M. (2014). Systemic lipopolysaccharide induces cochlear inflammation and exacerbates the synergistic ototoxicity of kanamycin and furosemide. *J. Assoc. Res. Otolaryngol.* 15, 555–570. doi: 10.1007/s10162-014-0458-8

Hirose, K., and Sato, E. (2011). Comparative analysis of combination kanamycin-furosemide versus kanamycin alone in the mouse cochlea. *Hear. Res.* 272, 108–116. doi: 10.1016/j.heares.2010.10.011

Jansen, T. T., Bremer, H. G., Topsakal, V., Hendriksen, F. G., Klis, S. F., and Grolman, W. (2013). Deafness induction in mice. *Otol. Neurotol.* 34, 1496–1502. doi: 10.1097/mao.0b013e318291c610

Kapić, D., Mornjaković, Z., Ćosović, E., and Šahinović, M. (2014). A histological study of the effect of exogenous melatonin on gentamicin induced structural alterations of proximal tubules in rats. *Bosn. J. Basic Med. Sci.* 14, 30–34. doi: 10.17305/bjbms.2014.2293

Kitahara, T., Li-Korotky, H. S., and Balaban, C. D. (2005). Regulation of mitochondrial uncoupling proteins in mouse inner ear ganglion cells in response to systemic kanamycin challenge. *Neuroscience* 135, 639–653. doi: 10.1016/j.neuroscience.2005.06.056

Koo, J. W., Wang, Q., and Steyger, P. S. (2011). Infection-mediated vasoactive peptides modulate cochlear uptake of fluorescent gentamicin. *Audiol. Neurootol.* 16, 347–358. doi: 10.1159/000322851

Koo, T. Y., Yan, J. J., and Yang, J. (2014). Protective effect of peptide GV1001 against renal ischemia-reperfusion injury in mice. *Transplant. Proc.* 46, 1117–1122. doi: 10.1016/j.transproceed.2013.12.019

Kyte, J. A., Gaudernack, G., Dueland, S., Trachsel, S., Julsrud, L., and Aamdal, S. (2011). Telomerase peptide vaccination combined with temozolomide: a clinical trial in stage IV melanoma patients. *Clin. Cancer Res.* 17, 4568–4580. doi: 10.1158/1078-0432.ccr-11-0184

Lee, S. A., Kim, B. R., Kim, B. K., Kim, D. W., Shon, W. J., Lee, N. R., et al. (2013). Heat shock protein-mediated cell penetration and cytosolic delivery of macromolecules by a telomerase-derived peptide vaccine. *Biomaterials* 34, 7495–7505. doi: 10.1016/j.biomaterials.2013.06.015

Lee, Y. K., Nata'atmaja, B. S., Kim, B. H., Pak, C. S., and Heo, C. Y. (2017). Protective effect of telomerase-based 16-mer peptide vaccine (GV1001) on inferior epigastric island skin flap survivability in ischaemia-reperfusion injury rat model. *J. Plast. Surg. Hand Surg.* 51, 210–216. doi: 10.1080/2000656x.2016.1235046

Martínez, P., and Blasco, M. A. (2011). Telomeric and extra-telomeric roles for telomerase and the telomere-binding proteins. *Nat. Rev. Cancer* 11, 161–176. doi: 10.1038/nrc3025

Maruyama, J., Miller, J. M., and Ulfendahl, M. (2008). Glial cell line-derived neurotrophic factor and antioxidants preserve the electrical responsiveness of the spiral ganglion neurons after experimentally induced deafness. *Neurobiol. Dis.* 29, 14–21. doi: 10.1016/j.nbd.2007.07.026

Mizutari, K., Fujioka, M., Hosoya, M., Bramhall, N., Okano, H. J., Okano, H., et al. (2013). Notch inhibition induces cochlear hair cell regeneration and recovery of hearing after acoustic trauma. *Neuron* 77, 58–69. doi: 10.1016/j.neuron.2012.10.032

Mukherjea, D., Rybak, L. P., Sheehan, K. E., Kaur, T., Ramkumar, V., Jajoo, S., et al. (2011). The design and screening of drugs to prevent acquired sensorineural hearing loss. *Expert Opin. Drug Discov.* 6, 491–505. doi: 10.1517/17460441.2011.562887

Nakagawa, T., Yamane, H., Takayama, M., Sunami, K., and Nakai, Y. (1998). Apoptosis of guinea pig cochlear hair cells following chronic aminoglycoside treatment. *Eur. Arch. Otorhinolaryngol.* 255, 127–131. doi: 10.1007/s004050050027

Park, H.-H., Lee, K.-Y., Kim, S., Lee, J. W., Choi, N.-Y., Lee, E.-H., et al. (2014). Novel vaccine peptide GV1001 effectively blocks β-amyloid toxicity by mimicking the extra-telomeric functions of human telomerase reverse transcriptase. *Neurobiol. Aging* 35, 1255–1274. doi: 10.1016/j.neurobiolaging.2013.12.015

Priuska, E. M., and Schacht, J. (1995). Formation of free radicals by gentamicin and iron and evidence for an iron/gentamicin complex. *Biochem. Pharmacol.* 50, 1749–1752. doi: 10.1016/0006-2952(95)02160-4

Rybak, L. P., and Ramkumar, V. (2007). Ototoxicity. *Kidney Int.* 72, 931–935. doi: 10.1038/sj.ki.5002434

Rybak, L. P., and Whitworth, C. A. (2005). Ototoxicity: therapeutic opportunities. *Drug Discov. Today* 10, 1313–1321. doi: 10.1016/s1359-6446(05)03552-x

Scimemi, R., Santarelli, R., Selmo, A., and Mammano, F. (2014). Auditory brainstem responses to clicks and tone bursts in C57 BL/6J mice. *Acta Otorhinolaryngol. Ital.* 34, 264–271.

Sha, S. H., Qiu, J. H., and Schacht, J. (2006). Aspirin to prevent gentamicin-induced hearing loss. *N Engl J. Med.* 354, 1856–1857. doi: 10.1056/NEJMc053428

Sha, S. H., and Schacht, J. (1999). Salicylate attenuates gentamicin-induced ototoxicity. *Lab. Invest.* 79, 807–813.

Sha, S.-H., Taylor, R., Forge, A., and Schacht, J. (2001). Differential vulnerability of basal and apical hair cells is based on intrinsic susceptibility to free radicals. *Hear. Res.* 155, 1–8. doi: 10.1016/s0378-5955(01)00224-6

Song, B. B., and Schacht, J. (1996). Variable efficacy of radical scavengers and iron chelators to attenuate gentamicin ototoxicity in guinea pig *in vivo*. *Hear. Res.* 94, 87–93. doi: 10.1016/0378-5955(96)00003-2

Song, B. B., Sha, S. H., and Schacht, J. (1998). Iron chelators protect from aminoglycoside-induced cochleo- and vestibulo-toxicity. *Free Radic. Biol. Med.* 25, 189–195. doi: 10.1016/s0891-5849(98)00037-9

Stender, R. N., Engler, W. J., Braun, T. M., and Hankenson, F. C. (2007). Establishment of blood analyte intervals for laboratory mice and rats by use of a portable clinical analyzer. *J. Am. Assoc. Lab. Anim. Sci.* 46, 47–52.

Tabuchi, K., Nishimura, B., Tanaka, S., Hayashi, K., Hirose, Y., and Hara, A. (2010). Ischemia-reperfusion injury of the cochlea: pharmacological strategies for cochlear protection and implications of glutamate and reactive oxygen species. *Curr. Neuropharmacol.* 8, 128–134. doi: 10.2174/157015910791233123

Tabuchi, K., Pak, K., Chavez, E., and Ryan, A. F. (2007). Role of inhibitor of apoptosis protein in gentamicin-induced cochlear hair cell damage. *Neuroscience* 149, 213–222. doi: 10.1016/j.neuroscience.2007.06.061

Wang, A., Hou, N., Bao, D., Liu, S., and Xu, T. (2012). Mechanism of alpha-lipoic acid in attenuating kanamycin-induced ototoxicity. *Neural Regen. Res.* 7, 2793–2800. doi: 10.3969/j.issn.1673-5374.2012.35.007

17

Interleukin-10 Attenuates Hypochlorous Acid-Mediated Cytotoxicity to HEI-OC1 Cochlear Cells

Martin Mwangi[1], Sung-Hee Kil[1], David Phak[1], Hun Yi Park[2], David J. Lim[1], Raekil Park[3] and Sung K. Moon[1]*

[1] *Department of Head and Neck Surgery, David Geffen School of Medicine, University of California, Los Angeles, Los Angeles, CA, United States,* [2] *Department of Otolaryngology, Ajou University School of Medicine, Suwon, South Korea,* [3] *Gwangju Institute of Science and Technology, Gwangju, South Korea*

Edited by:
Lisa Cunningham,
National Institutes of Health (NIH), United States

Reviewed by:
Meiyan Jiang,
Oregon Health and Science University, United States
Tejbeer Kaur,
Washington University in St. Louis, United States

***Correspondence:**
Sung K. Moon
skmoon@mednet.ucla.edu

Inflammatory reaction plays a crucial role in the pathophysiology of acquired hearing loss such as ototoxicity and labyrinthitis. In our earlier work, we showed the pivotal role of otic fibrocytes in cochlear inflammation and the critical involvement of proinflammatory cytokines in cisplatin ototoxicity. We also demonstrated that otic fibrocytes inhibit monocyte chemoattractant protein 1 (CCL2) upregulation in response to interleukin-10 (IL-10) via heme oxygenase 1 (HMOX1) signaling, resulting in suppression of cochlear inflammation. However, it is still unclear how IL-10 affects inflammation-mediated cochlear injury. Here we aim to determine how hypochlorous acid, a model inflammation mediator affects cochlear cell viability and how IL-10 affects hypochlorous acid-mediated cochlear cell injury. NaOCl, a sodium salt of hypochlorous acid (HOCl) was found to induce cytotoxicity of HEI-OC1 cells in a dose-dependent manner. Combination of hydrogen peroxide and myeloperoxidase augmented cisplatin cytotoxicity, and this synergism was inhibited by N-Acetyl-L-cysteine and ML-171. The rat spiral ligament cell line (RSL) appeared to upregulate the antioxidant response element (ARE) activities upon exposure to IL-10. RSL cells upregulated the expression of NRF2 (an ARE ligand) and NR0B2 in response to CoPP (a HMOX1 inducer), but not to ZnPP (a HMOX1 inhibitor). Adenovirus-mediated overexpression of NR0B2 was found to suppress CCL2 upregulation. IL-10-positive cells appeared in the mouse stria vascularis 1 day after intraperitoneal injection of lipopolysaccharide (LPS). Five days after injection, IL-10-positive cells were observed in the spiral ligament, spiral limbus, spiral ganglia, and suprastrial area, but not in the stria vascularis. IL-10R1 appeared to be expressed in the mouse organ of Corti as well as HEI-OC1 cells. HEI-OC1 cells upregulated Bcl-xL expression in response to IL-10, and IL-10 was shown to attenuate NaOCl-induced cytotoxicity. In addition, HEI-OC1 cells upregulated IL-22RA upon exposure to cisplatin, and NaOCl cytotoxicity was inhibited by IL-22. Taken together, our findings suggest that hypochlorous acid is involved in cochlear injury and that IL-10 potentially reduces cochlear injury through not only inhibition of inflammation but also enhancement of cochlear cell viability. Further studies are needed to determine immunological characteristics of intracochlear IL-10-positive cells and elucidate molecular mechanisms involved in the otoprotective activity of IL-10.

Keywords: oto-protection, IL-10, IL-22, hypochlorous acid, HMOX1, Nrf2, NR0B2

INTRODUCTION

Inflammation is a tightly controlled process because excessive inflammation potentially leads to unintended tissue injury. In the cochlea, inflammation is increasingly recognized to contribute to the pathophysiology of acquired sensorineural hearing loss (SNHL) such as ototoxicity, given that lipopolysaccharide (LPS)-induced inflammatory response aggravates cisplatin ototoxicity as well as the synergistic ototoxicity of kanamycin and furosemide (Oh et al., 2011; Hirose et al., 2014). Yet, it has not been fully understood how inflammatory reaction itself induces cochlear injury.

Pro-inflammatory cytokines such as TNF-α are known to critically mediate cisplatin ototoxicity (So et al., 2007, 2008), but the cochlear sensory cells appeared to be damaged only by the extremely high concentrations of TNF-α in animal experiments (Dinh et al., 2008; Keithley et al., 2008), indicating the involvement of multiple factors in inflammation-mediated cochlear injury. Among a number of inflammatory mediators, hypochlorous acid (HOCl) has gained attention due to the essential contribution to tissue injury (Johnson et al., 1987; Hammerschmidt and Wahn, 1997). Hypochlorous acid is a potent oxidant, released from activated phagocytes during the respiratory burst for the destruction of invading pathogens. Due to its powerful oxidative property, there is a risk of host tissue injuries when associated with excessive inflammatory reactions (Pullar et al., 2000). However, it is unclear whether hypochlorous acid is ototoxic and contributes to inflammation-mediated cochlear injury.

In our earlier work, downregulation of proinflammatory cytokines appeared to attenuate cisplatin ototoxicity (So et al., 2008), which led us to focus on the anti-inflammatory cytokine, IL-10. Otic fibrocytes were shown to inhibit monocyte chemoattractant protein-1 (CCL2) upregulation in response to IL-10 *via* heme oxygenase 1 (HMOX1) signaling, resulting in suppression of cochlear inflammation. However, it is unclear how IL-10 maintains HMOX1 upregulation because IL-10 paradoxically inhibits p38 MAPK that is required for HMOX1 upregulation (Kontoyiannis et al., 2001). Based on the finding showing the involvement of NRF2 (also known as NFE2L2) in HMOX1 regulation in cisplatin ototoxicity (So et al., 2006), we aim to elucidate an NRF2-mediated alternative pathway maintaining IL-10-induced HMOX1 regulation. Furthermore, NRF2 is involved in the regulation of NR0B2 (Huang et al., 2010), an orphan nuclear receptor involved in negative regulation of inflammatory reactions through inhibition of NF-κB (Yuk et al., 2011). Thus, we hypothesize that NR0B2 contributes to the anti-inflammatory effect of IL-10 on cochlear inflammation.

Besides the anti-inflammatory activity, there is accumulating evidence showing the cytoprotective activity of the IL-10 family cytokines. It has been reported that IL-10 upregulates anti-apoptotic factors such as Bcl-2 and Bcl-xL (Levy and Brouet, 1994; Stassi et al., 2000) and enhances cell viability of cortical neurons and retinal ganglion cells (Boyd et al., 2003; Sharma et al., 2011). Moreover, IL-22, which shares IL-10R2 with IL-10 for forming an active IL-22R complex, promotes the survival of hepatocytes (Radaeva et al., 2004) and even upregulates IL-10 in colon epithelial cells (Nagalakshmi et al., 2004). Moreover, IL-22 contributes to mucosal wound healing and intestinal epithelial regeneration via STAT3 signaling (Pickert et al., 2009; Lindemans et al., 2015). Based on these findings, we aim to determine cytoprotective activities of IL-10 and IL-22, inhibiting cochlear injury through promoting cochlear cell viability.

Here, we demonstrate that hypochlorous acid not only reduces cochlear cell viability but also exacerbates cisplatin ototoxicity, and that IL-10 is protective for hypochlorous acid-induced cytotoxicity. We found cochlear localization of IL-10-expressing cells and IL-10R1 expression in the organ of Corti. Moreover, it was shown that NRF2 and NR0B2 contribute to the IL-10 signaling network and that HEI-OC1 cells upregulate Bcl-xL expression in response to IL-10. This study may enable us to better understand the molecular pathogenesis involved in inflammation-mediated cochlear injury and would provide a scientific basis for the development of therapeutic tools to manage acquired SNHL.

METHODS

Reagents

Sodium hypochlorite (NaOCl), cisplatin (*cis*-[$Pt(NH_3)_2(Cl)_2$]), protoporphyrin IX cobalt chloride ($C_{34}H_{32}CoN_4O_4Cl$, CoPP), protoporphyrin IX zinc(II) ($C_{34}H_{32}N_4O_4Zn$, ZnPP), N-Acetyl-L-cysteine, LPS, recombinant IL-10, IL-22, and myeloperoxidase were purchased from Sigma-Aldrich (St. Louis, MO). ML-171 was purchased from Tocris (Minneapolis, MN). TaqMan primers and probes for rat CCL2 (Rn00580555_m1), rat HMOX1 (Rn01536933_m1), rat NRF2 (Rn00582415_m1), rat NR0B2 (Rn00589173_m1), and rat GAPDH (4352338E) were purchased from Life Technologies (Grand Island, NY).

Animals and Immunolabeling

Young adult C57BL/6 mice (The Jackson Laboratory, Bar Harbor, ME) were used. All animal experiments were approved by the Institutional Animal Care and Use Committee of University of California, Los Angeles. To induce cochlear inflammation, animals were injected i.p. with a non-septic dose (1 mg/kg) of LPS (Sigma-Aldrich) and euthanized 1 or 5 d after injection. Control animals were given with normal saline. For temporal bone sections, mouse temporal bones were dissected after decapitation. After fixation, decalcification and embedding in paraffin, serial sections (~10 μm thickness) were prepared through the mid-modiolar plane and were used for immunolabeling of IL-10 or IL-10R1. For whole mount preparation, bony otic capsules were carefully removed, and cochlear lateral wall tissues were dissected as described (Moon et al., 2007) and were further used for IL-10 immunolabeling. Cochlear lateral tissues were fixed in 4% paraformaldehyde overnight at 4°C and permeabilized in 0.5% Triton X-100 (Sigma-Aldrich) for 1 h. After immunoblocking with 10% goat serum, samples were incubated with a rat antibody against IL-10 (1:100, Santa Cruz Biotechnology, Dallas, TX) or IL-10R1 (1:200, Thermo Scientific, Waltham, MA) overnight at 4°C. After washing, sections were incubated with rhodamine-conjugated goat anti-rat IgG (1:200, Life Technologies). Mounted with anti-fade mounting media (Life Technologies), samples were viewed and photographed using a TCS SP5 confocal microscope (Leica, Buffalo Grove, IL).

Cell Culture, Cell Viability Assays, and Quantitative RT-PCR

Rat spiral ligament fibrocyte cell line (RSL) were maintained in DMEM supplemented with 10% FBS, penicillin (100 U/ml), and streptomycin (0.1 mg/ml; Life Technologies) at 37°C in a humidified atmosphere of 5% CO_2 and 95% air as described (Yian et al., 2006). HEI-OC1 cells were cultured under a permissive condition (33°C, 10% CO_2) in high-glucose DMEM containing 10% FBS without antibiotics as described (Kalinec et al., 2003). For cell viability, HEI-OC1 cells were exposed to cytotoxic agents such as NaOCl (1:50~1:1000), cisplatin (100 μM), hydrogen peroxide (100 μM) and myeloperoxidase (1μg/ml) for 8 or 16 h, and MTT assays were carried out using a Cell Proliferation Kit I (Roche, Indianapolis, IN), according to the manufacturer's instructions. After solubilization of formazan crystals, spectrophotometrical absorbance of samples was measured at 550 nm using a microplate reader. For quantitative RT-PCR, RSL cells were exposed to reagents such as IL-10 (50 ng/ml), CoPP (10 μM), or ZnPP (20 μM) for 6 h, and total RNA was extracted using TRIzol (Life Technologies). After cDNA was synthesized using TaqMan reverse transcription kit (Life Technologies), multiplex PCR was performed using the ABI 7500 Real-Time PCR system (Applied Biosystems, Foster City, CA) with gene-specific primers (FAM-conjugated probes for NRF2, NR0B2, HMOX1, and CCL2) and control primers (a VIC-conjugated probe for GAPDH). The cycle threshold (CT) values were determined according to the manufacturer's instructions. The relative quantity of mRNA was determined using the $2^{\Delta\Delta CT}$ method (Livak and Schmittgen, 2001). CT values were normalized to the internal control (GAPDH), and the results were expressed as a fold change in mRNA, with the mRNA levels in the non-treated group set as 1. For conventional PCR, primers were used as follows: mouse Bcl-xL (228 bp), 5′-TCCTGGAAGAGAATCGCTAAAC-3′ and 5′-CCCTCTCTG CTTCAGTTTCTT-3′; mouse IL-10R2 (256 bp), 5′-GGACAG GCAATGACGAAATAAC-3′ and 5′-GGGAAGGAGAACAGC AGAAA-3′; mouse IL-22RA (294 bp), 5′-CATGACCTGTTC TACCGCTTAG-3′ and 5′-AGGTGGCTTGGTGATGTATTT-3′; and 18S rRNA (200 bp), 5′-GTGGAGCGATTTGTCTGGTT-3′ and 5′-CGCTGAGCCAGTCAGTGTAG-3′. PCR products were analyzed by electrophoresis on 1.5% agarose gels, viewed after staining with GelRed Nucleic Acid Stain (Biotium, Hayward, CA) and photographed using ChemiDoc (Bio-Rad, Hercules, CA).

Adenoviral Vector, Plasmid, Transfection, and Luciferase Assays

To overexpress NR0B2, RSL cells were transfected with the adenoviral vector expressing NR0B2, kindly provided by Dr. Eun-Kyeong Jo (Chungnam National University, South Korea; Yuk et al., 2011). For luciferase assays, RSL cells were transfected with the luciferase-expressing vector with an antioxidant response element (ARE), a gift from Dr. Raekil Park (GIST, South Korea; So et al., 2006), at 60% confluence using the Transit-LT1 transfection reagent (Mirus, Madison, WI), according to the manufacturer's instructions. The pRL-TK vector (Promega, Madison, WI) was cotransfected to normalize for transfection efficiency. Transfected cells were starved overnight in serum-free DMEM and harvested after exposure to IL-10 (50 ng/ml) for 16 and 42 h. Luciferase activity was measured using a luminometer after adding the necessary luciferase substrate (Promega). Results were expressed as a fold change in luciferase activity, taking the value of the non-treated group as 1.

Statistics

For technical and independent replicates, all experiments were carried out in triplicate and repeated twice independently. For quantitative RT-PCR analysis and luciferase assays, results were analyzed with the Student *t*-test and one-way ANOVA followed by the Tukey *post-hoc* test using R2.14.0 software for Windows (The R Foundation for Statistical Computing). A p-value < 0.05 was considered significant.

RESULTS

Hypochlorous Acid is Involved in Cochlear Injury

Hypochlorous acid, generated by myeloperoxidase-mediated peroxidation of chloride ions, is cytotoxic to various mammalian cells such as epithelial cells and red blood cells. To determine whether hypochlorous acid is cytotoxic to cochlear cells *in vitro*, we performed cell viability assays with HEI-OC1, an organ of Corti cell line after exposure to NaOCl, a sodium salt of hypochlorous acid, used as bleaches and deodorants. As shown in **Figure 1A**, NaOCl reduced cell viability of HEI-OC1 cells in a dose-dependent manner. HEI-OC1 cells were viable in a 1:1000 dilution of NaOCl whereas its 1:100 dilution showed significant cytotoxicity. Furthermore, combination of a recombinant myeloperoxidase with hydrogen peroxide was not cytotoxic to HEI-OC1 cells but appeared to potentiate cisplatin cytotoxicity (**Figure 1B**). However, hydrogen peroxide or myeloperoxidase alone insignificantly affect cisplatin cytotoxicity (data not shown). Then, we sought to determine an effect of antioxidants on hypochlorous acid-induced cytotoxicity.

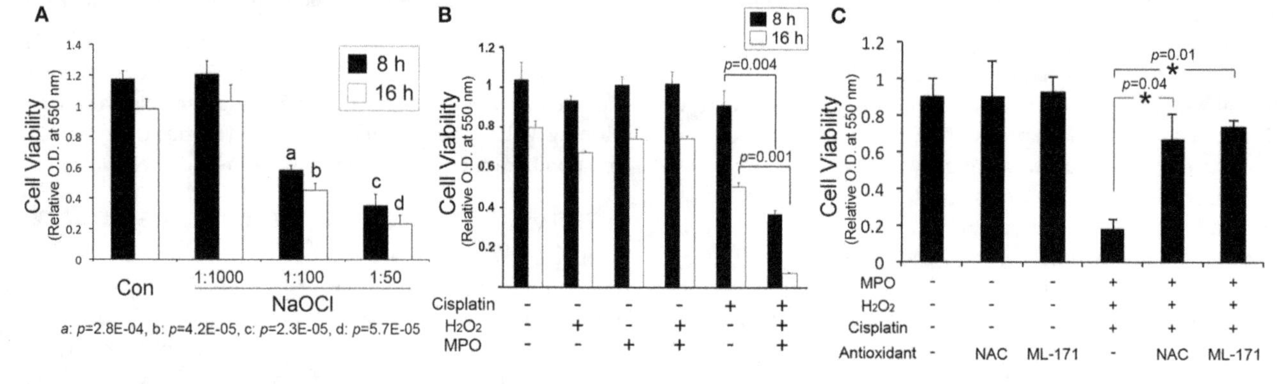

FIGURE 1 | Hypochlorous acid contributes to cochlear injury. **(A)** MTT assays show that sodium hypochlorite (NaOCl) inhibits the viability of HEI-OC1 cells in a dose-dependent manner. **(B)** Combination of hydrogen peroxide (H_2O_2) and myeloperoxidase (MPO) augments cisplatin cytotoxicity to HEI-OC1 cells. **(C)** N-Acetyl-L-cysteine (NAC) and ML-171 inhibit the enhancement of cisplatin cytotoxicity by the combination of H_2O_2 and MPO. Data are mean ± *SD* ($n = 3$). $^{*}p < 0.05$.

It was found that hypochlorous acid-mediated augmentation of cisplatin cytotoxicity is inhibited by N-Acetyl-L-cysteine and ML-171 (a NADPH oxidase 1 inhibitor) (**Figure 1C**). Taken together, it is suggested that hypochlorous acid, when it is excessively released by uncontrolled inflammatory reactions, potentially contributes to induction and exacerbation of cochlear injury.

NRF2 and NR0B2 Contribute to the Inhibitory Effect of IL-10 on Chemokine Production in Otic Fibrocytes

In our prior study, otic fibrocytes were shown to play a pivotal role in cochlear inflammation (Moon et al., 2007; Oh et al., 2012). It is unclear how IL-10 maintains HMOX1 upregulation in otic fibrocytes despite the inhibition of p38 MAPK required for HMOX1 upregulation (Kontoyiannis et al., 2001). In addition to p38 MAPK, NRF2 appeared to be involved in HMOX1 regulation in HEI-OC1 cells (So et al., 2006), which is a basic leucine zipper protein involved in the regulation of antioxidant genes. Therefore, we investigated an effect of IL-10 on the ARE/NRF2 system in otic fibrocytes. Luciferase assays were conducted with a luciferase vector containing ARE. As shown in **Figure 2A**, RSL cells appeared to upregulate ARE activity after exposure to IL-10. CoPP (a HMOX1 inducer), not ZnPP (a HMOX1 inhibitor), was found to upregulate NRF2 expression (**Figure 2B**), and HMOX1 expression was upregulated by IL-10 (**Figure 2C**). These findings indicate an existence of the NRF2-mediated positive feedback loop in otic fibrocytes, which may be required for maintaining IL-10-induced HMOX1 upregulation, through bypassing the p38 MAPK pathway.

In addition, we sought to determine the involvement of NR0B2 in the inhibitory effect of IL-10 on chemokine production because NR0B2, similar to IL-10 and carbon monoxide (CO) (Woo et al., 2015), suppresses inflammatory reactions through inhibition of NF-κB (Yuk et al., 2011). Quantitative RT-PCR analysis showed that RSL cells upregulate NR0B2 expression ~12-fold in response to CoPP, but ~3-fold to ZnPP (**Figure 2D**). Furthermore, adenoviral vector-mediated overexpression of NR0B2 was found to inhibit IL-1β-induced CCL2 upregulation in RSL cells (**Figure 2E**), which suggests the involvement of NR0B2 in the anti-inflammatory effect of IL-10.

Cochlear Localization of IL-10-Expressing Cells

Inner ear IL-10 expression is upregulated in experimental tympanogenic cochlear inflammation at the mRNA and protein levels (Trune et al., 2015); however, an intra-cochlear source of IL-10 still remains unclear. To determine cochlear localization of IL-10-expressing cells, immunolabeling of the mouse temporal bone sections were carried out. IL-10-positive cells first appeared in the stria vascularis on 1 d after LPS injection (**Figure 3A**). Consistently, surface preparation of the cochlear lateral wall showed the localization of IL-10-positive cells in the stria vascularis (**Figure 3D**). In addition, IL-10 was labeled in the suprastrial area and the lower part of the spiral ligament. On 5 d after injection, IL-10-positive cells were broadly found in the spiral ligament, spiral limbus and spiral ganglion (**Figure 3C**), but not in the stria vascularis (**Figure 3B**). IL-10 was not significantly labeled in the saline-injected control mice (data not shown). Altogether, these findings suggest that there are two groups of IL-10-expressing cells in the cochlea: recruited cells and resident cells, but their immunological characteristics remain to be revealed.

IL-10R Expression in the Organ of Corti Cells

The IL-10R complex is a tetramer composed of two subunits, IL-10R1 and IL-10R2. Previously, we have demonstrated the inducible expression of IL-10R1 and constitutive expression of IL-10R2 in otic fibrocytes (Woo et al., 2015), but it is unclear if other cochlear cells express IL-10Rs. To determine whether the organ of Corti cells express IL-10R1 enabling them to respond to IL-10, we performed immunolabeling with an anti-IL-10R1 antibody. As shown in **Figure 4A**, HEI-OC1 cells appeared to express IL-10R1. Moreover, IL-10R1 labeling was noted in the mouse organ of Corti cells such as inner and outer hair cells as

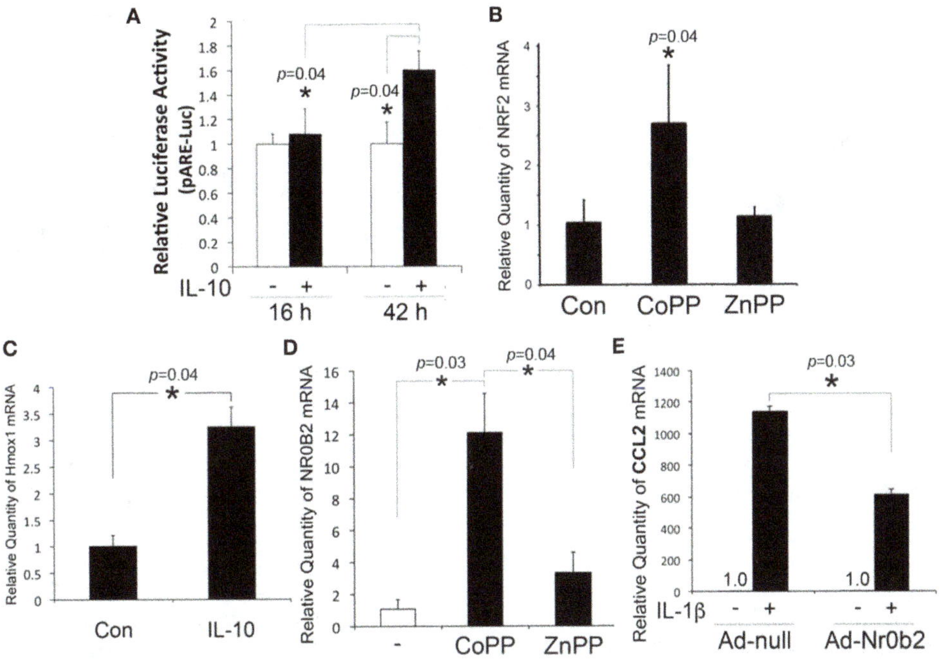

FIGURE 2 | Involvement of NRF2 and NR0B2 in the inhibitory effect of IL-10 on CCL2 regulation. **(A)** Luciferase assays show that IL-10 upregulates ARE activity in RSL cells. Quantitative RT-PCR analysis shows that RSL cells upregulate NRF2 upon exposure to CoPP **(B)** and HMOX1, to IL-10 **(C)**. NR0B2 is upregulated in response to CoPP in RSL cells **(D)**, and transfection of the adenoviral vector expressing NROB2 (Ad-Nr0b2) inhibits IL-1β-induced monocyte chemoattractant protein-1 (CCL2) upregulation **(E)**. Ad-null: a negative control vector. Data are mean ± *SD* (*n* = 3). $^*p < 0.05$.

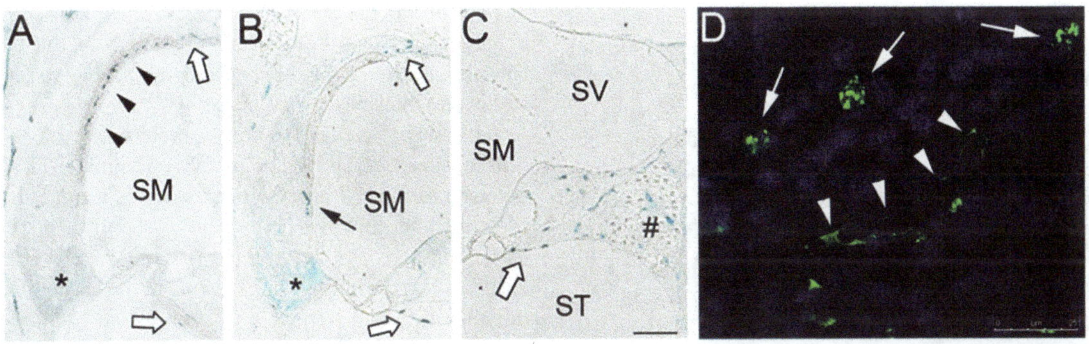

FIGURE 3 | Localization of IL-10-expressing cells in the mouse cochlea. **(A)** Immunolabeling shows appearance of IL-10-positive cells (black arrowheads) in the stria vascularis 1 d after LPS injection. IL-10 labeling is also noted in the lower part of the spiral ligament (asterisk). **(B,C)** On 5 d after LPS injection, IL-10-positive cells are observed in the spiral ligament (black arrow), but not in the stria vascularis. IL-10-positive cells are distributed in the spiral limbus, spiral ganglion area (#), suprastrial area and osseous spiral lamina (white block arrows). SM, scala media; ST, scala tympani; SV, scala vestibule. Scale bar: 100 μm. **(D)** Surface preparation showing IL-10-positive cells (white arrows) in the cochlear lateral wall tissue. IL-10 is also labeled in a capillary-like structure. Scale bar: 25 μm.

well as pillar cells (**Figures 4B–D**), but further studies are needed to characterize IL-10R-expressing cells in the organ of Corti.

IL-10 is Protective for Cochlear Cell Injury

In addition to the anti-inflammatory function, there is substantial evidence of the cytoprotective effect of IL-10 (Boyd et al., 2003; Zhou et al., 2009), but it is unclear whether IL-10 is protective for cochlear cell injury. HEI-OC1 cells were exposed to IL-10, and RT-PCR analysis was carried out. HEI-OC1 cells appeared to express Bcl-xL higher in response to IL-10 (**Figure 5A**), but further quantitative analysis would be needed to show IL-10-induced Bcl-xL regulation. MTT assays showed that IL-10 enhances the viability of HEI-OC1 cells against NaOCl-induced cytotoxicity (**Figure 5B**), but cisplatin cytotoxicity was not affected by IL-10 (data not shown). In addition to IL-10, we sought to determine a cytoprotective activity of IL-22, a member of the IL-10 superfamily because it uses an IL-10R2 subunit for forming an active IL-22R complex. Conventional RT-PCR analysis showed cisplatin-treated HEI-OC1 cells express IL-22RA (**Figure 5C**). Similar to IL-10, IL-22 was found to reduce NaOCl

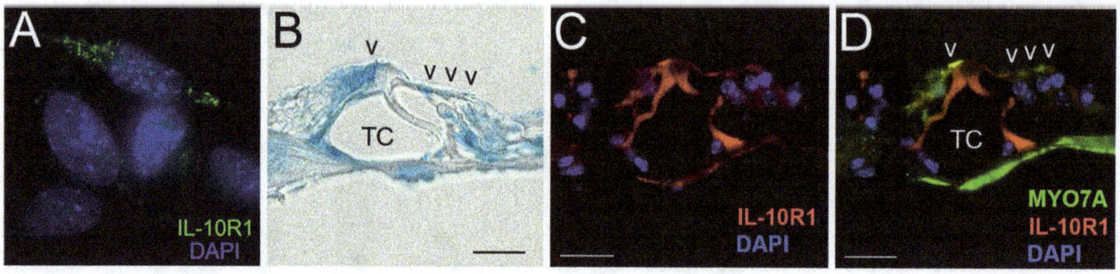

FIGURE 4 | Immunolabeling showing IL-10R1 expression in the HEI-OC1 cells **(A)** and mouse organ of Corti **(B–D)**. Note IL-10R1 labeling in the inner and outer hair cells as well as pillar cells. TC, Tunnel of Corti; V, auditory sensory cells. Scale bar: 25 μm.

cytotoxicity to HEI-OC1 cells (**Figure 5D**). Taken together, it is suggested that IL-10R2 ligands such as IL-10 and IL-22 have a protective effect on cochlear injury, mediated by regulation of anti-apoptotic factors.

DISCUSSION

Acquired SNHL is associated with postnatal cochlear injuries induced by a variety of causes including ototoxic drugs. This type of hearing loss is clinically important because it is potentially preventable and manageable if cochlear sensorineural tissues are preserved before they are irreversibly damaged. Multiple mechanisms are involved in the damage and survival of the cochlear sensorineural tissue (Wong and Ryan, 2015), and understanding those mechanisms would facilitate the development of a novel clinical tool for the management of acquired SNHL.

Tissue injury, in the absence of infection, is able to trigger inflammatory response to scavenge damaged tissues, but uncontrolled excessive inflammation rather leads to inadvertent tissue injury. Cochlear inflammation is like a double-edged sword; it is either harmful or beneficial to hosts. For instance, cochlear infiltration of macrophages is protective for the survival of spiral ganglion neurons after cochlear sensory cell death (Kaur et al., 2015). On the contrary, cochlear inflammation was found to not only mediate and but also aggravate ototoxic injury (So et al., 2007; Oh et al., 2011; Hirose et al., 2014). In this study, we showed hypochlorous acid, an inflammatory mediator released from activated phagocytes, is able to reduce the viability of cochlear cells *in vitro*. Further animal studies are needed to reveal how inflammatory mediators contribute to inflammation-mediated cochlear injury in a complex *in vivo* system.

Hypochlorous acid is a powerful oxidizing agent reacting with a wide variety of biomolecules such as proteins, nucleotides, and lipids, enabling it to kill pathogens (Pullar et al., 2000). For instance, hypochlorous acid inactivates proteins containing sulfhydryl groups, such as glutathione, by formation of disulfide bonds that result in crosslinking of proteins. Hypochlorous acid also reacts with NADH and the NH-groups of pyrimidines, leading to DNA denaturation. Reacting with lipids, hypochlorous acid induces formation of a chlorohydrin that can disrupt lipid bilayers and increase permeability. Consequently, hypochlorous acid, forming a significant cell stress, reduces the viability of various mammalian cells through apoptotic and necrotic cell death (Yap et al., 2006; Yang et al., 2012). Hypochlorous acid is known to induce Bax-dependent mitochondrial permeabilisation in chondrocytes, resulting in caspase-independent cell death (Whiteman et al., 2007). Similarly, hydrogen peroxide-induced oxidative stress appeared to lead to mitochondrial damage in cochlear sensory cells (Baker and Staecker, 2012), but it is yet to be elucidated how hypochlorous acid induces cochlear sensory cell death. Hypochlorous acid also appeared to enhance cisplatin cytotoxicity to HEI-OC1 cells, and this enhancement was inhibited by antioxidants. These findings suggest the potential involvement of hypochlorous acid-generating leukocytes. In cisplatin nephrotoxicity, there is an extensive renal infiltration of neutrophils (Tadagavadi et al., 2015), but it seems not to be apparent in cisplatin ototoxicity. This may be due to the blood-labyrinth barrier, but further studies are needed to reveal a role of leukocytes in cisplatin ototoxicity.

Otic fibrocytes, representing a heterogeneous population of cells localized in the spiral ligament and limbus, are importantly involved in normal hearing physiology as a route for potassium recycling and the formation of the mechanical anchorage for the basilar and tectorial membranes. In addition, otic fibrocytes were found to play an immunological role in the induction of cochlear inflammation and were able to suppress chemokine production in response to IL-10 (Moon et al., 2007; Oh et al., 2012; Woo et al., 2015). Similarly, circulating fibrocytes, which comprise <0.5% of blood cells, have been implicated in the pathophysiology of various inflammatory diseases through antigen presentation and secretion of inflammatory mediators (Galligan and Fish, 2013). Unlike otic fibrocytes originated from the periotic mesenchyme, circulating fibrocytes are derived from the bone marrow and are frequently transformed to activated fibroblast as observed in rheumatoid arthritis. Bone marrow cells were shown to contribute to the turnover of otic fibrocytes (Lang et al., 2006), but the involvement of circulating fibrocytes remains to be revealed.

In this study, we showed that our *in vitro* model of otic fibrocytes preserves the NRF2/CO-mediated feedback loop and CO-mediated NR0B2 regulatory pathway, involved in the anti-inflammatory activity of IL-10 (**Figure 6**). These findings suggest a therapeutic potential of CO releasers and NR0B2 inducers

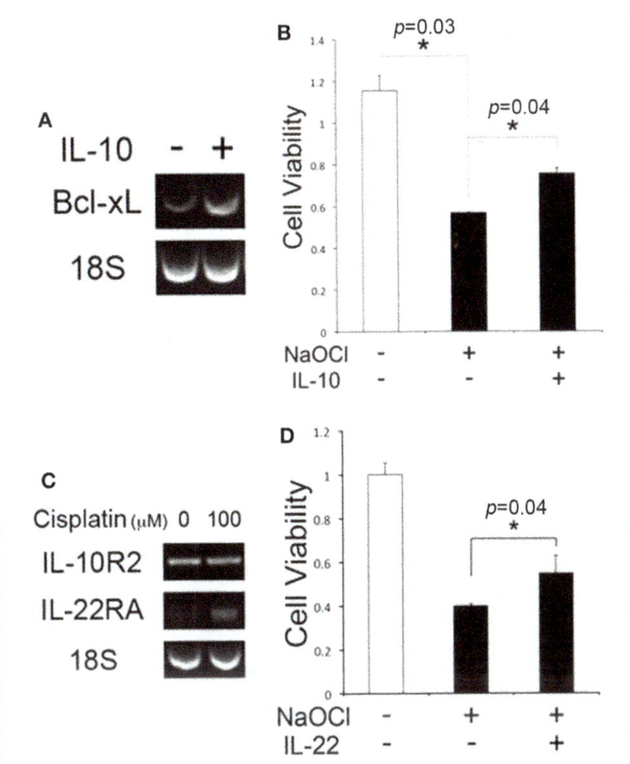

FIGURE 5 | IL-10 and IL-22 are protective against NaOCl cytotoxicity to HEI-OC1 cells. **(A)** Conventional RT-PCR analysis showing the Bcl-xL regulation in HEI-OC1 cells upon exposure to IL-10. 18S: 18S rRNA. **(B)** IL-10 enhances cell viability of HEI-OC1 cells against NaOCl cytotoxicity. **(C)** Conventional RT-PCR analysis showing the IL-22RA expression in cisplatin-treated HEI-OC1 cells. **(D)** MTT assays showing a protective effect of IL-22 on HEI-OC1 cells against NaOCl cytotoxicity. Data are mean ± *SD* ($n = 3$). $^{*}p < 0.05$.

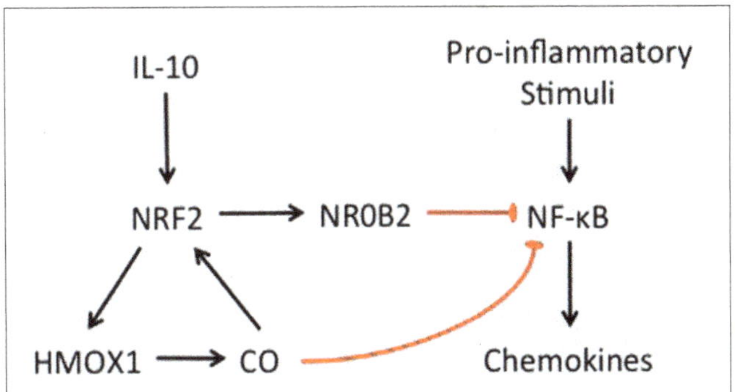

FIGURE 6 | Schematic illustration showing the involvement of NRF2 and NR0B2 in the anti-inflammatory activity of IL-10 in otic fibrocytes.

for the management of inflammation-mediated cochlear injury. For instance, ruthenium-based CO releasers not only suppress inflammatory responses *in vitro* (Sawle et al., 2005) but also ameliorate experimental acute pancreatitis (Xue and Habtezion, 2014). In addition, fenofibrate, a drug clinically used for hyperlipidemia, was found to attenuate experimental sepsis through NR0B2 upregulation (Yang et al., 2013). However, it remains to be revealed whether and how those pharmaceuticals affect inflammation-mediated cochlear injury.

IL-10 is predominantly produced by immune cells such as regulatory T cells, macrophages, and dendritic cells. For decades, the mammalian cochlea has been considered an immune-privileged organ. However, there is evidence supporting the presence of resident and recruited immune cells in the mammalian cochlea (Hirose et al., 2005; Okano et al., 2008). There are at least two types of resident macrophages in the cochlear lateral wall, including cochlear macrophages in the spiral ligament and perivascular macrophage-like melanocytes in the stria vascularis (Okano et al., 2008; Zhang et al., 2012). This study emphasized IL-10 expression in the recruited cells while our previous work showed the IL-10 expression in the isolated mouse cochlear lateral wall tissue, indicating its expression in the resident cells (Woo et al., 2015). Altogether, these findings suggest the involvement of both recruited cells and resident cells in IL-10 production in the cochlea, but further studies are necessary to elucidate their immunological characteristics.

In addition to the anti-inflammatory activity, there is accumulating evidence showing a cytoprotective effect of IL-10 on various mammalian cells such as neuronal cells (Molina-Holgado et al., 2001; Zhou et al., 2009; Lin et al., 2015). Cisplatin-induced acute renal injury also appeared to be reduced by systemic administration of IL-10 (Deng et al., 2001). Consistently, IL-10 deficiency and NRF2 depletion were shown to exacerbate experimental cisplatin nephrotoxicity (Liu et al., 2009; Tadagavadi and Reeves, 2010). In the cochlea, IL-10 has been reported to attenuate autoimmune hearing loss in experimental animals (Zhou et al., 2012). In agreement, we demonstrated the IL-10R1 expression in the organ of Corti as well as IL-10-mediated cytoprotection against hypochlorous acid-induced cytotoxicity. IL-10 also appeared to increase Bcl-xL expression, and Bcl-xL is suggested to inhibit hypochlorous acid cytotoxicity by retrotranslocation of Bax from the mitochondria into the cytosol (Edlich et al., 2011). IL-22, one of the IL-10 family cytokines also showed a meaningful cytoprotective activity, but further studies are needed to determine if combination of IL-10 and IL-22 synergistically upregulates IL-10R2/STAT3-mediated Bcl-xL expression and is effective for more potent ototoxic drugs. Moreover, animal studies are required to reveal how IL-10 affects cochlear inflammation and injury *in vivo*. Altogether, our results indicate the feasibility of an IL-10-based approach to manage inflammation-mediated cochlear injury.

Collectively, it is suggested that the IL-10/IL-10R axis is crucially involved in the modulation of cochlear inflammation in otic fibrocytes and the protection against inflammation-mediated cochlear injury in the organ of Corti. Understanding the complex network in IL-10 signaling would provide a new therapeutic target for the management of cochlear injury resulting in acquired SNHL.

AUTHOR CONTRIBUTIONS

MM and SK carried out the majority of the experiments and equally contributed to this work. DP and HP were involved in cell viability assays, immunolabeling, and statistical analysis. DL and RP were involved in histological analysis, data analysis, and preparation of the manuscript. SM designed the experiments, analyzed the results, and prepared the manuscript.

National Institute on Deafness and Other Communication Disorders (NIH) DC011862 (DL), and UCLA Faculty Research Grant (SM).

ACKNOWLEDGMENTS

We thank Dr. Eun-Kyeong Jo for providing the NR0B2-expressiong adenoviral vector and Dr. Jeong-Im Woo for offering technical support.

REFERENCES

Baker, K., and Staecker, H. (2012). Low dose oxidative stress induces mitochondrial damage in hair cells. *Anat. Rec.*295, 1868–1876. doi: 10.1002/ar.22594

Boyd, Z. S., Kriatchko, A., Yang, J., Agarwal, N., Wax, M. B., and Patil, R. V. (2003). Interleukin-10 receptor signaling through STAT-3 regulates the apoptosis of retinal ganglion cells in response to stress. *Invest. Ophthalmol. Vis. Sci.* 44, 5206–5211. doi: 10.1167/iovs.03-0534

Deng, J., Kohda, Y., Chiao, H., Wang, Y., Hu, X., Hewitt, S. M., et al. (2001). Interleukin-10 inhibits ischemic and cisplatin-induced acute renal injury. *Kidney Int.* 60, 2118–2128. doi: 10.1046/j.1523-1755.2001.00043.x

Dinh, C. T., Haake, S., Chen, S., Hoang, K., Nong, E., Eshraghi, A. A., et al. (2008). Dexamethasone protects organ of corti explants against tumor necrosis factor-alpha-induced loss of auditory hair cells and alters the expression levels of apoptosis-related genes. *Neuroscience* 157, 405–413. doi: 10.1016/j.neuroscience.2008.09.012

Edlich, F., Banerjee, S., Suzuki, M., Cleland, M. M., Arnoult, D., Wang, C., et al. (2011). Bcl-x(L) retrotranslocates Bax from the mitochondria into the cytosol. *Cell* 145, 104–116. doi: 10.1016/j.cell.2011.02.034

Galligan, C. L., and Fish, E. N. (2013). The role of circulating fibrocytes in inflammation and autoimmunity. *J. Leukoc. Biol.* 93, 45–50. doi: 10.1189/jlb.0712365

Hammerschmidt, S., and Wahn, H. (1997). Comparable effects of HOCl and of FMLP-stimulated PMN on the circulation in an isolated lung model. *Am. J. Respir. Crit. Care Med.* 156, 924–931. doi: 10.1164/ajrccm.156.3.9608032

Hirose, K., Discolo, C. M., Keasler, J. R., and Ransohoff, R. (2005). Mononuclear phagocytes migrate into the murine cochlea after acoustic trauma. *J. Comp. Neurol.* 489, 180–194. doi: 10.1002/cne.20619

Hirose, K., Li, S. Z., Ohlemiller, K. K., and Ransohoff, R. M. (2014). Systemic lipopolysaccharide induces cochlear inflammation and exacerbates the synergistic ototoxicity of kanamycin and furosemide. *J. Assoc. Res. Otolaryngol.* 15, 555–570. doi: 10.1007/s10162-014-0458-8

Huang, J., Tabbi-Anneni, I., Gunda, V., and Wang, L. (2010). Transcription factor Nrf2 regulates SHP and lipogenic gene expression in hepatic lipid metabolism. *Am. J. Physiol. Gastrointest. Liver Physiol.* 299, G1211–G1221. doi: 10.1152/ajpgi.00322.2010

Johnson, R. J., Couser, W. G., Chi, E. Y., Adler, S., and Klebanoff, S. J. (1987). New mechanism for glomerular injury. Myeloperoxidase-hydrogen peroxide-halide system. *J. Clin. Invest.* 79, 1379–1387. doi: 10.1172/JCI112965

Kalinec, G. M., Webster, P., Lim, D. J., and Kalinec, F. (2003). A cochlear cell line as an *in vitro* system for drug ototoxicity screening. *Audiol. Neurootol.* 8, 177–189. doi: 10.1159/000071059

Kaur, T., Zamani, D., Tong, L., Rubel, E. W., Ohlemiller, K. K., Hirose, K., et al. (2015). Fractalkine signaling regulates macrophage recruitment into the cochlea and promotes the survival of spiral ganglion neurons after selective hair cell lesion. *J. Neurosci.* 35, 15050–15061. doi: 10.1523/JNEUROSCI.2325-15.2015

Keithley, E. M., Wang, X., and Barkdull, G. C. (2008). Tumor necrosis factor alpha can induce recruitment of inflammatory cells to the cochlea. *Otol. Neurotol.* 29, 854–859. doi: 10.1097/MAO.0b013e31818256a9

Kontoyiannis, D., Kotlyarov, A., Carballo, E., Alexopoulou, L., Blackshear, P. J., Gaestel, M., et al. (2001). Interleukin-10 targets p38 MAPK to modulate ARE-dependent TNF mRNA translation and limit intestinal pathology. *EMBO J.* 20, 3760–3770. doi: 10.1093/emboj/20.14.3760

Lang, H., Ebihara, Y., Schmiedt, R. A., Minamiguchi, H., Zhou, D., Smythe, N., et al. (2006). Contribution of bone marrow hematopoietic stem cells to adult mouse inner ear: mesenchymal cells and fibrocytes. *J. Comp. Neurol.* 496, 187–201. doi: 10.1002/cne.20929

Levy, Y., and Brouet, J. C. (1994). Interleukin-10 prevents spontaneous death of germinal center B cells by induction of the bcl-2 protein. *J. Clin. Invest.* 93, 424–428. doi: 10.1172/JCI116977

Lin, L., Chen, H., Zhang, Y., Lin, W., Liu, Y., Li, T., et al. (2015). IL-10 protects neurites in oxygen-glucose-deprived cortical neurons through the PI3K/Akt pathway. *PLoS ONE* 10:e0136959. doi: 10.1371/journal.pone.0136959

Lindemans, C. A., Calafiore, M., Mertelsmann, A. M., O'connor, M. H., Dudakov, J. A., Jenq, R. R., et al. (2015). Interleukin-22 promotes intestinal-stem-cell-mediated epithelial regeneration. *Nature* 528, 560–564. doi: 10.1038/nature16460

Liu, M., Grigoryev, D. N., Crow, M. T., Haas, M., Yamamoto, M., Reddy, S. P., et al. (2009). Transcription factor Nrf2 is protective during ischemic and nephrotoxic acute kidney injury in mice. *Kidney Int.* 76, 277–285. doi: 10.1038/ki.2009.157

Livak, K. J., and Schmittgen, T. D. (2001). Analysis of relative gene expression data using real-time quantitative PCR and the $2^{-\Delta\Delta CT}$ method. *Methods* 25, 402–408. doi: 10.1006/meth.2001.1262

Molina-Holgado, E., Vela, J. M., Arevalo-Martin, A., and Guaza, C. (2001). LPS/IFN-gamma cytotoxicity in oligodendroglial cells: role of nitric oxide and protection by the anti-inflammatory cytokine IL-10. *Eur. J. Neurosci.* 13, 493–502. doi: 10.1046/j.0953-816x.2000.01412.x

Moon, S. K., Woo, J. I., Lee, H. Y., Park, R., Shimada, J., Pan, H., et al. (2007). Toll-like receptor 2-dependent NF-kappaB activation is involved in nontypeable *Haemophilus influenzae*-induced monocyte chemotactic protein 1 up-regulation in the spiral ligament fibrocytes of the inner ear. *Infect. Immun.* 75, 3361–3372. doi: 10.1128/IAI.01886-06

Nagalakshmi, M. L., Rascle, A., Zurawski, S., Menon, S., and de Waal Malefyt, R. (2004). Interleukin-22 activates STAT3 and induces IL-10 by colon epithelial cells. *Int. Immunopharmacol.* 4, 679–691. doi: 10.1016/j.intimp.2004.01.008

Oh, G. S., Kim, H. J., Choi, J. H., Shen, A., Kim, C. H., Kim, S. J., et al. (2011). Activation of lipopolysaccharide-TLR4 signaling accelerates the ototoxic potential of cisplatin in mice. *J. Immunol.* 186, 1140–1150. doi: 10.4049/jimmunol.1002183

Oh, S., Woo, J. I., Lim, D. J., and Moon, S. K. (2012). ERK2-dependent activation of c-Jun is required for nontypeable *Haemophilus influenzae*-induced CXCL2 upregulation in inner ear fibrocytes. *J. Immunol.* 188, 3496–3505. doi: 10.4049/jimmunol.1103182

Okano, T., Nakagawa, T., Kita, T., Kada, S., Yoshimoto, M., Nakahata, T., et al. (2008). Bone marrow-derived cells expressing Iba1 are constitutively present as resident tissue macrophages in the mouse cochlea. *J. Neurosci. Res.* 86, 1758–1767. doi: 10.1002/jnr.21625

Pickert, G., Neufert, C., Leppkes, M., Zheng, Y., Wittkopf, N., Warntjen, M., et al. (2009). STAT3 links IL-22 signaling in intestinal epithelial cells to mucosal wound healing. *J. Exp. Med.* 206, 1465–1472. doi: 10.1084/jem.20082683

Pullar, J. M., Vissers, M. C., and Winterbourn, C. C. (2000). Living with a killer: the effects of hypochlorous acid on mammalian cells. *IUBMB Life* 50, 259–266. doi: 10.1080/15216540051080958

Radaeva, S., Sun, R., Pan, H. N., Hong, F., and Gao, B. (2004). Interleukin 22 (IL-22) plays a protective role in T cell-mediated murine hepatitis: IL-22 is a survival factor for hepatocytes via STAT3 activation. *Hepatology* 39, 1332–1342. doi: 10.1002/hep.20184

Sawle, P., Foresti, R., Mann, B. E., Johnson, T. R., Green, C. J., and Motterlini, R. (2005). Carbon monoxide-releasing molecules (CO-RMs) attenuate the inflammatory response elicited by lipopolysaccharide in RAW264.7 murine macrophages. *Br. J. Pharmacol.* 145, 800–810. doi: 10.1038/sj.bjp.0706241

Sharma, S., Yang, B., Xi, X., Grotta, J. C., Aronowski, J., and Savitz, S. I. (2011). IL-10 directly protects cortical neurons by activating PI-3 kinase and STAT-3 pathways. *Brain Res.* 1373, 189–194. doi: 10.1016/j.brainres.2010.11.096

So, H., Kim, H., Kim, Y., Kim, E., Pae, H. O., Chung, H. T., et al. (2008). Evidence that cisplatin-induced auditory damage is attenuated by downregulation of pro-inflammatory cytokines via Nrf2/HO-1. *J. Assoc. Res. Otolaryngol.* 9, 290–306. doi: 10.1007/s10162-008-0126-y

So, H., Kim, H., Lee, J. H., Park, C., Kim, Y., Kim, E., et al. (2007). Cisplatin cytotoxicity of auditory cells requires secretions of proinflammatory cytokines via activation of ERK and NF-kappaB. *J. Assoc. Res. Otolaryngol.* 8, 338–355. doi: 10.1007/s10162-007-0084-9

So, H. S., Kim, H. J., Lee, J. H., Lee, J. H., Park, S. Y., Park, C., et al. (2006). Flunarizine induces Nrf2-mediated transcriptional activation of heme oxygenase-1 in protection of auditory cells from cisplatin. *Cell Death Differ.* 13, 1763–1775. doi: 10.1038/sj.cdd.4401863

Stassi, G., Di Liberto, D., Todaro, M., Zeuner, A., Ricci-Vitiani, L., Stoppacciaro, A., et al. (2000). Control of target cell survival in thyroid autoimmunity by T helper cytokines via regulation of apoptotic proteins. *Nat. Immunol.* 1, 483–488. doi: 10.1038/82725

Tadagavadi, R. K., Gao, G., Wang, W. W., Gonzalez, M. R., and Reeves, W. B. (2015). Dendritic cell protection from cisplatin nephrotoxicity is independent of neutrophils. *Toxins* 7, 3245–3256. doi: 10.3390/toxins7083245

Tadagavadi, R. K., and Reeves, W. B. (2010). Endogenous IL-10 attenuates cisplatin nephrotoxicity: role of dendritic cells. *J. Immunol.* 185, 4904–4911. doi: 10.4049/jimmunol.1000383

Trune, D. R., Kempton, B., Hausman, F. A., Larrain, B. E., and Macarthur, C. J. (2015). Correlative mRNA and protein expression of middle and inner ear inflammatory cytokines during mouse acute otitis media. *Hear. Res.* 326, 49–58. doi: 10.1016/j.heares.2015.04.006

Whiteman, M., Chu, S. H., Siau, J. L., Rose, P., Sabapathy, K., Schantz, J. T., et al. (2007). The pro-inflammatory oxidant hypochlorous acid induces Bax-dependent mitochondrial permeabilisation and cell death through AIF-/EndoG-dependent pathways. *Cell. Signal.* 19, 705–714. doi: 10.1016/j.cellsig.2006.08.019

Wong, A. C., and Ryan, A. F. (2015). Mechanisms of sensorineural cell damage, death and survival in the cochlea. *Front. Aging Neurosci.* 7:58. doi: 10.3389/fnagi.2015.00058

Woo, J. I., Kil, S. H., Oh, S., Lee, Y. J., Park, R., Lim, D. J., et al. (2015). IL-10/HMOX1 signaling modulates cochlear inflammation via negative regulation of MCP-1/CCL2 expression in cochlear fibrocytes. *J. Immunol.* 194, 3953–3961. doi: 10.4049/jimmunol.1402751

Xue, J., and Habtezion, A. (2014). Carbon monoxide-based therapy ameliorates acute pancreatitis via TLR4 inhibition. *J. Clin. Invest.* 124, 437–447. doi: 10.1172/JCI71362

Yang, C. S., Yuk, J. M., Kim, J. J., Hwang, J. H., Lee, C. H., Kim, J. M., et al. (2013). Small heterodimer partner-targeting therapy inhibits systemic inflammatory responses through mitochondrial uncoupling protein 2. *PLoS ONE* 8:e63435. doi: 10.1371/journal.pone.0063435

Yang, Y. T., Whiteman, M., and Gieseg, S. P. (2012). HOCl causes necrotic cell death in human monocyte derived macrophages through calcium dependent calpain activation. *Biochim. Biophys. Acta* 1823, 420–429. doi: 10.1016/j.bbamcr.2011.09.019

Yap, Y. W., Whiteman, M., Bay, B. H., Li, Y., Sheu, F. S., Qi, R. Z., et al. (2006). Hypochlorous acid induces apoptosis of cultured cortical neurons through activation of calpains and rupture of lysosomes. *J. Neurochem.* 98, 1597–1609. doi: 10.1111/j.1471-4159.2006.03996.x

Yian, C., Moon, S. K., Jin, S., Webster, P., Rhim, J. S., Andalibi, A., et al. (2006). Characterization of rat spiral ligament cell line immortalized by adenovirus 12-simian virus 40 hybrid virus. *Ann. Otol. Rhinol. Laryngol.* 115, 930–938. doi: 10.1177/000348940611501213

Yuk, J. M., Shin, D. M., Lee, H. M., Kim, J. J., Kim, S. W., Jin, H. S., et al. (2011). The orphan nuclear receptor SHP acts as a negative regulator in inflammatory signaling triggered by Toll-like receptors. *Nat. Immunol.* 12, 742–751. doi: 10.1038/ni.2064

Zhang, W., Dai, M., Fridberger, A., Hassan, A., Degagne, J., Neng, L., et al. (2012). Perivascular-resident macrophage-like melanocytes in the inner ear are essential for the integrity of the intrastrial fluid-blood barrier. *Proc. Natl. Acad. Sci. U.S.A.* 109, 10388–10393. doi: 10.1073/pnas.1205210109

Zhou, B., Kermany, M. H., Cai, Q., Cai, C., Zhou, Y., Nair, U., et al. (2012). Experimental autoimmune hearing loss is exacerbated in IL-10-deficient mice and reversed by IL-10 gene transfer. *Gene Ther.* 19, 228–235. doi: 10.1038/gt.2011.88

Zhou, Z., Peng, X., Insolera, R., Fink, D. J., and Mata, M. (2009). Interleukin-10 provides direct trophic support to neurons. *J. Neurochem.* 110, 1617–1627. doi: 10.1111/j.1471-4159.2009.06263.x

18

Protein Synthesis Inhibition and Activation of the c-Jun N-Terminal Kinase are Potential Contributors to Cisplatin Ototoxicity

*Brian D. Nicholas†, Shimon Francis†, Elizabeth L. Wagner, Sibo Zhang and Jung-Bum Shin**

Department of Neuroscience, University of Virginia, Charlottesville, VA, United States

Edited by:
Jian Zuo,
St. Jude Children's Research Hospital, United States

Reviewed by:
Jonathan E. Gale,
University College London, United Kingdom
Tatsuro Mutoh,
Fujita Health University, Japan

***Correspondence:**
Jung-Bum Shin
js2ee@virginia.edu

Cisplatin has been regarded as an effective and versatile chemotherapeutic agent for nearly 40 years. Though the associated dose-dependent ototoxicity is known, the cellular mechanisms by which cochleovestibular hair cell death occur are not well understood. We have previously shown that aminoglycoside ototoxicity is mediated in part by cytosolic protein synthesis inhibition. Despite a lack of molecular similarity, aminoglycosides were shown to elicit similar stress pathways to cisplatin. We therefore reasoned that there may be some role of protein synthesis inhibition in cisplatin ototoxicity. Employing a modification of the bioorthogonal noncanonical amino acid tagging (BONCAT) method, we evaluated the effects of cisplatin on cellular protein synthesis. We show that cisplatin inhibits cellular protein synthesis in organ of Corti explant cultures. Similar to what was found after gentamicin exposure, cisplatin activates both the c-Jun N-terminal kinase (JNK) and mammalian target of rapamycin (mTOR) pathways. In contrast to aminoglycosides, cisplatin also inhibits protein synthesis in all cochlear cell types. We further demonstrate that the multikinase inhibitor sorafenib completely prevents JNK activation, while providing only moderate hair cell protection. Simultaneous stimulation of cellular protein synthesis by insulin, however, significantly improved hair cell survival in culture. The presented data provides evidence for a potential role of protein synthesis inhibition in cisplatin-mediated ototoxicity.

Keywords: Cisplatin, ototoxicity, inner ear, hair cell, protein synthesis, BONCAT, JNK, mTOR

INTRODUCTION

Cisplatin is a long-established therapeutic agent for a variety of malignant diseases (Rybak, 2007; Langer et al., 2013; Landier, 2016). It is associated with dose-dependent nephro- and ototoxicity, though the cellular mechanisms by which these processes occur are poorly understood (Humes, 1999; Karasawa and Steyger, 2015). Within the cochlea, cisplatin uptake results in the degradation of outer hair cells with subsequent loss of inner hair cells and supporting cells within the organ of Corti at higher doses (Hawkins, 1976). A similar loss of sensory hair cells within the vestibular end organs has been noted after exposure to cisplatin (Black et al., 1982; Zhang et al., 2003; Baker et al., 2015). The incidence of ototoxicity among those receiving cisplatin ranges from 35% to 100% (Benedetti Panici et al., 1993; Nitz et al., 2013; Malgonde et al., 2015).

Reflecting the incomplete understanding of the cellular mechanisms underlying cisplatin ototoxicity, clinical trials employing empiric strategies for otoprotection have resulted in mostly mixed results (Marina et al., 2005; Gurney et al., 2014; Yoo et al., 2014).

Protein synthesis and cellular degradation are tightly regulated processes that allow for cells to adapt to a range of environmental conditions. A universal stress response within the cell has been described and nutritional, chemical and ischemic stresses to the cell can alter intracellular protein homeostasis (Gebauer and Hentze, 2004; Sonenberg and Hinnebusch, 2009). In addition to serving as a response to stress conditions, the regulation of protein synthesis and proteolysis, itself, can alter the viability of the cell. An arrest of translation or disruption of protein degradation has been shown to result in neurodegenerative and ototoxic disease processes (Keller, 2006; Kim et al., 2017). The relationship between protein synthesis inhibition and apoptosis, however, is complex. While known inhibitors of protein synthesis such as ricin and anisomycin have been shown to induce apoptosis (Kageyama et al., 2002; Croons et al., 2009), the apoptotic process itself is dependent on cellular protein synthesis (Lockshin and Zakeri, 1992; Mesner et al., 1992). In this way, translational arrest can either promote or inhibit programmed cell death (Rehen et al., 1996), depending on how the balance of pro-survival and pro-death factors is influenced by protein synthesis inhibition in that particular cell type or tissue.

We have previously shown that gentamicin-induced ototoxicity is associated with cellular protein synthesis inhibition (Francis et al., 2013). This is correlated with activation of both the c-Jun N-terminal kinase (JNK) and mammalian target of rapamycin (mTOR) pathways (Francis et al., 2013). There appears to be significant similarity between cellular processes associated with aminoglycoside and cisplatin ototoxity (Schacht et al., 2012). The goal of the present study, then, was to determine if cisplatin ototoxicity is associated with an inhibition of cellular protein synthesis. In addition, we sought to test whether modulation of correlated cell signaling events such as the JNK and mTOR pathways, and/or stimulation of protein synthesis might mitigate cisplatin-induced sensory hair cell loss.

In order to test our hypothesis, we utilized the biorthogonal non-canonical amino acid tagging (BONCAT) method (Dieterich et al., 2007), in which the incorporation of methionine analogs into newly formed proteins serves as a measure for overall cellular protein synthesis activity. We recently modified this method to allow for a cell-by-cell analysis of protein synthesis (Francis et al., 2013). The effects of varying concentrations of cisplatin on cellular protein synthesis in organ of Corti explant cultures were detailed. As seen previously with gentamicin, cisplatin inhibits cellular protein synthesis. We further demonstrate an associated activation of the JNK and mTOR pathways after exposure to cisplatin, which in turn is prevented by the multikinase inhibitor sorafenib. While sorafenib alone only moderately improves hair cell survival, combination with insulin, employed here for its ability to stimulate cellular protein synthesis, significantly improves hair cell survival after cisplatin exposure.

MATERIALS AND METHODS

Animal Care and Handling

This study involves the use of mice. The protocol for care and use of animals was approved by the University of Virginia Animal Care and Use Committee. The University of Virginia is accredited by the American Association for the Accreditation of Laboratory Animal Care. All mouse experiments were performed using the CBA/J inbred mouse strain. Neonatal mouse pups (postnatal day 3 (P3)–P4) were killed by rapid decapitation, and mature mice were killed by CO_2 asphyxiation followed by cervical dislocation.

Organotypic Explant Cultures

Mouse cochleae and utricles were dissected in Hank's balanced salt solution (HBSS, Invitrogen, MA, USA) containing 25 mM HEPES, pH 7.5. The organ of Corti was separated from the spiral lamina and the spiral ligament using fine forceps and attached to the bottom of sterile 35 mm Petri dishes (BD Falcon, NY), with the hair bundle side facing up. The dissection medium was then replaced by two exchanges with culture medium (complete high-glucose DMEM containing 1% FBS, supplemented with ampicillin and ciprofloxacin). Prior to experimental manipulation, explants were pre-cultured for 24 h, to allow acclimatization to the culture conditions (Francis et al., 2013). Cisplatin (TEVA, MD NDC 0703-5748-11, injectable solution, 1 mg/ml) and gentamicin (Sigma, St. Louis, MO, USA) were dissolved in water. Sorafenib and rapamycin (Selleckchem, TX, USA) were dissolved in DMSO (1 mM stock solutions). The organ of Corti was cultured as a whole. Number of experiments (*n*) for quantification of hair cell numbers, activated caspase-3 positive cells and Azidohomoalanine (AHA) uptake indicates number of organs.

BONCAT and Click-Chemistry Reaction

AHA, incorporated into new proteins, was conjugated via click-chemistry reaction with a biotin moiety, which in turn was detected using streptavidin (SA)-horseradish peroxidase (HRP) for immunoblots and SA-fluorophore for fluorescence microscopy. In contrast to a more complex protocol used in a previous study (Francis et al., 2013), we here used a copper-free version of the click-chemistry reaction (strain-promoted click chemistry; Agard et al., 2004). Here, the azide group on AHA is reacted with a dibenzylcyclooctyne (DBCO)-conjugated biotin (instead of alkyne-biotin) in aqueous solution that does not require copper catalysis. Organotypic explants were cultured for various times in methionine-free medium containing AHA (Invitrogen, catalog #C10102, or Anaspec, Fremont, CA, USA) at a final concentration of 400 μM. After the desired culture time, organs were washed in HBSS for 15 min at 37°C to remove unincorporated AHA. For immunoblots, protein lysates were prepared (10 mg/ml) in protein extraction buffer, and incubated in 50 mM Tris/HCl, pH 7.5, containing 10 μM sulfo-DBCO-biotin conjugate (Click Chemistry Tools, AZ, USA;

catalog #A115-10) for 1 h. Proteins were precipitated using methanol/chloroform protein extraction. The protein pellet was resolubilized into 100 μl Laemmli buffer, and 10 μl was run on the gels. For copper-free click reaction in fixed whole-mount organs to be imaged by fluorescence microscopy, explants that have incorporated AHA were fixed, permeabilized and washed in 50 mM Tris/HCl, pH 7.5. Organs were then incubated in 50 mM Tris/HCl, pH 7.5, 0.2% saponin, containing 10 μM sulfo-DBCO-biotin conjugate (Click Chemistry Tools, catalog #A115-10) for 1 h and washed three times in PBS. Biotin was then detected using fluorophore-conjugated SA.

Quantification of AHA Signal

For a relative quantification of AHA incorporation, the fluorescence intensity of the AHA-biotin-fluorophore conjugate was normalized to Myosin 7a (MYO7A) immunoreactivity, because it was consistent, strong and not affected by cisplatin exposure in the time frame relevant for AHA uptake measurements (4 h; see **Figure 1F**). For hair cells, the AHA signal was normalized to MYO7A of the same cell, and for supporting cells, AHA immunofluorescence was normalized to MYO7A of the adjacent hair cell. Staining procedures and confocal microscopy settings (gain, offset, laser power, magnification and z-stack numbers) were kept identical for all comparative experiments. For each experimental group, four organ of Corti were analyzed, with a minimum of 40 cells quantified per organ (mid frequency region).

Immunoblots

Organs were homogenized in reducing SDS-PAGE sample buffer, heated to 70°C for 5 min, and microcentrifuged for 5 min to remove insoluble debris. Proteins were resolved using Bis-Tris SDS PAGE gel (Novex 4%–12%, Invitrogen, and TGX gels from Bio-Rad, CA, USA), transferred to PVDF membranes and stained with India Ink (total protein stain). Blots were then blocked in blocking buffer (ECL prime blocking reagent; GE Healthcare, UK) for 1 h and probed with the following primary antibodies overnight at 4°C: mouse anti phospho-JNK antibody (Thr183/Tyr185; catalog #9255, Cell Signaling, 1:1000), rabbit anti phospho-rpS6 antibody (Ser235/236; catalog #2211, Cell Signaling, 1:1000), rabbit anti-phospho-cJun (Ser73; cat #3270, 1:1000). After three 5 min washes in PBS/0.3% Tween 20, blots were incubated with HRP conjugated goat anti-rabbit secondary antibody (Cell Signaling Technology, Danvers, MA, USA) for 1 h, and bands were visualized by ECL reagent (Pierce Biotechnology, IL, USA; ECL Western blotting substrate and GE Healthcare GE ECL prime Western blotting reagent). Chemiluminescence was detected using an ImageQuant LAS4000 mini imager (GE Healthcare). The immunoblot for AHA incorporation (**Figure 2B**) was quantified by normalizing gray values from the AHA-biotin-SA-HRP signal to the gray value of corresponding india ink stain, which is a measure for total protein loading. Triplicate measurements were performed.

Immunocytochemistry

Tissues were fixed for 25 min in 3% formaldehyde, washed three times for 5 min each in PBS, and incubated in blocking buffer (PBS containing 1% bovine serum albumin, 3% normal donkey serum and 0.2% saponin) for 1 h. Organs were then incubated with primary antibody overnight at room temperature in blocking buffer. Organs were washed three times for 5 min each with PBS and incubated with secondary antibodies (fluorophore-conjugated IgGs at 1:100; Invitrogen) and 0.25 μM phalloidin-Alexa 488 (Invitrogen) in the blocking solution for 1–3 h. Finally, organs were washed five times in PBS and mounted in Vectashield (Vector Laboratories, CA, USA). Samples were imaged using Zeiss LSM700 confocal microscopes. The following antibodies were used in this study: mouse anti-MYO7A antibody (Developmental Studies Hybridoma Bank, IA, USA, 1:100), mouse anti phosphorylated JNK (p-JNK) antibody (Thr183/Tyr185; catalog #9255, Cell Signaling, 1:100), rabbit anti phosphorylated ribosomal protein S6 (p-rpS6) antibody (Ser235/236; catalog #2211, Cell Signaling, 1:100), mouse anti gentamicin antibody (QED Biosciences, CA, USA, 1:100), rabbit anti cleaved caspase-3 antibody (Asp175; catalog #9661, Cell Signaling, 1:200).

Hair Cell Counts

Hair cells were counted based on MYO7A or Phalloidin (in case MYO7A immunoreactivity was abolished despite presence of hair cell/bundle staining, as in **Figures 3**, **4**) staining over a length of 100 μm of the basal turn of the cochlea, omitting the last 100 μm of the basal tip, which was often damaged during dissection. Activated caspase-3 immunoreactivity was counted over a stretch of 200 μm of the basal turn. For each experimental condition, at least four organ of Corti were analyzed. Exact numbers of organs (n) are indicated in the legends.

Statistical Analysis

For statistical analysis, GraphPad Prism was used. One-way analysis of variance (ANOVA) was used to determine statistically significant differences between the means of the experimental groups. For pair-wise comparisons, a Tukey *post hoc* analysis was performed. P values smaller than 0.05 were considered significant. All n in statistical analyses refer to number of organs per experimental condition. All error bars indicate SEM.

RESULTS

Cisplatin Inhibits Protein Synthesis in Organ of Corti Explants

We first sought to visualize and quantify, with cellular resolution, the effect of cisplatin on overall protein synthesis in organ of Corti explant cultures. This was achieved using the previously described BONCAT method (Dieterich et al., 2006), in which the incorporation of the methionine analog AHA into newly synthesized proteins serves as a proxy for overall protein synthesis activity. **Figure 1A** illustrates the molecular structure of AHA as it compares to methionine. **Figure 1B** illustrates the BONCAT technique using either cell lysates for immunoblot or fixed organs for fluorescence microscopy. Organ of Corti explants from 3 to 4 day old mice were cultured in growth medium containing AHA, in the presence of varying cisplatin

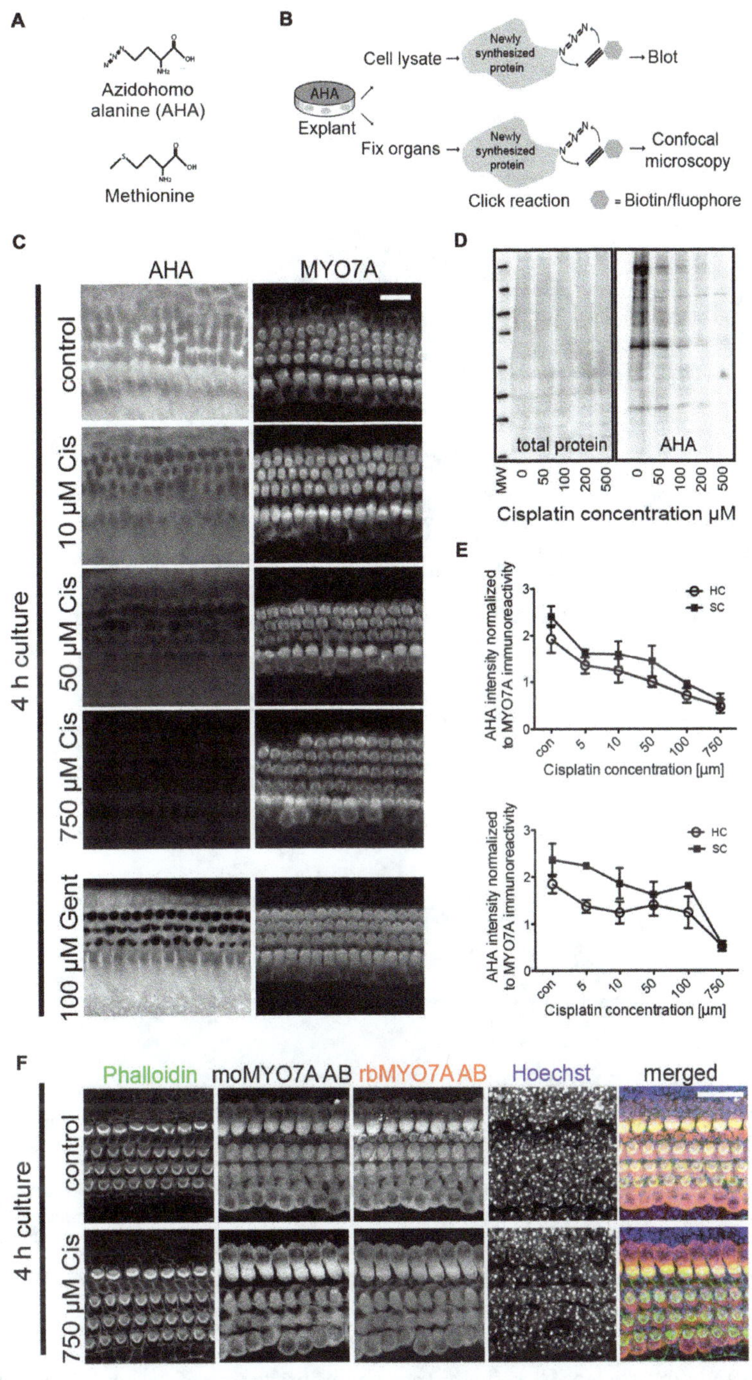

FIGURE 1 | Bioorthogonal noncanonical amino acid tagging (BONCAT) to study protein synthesis within sensory hair cells of mouse explant cultures. **(A)** Chemical structure of methionine and its utilized analog, azidohomoalanine (AHA). **(B)** Schematic of the BONCAT technique using either cell lysates for immunoblot or fixed organs for fluorescence microscopy. **(C)** AHA-biotin immunoreactivity demonstrates dose-dependent inhibition of protein synthesis on a cell-by-cell basis after treatment with cisplatin. P3–4 organ of Corti explants were cultured in growth medium containing AHA, in the presence of varying cisplatin concentrations. After 4 h, prior to the onset of cisplatin-induced cell death or changes in Myosin 7a (MYO7A) levels, explants were fixed and processed for click-chemistry reaction and imaged using confocal microscopy. Protein synthesis is inhibited in both hair cells and supporting cells. Gentamicin induced inhibition of cellular protein synthesis shown to involve only hair cells (bottom panels). Scale bar 20 µm. **(D)** Immunoblot showing a decrease in cellular protein synthesis within organ of Corti explant lysates. AHA-biotin was detected with streptavidin (SA)-horseradish peroxidase (HRP). **(E)** Quantification of AHA uptake relative to immunoreactivity of MYO7A within mouse cochleae and utricles (n = 4). There is a marked dose-dependent reduction in AHA uptake in both sensory hair cells (HC) and supporting cells (SC). Error bars indicate SEM (standard error of the mean). **(F)** MYO7A immunoreactivity and nuclear morphology is not affected by short exposure (4 h) to high concentrations of cisplatin, demonstrating the appropriateness of using MYO7A staining to normalize the AHA signal.

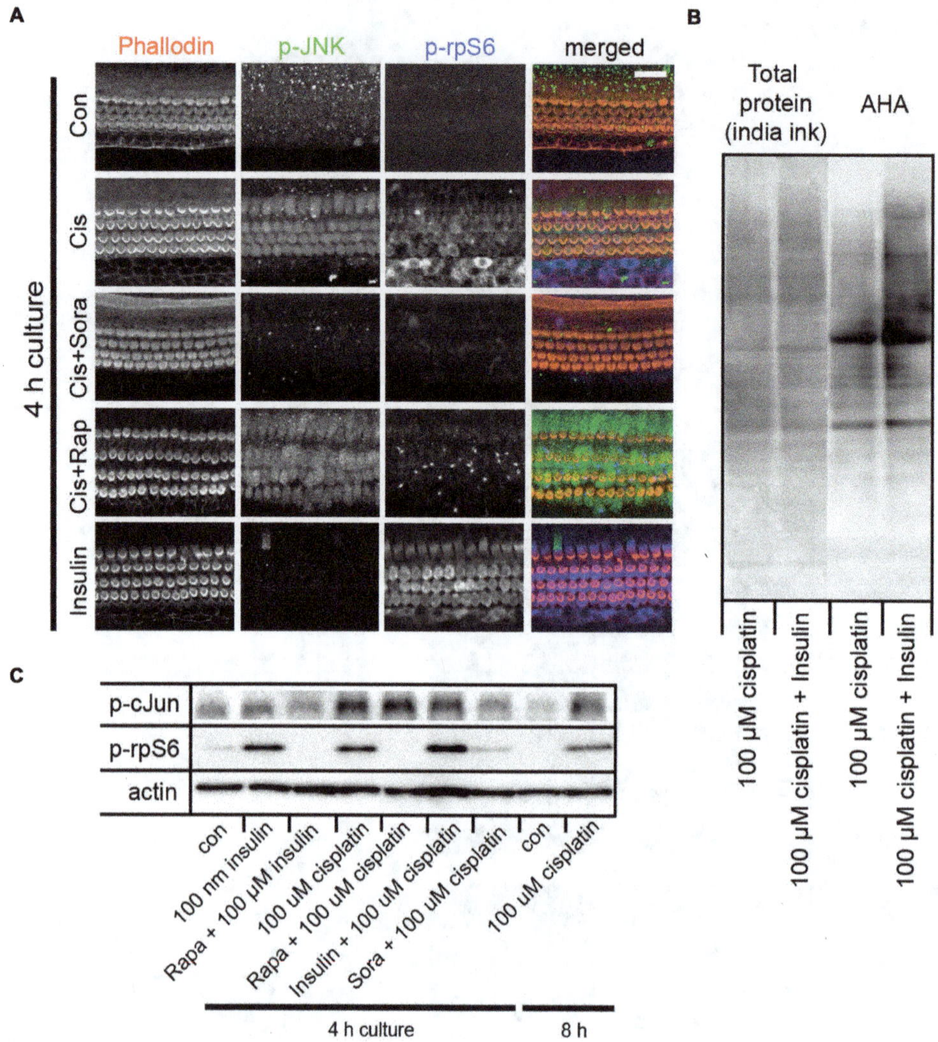

FIGURE 2 | Cisplatin exposure activates both the c-Jun N-terminal kinase (JNK) and mammalian target of rapamycin (mTOR) pathways in sensory hair cells. **(A)** Cisplatin exposure resulted in a coordinated increase in phosphorylated JNK (p-JNK) and phosphorylated ribosomal protein S6 (p-rpS6) immunoreactivity, indicating an activation of the JNK and mTOR pathways. When explant cultures were exposed to both cisplatin and the multikinase inhibitor sorafenib (500 nM), the activation of JNK and mTOR pathways were inhibited. Rapamycin exposure did not alter the cisplatin-induced activation of JNK, but prevented activation of mTOR. When cultures were incubated with 100 nM insulin for 4 h, it resulted in robust activation of mTOR but not the JNK pathway (bottom panel). **(B)** AHA-biotin immunoblot showing that when administered with cisplatin, insulin lead to a 34% increase (*p*-value 0.004) in overall cellular protein synthesis, when compared to cisplatin alone. **(C)** Immunoblot confirming cisplatin-induced activation of the JNK pathway (as measured by p-c-Jun) and mTOR (as measured by p-rpS6), and the modulation of this response by sorafenib, rapamycin and insulin. Scale bar 20 μm.

concentrations. After 4 h, prior to onset of cisplatin-induced cell death, explants were fixed and processed for click-chemistry reaction and imaged using confocal microscopy. As evident in **Figure 1C**, cisplatin inhibits AHA incorporation, thus protein synthesis, in a concentration-dependent manner (quantified in **Figure 1E**). Cisplatin inhibited protein synthesis in all cell types in the organ of Corti, including hair cells and supporting cells. This is in contrast to the pattern of protein synthesis inhibition elicited by aminoglycosides, which is restricted to hair cells (**Figure 1C**, bottom panels). As shown in **Figure 1F**, cochlear hair cells display normal nuclear morphology and MYO7A immunoreactivity after 4 h of culture, even at very high cisplatin concentrations (750 μM), demonstrating the appropriateness of using MYO7A levels for normalizing the AHA signal. A similar effect of cisplatin on protein synthesis was seen in utricle explants (no images shown, quantification in **Figure 1E**, bottom). The reduction of protein synthesis was also evident in immunoblot experiments of organ of Corti explant lysates, in which AHA-biotin was detected with SA-HRP (**Figure 1D**). In summary, we demonstrated that cisplatin inhibits protein synthesis in a dose-dependent manner in all cell types under organ of Corti explant culture conditions, including hair cells and surrounding supporting cells.

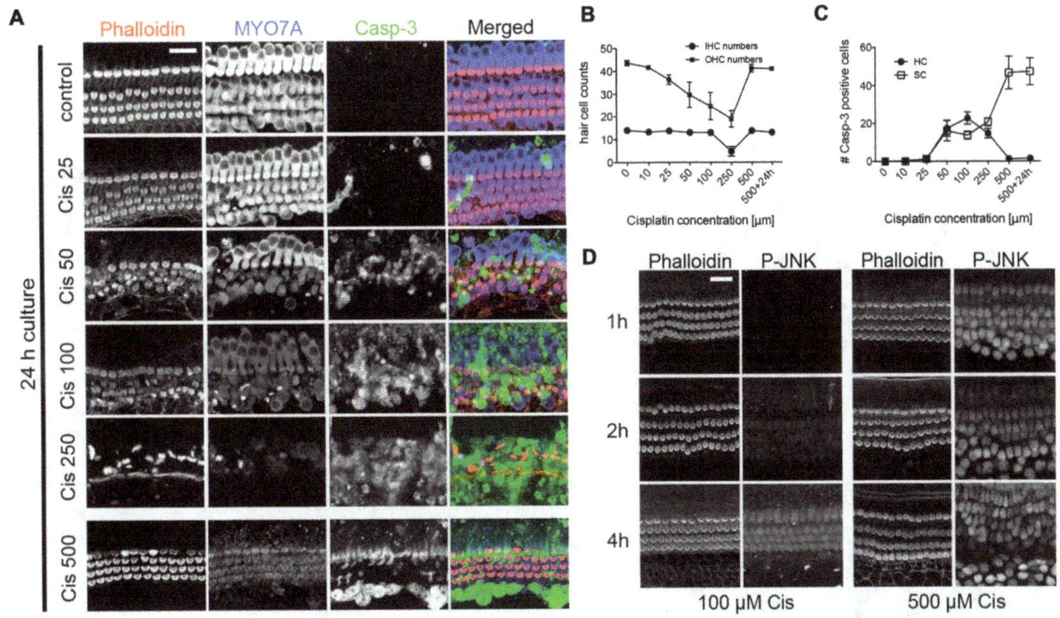

FIGURE 3 | Cisplatin-induced hair cell death and dose-response curve. **(A–C)** Immunoreactivity of MYO7A and cleaved caspase-3 in organ of Corti explants with varying concentrations of cisplatin. Increasing cisplatin (cis) concentrations of up to 250 μM lead to an increase in hair cell death and caspase-3 positive hair cells. At very high concentrations (>500 μM) of cisplatin, however, there is a near complete protection of hair cells and an absence of cleaved caspase-3 staining in hair cells. Supporting cells exhibited strong caspase-3 immunoreactivity at higher concentrations. Outer hair cell (OHC) numbers were counted over a length of 100 μm in the basal turn. Caspase-3 positive cells were counted over a length of 200 μm of the basal turn. Error bars indicate SEM (standard error of the mean). $n = 4$ organs per experimental group. **(D)** Both moderate (100 μM) and high (500 μM) dose cisplatin activate JNK in hair cells (with different kinetics), suggesting that even at high doses, cisplatin uptake is not inhibited. Scale bar 20 μm.

Cisplatin Activates JNK and mTOR Pathways, While Insulin Activates mTOR and Stimulates Cellular Protein Synthesis

We previously demonstrated that aminoglycoside antibiotics activate the JNK and mTOR pathways (Francis et al., 2013). This activation was also noted to have correlated with the inhibition of cellular protein synthesis. The activation of the mTOR pathway was proposed to be a compensatory response to protein synthesis inhibition (Francis et al., 2013). To test whether cisplatin resulted in a similar stress response, mouse organ of Corti explant cultures were exposed to 100 μM cisplatin, and JNK and mTOR activation was detected by p-JNK and p-rpS6 immunoreactivity, respectively. As was found with gentamicin, cisplatin exposure resulted in a coordinated increase in p-JNK and p-rpS6 immunoreactivity, indicating an activation of the JNK and mTOR pathways (**Figure 2A**). We next tested whether activation of JNK and mTOR is modulated by pharmaceutical compounds. Sorafenib is an FDA-approved drug used as an adjunct in chemotherapeutic strategies for renal cell, hepatocellular and thyroid carcinomas (Blair and Plosker, 2015; Gadaleta-Caldarola et al., 2015). It is a multikinase inhibitor and is known to inhibit VEGFR, PDGFR as well as the MAP3K and MLK7. MLK7 (aka ZAK) has been shown to be activated in apoptosis associated with the ribotoxic stress response (Wang et al., 2005; Jandhyala et al., 2008; Sauter et al., 2010). We have previously demonstrated that aminoglycosides elicit a similar ribotoxic stress response within sensory hair cells and that sorafenib inhibits JNK activation. Sorafenib was also found to confer a partial protection from gentamicin-induced hair cell death (Francis et al., 2013). To determine if cisplatin-induced JNK activation can be prevented by sorafenib, we incubated mouse cochlea cultures in 500 nM sorafenib for 1 h, prior to incubation in 100 μM cisplatin. Strikingly, sorafenib nearly completely prevented cisplatin-induced JNK phosphorylation (**Figure 2A**). In addition to the prevention of JNK activation, sorafenib also inhibited the phosphorylation of rpS6 (**Figure 2A**). We then tested whether the prototypical mTOR inhibitor, rapamycin, inhibits JNK and/or mTOR activation. As expected, rapamycin inhibited the phosphorylation of rpS6 (**Figure 2A**). However, unlike sorafenib, rapamycin did not alter cisplatin-induced activation of the JNK pathway (**Figure 2A**), indicating JNK activation occurs upstream of mTOR. Cisplatin-induced activation of the JNK pathway (as measured by p-c-Jun) and mTOR (as measured by p-rpS6), and the modulation of this response by sorafenib, rapamycin and insulin, were validated in immunoblot experiments (**Figure 2C**).

Next, we sought a way to counteract cisplatin-induced protein synthesis inhibition using pharmacological means. It is well established that insulin activates mTOR and cellular protein synthesis (Proud, 2006). Indeed, when cultures were incubated with 100 nM insulin for 4 h, we observed a robust activation of the mTOR pathway (**Figure 2A**, bottom). Insulin

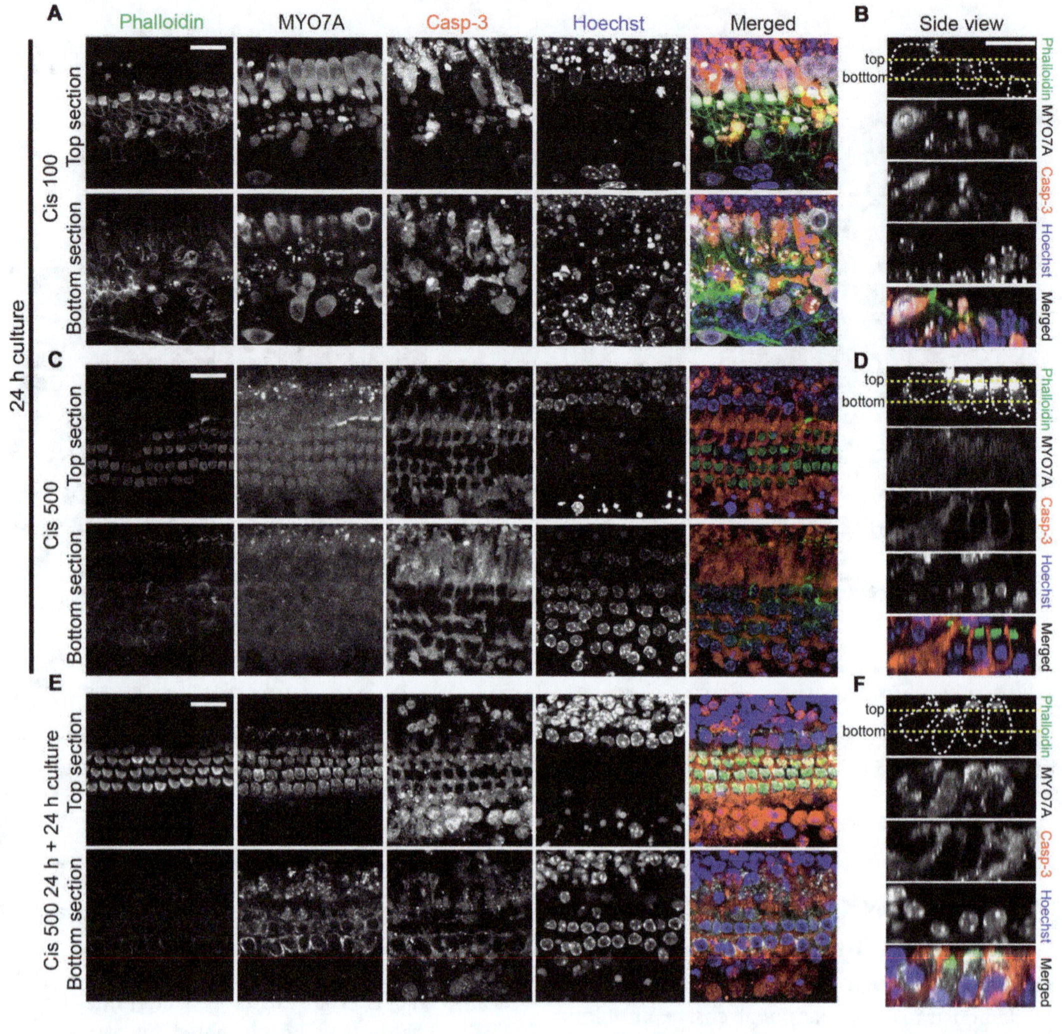

FIGURE 4 | Analysis of hair cell integrity after exposure to high cisplatin concentrations. Explants were treated as follows: 24 h in 100 μM cisplatin **(A,B)**, 24 h in 500 μM cisplatin **(C,D)** or 24 h in 500 μM, followed by 24 h in normal growth medium **(E,F)**. Organs were then co-stained for F-actin (phalloidin, green), MYO7A (gray), cleaved casp-3 (red) and Hoechst (blue), colors are used in merged images only. In the merged images of **(C,D)**, the MYO7A (gray) signal, for which a high image gain was used for better visibility, was omitted. **(A,C,E)** are optical sections at the level of hair bundles (top section) and outer hair cell nuclei (bottom section). **(B,D,F)** are side views (generated by Reslice function in ImageJ), with the yellow dotted lines indicating the level of optical sections used in **(A,C,E)**. The protected hair cells at high cisplatin concentrations (500 μM) display normal nuclear morphology. Continuing the culture for 24 h in normal growth medium leads to near complete recovery of MYO7A immunoreactivity in hair cells initially exposed to 500 μM cisplatin. Scale bar 20 μm.

did not, however, activate the JNK pathway (**Figure 2A**, bottom). At the same time, insulin induced an increase in overall cellular protein synthesis, as demonstrated in an AHA-biotin immunoblot experiment (**Figure 2B**; 34% increase of AHA-biotin signal in cultures treated with cisplatin and insulin, compared to cultures treated with cisplatin alone). In summary, we showed that cisplatin activates both the JNK and the mTOR pathways. Inhibition of JNK by sorafenib prevents both JNK and mTOR activation, while rapamycin only prevents mTOR activation, demonstrating that mTOR is downstream of JNK in this particular stress pathway. Furthermore, we show that insulin activates mTOR and stimulates protein synthesis, independent of the JNK pathway.

Cisplatin-Induced Hair Cell Death and Dose-Response Curve

Next, we analyzed hair cell death in organ of Corti explants exposed to cisplatin. Explant cultures were exposed to concentrations of cisplatin ranging from 10 μM to 500 μM, over 24 h. Hair cells were counted using MYO7A and phalloidin reactivity. Apoptotic events were visualized using cleaved caspase-3 immunoreactivity. We observed a surprising dose-response relationship (**Figures 3A–C**): increasing cisplatin concentrations of up to 250 μM lead to an increase in hair cell death and caspase-3 positive hair cells. At very high concentrations (>500 μM) of cisplatin, however, we observed a near complete inhibition of hair cell loss and absence of cleaved caspase-3 staining in hair cells, while supporting cells

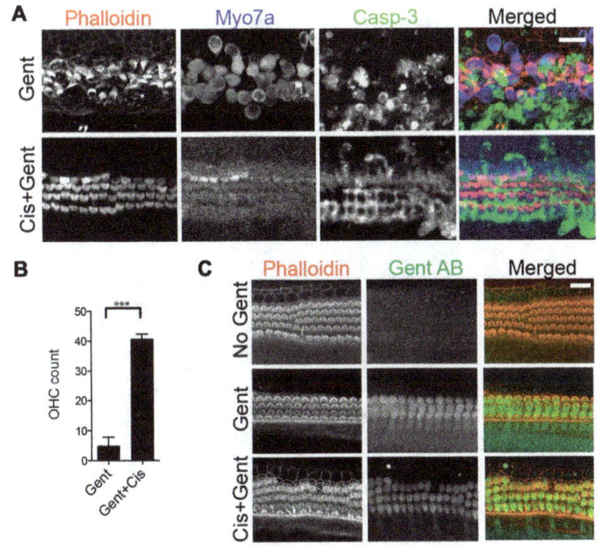

FIGURE 5 | High-dose cisplatin cross-preserves hair cells exposed to toxic doses of gentamicin. **(A)** Mouse organ of Corti explant cultures exposed to 100 μM gentamicin (Gent) for 24 h results in significant hair cell loss (top panels). Additional supplementation of 500 μM cisplatin to the toxic concentration of gentamicin rescues the hair cells, albeit with severely reduced MYO7A immunoreactivity (bottom panels). **(B)** Outer hair cell counts per 100 μm (basal turn) after exposure to gentamicin with or without high dose cisplatin (Unpaired *t*-test, *p*-value: < 0.0001, *n* = 6 organs). **(C)** Gentamicin uptake into cochlear cells was visualized by immunocytochemistry using a gentamicin-specific antibody. There was no difference in gentamicin immunoreactivity within the cochlear hair cells between gentamicin alone or with high dose cisplatin. Scale bar 20 μm.

exhibited strong caspase-3 immunoreactivity. This pattern of seemingly paradoxical hair cell protection with very high doses of cisplatin is similar to a previously reported finding (Ding et al., 2011). Next, we sought to demonstrate that rescue of hair cells at very high concentrations is not caused by a reduced uptake of cisplatin into cochlear cells. As demonstrated in **Figure 2**, cisplatin causes a robust, dose-dependent activation of the JNK pathway, as visualized by detection of p-JNK. We employed this phenomenon as a surrogate marker for cisplatin entry into cells. We examined the time-dependent activation of JNK at moderate cisplatin concentration, as well as very high cisplatin concentrations. At lower cisplatin concentrations (100 μM), JNK is activated preferentially in hair cells, increasing over a time period of 2–4 h. At 500 μM, however, JNK immunoreactivity can be found broadly in hair cells and supporting cells after only 1 h, remaining at high levels up to 4 h (**Figure 3D**). This is consistent with a model in which cisplatin uptake increases with its dose, and hair cells more readily take up cisplatin compared to supporting cells. Our data thus suggests that uptake of cisplatin into organ of Corti cells is likely not inhibited at very high cisplatin concentrations.

Next, we further investigated the nature of the hair cells surviving at high cisplatin concentrations, by correlating MYO7A and caspase-3 immunoreactivity with appearance of nuclei. Significant hair cell loss is observed at moderate cisplatin concentrations (100 μM), accompanied by cleaved caspase-3 immunoreactivity and nuclear fragmentation in hair cells (**Figures 4A,B**). At very high cisplatin concentrations, however, hair cells are free of caspase-3 immunoreactivity, and the hair cell nuclei display normal morphology, while supporting cells exhibit strong caspase-3 immunoreactivity and fragmented nuclei (**Figures 4C,D**). Moreover, when the culture was continued in normal growth medium for another 24 h (without cisplatin), the hair cells remained seemingly healthy, free of caspase-3 and of normal nuclear appearance (**Figures 4E,F**, quantified in **Figures 3B,C**).

Several other observations are worth noting. Hair cell death was preceded by a weakening of MYO7A immunoreactivity, starting with outer hair cells, and at higher cisplatin concentrations, also affecting the inner hair cells (**Figure 3A**). This suggests that MYO7A level in hair cells is affected by the protein synthesis inhibition. At very high cisplatin concentrations (500 μM, 24 h culture), the MYO7A immunoreactivity has weakened to a degree that hair cells are barely detectably based on MYO7A staining (**Figures 4C,D**). However, hair cell bodies are clearly present, as evident in the phalloidin and MYO7A signal (at higher image gain) and the presence of nuclei (Hoechst staining; **Figures 4C,D**). Interestingly, these hair cells nearly fully recovered their MYO7A immunoreactivity when cultured without cisplatin for another 24 h (**Figures 4E,F**), suggesting that these hair cells retain a survival benefit. In summary, we report that moderate cisplatin concentrations cause hair cell death and removal (possibly by supporting cells), but that very high concentrations of cisplatin abolishes this effect, preventing hair cell death and removal.

High-Dose Cisplatin Cross-Protects Against Gentamicin Ototoxicity in Sensory Hair Cells

What would cause the rescue of hair cells at very high concentrations of cisplatin? Previous studies have shown that high concentrations of protein synthesis inhibitors such as cycloheximide can prevent hair cell death (Matsui et al., 2002), possibly due to the fact that regulated forms of cell death themselves depend on proteinaceous factors, such that complete shutdown of protein synthesis even prevents apoptotic cell death. If this was true, we reasoned that high concentrations of cisplatin should also prevent the cell death and removal of hair cells caused by other ototoxins such as aminoglycosides. This was indeed the case; exposure to 100 μM gentamicin for 24 h causes significant hair cell loss, while additional supplementation of 500 μM cisplatin rescues the hair cells, albeit with severely reduced MYO7A immunoreactivity (**Figures 5A,B**). One potential explanation for this apparent broad hair cell protection was the possibility that gentamicin uptake into hair cells is inhibited by cisplatin. To test this, gentamicin taken up into cochlear cells was detected using a gentamicin-specific antibody. There was no difference in gentamicin immunoreactivity within the cochlear hair cells between gentamicin alone or with high dose cisplatin (**Figure 5C**). This indicates that, although high dose cisplatin confers a protective effect from gentamicin toxicity, this is not a result of prevention of gentamicin uptake. We suggest that the protective effect of high cisplatin concentrations is directly caused by a complete shutdown of protein synthesis (discussed later).

Preventing JNK Activation and Stimulating Protein Synthesis Ameliorates Cisplatin-Induced Hair Cell Death

Next, we explored whether drug-mediated modulation of the JNK and/or mTOR pathway, in conjunction with a stimulation of cellular protein synthesis, could be used to alleviate cisplatin ototoxicity in culture. We have previously shown that while sorafenib inhibits gentamicin-induced activation of JNK, it provides only partial protection from hair cell loss (Francis et al., 2013). This suggests that there are other pathways contributing to cellular apoptosis in addition to JNK. We sought to determine whether combinatorial prevention of JNK activation (using sorafenib), inhibition of mTOR (using rapamycin) and stimulation of overall protein synthesis (using insulin) might result in the protection from cisplatin-induced hair cell death. As expected, exposure to cisplatin caused significant hair cell death (**Figure 6A**). When the cisplatin-exposed organs were co-cultured with either insulin or sorafenib, there was a small increase in the number of surviving outer hair cells. Simultaneous application of both sorafenib and insulin, however, lead to a significant rescue of cisplatin-exposed hair cells (**Figure 6A**, 5th row). This preservation also correlated with the number of caspase-3 positive cells (**Figure 6C**). To determine if the added hair cell protection conferred by insulin was related to activation of the mTOR pathway, cisplatin-exposed organ of Corti were co-cultured with sorafenib, insulin and rapamycin. The addition of rapamycin did not alter the hair cell preservation seen with sorafenib and insulin (**Figures 6A,B**). This suggests that the combined protective effects of sorafenib and insulin are independent of the mTOR pathway. Finally, we tested whether the protective effect of insulin and sorafenib persisted when removed from the culture medium. Unlike the continued protection of hair cells after exposure to very high cisplatin concentrations (>500 μM; **Figures 3, 4**), the protection conveyed by combined application of insulin and sorafenib was not sustained when the cultures were continued in normal growth medium (**Figure 6A**, bottom row, and **Figures 6B–E**). In summary, we demonstrate that cisplatin-induced ototoxicity in culture is alleviated by simultaneous inhibition of JNK activation and stimulation of protein synthesis. Both manipulations have an additive, otoprotective effect, suggesting the respective pathways operate independently.

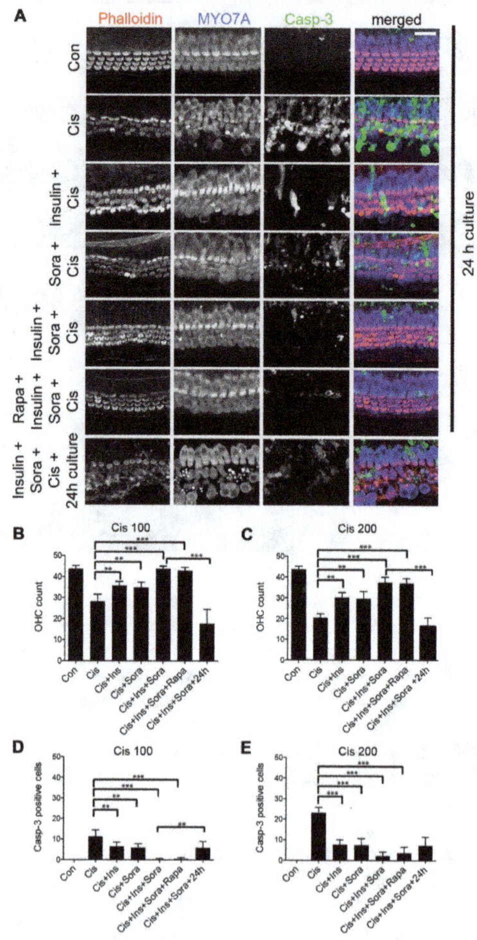

FIGURE 6 | Inhibition of JNK activation with simultaneous stimulation of protein synthesis results in protection from cisplatin ototoxicity. **(A)** Cisplatin exposure (100 μM) results in significant loss of outer hair cells (second row). Co-incubation of cisplatin with either insulin or sorafenib results in a small, but significant protection of outer hair cells (3rd, 4th rows). Combined incubation with cisplatin, insulin and sorafenib provided strong protection of cochlear hair cells (5th row). This protection, however, did not persist when organs were cultured for another 24 h in normal growth medium (7th row). Addition of rapamycin, a known inhibitor of the mTOR pathway, did not reverse the protection seen with sorafenib and insulin (6th row). **(B)** Quantification of outer hair cell numbers demonstrating the protective effect of insulin (Ins), sorafenib (Sora) and the combination of the two after 100 μM cisplatin (Cis) exposure. *P*-values for analysis of variance (ANOVA) with *post hoc* test (Tukey): Con to Cis: < 0.0001, Cis to Cis+Ins and Cis+Sora: < 0.001, Cis to Cis+Ins+Sora: < 0.0001. **(C)** Same as **(B)**, but after 200 μM cisplatin exposure. *P*-values for ANOVA with *post hoc* test (Tukey): Con to Cis: < 0.0001, Cis to Cis+Ins and Cis+Sora: < 0.001, Cis to Cis+Ins+Sora: < 0.0001. **(D)** Quantification of cleaved Caspase-3 (Casp-3)-positive cells, demonstrating the protective effect of insulin (Ins), sorafenib (Sora) and the combination of the two after 100 μM cisplatin (Cis) exposure. *P*-values for ANOVA with *post hoc* test (Tukey): Con to Cis: < 0.001, Cis to Cis+Ins and Cis+Sora: < 0.001, Cis to Cis+Ins+Sora: < 0.0001. **(E)** Same as **(D)**, but after 200 μM cisplatin exposure. *P*-values for ANOVA with *post hoc* test (Tukey): Con to Cis: < 0.0001, Cis to Cis+Ins and Cis+Sora: < 0.0001, Cis to Cis+Ins+Sora: < 0.0001. Asterisks in plots indicate *p*-values (*** < 0.0001, ** < 0.001). To reduce unnecessary complexity in the plots, only a subset of the *p*-values of the pair-wise *post hoc* tests are displayed. Inner hair cells were not affected in all experimental groups (not included in quantification). Scale bar 20 μm.

Pre- and Post-Treatment with Sorafenib and Insulin Provide Equal Hair Cell Protection

Finally, to determine whether the timing of treatment with sorafenib and insulin relative to cisplatin exposure altered their protective effects, we compared pre- and post-treatment paradigms. In the former, organ of Corti explants were cultured with sorafenib and insulin 1 h prior to being

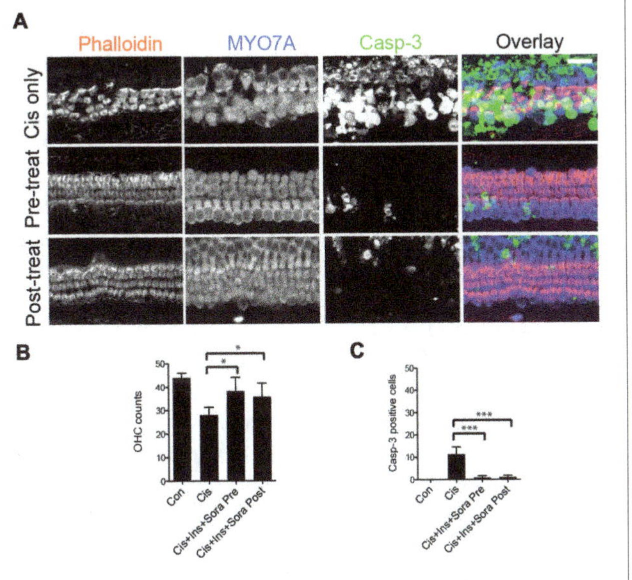

FIGURE 7 | Effects of timing of treatment with sorafenib and insulin on hair cell protection from cisplatin-induced cell death. **(A–C)** Cisplatin exposure results in marked immunoreactivity of caspase-3 and loss of outer hair cells. There is significant protection of outer hair cells and limited immunoreactivity of caspase-3 with either pre- (1 h treatment prior to 200 μM cisplatin) or post-treatment (added after 1 h exposure to cisplatin) with 500 nM sorafenib and 100 nM insulin. Differences between pre- and post-treatment paradigms were not significant, though each were significantly different from cisplatin alone. ANOVA with *post hoc* test (Tukey) was performed for statistical analysis. Asterisks in plots indicate *p*-values (*** < 0.0001, * < 0.01). Inner hair cells were not affected in all experimental groups (not included in quantification). Scale bar 20 μm.

incubated with cisplatin. In the post-treatment group, the organs were incubated first with cisplatin, followed 1 h later with sorafenib and insulin. Both pre- and post-treatment with sorafenib and insulin resulted in a similar degree of hair cell protection, indicating both paradigms are effective in inhibiting cisplatin-induced hair cell death (**Figures 7A–C**).

DISCUSSION

Despite the lack of similarity in molecular structure, aminoglycosides and cisplatin exhibit significant overlap in the stress response they elicit in sensory hair cells: to mention a few, both elicit oxidative stress (Lautermann et al., 1995; Clerici et al., 1996; Hirose et al., 1997; Kopke et al., 1997; Dehne et al., 2000), activate p53 (Zhang et al., 2003; Coffin et al., 2013; Benkafadar et al., 2017) and the JNK pathway (Wang et al., 2004; Francis et al., 2013). A comprehensive summary for the commonalities and differences in aminoglycoside and cisplatin ototoxicity is presented in the review by Schacht et al. (2012). We have previously demonstrated that aminoglycosides cause a stress response reminiscent of ribotoxic stress, involving activation of the JNK and mTOR pathways and inhibition of cellular protein synthesis (Francis et al., 2013). In this study, we demonstrate that, like aminoglycosides, cisplatin causes a significant reduction in cellular protein synthesis within sensory hair cells in culture. In contrast to aminoglycosides, cisplatin inhibits protein synthesis in all cochlear cell types. We suggest this is due to differences in uptake specificity. Aminoglycosides are highly preferentially taken up by hair cells through the mechanotransduction channel (Marcotti et al., 2005; Waguespack and Ricci, 2005; Wang and Steyger, 2009; Alharazneh et al., 2011), while cisplatin might enter cells through a more generic pathway (Sinani et al., 2007; Ding et al., 2011; Ciarimboli, 2014). It should be noted, however, that cisplatin also displays a slight preference for hair cells compared to supporting cells: while high concentrations of cisplatin (500 μM) activate JNK in hair cells and supporting cells, lower doses of cisplatin (100 μM) activate JNK in hair cells only (**Figure 3D**), This is consistent with a previous report suggesting that cisplatin also enters the hair cell through the mechanotransduction channel (Thomas et al., 2013). Nevertheless, we suggest that compared to aminoglycosides, cisplatin affects various cell types in a broader manner. We believe that the difference in cellular damage profile is highly relevant for developing therapeutic strategies, in that prevention of aminoglycoside ototoxicity might be primarily directed to hair cells, while addressing cisplatin ototoxicity should require a broader protective effort.

Cisplatin's effect on blocking protein synthesis might also offer an explanation for a curious dose-response curve, first reported by the Salvi lab (Ding et al., 2011), and also confirmed in our present study. Cisplatin caused an increasing loss of hair cells up to a concentration of 250 μM. At very high concentrations of cisplatin, however, there appeared to be a protective effect on sensory hair cells. Ding et al. (2011) postulated that this may be caused by the complex interplay of various copper transporters, which enable cisplatin uptake into hair cells. We suggest that additional mehanisms could contribute to this phenomenon; at moderate concentrations (below 250 μM), cisplatin causes the expected stress and cell death response. At concentrations above that level, hair cells experience a complete arrest of protein synthesis, inhibiting all cellular processes, including cell death programs. The strongest indication for a general arrest of cell death programs is presented in our observation that very high concentrations of cisplatin cross-protects against aminoglycoside ototoxicity, suggesting this protection is not specific to cisplatin.

What is the nature of the hair cells surviving at high cisplatin concentrations? One possibility is that the supposedly rescued hair cells are in fact committed to cell death, but fail to initiate or complete the cell death program. These hair cells would be retained in the epithelium, since supporting cells at such high cisplatin levels undergo apoptosis (as evident in strong cleaved caspase-3 immunoreactivity in **Figures 3A, 4C–F**) and might loose their ability to phagocytose dying hair cell (Monzack et al., 2015). Experiments detailed in **Figure 4**, however, demonstrate that the hair cells exposed to high cisplatin doses remain healthy after cisplatin is washed out, at least for 24 h in continued culture. We therefore have to assume that these hair cells sustain a survival benefit in absence of high cisplatin doses. The significance and therapeutic usefulness of this protection is unclear. First, such high cisplatin concentrations (>500 μM) are irrelevant for clinical considerations, with typical plasma concentrations ranging between 600 nM and 20 μM (Urien et al., 2005). Possibly more detrimental, such high cisplatin concentrations induce apoptosis in supporting cells, which will inevitably affect the function and survival of the sensory epithelium. Neverthelss, learning the basis of this curious protection will provide important clues for understanding basic mechanisms of cisplatin ototoxicity.

What is the mechanism by which cisplatin inhibits protein synthesis? We have previously shown that the usual pathways affecting protein synthesis, most notably stress responses like the unfolded protein response or an inhibition of the mTOR pathway, are not causative with aminoglycoside-induced protein synthesis inhibition (Francis et al., 2013). Instead, we provided evidence that aminoglycosides directly bind and inhibit ribosomal RNA (Scheunemann et al., 2010; Francis et al., 2013). Such binding activity, negligible in most other cell types, reaches toxic levels in hair cells, which possess the unfortunate property of accumulating aminoglycosides. Despite differences in molecular structure between aminoglycoside antibiotics and cisplatin, there is some evidence that also cisplatin might bind to RNA; Heminger et al. (1997) demonstrated that cisplatin crosslinks mRNA and rRNA, causing translational arrest in reticulocytes. And just recently, the crystal structure of cisplatin bound to RNA was reported (Melnikov et al., 2016). It is therefore conceivable that cisplatin elicits a ribotoxic stress response similar to toxins such as ricin, and as we proposed in our previous study, aminoglycoside antibiotics. Cisplatin could, however, also affect protein synthesis through its canonical DNA-crosslinking activity, accepted to be the main mechanism underlying its cytotoxic effect (Eastman, 1987). DNA crosslinking causes genotoxicity, which is a well-established cause for protein synthesis inhibition (Sheikh and Fornace, 1999; Braunstein et al., 2009). In summary, we believe that cisplatin behaves like a "dirty bomb", affecting protein synthesis through various ways, but also eliciting other stress signaling such as the JNK pathway; all of which contribute to the overall ototoxicity. While such multi-faceted toxicity is a boon for killing cancer cells, it represents a great challenge when it comes to preventing toxic side effects, necessitating a multi-pronged approach. Our present study points to several potential avenues for intervention, all of which might have to be targeted simultaneously.

JNK Pathway

It is well documented that various ototoxic stressors, including cisplatin, result in activation the JNK pathway (Zine and Romand, 1996; Pirvola et al., 2000; Matsui et al., 2004). Despite a proposed role of JNK activation in initiating apoptosis, whether JNK is necessary for, or causal of, apoptosis is controversial (Liu and Lin, 2005). In the case of cisplatin ototoxicity, a previous study has shown that inhibition of the JNK pathway does not result in protection of auditory hair cells (Wang et al., 2004). Our results confirmed that near complete blockade of JNK with sorafenib does not provide an equal benefit for hair cell survival. However, our study suggests that JNK inhibition can synergize with other protective measures.

Protein Synthesis

If protein synthesis inhibition is indeed a significant contributor to ototoxicity, how does this knowledge guide the development of preventative or ameliorative strategies? Our success using insulin, a general stimulating agent of protein synthesis, points in one potentially beneficial direction. Future strategies must be based on the understanding that protein synthesis inhibition, like so many other stress responses, is a double-edged sword, and that finding the right balance is the key. Blocking the synthesis of new proteins will most affect proteins with high turnover (Adams and Cooper, 2007). Therefore, to tip the balance of pro-survival and pro-death factors to the former, it is crucial to understand the overall proteostasis (sum of synthesis and degradation) of cell stress and death factors, with expected differences in different cell types.

Protein synthesis is regulated on so many levels, and affects so many aspects of cellular signaling that its targeted and isolated manipulation is intractable. The otoprotective effect of insulin, for example, might be mediated by mechanisms independent from protein synthesis stimulation. Several previous reports have described that growth factors such as IGF-1, EGF, TGF alpha and insulin protect against various ototoxic insults (Romand and Chardin, 1999; Iwai et al., 2006; Lou et al., 2015; Yamahara et al., 2015). In the case of IGF-1, protection was mediated by supporting cells (Yamahara et al., 2015). Insulin also activates phosphatidylinositol-4,5-bisphosphate 3-kinase (PI3K)- protein kinase B (Akt) signaling, which has been shown to be protective against both aminoglycoside and cisplatin ototoxicity, potentially through activation of pro-survival MAPK signaling and/or inactivation or downregulation of pro-apoptotic proteins (Lizcano and Alessi, 2002; Chung et al., 2006; Brand et al., 2011; Jadali and Kwan, 2016; Jadali et al., 2017). In addition, insulin-activated Akt is known to inhibit glycogen synthase kinases (GSKs), and inhibition of GSK-3 activity has been shown to inhibit cisplatin ototoxicity in auditory cells (Park et al., 2009; Kim et al., 2014; Hermida et al., 2017). Alternatively, insulin also inhibits AMP-activated protein kinase (AMPK) activity (Towler and Hardie, 2007). AMPK has been shown to play a role in noise-induced hearing loss, and inhibition of AMPK activation protects hair cells and ribbon synapses against acoustical overstimulation (Nagashima et al., 2011; Zheng et al., 2014; Hill et al., 2016). Further studies are required to obtain a full understanding of the mechanisms by which insulin confers otoprotection against cisplatin, and how much of this protection is attributable to an increase in protein synthesis. It should be noted, however, that the mTOR stimulating effect of insulin does not seem to play a role in the protective effect, since mTOR inhibition by rapamycin did not reverse insulin-mediated hair cell protection (**Figure 6**).

Countless other pathways and corresponding protective interventions have been reported and reviewed extensively (Rybak et al., 2008, 2007; Schacht et al., 2012; Waissbluth and Daniel, 2013; Karasawa and Steyger, 2015), underscoring the notion that no single "magic bullet" will achieve the clinically relevant level of protection, and that a combination of interventions, accompanied by a thorough understanding of the underlying mechanisms, must be sought.

CONCLUSION

We found that cisplatin inhibits cellular protein synthesis in organ of Corti explant cultures. Similar to gentamicin, cisplatin also activates the JNK. Simultaneous stimulation of cellular protein synthesis by insulin, and inhibition of JNK activation by sorafenib, significantly improved hair cell survival in culture. The presented data thus suggest that protein synthesis inhibition might be a potential contributor to cisplatin-mediated ototoxicity.

AUTHOR CONTRIBUTIONS

This study was designed by BDN, SF and J-BS. Experiments were performed by BDN, SF, ELW, SZ and J-BS; data was analyzed by BDN and J-BS; this article was written by BDN, SF and J-BS.

ACKNOWLEDGMENTS

Work described here was in part supported by National Institutes of Health (NIH) grant R01 DC014254 (to J-BS).

REFERENCES

Adams, K. W., and Cooper, G. M. (2007). Rapid turnover of mcl-1 couples translation to cell survival and apoptosis. *J. Biol. Chem.* 282, 6192–6200. doi: 10.1074/jbc.m610643200

Agard, N. J., Prescher, J. A., and Bertozzi, C. R. (2004). A strain-promoted [3 + 2] azide–alkyne cycloaddition for covalent modification of biomolecules in living systems. *J. Am. Chem. Soc.* 126, 15046–15047. doi: 10.1021/ja044996f

Alharazneh, A., Luk, L., Huth, M., Monfared, A., Steyger, P. S., Cheng, A. G., et al. (2011). Functional hair cell mechanotransducer channels are required for aminoglycoside ototoxicity. *PLoS One* 6:e22347. doi: 10.1371/journal.pone.0022347

Baker, T. G., Roy, S., Brandon, C. S., Kramarenko, I. K., Francis, S. P., Taleb, M., et al. (2015). Heat shock protein-mediated protection against cisplatin-induced hair cell death. *J. Assoc. Res. Otolaryngol.* 16, 67–80. doi: 10.1007/s10162-014-0491-7

Benedetti Panici, P., Greggi, S., Scambia, G., Baiocchi, G., Lomonaco, M., Conti, G., et al. (1993). Efficacy and toxicity of very high-dose cisplatin in advanced ovarian carcinoma: 4-year survival analysis and neurological follow-up. *Int. J. Gynecol. Cancer* 3, 44–53. doi: 10.1046/j.1525-1438.1993.03010044.x

Benkafadar, N., Menardo, J., Bourien, J., Nouvian, R., François, F., Decaudin, D., et al. (2017). Reversible p53 inhibition prevents cisplatin ototoxicity without blocking chemotherapeutic efficacy. *EMBO Mol. Med.* 9, 7–26. doi: 10.15252/emmm.201606230

Black, F. O., Myers, E. N., Schramm, V. L., Johnson, J., Sigler, B., Thearle, P. B., et al. (1982). Cisplatin vestibular ototoxicity: preliminary report. *Laryngoscope* 92, 1363–1368. doi: 10.1288/00005537-198212000-00003

Blair, H. A., and Plosker, G. L. (2015). Sorafenib: a review of its use in patients with radioactive iodine-refractory, metastatic differentiated thyroid carcinoma. *Target. Oncol.* 10, 171–178. doi: 10.1007/s11523-015-0363-z

Brand, Y., Setz, C., Levano, S., Listyo, A., Chavez, E., Pak, K., et al. (2011). Simvastatin protects auditory hair cells from gentamicin-induced toxicity and activates Akt signaling *in vitro*. *BMC Neurosci.* 12:114. doi: 10.1186/1471-2202-12-114

Braunstein, S., Badura, M. L., Xi, Q., Formenti, S. C., and Schneider, R. J. (2009). Regulation of protein synthesis by ionizing radiation. *Mol. Cell. Biol.* 29, 5645–5656. doi: 10.1128/MCB.00711-09

Chung, W.-H., Pak, K., Lin, B., Webster, N., and Ryan, A. F. (2006). A PI3K pathway mediates hair cell survival and opposes gentamicin toxicity in neonatal rat organ of Corti. *J. Assoc. Res. Otolaryngol.* 7, 373–382. doi: 10.1007/s10162-006-0050-y

Ciarimboli, G. (2014). Membrane transporters as mediators of cisplatin side-effects. *Anticancer Res.* 34, 547–550.

Clerici, W. J., Hensley, K., DiMartino, D. L., and Butterfield, D. A. (1996). Direct detection of ototoxicant-induced reactive oxygen species generation in cochlear explants. *Hear. Res.* 98, 116–124. doi: 10.1016/0378-5955(96)00075-5

Coffin, A. B., Rubel, E. W., and Raible, D. W. (2013). Bax, Bcl2, and p53 differentially regulate neomycin- and gentamicin-induced hair cell death in the zebrafish lateral line. *J. Assoc. Res. Otolaryngol.* 14, 645–659. doi: 10.1007/s10162-013-0404-1

Croons, V., Martinet, W., Herman, A. G., Timmermans, J.-P., and De Meyer, G. R. Y. (2009). The protein synthesis inhibitor anisomycin induces macrophage apoptosis in rabbit atherosclerotic plaques through p38 mitogen-activated protein kinase. *J. Pharmacol. Exp. Ther.* 329, 856–864. doi: 10.1124/jpet.108.149948

Dehne, N., Lautermann, J., ten Cate, W.-J. F., Rauen, U., and de Groot, H. (2000). *In vitro* effects of hydrogen peroxide on the cochlear neurosensory epithelium of the guinea pig. *Hear. Res.* 143, 162–170. doi: 10.1016/s0378-5955(00)00036-8

Dieterich, D. C., Lee, J. J., Link, A. J., Graumann, J., Tirrell, D. A., and Schuman, E. M. (2007). Labeling, detection and identification of newly synthesized proteomes with bioorthogonal non-canonical amino-acid tagging. *Nat. Protoc.* 2, 532–540. doi: 10.1038/nprot.2007.52

Dieterich, D. C., Link, A. J., Graumann, J., Tirrell, D. A., and Schuman, E. M. (2006). Selective identification of newly synthesized proteins in mammalian cells using bioorthogonal noncanonical amino acid tagging (BONCAT). *Proc. Natl. Acad. Sci. U S A* 103, 9482–9487. doi: 10.1073/pnas.0601637103

Ding, D., He, J., Allman, B. L., Yu, D., Jiang, H., Seigel, G. M., et al. (2011). Cisplatin ototoxicity in rat cochlear organotypic cultures. *Hear. Res.* 282, 196–203. doi: 10.1016/j.heares.2011.08.002

Eastman, A. (1987). The formation, isolation and characterization of DNA adducts produced by anticancer platinum complexes. *Pharmacol. Ther.* 34, 155–166. doi: 10.1016/0163-7258(87)90009-x

Francis, S. P., Katz, J., Fanning, K. D., Harris, K. A., Nicholas, B. D., Lacy, M., et al. (2013). A novel role of cytosolic protein synthesis inhibition in aminoglycoside ototoxicity. *J. Neurosci.* 33, 3079–3093. doi: 10.1523/JNEUROSCI.3430-12.2013

Gadaleta-Caldarola, G., Infusino, S., Divella, R., Ferraro, E., Mazzocca, A., De Rose, F., et al. (2015). Sorafenib: 10 years after the first pivotal trial. *Future Oncol.* 11, 1863–1880. doi: 10.2217/fon.15.85

Gebauer, F., and Hentze, M. W. (2004). Molecular mechanisms of translational control. *Nat. Rev. Mol. Cell Biol.* 5, 827–835. doi: 10.1038/nrm1488

Gurney, J. G., Bass, J. K., Onar-Thomas, A., Huang, J., Chintagumpala, M., Bouffet, E., et al. (2014). Evaluation of amifostine for protection against cisplatin-induced serious hearing loss in children treated for average-risk or high-risk medulloblastoma. *Neuro Oncol.* 16, 848–855. doi: 10.1093/neuonc/not241

Hawkins, J. (1976). "Drug ototoxicity," in *Handbook of Sensory Physiology*, eds W. B. Keidel and W. B. Neff (Berlin: Springer Verlag), 707–748.

Heminger, K. A., Hartson, S. D., Rogers, J., and Matts, R. L. (1997). Cisplatin inhibits protein synthesis in rabbit reticulocyte lysate by causing an arrest in elongation. *Arch. Biochem. Biophys.* 344, 200–207. doi: 10.1006/abbi.1997.0198

Hermida, M. A., Dinesh Kumar, J., and Leslie, N. R. (2017). GSK3 and its interactions with the PI3K/AKT/mTOR signalling network. *Adv. Biol. Regul.* 65, 5–15. doi: 10.1016/j.jbior.2017.06.003

Hill, K., Yuan, H., Wang, X., and Sha, S.-H. (2016). Noise-induced loss of hair cells and cochlear synaptopathy are mediated by the activation of AMPK. *J. Neurosci.* 36, 7497–7510. doi: 10.1523/JNEUROSCI.0782-16.2016

Hirose, K., Hockenbery, D. M., and Rubel, E. W. (1997). Reactive oxygen species in chick hair cells after gentamicin exposure *in vitro*. *Hear. Res.* 104, 1–14. doi: 10.1016/s0378-5955(96)00169-4

Humes, H. D. (1999). Insights into ototoxicity. Analogies to nephrotoxicity. *Ann, N Y Acad. Sci.* 884, 15–18. doi: 10.1111/j.1749-6632.1999.tb00278.x

Iwai, K., Nakagawa, T., Endo, T., Matsuoka, Y., Kita, T., Kim, T.-S., et al. (2006). Cochlear protection by local insulin-like growth factor-1 application using biodegradable hydrogel. *Laryngoscope* 116, 529–533. doi: 10.1097/01.mlg.0000200791.77819.eb

Jadali, A., and Kwan, K. Y. (2016). Activation of PI3K signaling prevents aminoglycoside-induced hair cell death in the murine cochlea. *Biol. Open* 5, 698–708. doi: 10.1242/bio.016758

Jadali, A., Ying, Y.-L. M., and Kwan, K. Y. (2017). Activation of CHK1 in supporting cells indirectly promotes hair cell survival. *Front. Cell. Neurosci.* 11:137. doi: 10.3389/fncel.2017.00137

Jandhyala, D. M., Ahluwalia, A., Obrig, T., and Thorpe, C. M. (2008). ZAK: a MAP3Kinase that transduces Shiga toxin- and ricin-induced proinflammatory cytokine expression. *Cell. Microbiol.* 10, 1468–1477. doi: 10.1111/j.1462-5822.2008.01139.x

Kageyama, A., Kusano, I., Tamura, T., Oda, T., and Muramatzu, T. (2002). Comparison of the apoptosis-inducing abilities of various protein synthesis inhibitors in U937 cells. *Biosci. Biotechnol. Biochem.* 66, 835–839. doi: 10.1271/bbb.66.835

Karasawa, T., and Steyger, P. S. (2015). An integrated view of cisplatin-induced nephrotoxicity and ototoxicity. *Toxicol. Lett.* 237, 219–227. doi: 10.1016/j.toxlet.2015.06.012

Keller, J. N. (2006). Interplay between oxidative damage, protein synthesis, and protein degradation in Alzheimer's disease. *J. Biomed. Biotechnol.* 2006:12129. doi: 10.1155/JBB/2006/12129

Kim, S.-J., Lim, J.-Y., Lee, J. N., Choe, S.-K., Kim, Y.-I. L., Song, S. R., et al. (2014). Activation of β-catenin by inhibitors of glycogen synthase kinase-3 ameliorates cisplatin-induced cytotoxicity and pro-inflammatory cytokine expression in HEI-OC1 cells. *Toxicology* 320, 74–82. doi: 10.1016/j.tox.2014.01.013

Kim, Y. J., Tian, C., Kim, J., Shin, B., Choo, O.-S., Kim, Y.-S., et al. (2017). Autophagic flux, a possible mechanism for delayed gentamicin-induced ototoxicity. *Sci. Rep.* 7:41356. doi: 10.1038/srep41356

Kopke, R. D., Liu, W., Gabaizadeh, R., Jacono, A., Feghali, J., Spray, D., et al. (1997). Use of organotypic cultures of Corti's organ to study the protective effects of antioxidant molecules on cisplatin-induced damage of auditory hair cells. *Am. J. Otol.* 18, 559–571.

Landier, W. (2016). Ototoxicity and cancer therapy. *Cancer* 122, 1647–1658. doi: 10.1002/cncr.29779

Langer, T., Am Zehnhoff-Dinnesen, A., Radtke, S., Meitert, J., and Zolk, O. (2013). Understanding platinum-induced ototoxicity. *Trends Pharmacol. Sci.* 34, 458–469. doi: 10.1016/j.tips.2013.05.006

Lautermann, J., McLaren, J., and Schacht, J. (1995). Glutathione protection against gentamicin ototoxicity depends on nutritional status. *Hear. Res.* 86, 15–24. doi: 10.1016/0378-5955(95)00049-a

Liu, J., and Lin, A. (2005). Role of JNK activation in apoptosis: a double-edged sword. *Cell Res.* 15, 36–42. doi: 10.1038/sj.cr.7290262

Lizcano, J. M., and Alessi, D. R. (2002). The insulin signalling pathway. *Curr. Biol.* 12, R236–R238. doi: 10.1016/S0960-9822(02)00777-7

Lockshin, R. A., and Zakeri, Z. F. (1992). Physiology and protein synthesis in programmed cell death. Early synthesis and DNA degradationa. *Ann. N Y Acad. Sci.* 663, 234–249. doi: 10.1111/j.1749-6632.1992.tb38667.x

Lou, X., Yuan, H., Xie, J., Wang, X., Yang, L., and Zhang, Y. (2015). Growth factors have a protective effect on neomycin-induced hair cell loss. *Cell Biol. Int.* 39, 65–73. doi: 10.1002/cbin.10347

Malgonde, M. S., Nagpure, P. S., and Kumar, M. (2015). Audiometric patterns in ototoxicity after radiotherapy and chemotherapy in patients of head and neck cancers. *Indian J. Palliat. Care* 21, 164–167. doi: 10.4103/0973-1075.156479

Marcotti, W., Van Netten, S. M., and Kros, C. J. (2005). The aminoglycoside antibiotic dihydrostreptomycin rapidly enters mouse outer hair cells through the mechano-electrical transducer channels. *J. Physiol.* 567, 505–521. doi: 10.1113/jphysiol.2005.085951

Marina, N., Chang, K. W., Malogolowkin, M., London, W. B., Frazier, A. L., Womer, R. B., et al. (2005). Amifostine does not protect against the ototoxicity of high-dose cisplatin combined with etoposide and bleomycin in pediatric germ-cell tumors: a children's oncology group study. *Cancer* 104, 841–847. doi: 10.1002/cncr.21218

Matsui, J. I., Gale, J. E., and Warchol, M. E. (2004). Critical signaling events during the aminoglycoside-induced death of sensory hair cells *in vitro*. *J. Neurobiol.* 61, 250–266. doi: 10.1002/neu.20054

Matsui, J. I., Ogilvie, J. M., and Warchol, M. E. (2002). Inhibition of caspases prevents ototoxic and ongoing hair cell death. *J. Neurosci.* 22, 1218–1227.

Melnikov, S. V., Söll, D., Steitz, T. A., and Polikanov, Y. S. (2016). Insights into RNA binding by the anticancer drug cisplatin from the crystal structure of cisplatin-modified ribosome. *Nucleic Acids Res.* 44, 4978–4987. doi: 10.1093/nar/gkw246

Mesner, P. W., Winters, T., and Green, S. (1992). Nerve growth factor withdrawal-induced cell death in neuronal PC12 cells resembles that in sympathetic neurons. *J. Cell Biol.* 119, 1669–1680. doi: 10.1083/jcb.119.6.1669

Monzack, E. L., May, L. A., Roy, S., Gale, J. E., and Cunningham, L. L. (2015). Live imaging the phagocytic activity of inner ear supporting cells in response to hair cell death. *Cell Death Differ.* 22, 1995–2005. doi: 10.1038/cdd.2015.48

Nagashima, R., Yamaguchi, T., Kuramoto, N., and Ogita, K. (2011). Acoustic overstimulation activates 5′-AMP-activated protein kinase through a temporary decrease in ATP level in the cochlear spiral ligament prior to permanent hearing loss in mice. *Neurochem. Int.* 59, 812–820. doi: 10.1016/j.neuint.2011.08.015

Nitz, A., Kontopantelis, E., Bielack, S., Koscielniak, E., Klingebiel, T., Langer, T., et al. (2013). Prospective evaluation of cisplatin- and carboplatin-mediated ototoxicity in paediatric and adult soft tissue and osteosarcoma patients. *Oncol. Lett.* 5, 311–315. doi: 10.3892/ol.2012.997

Park, H.-J., Kim, H.-J., Bae, G.-S., Seo, S.-W., Kim, D.-Y., Jung, W.-S., et al. (2009). Selective GSK-3β inhibitors attenuate the cisplatin-induced cytotoxicity of auditory cells. *Hear. Res.* 257, 53–62. doi: 10.1016/j.heares.2009.08.001

Pirvola, U., Xing-Qun, L., Virkkala, J., Saarma, M., Murakata, C., Camoratto, A. M., et al. (2000). Rescue of hearing, auditory hair cells, and neurons by CEP-1347/KT7515, an inhibitor of c-Jun N-terminal kinase activation. *J. Neurosci.* 20, 43–50.

Proud, C. G. (2006). Regulation of protein synthesis by insulin. *Biochem. Soc. Trans.* 34, 213–216. doi: 10.1042/BST20060213

Rehen, S. K., Varella, M. H., Freitas, F. G., Moraes, M. O., and Linden, R. (1996). Contrasting effects of protein synthesis inhibition and of cyclic AMP on apoptosis in the developing retina. *Development* 122, 1439–1448.

Romand, R., and Chardin, S. (1999). Effects of growth factors on the hair cells after ototoxic treatment of the neonatal mammalian cochlea *in vitro*. *Brain Res.* 825, 46–58. doi: 10.1016/s0006-8993(99)01211-1

Rybak, L. P. (2007). Mechanisms of cisplatin ototoxicity and progress in otoprotection. *Curr. Opin. Otolaryngol. Head Neck Surg.* 15, 364–369. doi: 10.1097/moo.0b013e3282eee452

Rybak, L. P., Talaska, A. E., and Schacht, J. (2008). "Drug-induced hearing loss," in *Auditory Trauma, Protection, and Repair*, eds J. Schacht, A. N. Popper, and R. R. Fay (New York, NY: Springer), 219–256.

Rybak, L. P., Whitworth, C. A., Mukherjea, D., and Ramkumar, V. (2007). Mechanisms of cisplatin-induced ototoxicity and prevention. *Hear. Res.* 226, 157–167. doi: 10.1016/j.heares.2006.09.015

Sauter, K. A. D., Magun, E. A., Iordanov, M. S., and Magun, B. E. (2010). ZAK is required for doxorubicin, a novel ribotoxic stressor, to induce SAPK activation and apoptosis in HaCaT cells. *Cancer Biol. Ther.* 10, 258–266. doi: 10.4161/cbt.10.3.12367

Schacht, J., Talaska, A. E., and Rybak, L. P. (2012). Cisplatin and aminoglycoside antibiotics: hearing loss and its prevention. *Anat. Rec. (Hoboken)* 295, 1837–1850. doi: 10.1002/ar.22578

Scheunemann, A. E., Graham, W. D., Vendeix, F. A. P., and Agris, P. F. (2010). Binding of aminoglycoside antibiotics to helix 69 of 23S rRNA. *Nucleic Acids Res.* 38, 3094–3105. doi: 10.1093/nar/gkp1253

Sheikh, M. S., and Fornace, A. J. (1999). Regulation of translation initiation following stress. *Oncogene* 18, 6121–6128. doi: 10.1038/sj.onc.1203131

Sinani, D., Adle, D. J., Kim, H., and Lee, J. (2007). Distinct mechanisms for Ctr1-mediated copper and cisplatin transport. *J. Biol. Chem.* 282, 26775–26785. doi: 10.1074/jbc.m703973200

Sonenberg, N., and Hinnebusch, A. G. (2009). Regulation of translation initiation in eukaryotes: mechanisms and biological targets. *Cell* 136, 731–745. doi: 10.1016/j.cell.2009.01.042

Thomas, A. J., Hailey, D. W., Stawicki, T. M., Wu, P., Coffin, A. B., Rubel, E. W., et al. (2013). Functional mechanotransduction is required for cisplatin-induced hair cell death in the zebrafish lateral line. *J. Neurosci.* 33, 4405–4414. doi: 10.1523/jneurosci.3940-12.2013

Towler, M. C., and Hardie, D. G. (2007). AMP-activated protein kinase in metabolic control and insulin signaling. *Circ. Res.* 100, 328–341. doi: 10.1161/01.res.0000256090.42690.05

Urien, S., Brain, E., Bugat, R., Pivot, X., Lochon, I., Vo Van, M. L., et al. (2005). Pharmacokinetics of platinum after oral or intravenous cisplatin: a phase 1 study in 32 adult patients. *Cancer Chemother. Pharmacol.* 55, 55–60. doi: 10.1007/s00280-004-0852-8

Waguespack, J. R., and Ricci, A. J. (2005). Aminoglycoside ototoxicity: permeant drugs cause permanent hair cell loss. *J. Physiol.* 567, 359–360. doi: 10.1113/jphysiol.2005.094474

Waissbluth, S., and Daniel, S. J. (2013). Cisplatin-induced ototoxicity: transporters playing a role in cisplatin toxicity. *Hear. Res.* 299, 37–45. doi: 10.1016/j.heares.2013.02.002

Wang, J., Ladrech, S., Pujol, R., Brabet, P., Van De Water, T. R., and Puel, J. L. (2004). Caspase inhibitors, but not c-Jun NH_2-terminal kinase inhibitor treatment, prevent cisplatin-induced hearing loss. *Cancer Res.* 64, 9217–9224. doi: 10.1158/0008-5472.can-04-1581

Wang, X., Mader, M. M., Toth, J. E., Yu, X., Jin, N., Campbell, R. M., et al. (2005). Complete inhibition of anisomycin and UV radiation but not cytokine induced JNK and p38 activation by an aryl-substituted dihydropyrrolopyrazole quinoline and mixed lineage kinase 7 small interfering RNA. *J. Biol. Chem.* 280, 19298–19305. doi: 10.1074/jbc.m413059200

Wang, Q., and Steyger, P. S. (2009). Trafficking of systemic fluorescent gentamicin into the cochlea and hair cells. *J. Assoc. Res. Otolaryngol.* 10, 205–219. doi: 10.1007/s10162-009-0160-4

Yamahara, K., Yamamoto, N., Nakagawa, T., and Ito, J. (2015). Insulin-like growth factor 1: a novel treatment for the protection or regeneration of cochlear hair cells. *Hear. Res.* 330, 2–9. doi: 10.1016/j.heares.2015.04.009

Yoo, J., Hamilton, S. J., Angel, D., Fung, K., Franklin, J., Parnes, L. S., et al. (2014). Cisplatin otoprotection using transtympanic L-N-acetylcysteine: a pilot randomized study in head and neck cancer patients. *Laryngoscope* 124, E87–E94. doi: 10.1002/lary.24360

Zhang, M., Liu, W., Ding, D., and Salvi, R. (2003). Pifithrin-α supresses p53 and protects cochlear and vestibular hair cells from cisplatin-induced apoptosis. *Neuroscience* 120, 191–205. doi: 10.1016/S0306-4522(03)00286-0

Zheng, H.-W., Chen, J., and Sha, S.-H. (2014). Receptor-interacting protein kinases modulate noise-induced sensory hair cell death. *Cell Death Dis.* 5:e1262. doi: 10.1038/cddis.2014.177

Zine, A., and Romand, R. (1996). Development of the auditory receptors of the rat: a SEM study. *Brain Res.* 721, 49–58. doi: 10.1016/0006-8993(96)00147-3

19

Partial Aminoglycoside Lesions in Vestibular Epithelia Reveal Broad Sensory Dysfunction Associated with Modest Hair Cell Loss and Afferent Calyx Retraction

David R. Sultemeier[1] *and Larry F. Hoffman*[1,2*]

[1] *Department of Head and Neck Surgery, David Geffen School of Medicine, University of California, Los Angeles, Los Angeles, CA, United States,* [2] *Brain Research Institute, David Geffen School of Medicine, University of California, Los Angeles, Los Angeles, CA, United States*

Edited by:
Peter S. Steyger,
Oregon Health & Science University, United States

Reviewed by:
James Phillips,
University of Washington, United States
Ian S. Curthoys,
University of Sydney, Australia

****Correspondence:***
Larry F. Hoffman
lfh@g.ucla.edu

Although the effects of aminoglycoside antibiotics on hair cells have been investigated for decades, their influences on the dendrites of primary afferent neurons have not been widely studied. This is undoubtedly due to the difficulty in disassociating pathology to dendritic processes from that resulting from loss of the presynaptic hair cell. This was overcome in the present investigation through development of a preparation using *Chinchilla laniger* that enabled direct perilymphatic infusion. Through this strategy we unmasked gentamicin's potential effects on afferent calyces. The pathophysiology of the vestibular neuroepithelia after post-administration durations of 0.5 through 6 months was assessed using single-neuron electrophysiology, immunohistochemistry, and confocal microscopy. Hair cell densities within cristae central zones (0.5-, 1-, 2-, and 6-months) and utricle peri- and extrastriola (6-months) regions were determined, and damage to calretinin-immunoreactive calyces was quantified. Gentamicin-induced hair cell loss exhibited a profile that reflected elimination of a most-sensitive group by 0.5-months post-administration (18.2%), followed by loss of a second group (20.6%) over the subsequent 5.5 months. The total hair cell loss with this gentamicin dose (approximately 38.8%) was less than the estimated fraction of type I hair cells in the chinchilla's crista central zone (approximately 60%), indicating that viable type I hair cells remained. Extensive lesions to afferent calyces were observed at 0.5-months, though stimulus-evoked modulation was intact at this post-administration time. Widespread compromise to calyx morphology and severe attenuation of stimulus-evoked afferent discharge modulation was found at 1 month post-administration, a condition that persisted in preparations examined through the 6-month post-administration interval. Spontaneous discharge was robust at all post-administration intervals. All calretinin-positive calyces had retracted at 2 and 6 months post-administration. We found no evidence of morphologic or physiologic recovery. These results indicate that gentamicin-induced partial lesions to vestibular epithelia include hair cell loss (ostensibly reflecting an *apoptotic effect*) that is far less extensive than the compromise to stimulus-evoked afferent discharge modulation and retraction of afferent calyces (reflecting *non-apoptotic effects*). Additionally, calyx retraction cannot be completely accounted for by loss of type I hair cells, supporting the possibility for direct action of gentamicin on the afferent dendrite.

Keywords: ototoxicity, primary afferent, stimulus–response coherence, spontaneous discharge

INTRODUCTION

The vestibulotoxic effects of aminoglycosides became apparent shortly after implementation of streptomycin therapy in the treatment of tuberculosis (Bignall et al., 1951; Robson and Goulding, 1952). Early investigations of aminoglycoside otopathology in animal models focused upon hair cells as the primary targets (Wersall and Hawkins, 1962; Lindeman, 1969a; Wersall et al., 1969; Watanuki et al., 1972). Since then, aminoglycosides have been widely used as research tools to lesion vestibular epithelia in investigations of the cellular and molecular mechanisms of hair cell regeneration (Weisleder and Rubel, 1992; Forge et al., 1993; Weisleder and Rubel, 1993; Lopez et al., 1999; Popper et al., 1999; Stone and Rubel, 2000; Dickman and Lim, 2004; Stone et al., 2004; Lyford-Pike et al., 2007; Haque et al., 2009; Kawamoto et al., 2009; Warchol, 2010b; Burns and Corwin, 2014; Warchol et al., 2017). Additionally, gentamicin is an agent commonly used in investigations of mammalian vestibular pathophysiology (Imamura and Adams, 2003a,b; Hirvonen et al., 2005; Hong et al., 2006; Day et al., 2007; Lue et al., 2009; Ding et al., 2010; Warchol, 2010a; Bremer et al., 2014; King et al., 2017). These studies have considerable translational value to enhance the understanding of gentamicin's use in ablative therapy for intractable vertigo associated with Mèniére's syndrome (Schuknecht, 1956, 1957; Nedzelski et al., 1993; Halmagyi et al., 1994; Minor, 1999; De Waele et al., 2002; Magnusson et al., 2007; Nguyen et al., 2009; Marques et al., 2015; Junet et al., 2016).

In most studies of aminoglycoside-induced vestibular pathophysiology, the lesions have been extensive with damage to hair cells, supporting cells, and afferent neurons. However, particular components of the mammalian vestibular neuroepithelia are believed to exhibit greater sensitivity to the deleterious effects of aminoglycosides than others. There is evidence suggesting that type I hair cells, particularly those in cristae central zones and utriclar striolae, are the most sensitive and are the first to be compromised or eliminated after aminoglycoside administration (Wersall and Hawkins, 1962; Lindeman, 1969b; Watanuki et al., 1972; Hirvonen et al., 2005). Lyford-Pike et al. (2007) provided evidence indicating that type I hair cells accumulated higher gentamicin concentrations than type II hair cells, supporting the notion that type I hair cells exhibit enhanced susceptibility to gentamicin toxicity than other constituents of the vestibular epithelia.

Although gentamicin toxicity to vestibular hair cells has been extensively investigated, few studies have focused upon the effects on Scarpa's ganglion neurons and their dendrites within the sensory epithelia. Imamura and Adams (2003b) found only weak anti-gentamicin immunolabeling in Scarpa's ganglion somata following both systemic or middle ear gentamicin administrations that produced strong immunolabeling in vestibular hair cells. Roehm et al. (2007) reported similar findings following gentamicin application to the round window in chinchillas (i.e., either by middle ear instillation or microcatheter delivery directed to the round window from an implanted osmotic pump). Harada et al. (1991) reported evidence of Scarpa's ganglion degeneration after a 5-day course of middle ear gentamicin administration. In another investigation transtympanic gentamicin application led to increased levels of oxidative stress markers in the calyceal afferent endings (Hong et al., 2006). Hirvonen et al. (2005) used similar transtympanic applications of gentamicin in chinchillas to produce preparations in which mean hair cell density was reduced by 57% while virtually all afferent calyces were lost [see also Lyford-Pike et al. (2007)]. The remarkable finding from Hirvonen et al. (2005) was that afferent spontaneous discharge was preserved while evoked discharge was nearly eliminated, indicating that viable hair cells exhibited dramatic functional compromise not associated with hair cell apoptosis or necrosis (Li et al., 1995; Forge and Li, 2000; Matsui et al., 2002, 2003, 2004; Cunningham et al., 2004; Ding et al., 2010; Zhang et al., 2012; Tao and Segil, 2015).

Because the investigations by Hirvonen et al. (2005) and Lyford-Pike et al. (2007) utilized gentamicin doses that resulted in hair cell losses approaching 60% [i.e., approximating the proportion of type I hair cells (Desai et al., 2005a,b)], it could not be determined whether degeneration of afferent calyces stemmed from type I hair cell loss and subsequent postsynaptic degeneration, or whether it reflected direct and/or independent effects on calyces. Furthermore, neither of these studies tracked the fate of the afferent parent axons following gentamicin administration. Both issues are critical to the development of a more complete understanding of the cellular targets of aminoglycoside ototoxicity. That is, if afferent calyx loss is secondary to hair cell loss, and if the parent axons degenerate following calyx loss, then the cellular mechanisms of the lesions are likely to involve terminal cellular pathways in both hair cells and afferent neurons. However, if calyx damage exhibits some independence from hair cell loss, and if the parent axons remain within the epithelium, there must be intermediate levels of pathology that do not necessarily involve terminal (e.g., apoptotic or necrotic) mechanisms. These may be referred to as *non-apoptotic* effects. If the latter alternative is true, identifying epithelial constituents that are generally labile to other ototoxic agents, then there is hope for rehabilitation of vestibular hypofunction resulting from toxicity secondary to systemic aminoglycoside or other therapies. These issues were addressed in the present study through the development of a novel preparation enabling the use of refined gentamicin dosing that resulted in less extensive yet highly repeatable lesions than achieved in previous studies. The goal of these preparations was to use lower gentamicin doses to produce partial lesions enabling the distinction of hair cell and afferent pathology. Pathophysiologic correlates of these lesions were determined through single-afferent electrophysiology and immunohistochemical methodologies.

MATERIALS AND METHODS

Experimental Animals, Surgical Preparation, and Gentamicin Administration

Adult male chinchillas (6–7 months of age, 0.4–0.6 kg body mass) were used for this study. These animals were acquired, cared for, and handled in accordance with the guidelines published in the NIH *Guide for the Care and Use of Laboratory Animals* (National Institutes of Health Publication revised 2011), and the principles presented in the *Guidelines for the Use of Animals in Neuroscience Research* by the Society for Neuroscience (available from the Society for Neuroscience). All procedures were approved by UCLA's institutional animal care and use committee.

For the surgical implantation of a perilymph access port enabling direct gentamicin infusion, animals were anesthetized and placed on a platform equipped with a servo-controlled heater for core temperature maintenance (approximately 36.5°C) throughout the surgical preparation and gentamicin administration. Two anesthesia protocols were utilized during this study. For the early preparations, the protocol included administration of an intramuscular cocktail of ketamine and xylazine (30 and 4 mg/kg, respectively), followed by maintenance doses that amounted to 25% of the initial dose administered only as needed. For later preparations, isoflurane anesthesia (2–2.5%) was used exclusively. Once a surgical plane of anesthesia was achieved, the head was placed within a custom holder. A midline scalp incision was made to expose the surface of the tympanic bulla, and the bulla's bony cap was removed to expose the middle ear. The chinchilla exhibits cavernous tympanic bullae with plenty of space between the prominent bony superior semicircular canal and the dorsal cap of the bulla. At the canal's dorsal-most aspect, a small fenestra was carefully made into the perilymphatic space surrounding the membranous superior canal, into which a 5 mm length of 27-gauge stainless steel tubing was fit and secured with cyanoacrylate cement. The fenestra was made to provide patent access to the perilymphatic space surrounding the semicircular canal, but was not so large to allow the tubing to completely enter the superior semicircular canal and potentially occlude the duct. Once the cyanoacrylate cement cured, an epoxy-like bonding agent (Cerebond, 39465030; Leica Microsystems, Bannockburn, IL, United States) was poured around the cannula to secure it in place and fix the entire preparation to the surrounding temporal bone, leaving the top 1 mm of cannula exposed. By the time the bonding agent cured (approximately 5 min), perilymph was generally visualized at the top of the cannula. The cannula was fit with polyethylene tubing (PE-20) leading to a precision syringe placed in an infusion pump. A fixed volume of treatment solution (2.5 μl, composed of either 0.4 μg gentamicin/μl in Hank's Balanced Saline Solution, HBSS, for lesioned specimens or HBSS alone for vehicle control specimens) was administered directly to the perilymphatic space over a 1-h period. Administration of 0.4 μg/μl gentamicin in 2.5 μl HBSS amounted to a total delivery of 1 μg gentamicin. The PE delivery tubing was then removed and the cannula sealed prior to replacing the bulla's bony cap. The scalp incision was then sutured, whereupon the animal was removed from anesthesia and closely monitored until it regained sternal posture (<30 min). Upon full recovery from anesthesia, a minority of gentamicin treated specimens ($n = 5/13$) exhibited a slight head tilt toward the lesioned side within 2–3 postoperative days, whereas no vehicle control specimens ($n = 3$) exhibited head tilt. The head tilt resolved within 2 weeks after drug administration. Spontaneous nystagmus was not observed in any animal subjects.

Vestibular Afferent Electrophysiology

The function of the vestibular epithelia in untreated, gentamicin-treated, or vehicle-control (i.e., HBSS only) preparations was assessed by electrophysiologic recording from individual afferent neurons following post-administration durations of 0.5, 1, 2, and 6 months. At the specified duration, animals were deeply anesthetized with a single intraperitoneal administration of sodium pentobarbital (50 mg/kg), which was sufficient to allow for cannulation of a jugular vein through which maintenance doses were administered as needed (0.05 cc, 50 mg/cc). A tracheotomy was performed for placement of an endotracheal tube into which a loosely fitting cannula delivering supplemental oxygen (100% O_2) was placed. Core body temperature was maintained at 38°C via rectal probe and a custom servo-controlled heating system. Each animal's head was held in a stereotyped position (10° right ear down, 15° nose down) by a custom holder fixed to a servo-controlled rotation table. This position was maintained for each experimental preparation. Heart and respiratory rates, as well as blood oxygen saturation, were recorded at regular intervals throughout the recording session.

Recordings from individual vestibular afferent neurons were made by exposing the right superior vestibular nerve in the region of Scarpa's ganglion through a fenestra made in the internal vestibular meatus, approximately 1mm medial to the superior and horizontal semicircular canal ampullae. Vestibular afferent discharge was recorded using glass microelectrodes pulled to impedances of approximately 40 MΩ when filled with 1 M KCl. With the animal restrained in the custom head holder, afferent discharge was recorded in the absence of head movement stimuli (i.e., spontaneous discharge) and during a broad repertoire of stimulus rotations. Afferents projecting from the horizontal and superior cristae and from the utricle could be recorded from this site in the superior vestibular nerve, which were easily distinguished in normal animals based upon their discharge modulation during manual turntable rotations. That is, in untreated preparations horizontal canal afferents were identified by increased discharge rate during turntable rotations producing utriculopetal relative endolymph flow, while superior canal afferents exhibited decreased discharge rate with similar rotations (this phase relationship is illustrated in **Figure 2**). Utricular afferents were identified as those that were unresponsive to turntable rotations, or responded at twice the stimulus frequency (i.e., increased or decreased discharge with rotations in either direction).

Spontaneous and stimulus-evoked spike trains were first analyzed using methods routine for studies of vestibular afferents neurons. For spontaneous discharge, interspike intervals (ISIs) were calculated during a 20 s recording epoch, from which the mean and standard deviation were determined. The coefficient of variation (CV) for each afferent was then computed as the ratio of ISI standard deviation to ISI mean. The perstimulus discharge spike trains were first analyzed using discrete Fourier analysis. However, upon finding that the responses in gentamicin-treated specimens were severely attenuated or non-existent, it became clear that methods were needed to objectively verify a statistical correlation between stimulus and response. To achieve greater measure of confidence in evaluating very weak responses, we adapted the frequency-domain measures for determining stimulus–response coherence computed directly from the spike trains (Jarvis and Mitra, 2001).

As in all experiments employing glass microelectrodes and axonal recordings, an inherent sampling bias exists toward the larger axons in the chinchilla's superior vestibular nerve. Despite this potential bias, our recordings from untreated specimens suggest that it is offset with methods (e.g., use of high-impedance electrodes) resulting in a proclivity for afferents with low values of CV, indicative of smaller caliber afferents (Baird et al., 1988). The inherent bias toward sampling afferents with larger axons, together with the implementation of methods with demonstrable capabilities for recording from smaller afferents, result in a paradigm designed for sampling the broad distribution of axon diameters that are found in the chinchilla's vestibular nerve (Hoffman and Honrubia, 2002).

Histology and Whole-Mount Immunohistochemistry

We utilized fluorescence immunohistochemistry and confocal microscopy to visualize the cytoarchitecture of chinchilla vestibular sensory epithelia. Vestibular endorgans were prepared as whole mounts and incubated with an antibody to calretinin (anti-CALB2) to immunolabel calyx-only afferents, and, in some specimens, an antibody to β3-tubulin (anti-TUBB3) to label all calyces and nerve fibers. In contrast to murine vestibular organs in which most hair cells are calretinin-immunopositive (CALB2+) (Desai et al., 2005a,b), only a subset of afferent calyces (i.e., those associated with calyx-only afferents) are CALB2+ in chinchilla vestibular epithelia (Desmadryl and Dechesne, 1992). We used CALB2 immunohistochemistry to delimit cristae central zones and utricular striola regions, and quantified gentamicin-induced modifications to hair cells and afferents in these regions which reportedly were most sensitive to gentamicin (Chen et al., 1999; Hilton et al., 2002).

After specified post-administration durations and electrophysiologic recording sessions, animals were euthanized (sodium pentobarbital overdose) and temporal bones were quickly dissected. Temporal bones were immediately infused with 4% paraformaldehyde (in 0.1 M phosphate buffer) through the oval window, after which the roof of the vestibule (floor of the subarcuate fossa) was removed prior to incubating in fixative overnight at 4°C. After three washes in 0.1 M phosphate buffered saline (PBS; pH 7.4), vestibular epithelia and nerve branches were microdissected. The tissues were incubated in blocking solution (0.25% Triton-X100, 1.0% BSA solution in PBS) for 2 h at room temperature, and then incubated 48–72 h at 4°C in a primary antibody cocktail that included combinations of the following antibodies diluted in blocking solution: 1:250 mouse anti-CALB2 (MAB1568; Millipore, Billerica, MA, United States) or 1:250 rabbit anti-CALB2 (AB5054; Millipore), 1:250 rabbit anti-Class III β-TUBB3 (PRB-435P; Covance, Princeton, NJ, United States), 1:250 rabbit anti-Myosin VI (MYOVI; 25-6791, Proteus Biosciences, Ramona, CA, United States). After washing in PBS, specimens were incubated for 2 h at room temperature in combinations of the following secondary antibodies and stains diluted in blocking solution: 1:500 Alexa Fluor 633 conjugated goat anti-mouse antibody (A-21050; Invitrogen, Carlsbad, CA, United States), 1:500 Alexa Fluor 546 goat anti-rabbit antibody (A-11010; Invitrogen), 1:150 NeuroTrace 500/525 green fluorescent Nissl stain (N-21480; Invitrogen). Tissue was mounted on glass slides with 1–2 spacers (S-24735; Invitrogen) in Vectashield Hard Set Mounting Medium (H-1500; Vector Laboratories, Burlingame, CA, United States).

Antibody Specificity

Secondary-only controls for all antibodies were processed alongside regular staining to ascertain background fluorescence. No immunolabeling was observed in any tissues processed without the addition of primary antibody (not shown).

The two anti-CALB2 antibodies utilized in the present study were generated against recombinant rat Calretinin (manufacturer's technical information). We confirmed antigen specificity of the antibodies by staining cryosections of mouse cerebellum (data not shown). In these controls we observed immunolabeling consistent with previous investigations (Miyata et al., 1999; Bearzatto et al., 2006), whereby anti-CALB2 antibody positively labeled granule cells but not Purkinje cells, the latter of which are positive for calbindin (a very similar but distinct calcium-binding protein). Furthermore, the staining pattern that we observed in the control chinchilla vestibular epithelia was consistent with that observed in previous studies (Desmadryl and Dechesne, 1992; Desai et al., 2005a,b).

The anti-TUBB3 antibody was produced against microtubules isolated from rat brain (manufacturer's technical information). This antibody has been widely used as a neuron specific marker and does not bind β-tubulin found in glia (manufacturer's technical information). Western blot analyses of the antibody against β3-tubulin demonstrated that this antibody recognized a doublet of bands in spiral ganglion extracts (Flores-Otero et al., 2007) consistent with a post-translational modification of β3-tubulin detected by this antibody (Cicchillitti et al., 2008). As previously reported, we did not observe staining of non-neuronal cells (i.e., support cells or hair cells).

The anti-MYOVI antibody was generated against amino acids 1049–1254 of porcine MYOVI (manufacturer's technical information). Anti-MYOVI is commonly used as a marker for hair cells including vestibular types I and II (Hasson et al., 1997). Consistent with this and other studies, we observed specific hair cell labeling with this antibody in chinchilla vestibular epithelia.

Confocal Microscopy and Analysis

Confocal images were captured on a Zeiss LSM 510 Meta confocal microscope implemented on an upright Axioplan 2 microscope using Zeiss LSM 510 software. The 488 nm (15% intensity), 543 nm (80–100% intensity) and 633 nm (10–20% intensity) laser lines were used for excitation. Bandpass filters of 505–530 nm, 560–615 nm, and a longpass filter 650 nm were used to capture separate emission channels. A Zeiss Plan-Neofluar 10X/0.3 NA objective was used to capture low-magnification images and high magnification images were obtained using a Zeiss Plan-Apochromat 63X/1.4 NA oil-immersion objective. Confocal stack micrographs were prepared for publication using Volocity software (Perkin Elmer, Waltham, MA, United States). Adobe Photoshop 7.0.1 (Adobe Systems Incorporated, San Jose, CA, United States) was used to compile figures.

Morphometric Analyses

Parent axons and calyces of CALB2+ afferents were counted using the neuron tracing application in *Neurolucida* (MBF Bioscience; Williston, VT, United States). Hair cell quantification and sensory epithelia area measurements were completed using automated and semi-automated methods implemented within the *Volocity* software environment (PerkinElmer/Improvision, Waltham, MA, United States). Hair cell nuclei were differentiated from support cell nuclei based on position within the sensory epithelium, morphology, and chromatin condensation (i.e., manifested in Nissl stain fluorescence intensity). Support cell nuclei were cuboidal, had compact chromatin, and formed a tightly packed monolayer over the basement membrane extending to the transitional epithelia at the ends of the sensory epithelia. In contrast, nuclei of hair cells were usually spherical, have less compact chromatin, and were located more toward the lumen compared to support cell nuclei.

Hair cell nuclei within crista central zones and utricular peri- and extrastriola regions were included in density measurements. Cristae central zones were approximated as the area of sensory epithelia innervated by CALB2+ afferents. Two – four confocal stacks were sampled from each crista. Four utricle peristriola regions were systematically evaluated along the rostral to caudal line of polarity reversal (LPR), and encompassed the striola, defined as the region harboring CALB2+ calyces, and immediately adjacent areas. Two confocal stacks each from the lateral and medial striola were used to estimate hair cell densities in these regions. The borders of these image stacks constituted the counting frames for quantification. Nuclei contacting either of two adjacent sides of the counting frames were excluded from quantification, while nuclei contacting the other two sides were included in the counts. This estimation procedure was implemented to compensate for incomplete counting units transected by the counting frame. Support cell densities were quantified using similar methods to evaluate the treatment-induced alterations of the epithelia surface areas.

We found that intraperilymphatic gentamicin administration resulted morphologic distortion in afferent calyces, and therefore established criteria on which to identify an "intact" calyx for quantification purposes. A CALB2+ calyx was counted if its height (i.e., along the base-neck hair cell axis) extended to or above the apical-most level of the Nissl-stained hair cell nucleus. Density measures were computed as fractions of contralateral control density, and are also presented as CALB2+ calyces or axons per 100 μm^2 of epithelium.

The areas of sensory epithelia used to determine densities of hair cells and CALB2+ parent axons and calyces were established by measuring the width along the support cell nuclei layer every 24 μm across the length of the cristae central zone (estimated by presence of CALB2+ parent axons) and utricle. The area was estimated as the product of the average width and the length.

Correlates between Afferent Electrophysiology and Vestibular Epithelia Morphology

It should be clarified that the characteristics of afferent electrophysiology and sensory epithelia morphology are intended to be representative of each metric within a given specimen. For most specimens, stimulus-evoked discharge modulation was lost or severely attenuated, and in all but a limited number of records (e.g., **Figures 3C, 4A-v,vi**) it was not possible to distinguish the epithelial origin of a given afferent. Furthermore, morphologic analyses were restricted to the central zones of the cristae. Direct associations between afferent discharge and morphologic characteristics of these crista regions were not made.

Retrograde Labeling of Vestibular Afferent Dendrites

To confirm the presence of putative boutons within crista central zones and utricular striolae, representing the intact components of dimorphic afferents, we performed extracellular injections of 2% TRITC-conjugated biotin (T12092, Molecular Probes Inc.) in two gentamicin-dosed specimens. This was accomplished through pneumatic injection of the label directly into the superior vestibular nerve in the vicinity of Scarpa's ganglion (i.e., approximately 2 mm medial to the superior and horizontal ampullae). The label was allowed to incubate for 6 h, after which normal fixation and tissue harvesting procedures were completed.

Statistical Analyses

Analyses and Comparisons of Afferent Discharge Characteristics

In this report most of the electrophysiologic data are represented as epochs of instantaneous discharge rates under the different gentamicin exposure conditions. The goal of these illustrations was to demonstrate the perstimulus discharge associated with the morphologic analyses. All instantaneous discharge rate waveforms were based upon spiketimes and derived from a Gaussian local rate filter using a 6.4 Hz corner frequency (Paulin and Hoffman, 2001). Mean spontaneous discharge rates (e.g., **Figure 4**) were computed as the reciprocal of ISI mean. Most perstimulus discharge records were obtained during 0.8 Hz, with the exception of **Figure 4B** for which the records were obtained during 0.4 Hz rotations.

Hirvonen et al. (2005) demonstrated that gentamicin eliminated the responses of vestibular afferents to head movement stimuli, while spontaneous discharge was preserved. As indicated above, our recording paradigm was conducted in head-fixed preparations on a turntable that precluded the ability to identify utricular afferents through the modulation of linear acceleration stimuli. In untreated preparations afferents projecting from the utricle were most often identified as those unresponsive to rotational stimuli. Therefore, the challenge in the present study was interpreting the absence of rotational responses as those resulting from the effects of gentamicin from a utricular afferent in our recording paradigm. We addressed this challenge by: (1) providing a perspective of the relatively low probability of recording a utricular afferent at the recording site; and (2) through analyses of previously published data of semicircular canal and utricular afferents (Baird et al., 1988; Goldberg et al., 1990).

For analyses of afferent discharge from gentamicin-treated vestibular epithelia it was important to have samples of untreated (normal) afferents that projected within the chinchilla's superior vestibular nerve accessible at the recording site. This included afferents from the horizontal and superior cristae and the utricle. Data for untreated cristae afferents came from our laboratory's database that included 431 neurons projecting from horizontal and superior cristae. In addition, the spontaneous discharge characteristics of canal and utricular afferents were obtained from earlier investigations (Baird et al., 1988; Goldberg et al., 1990). Using image analysis software (ImageJ 1.38g), we reconstituted CV and mean ISI values of 438 semicircular canal afferents (Baird et al., 1988), and 342 utricular afferents (Goldberg et al., 1990). The reconstituted values were compared to reported summaries of the original data. For example, the mean discharge rate of 251 *regular* afferents of the original utricular afferent dataset (i.e., those with $CV^* < 0.1$) was reported to be 54.2 ± 1.0 spikes·s^{-1} [standard error as originally reported; (Goldberg et al., 1990)], and the reconstituted dataset of 238 regular afferents exhibited a similar mean discharge rate (±standard error) of 54.6 ± 1.07 spikes·s^{-1}. These analyses indicated that reconstitution of the published datasets produced a representative facsimile of the published data.

As specified above, coherence analyses were used to statistically verify stimulus-evoked discharge modulation. These measures were based upon multitaper spectral analyses (Jarvis and Mitra, 2001), and were primarily used to determine whether the perstimulus discharge of afferents in gentamicin-treated specimens represented statistically verifiable responses to discrete sine rotational stimuli. Coherence measures of the discharge from untreated afferents were also conducted to illustrate the sensitivity and veracity of this analytical strategy in identifying stimulus-evoked responses from challenging perstimulus discharge data (e.g., those exhibiting low sensitivity measures during low stimulus magnitudes).

The distributions of spontaneous discharge characteristics were compared by computing Kullback–Leibler divergences (KLDs). KLD is a non-symmetrical measure of the difference between two probability distributions. For two discrete probability distributions P and Q, KLD is computed from the formula (Mackay, 2003):

$$\mathrm{KLD}(P||Q) = \sum_i P_i \log \frac{P_i}{Q_i}$$

Therefore, in the present study we established the convention that distributions representing semicircular canal afferents conformed to P, while the compared distributions conformed to Q. A resampling strategy was implemented to test hypotheses that the KLD between two original distributions could have been derived from random sampling from the combined distributions (i.e., no difference between the original distributions). Software scripts used to compute KLD and manage the bootstrap resampling were written in the *Igor* environment (Wavemetrics Inc., Lake Oswego, OR, United States). The resampling strategy was based upon one million resamples and subsequent KLD calculations. Probabilities to support the null hypothesis (specified above) were determined explicitly, except when the KLDs from the original distributions were outside the range of the distribution of KLDs generated from one million random resamples. In these cases, the probability is expressed as an inequality (i.e., $p < 10^6$). Values less than 0.05 support rejection of the null hypothesis stated above, indicating that the two distributions could not be derived by random sampling from a dataset constituted from the combined distributions (i.e., they were different).

Comparisons of Morphometric Parameters

Statistical comparisons of the different treatment groups were done by analysis of variance (single and multifactor ANOVA) with a Newman–Keuls *post hoc* test and performed using GraphPad Prism 6.0 software (GraphPad Software, San Diego, CA, United States). Data are presented as mean ± standard deviation (SD). Observed significance levels (p-value) are indicated in the figures with asterisks coded as follows: single asterisk (*) reflects $p < 0.05$, double asterisks (**) reflect $p < 0.01$, and triple asterisks (***) reflect $p < 0.001$.

RESULTS

Morphology and Physiology of Non-lesioned Crista Epithelia and Afferent Dendrites

Cytoarchitecture of the Chinchilla Crista Central Zones

The cytoarchitecture of central zone epithelia from non-lesioned chinchilla cristae are presented first to provide the histologic perspective for the balance of the physiologic and morphologic correlates presented in this investigation. This was achieved

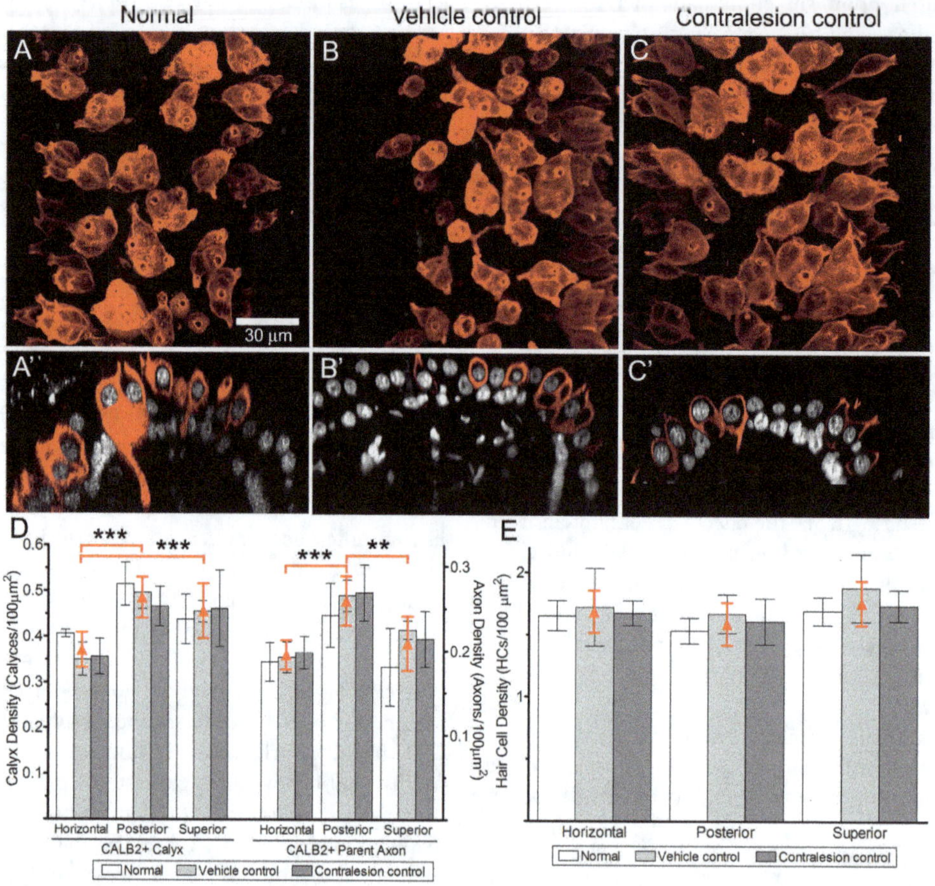

FIGURE 1 | Comparison of CALB2+ calyces within cristae central zones from Normal, Vehicle Control, and Contralesion control specimens. The micrographs represent maximum intensity projections **(A–C)** and orthogonal optical sections **(A′–C′)** of whole-mounted horizontal semicircular canal cristae labeled with anti-CALB2 (red) and Nissl stain (grayscale). Calyx morphology was similar in all control specimens, and exhibited narrow fluted necks at their apex closely conforming to the type I hair cell morphology. Scale bar shown in **(A)** applies to all micrographs. **(D)** CALB2+ calyx and parent axon densities expressed as counts/100 μm^2 epithelial area for horizontal, posterior, and superior cristae in all control specimens. See text for a discussion of the differences across epithelia. CALB2+ calyx densities were similar across all control conditions. **(E)** Central zone hair cell densities were similar across crista type and control conditions. The three control conditions were similar within any epithelium for each measure, and therefore the red triangles (and error bars) represent the mean control densities (±*SD*) over all conditions.

through quantitative morphometry of normal (untreated), vehicle control (HBSS-infused) and contralesion control (epithelia contralateral to gentamicin infusion) cristae. In addition, these data provided the basis to determine whether the intraperilymphatic administration procedure induced histologic or physiologic changes that could have influenced our analyses independent of gentamicin's effects. Maximum intensity projections of confocal image stacks from the central zones of CALB2-immunolabeled horizontal cristae, representing the three control groups, are shown in **Figures 1A–C**. In each control condition similar simple and complex calyx arbor morphologies (Fernandez et al., 1988) were observed. Also shown are corresponding orthogonal optical sections through each confocal stack (**Figures 1A′–C′**) to further illustrate similarities in CALB2+ calyx morphology among these control groups. These micrographs demonstrate that CALB2+ calyces in non-lesioned epithelia were strongly labeled from the parent axons to the fluted calyceal necks, which extended well above the nuclei of encapsulated hair cells.

Quantitative estimates of the distributions of CALB2+ calyces, CALB2+ parent axons, and hair cells were expressed as densities (count per 100 μm^2 area of the crista central zone), and compared (two-factor repeated measures ANOVA) across control condition (i.e., untreated normal, vehicle control, and contralesion control) and crista identity (i.e., horizontal, posterior, and superior). We found that the densities of each epithelial component were similar across control conditions as shown in **Figures 1D,E** and **Tables 1, 2** ($p > 0.5$). The similarities between vehicle controls and normal epithelia indicate that the chronic placement of the perilymph access port and HBSS infusion did not result in alterations of the morphologic parameters analyzed. Furthermore, despite the presence of a patent vestibular aqueduct in the chinchilla (Roehm et al., 2007) the similarities between contralesion controls and

TABLE 1 | CALB2+ parent axon and calyx densities.

Treatment	Density (units/100 μm²)					
	CALB2+ calyx			CALB2+ parent axon		
	Horizontal	Posterior	Superior	Horizontal	Posterior	Superior
Normal	0.41 ± 0.009 (N = 3)	0.47 ± 0.027 (N = 3)	0.44 ± 0.054 (N = 3)	0.19 ± 0.023 (N = 3)	0.24 ± 0.038 (N = 3)	0.18 ± 0.046 (N = 3)
Vehicle control	0.35 ± 0.036 (N = 3)	0.50 ± 0.035 (N = 3)	0.46 ± 0.023 (N = 3)	0.19 ± 0.018 (N = 3)	0.27 ± 0.019 (N = 3)	0.23 ± 0.011 (N = 3)
Contralesion control	0.36 ± 0.039 (N = 5)	0.47 ± 0.043 (N = 8)	0.46 ± 0.084 (N = 5)	0.20 ± 0.019 (N = 5)	0.27 ± 0.033 (N = 8)	0.21 ± 0.033 (N = 5)
Combined control	0.37 ± 0.039 (N = 11)	0.48 ± 0.045 (N = 14)	0.45 ± 0.060 (N = 11)	0.19 ± 0.019 (N = 11)	0.26 ± 0.031 (N = 14)	0.21 ± 0.035 (N = 11)
0.5 month	0.12 ± 0.210* (N = 3)	0.19 ± 0.320*** (N = 3)	0.18 ± 0.311** (N = 3)	0.20 ± 0.032 (N = 3)	0.26 ± 0.014 (N = 3)	0.21 ± 0.021 (N = 3)
1 month	0.11 ± 0.186 (N = 3)	0.11 ± 0.172** (N = 3)	0.12 ± 0.200* (N = 3)	0.17 ± 0.044 (N = 3)	0.23 ± 0.031 (N = 3)	0.20 ± 0.028 (N = 3)
2 months	0.00 ± 0.000*** (N = 3)	0.00 ± 0.000*** (N = 3)	0.00 ± 0.000*** (N = 2)	0.15 ± 0.009 (N = 3)	0.22 ± 0.035 (N = 3)	0.20 ± 0.037 (N = 2)
6 months	0.00 ± 0.000*** (N = 3)	0.00 ± 0.000*** (N = 4)	0.01 ± 0.015*** (N = 4)	0.19 ± 0.019 (N = 3)	0.23 ± 0.027 (N = 4)	0.17 ± 0.054 (N = 4)

All values are means ± SD. N, number of specimens. Significance values represent comparisons with combined controls. These data complement the relative densities depicted in ***Figure 8****. Asterisks correspond to:* $*p < 0.05$; $**p < 0.01$; $***p < 0.001$.

normal epithelia indicated that administration of HBSS, and low gentamicin doses as compared later, did not alter these morphologic indices in the contralateral epithelia. This supports the use of contralesion control specimens for direct comparison of the lesions induced by the intraperilymphatic gentamicin administration.

Though not a principal objective of this investigation, our analyses revealed differences in CALB2+ calyx and parent axon densities across cristae type (**Figure 1D** and **Table 1**). While CALB2+ calyx densities (calyces/100 μm^2) were similar in the posterior (0.48 ± 0.045; $N = 14$) and superior (0.45 ± 0.06; $N = 11$) cristae, mean CALB2+ calyx density of the horizontal cristae (0.37 ± 0.039; $N = 11$) was approximately 20% less than the vertical cristae ($p < 0.001$). Additionally, CALB2+ axon density (axons/100 μm^2) was approximately 25% higher in posterior canal cristae (0.26 ± 0.031; $N = 14$) than in horizontal (0.19 ± 0.019, $N = 11$; $p < 0.001$) and superior (0.21 ± 0.035, $N = 11$; $p < 0.01$) cristae. In contrast to these differences in CALB2+ afferent innervation, mean central zone hair cell densities (HCs/100 μm^2) were similar across all control cristae ($p > 0.05$; **Figure 1E** and **Table 2**). These data suggest that the chinchilla superior cristae receive putative calyx-only afferents with a larger number of complex calyces compared to horizontal cristae. Additionally, the increased number of CALB2+ calyces in the posterior cristae, accompanied by an increase in parent axon density, reflects a greater number of putative calyx-only afferents.

Afferent Electrophysiology in Non-lesioned Specimens

The electrophysiology of non-lesioned chinchilla vestibular afferent neurons provides the background for evaluating the alterations concomitant with low-dose gentamicin administration. This background is provided primarily by our laboratory's database of afferents recorded in normal, untreated specimens (**Figures 2A,B** *Untreated*). In addition, a population of non-lesioned afferents were derived from the vehicle-control specimens described above. These serve to test whether the surgical implantation of the perilymph port into the bony superior semicircular canal or the infusion of HBSS resulted in deleterious effects upon the physiology of superior and horizontal semicircular canal afferents. As discussed above, no differences were found in the morphology of CALB2+ calyces and hair cell densities in these specimens.

Our experience in recording from over 400 semicircular canal afferents in normal, untreated specimens also served as the basis for establishing the probability of encountering afferents at the recording site within the superior vestibular nerve that projected to specific epithelia (i.e., the superior and horizontal cristae and the utricle, **Figure 2A**). In untreated specimens, the recording procedures utilized herein revealed afferent discharge characteristics similar to those previously reported (Baird et al., 1988; Hullar and Minor, 1999), including high levels of spontaneous discharge around which modulation was induced by turntable rotation. It is important to note that in our recording configuration the animals' heads were held in a fixed position (15° nose down, 10° recorded-ear

TABLE 2 | Hair cell densities in the cristae central zones.

Treatment	Hair cell density (hair cell nuclei/100 μm²)			
	Horizontal	**Posterior**	**Superior**	**Average**
Normal	1.65 ± 0.122 (*N* = 3)	1.53 ± 0.102 (*N* = 3)	1.69 ± 0.112 (*N* = 3)	1.62 ± 0.071 (*N** = 3)
Vehicle control	1.72 ± 0.311 (*N* = 3)	1.67 ± 0.156 (*N* = 2)	1.88 ± 0.272 (*N* = 3)	1.79 ± 0.153 (*N** = 3)
Contralesion control	1.67 ± 0.100 (*N* = 5)	1.61 ± 0.184 (*N* = 8)	1.74 ± 0.130 (*N* = 5)	1.69 ± 0.066 (*N** = 5)
Combined control	1.68 ± 0.165 (*N* = 11)	1.60 ± 0.160 (*N* = 13)	1.77 ± 0.172 (*N* = 11)	1.70 ± 0.107 (*N** = 11)
0.5 month	1.43 ± 0.167 (*N* = 3)	1.40 ± 0.226 (*N* = 3)	1.32 ± 0.321 (*N* = 3)	1.39 ± 0.231** (*N* = 3)
1 month	1.34 ± 0.388 (*N* = 3)	1.24 ± 0.146 (*N* = 3)	1.18 ± 0.244 (*N* = 3)	1.24 ± 0.276** (*N* = 3)
2 months	1.14 ± 0.066 (*N* = 3)	1.24 ± 0.121 (*N* = 3)	1.17 ± 0.035 (*N* = 2)	1.17 ± 0.032*** (*N* = 3)
6 months	1.03 ± 0.255 (*N* = 3)	1.06 ± 0.208 (*N* = 4)	1.05 ± 0.113 (*N* = 3)	1.04 ± 0.171*** (*N* = 4)

All values are means ± SD. N, number of specimens; N, number of specimens with >2 cristae counted. Average represents hair cell density calculated when cristae from a specimen were treated as a single epithelium. Significance values represent comparisons with combined controls. These data complement that depicted in* ***Figure 9****. Asterisks correspond to: **p < 0.01; ***p < 0.001.*

down) so that turntable rotation evokes a clear modulation in afferents projecting from both horizontal and superior semicircular canal cristae. Even afferent discharge modulated by 1–2 spikes·s^{-1} are unambiguously identified and characterized with these methods and subsequent analyses. In untreated specimens, a relatively small fraction of afferents was encountered in each preparation whose discharge did not modulate with turntable rotation, which was consistent with afferents projecting from the utricle. These afferents were not further explored as our experimental configuration precluded the application of linear acceleration stimuli, even in a paradigm of eccentric rotation. Furthermore, since the head was held in a static tilt, resultant discharge from most utricular afferents could not be considered "spontaneous," their discharge reflecting head position in a static tilt. These data indicated that when recording from the site described above in section "Materials and Methods" the majority of afferents encountered projected from the cristae, while only approximately 20% projected from the utricle. This observation is important in the context of evaluating afferents in gentamicin-treated specimens.

The balance of afferents probed at the recording site exhibited discharge that was clearly modulated during turntable rotations, as exemplified in **Figure 2B**. The afferents from *Untreated* preparations were selected to illustrate the high fidelity of responses to sinusoidal stimuli despite the low sensitivity measures (e.g., ±5 spikes·s^{-1} during sinusoidal stimuli of ±30°·s^{-1} peak velocity). In addition, robust stimulus-evoked responses were also recorded from superior and horizontal semicircular canal afferents in *Vehicle Control* specimens (right). Like the *Untreated* specimens, semicircular canal afferents in these controls were clearly modulated in response to sinusoidal turntable rotation, indicating that perilymphatic port implantation and infusion of HBSS did not lead to deleterious outcomes with respect to afferent electrophysiologic measures. High measures of stimulus–response coherence (>0.85) were observed in these two afferent groups, even under conditions of modest discharge modulation (±5 spikes·s^{-1}). Measures of stimulus–response coherence remained high in these controls.

Early Periods Following Gentamicin Administration Reveal Independence of Hair Cell and Afferent Neuron Pathotypes

Lesions to the peripheral vestibular receptors may involve hair cells, support cells, and afferent dendrites, inducing alterations in cellular function that may eventually lead to pathophysiologic changes in afferent discharge transmitted to the central nervous system. We refer to each general morphologic and physiologic component of the lesion as a *pathotype*, representing the different forms or "types" of pathology to specific components within the sensory epithelia. The goal of the present investigation was to refine production of the lesions so that unique pathotypes could be distinguished. Rather than strictly examine the lesions at the final mature stage, we envisioned that hair cell and afferent pathotypes might be distinguished if they exhibited differential temporal sensitivities to low-dose gentamicin. Therefore, we examined specimens at 0.5 and 1 months following gentamicin administration.

The early post-administration periods provided insight into the progression of the lesions to the stable state observed at later post-administration times. The morphologic and physiologic pathotypes of specimens analyzed at 0.5 and 1 months are represented in **Figure 3**, and illustrate the heterogeneity in calyx morphology and associated physiology observed at these times. The morphologic and physiologic data shown in these figures were selected to be representative of the specimens, and direct associations between the afferent discharge records and the crista region highlighted in the micrographs cannot be made (i.e., without intracellular labeling and tract tracing). **Figures 3A,B** show maximum intensity projection and orthogonal views (respectively) of the horizontal crista from a 0.5-month specimen exhibiting severe pathology to CALB2+ calyces. All CALB2+ calyces in this specimen were retracted, characterized by CALB2+ parent axons without calyces or drastically malformed partial calyces (**Figure 3B**). The central zones of the three cristae from this specimen exhibited a mean decrease in hair cell density of approximately 24%. In the chinchilla crista central zone 60% of hair cells are type I (Desai et al., 2005a), indicating that even if the hair cell loss was restricted to type I in this specimen a large

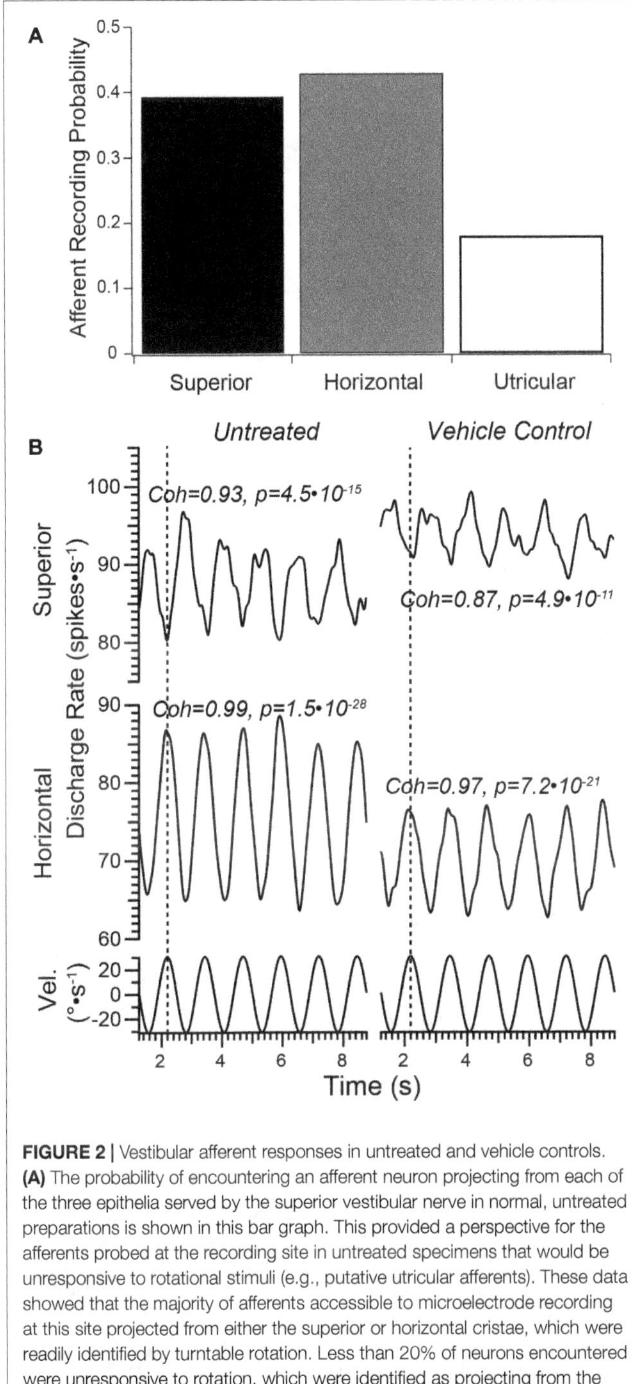

FIGURE 2 | Vestibular afferent responses in untreated and vehicle controls. **(A)** The probability of encountering an afferent neuron projecting from each of the three epithelia served by the superior vestibular nerve in normal, untreated preparations is shown in this bar graph. This provided a perspective for the afferents probed at the recording site in untreated specimens that would be unresponsive to rotational stimuli (e.g., putative utricular afferents). These data showed that the majority of afferents accessible to microelectrode recording at this site projected from either the superior or horizontal cristae, which were readily identified by turntable rotation. Less than 20% of neurons encountered were unresponsive to rotation, which were identified as projecting from the utricle. **(B)** Afferents recorded from *Vehicle Control* specimens exhibited stimulus-evoked modulation similar to *Normal* (untreated) controls. Representative afferents that projected from the superior and horizontal cristae in one preparation are shown demonstrating robust modulation in response to sinusoidal turntable rotation (sinusoidal angular velocity stimulus trajectories, in $°s^{-1}$, represented in the bottom traces). The scale of the vertical axes are similar in absolute range. Note the responses of the superior and horizontal afferents were approximately 180° out of phase (denoted by the dashed vertical line along each horizontal axis), illustrating the distinguishing characteristic of afferents projecting from these neuroepithelia. Afferents projecting from each crista in *Vehicle Control* specimens exhibited similarly robust modulation. Coherence and associated *p*-values for each full record are shown.

fraction of the phenotype remained. Therefore, while the lesion involved both hair cells and afferent calyces, the pathology to central zone CALB2+ calyces was more severe than central zone hair cell loss.

The discharge characteristics of afferents projecting to cristae of the preparation represented in **Figures 3A,B** are illustrated in **Figure 3C**, where the instantaneous discharge of afferents projecting to the horizontal and superior cristae during sinusoidal turntable velocity (**Figure 3C**, bottom) is shown. These records demonstrated that despite the histopathology exhibited by the crista epithelia (i.e., complete central zone calyx retraction and decreased hair cell density) afferent discharge was clearly modulated in response to sinusoidal stimuli. Additionally, stimulus-evoked discharge modulation (approximately $\pm$7–10 spikes$\cdot s^{-1}$) is superimposed upon spontaneous discharge (40–45 spikes$\cdot s^{-1}$), indicating that spontaneous discharge is preserved in these specimens that exhibited significant pathology. Coherence measures were comparable to that observed in untreated and vehicle control specimens (**Figure 2B**).

The histologic and physiologic results from a preparation examined at 1 month post-administration is shown in **Figures 3D–F**, illustrating a unique histopathologic variant while the physiology of vestibular afferents demonstrated more severe functional compromise than shown in **Figure 3C**. Two of the three 1-month preparations exhibited complete calyx retraction, similar to that depicted by the micrographs in **Figures 3A,B**. The third preparation is shown in **Figures 3D,E**, illustrating CALB2+ calyces within the horizontal crista central zone that have lost the narrow fluted necks characteristic of untreated central zone calyces (**Figure 1**). The apical openings of most calyces in this specimen were widened. The inset micrograph, showing a volume reconstruction of the area enclosed by the dashed box (**Figure 3D**, bottom), illustrates that the calyx opening was sufficiently large to enable visualization of the enclosed hair cell nuclei (yellow). Because these calyces extended above the hair cell nucleus, they were counted as intact calyces (i.e., conforming to the specified criteria) despite the obvious morphologic anomaly.

The consistent electrophysiologic feature among all afferents recorded from 1-month post-administration preparations was the absence of responses to sinusoidal rotation. These are represented by the instantaneous discharge records shown in **Figure 3F**, which were recorded from the same preparation that yielded **Figures 3D,E**. These traces are shown to be representative of the unresponsive afferents recorded in this preparation, and they are not meant to be directly associated with the horizontal crista represented in the micrograph. The absence of stimulus-evoked discharge modulation precludes us from drawing the direct correlate. The stimulus–response coherence measures are shown for each trace, indicating the absence of discharge modulation to the stimulus (**Figure 3F**, bottom). However, these afferents exhibited robust spontaneous discharge. This preparation is remarkable in that full calyx retraction had yet to dominate the crista landscape, yet afferent discharge reflected the severe response attenuation characteristic of other specimens evaluated at 1 month post-administration

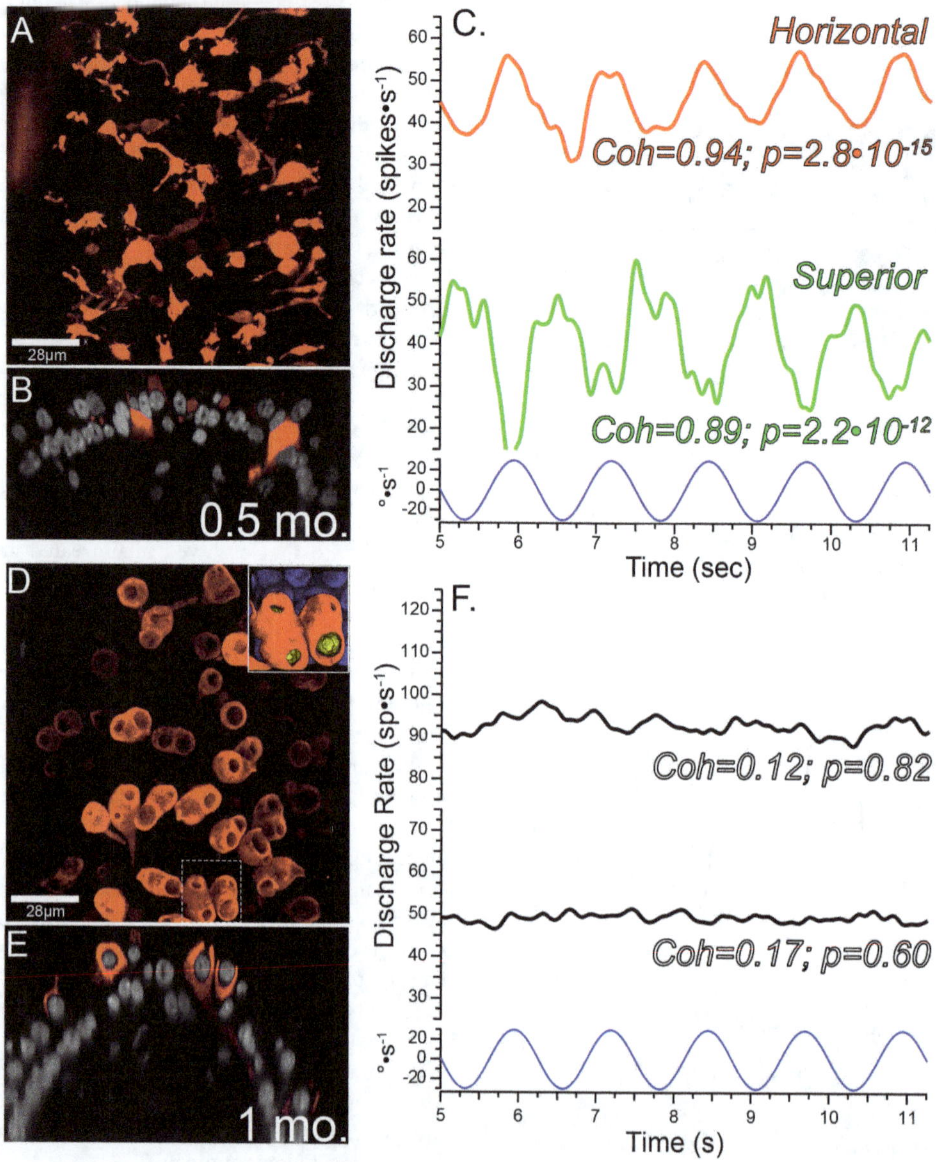

FIGURE 3 | Pathophysiologic correlates in the 1st month following intraperilymphatic gentamicin administration. Micrographs of horizontal crista epithelia at 0.5 **(A,B)** and 1 **(D,E)** month following gentamicin administration illustrate the variability in the histopathology at these early post-administration periods. The discharge of two afferents from each preparation are shown to demonstrate the physiologic status of each (i.e., **C** corresponds to the micrographs in **A** and **B**; **F** corresponds to **D** and **E**). **(A,B)** Maximum intensity projection **(A)** and orthogonal optical section **(B)** views of CALB2+ afferents in the horizontal crista central zone 0.5 months after 1 μg gentamicin administration. All calyces retracted in this specimen, while remnant CALB2+ endings of parent axons and fine branches are observed. **(C)** In this preparation both horizontal and superior afferents exhibited robust responses to rotational stimuli despite the widespread central zone calyx retraction and very modest hair cell loss in this specimen (not shown). The 0.8 Hz stimulus trajectory ($\pm 30^{\circ}\cdot s^{-1}$) is represented by the bottom trace (blue). The coherence measures (*Coh*) demonstrated the high fidelity between stimulus and response that was retained at this early post-administration time. **(D,E)** Maximum intensity projection **(D)** and orthogonal optical section **(E)** views illustrating CALB2+ calyces in a horizontal crista central zone from a specimen harvested 1 month following 1 μg intraperilymphatic gentamicin. The fluted and narrow apical extensions seen in untreated calyces (see **Figure 1**) were absent in the majority of these calyces and appear to have retracted to exhibit wide openings in this treated specimen. This is illustrated in the orthogonal view **(E)** illustrating a calyx whose apical portion – just higher than the hair cell nucleus – is not observed. A 3D volume reconstruction of the boxed region (**D**, bottom) is shown at higher magnification in the inset (top right in **D**), for which the hair cell nuclei within the CALB2+ calyces were clearly visible through the widened apical openings of the calyces (recolored yellow).
(F) Representative instantaneous discharge traces for two afferents recorded from the preparation represented in **(D,E)**. These afferents were unresponsive to the sinusoidal rotation (0.8 Hz, $30^{\circ}\cdot s^{-1}$, bottom), confirmed by the low coherence values (*Coh*) shown for each perstimulus discharge record.

(e.g., **Figure 7F**). This contrasts the clear stimulus-evoked discharge modulation in the 0.5 month specimen recorded in afferents projecting to cristae where central zone calyces have fully retracted (**Figures 3A–C**). These observations supporting the conclusions that severe attenuation in stimulus-evoked afferent discharge modulation did not depend upon full calyx

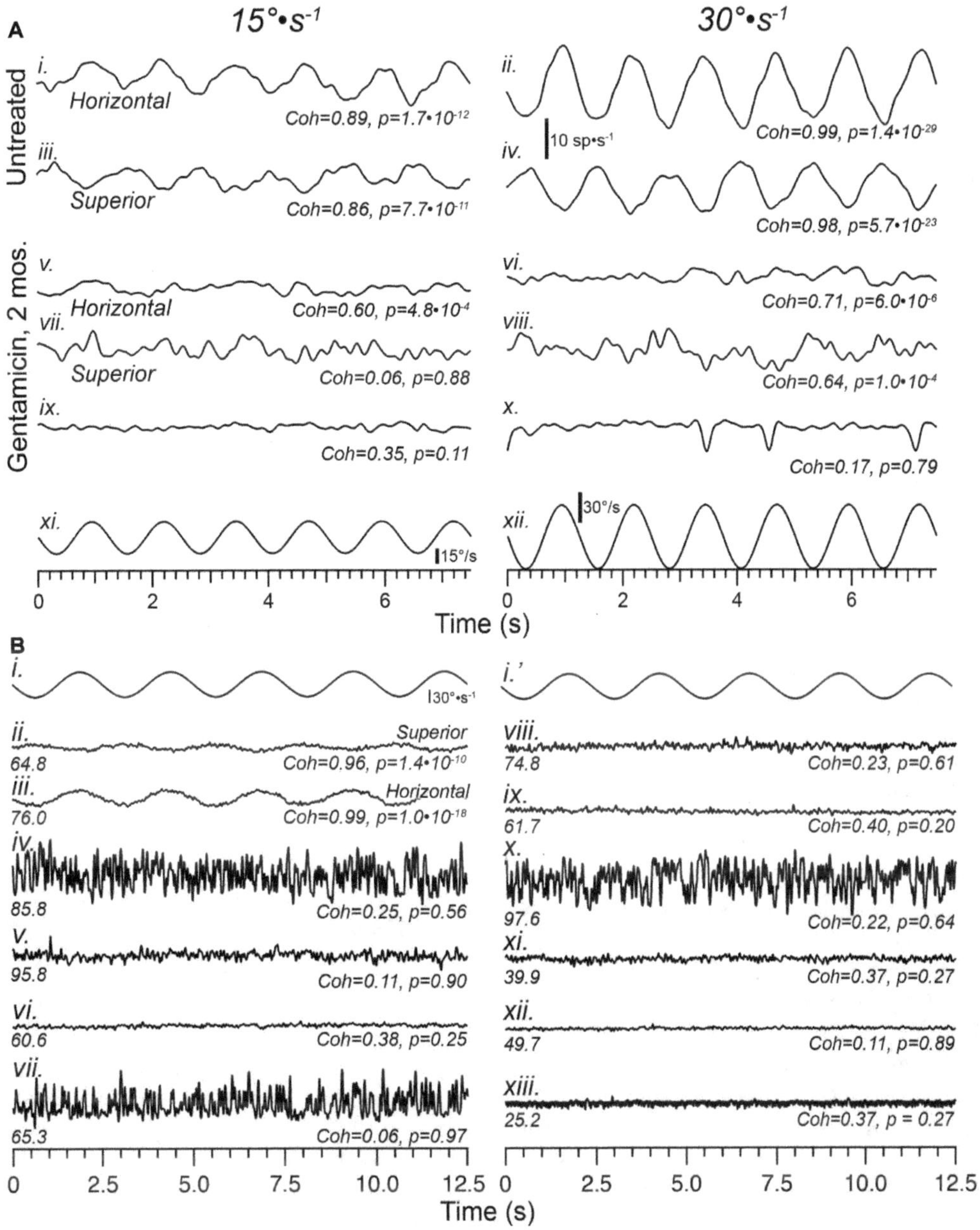

FIGURE 4 | Sensory function is severely compromised by 2 months, and continues through 6 months, following intraperilymphatic gentamicin. **(A)** Representative responses of horizontal and superior semicircular canal afferents recorded from Untreated **(i–iv)** and gentamicin-treated **(v–x)** specimens in response to 0.8 Hz sinusoidal rotations of 15 (left) and $30°\cdot s^{-1}$ (right) peak velocity (bottom traces in **A**). Among afferents recorded in three preparations at 2 months post-administration, most exhibited no response to rotation, similar to the traces in **(ix,x)** (verified by the low coherence values at each stimulus magnitude). However, in the gentamicin-treated preparation represented in this figure meager response were recorded in a few horizontal and superior afferents, shown in traces labeled **(v–viii)**. Though the coherence values were lower than those typically measured in untreated preparations, the responses were verified for the horizontal afferent at both stimulus magnitudes, and the superior afferent only at $30°\cdot s^{-1}$ magnitude. The third afferent from this preparation was unresponsive **(ix,x)**. The discharge rate scale shown beneath the untreated horizontal afferent ($30°\cdot s^{-1}$) applies to all traces in **(A)**. **(B)** Instantaneous discharge records of afferents during sinusoidal rotation (0.4 Hz, $30°\cdot s^{-1}$; **i,i'**) obtained 6 months following gentamicin administration are shown. For comparison, representative perstimulus discharge records of afferents projecting from the superior **(ii)** and horizontal **(iii)** cristae in an untreated specimen are shown. The mean spontaneous discharge rates are provided at the left underneath each record, while stimulus–response coherence measures (*Coh*) and corresponding *p*-values (*p*) are shown at right. Note the high coherence values for afferents from the untreated specimen, even the superior afferent in which the stimulus-evoked modulation is very modest. The 10 afferents from the treated specimen **(iv–xiii)** were recorded in succession during the experimental session, and all exhibited low coherence measures that corresponded with probabilities greater than 0.2 that this measure could have arisen randomly. The low coherence measures confirmed that these afferents were unresponsive to the sinusoidal rotational stimulus. See text for more detailed interpretation.

retraction, and that these two pathotypes are associated with independent mechanisms.

Sensory Dysfunction Appears Permanent

As illustrated in **Figure 3**, stimulus-evoked modulation was severely attenuated in all afferents recorded 1-month following gentamicin administration. **Figure 4** demonstrates that this sensory dysfunction persists into post-administration times of 2 and 6 months. Detailed responses of afferents recorded from a 2-month preparation are shown in **Figure 4A**, illustrating paired perstimulus discharge from the same afferents during presentation of 0.8 Hz rotational sinusoids at 15 (left: **Figures 4A-i,iii,v,vii,ix**) and $30°\cdot s^{-1}$ (right; **Figures 4A-ii,iv,vi,viii,x**) peak stimulus velocities. The trajectories of these stimuli are illustrated by the bottom waveforms (**Figures 4A-xi,xii**), and representative responses of horizontal (**Figures 4A-i,ii**) and superior (**Figures 4A-ii,iv**) semicircular canal afferents from untreated specimens are shown at the top. The responses of three afferents from the same preparation are shown in **Figures 4A-v–A-x**, and illustrate the heterogeneity in the severe compromise found in this preparation. The histopathology of this horizontal crista is illustrated in **Figure 7G**, where complete loss of CALB2+ calyces was observed. **Figures 4A-v,vi** represent the discharge of a horizontal canal afferent exhibiting severely compromised responses to both 15 and $30°\cdot s^{-1}$ stimulus intensities, but coherence analyses confirmed statistically verifiable responses ($p = 4.8\cdot10^{-4}$ and $6.0\cdot10^{-6}$, respectively). The perstimulus discharge records of the superior canal afferent (**Figures 4A-iii,vii**) illustrated the case where coherence analysis indicated the absence of a response in the discharge at $15°\cdot s^{-1}$, but the discharge during the $30°\cdot s^{-1}$ peak velocity stimulus did evoke a verifiable response ($p = 1.0\cdot10^{-4}$). The perstimulus discharge of the third afferent (**Figures 4A-ix,x**), however, did not exhibit modulation by either stimulus magnitude ($p = 0.11$). These data demonstrate that severe response attenuation, and not solely response elimination, was a potential outcome of gentamicin administration at this post-administration time. In addition, these data illustrate the value in computing stimulus–response coherence as a firm metric to analyze these severely attenuated responses.

The physiologic ramifications of intraperilymphatic administration of 1 μg gentamicin at 6 months post-administration are shown in **Figure 4B**. These data depict 12.5 s epochs of perstimulus discharge (in $spikes\cdot s^{-1}$) from 10 afferents recorded consecutively in a single preparation during presentation of 0.4 Hz sinusoidal rotations ($30°\cdot s^{-1}$ peak velocity; **Figures 4B-i,i′**). For reference, representative response discharge recordings from superior and horizontal semicircular canal afferents in an untreated preparation at this stimulus intensity are shown in **Figures 4B-ii,iii**, respectively. The coherence values associated with these two responses were 0.96 and 0.99, with associated p-values of $1.4\cdot10^{-10}$.and $1.0\cdot10^{-18}$, respectively. Particularly notable is the high coherence of the superior canal afferent (**Figures 4B-ii**) despite the very low sensitivity and small modulation depth, indicating the coherence measures remain very high even in afferents for which the discharge modulation is extremely low.

The discharge characteristics representative of afferents recorded 6 months after receiving 1 μg intraperilymphatic gentamicin are represented in **Figures 4B-iv–B-xiii**, illustrating the perstimulus discharge during 0.4 Hz rotation ($30°\cdot s^{-1}$ peak velocity, **Figures 4B-i,i′**; the same stimulus is shown in the interest of providing temporal correlation with the discharge records beneath). These data demonstrate three fundamental features of the electrophysiologic pathotype. First, coherence analyses verify the absence of rotational responses in all 10 perstimulus discharge records (Coh < 0.38; $p > 0.2$). While some of these afferents may have projected to the utricle (which, under normal conditions, would be unresponsive to rotation), the probability that all ten afferents would project to the utricle is extremely low. Therefore, the absence of a response in all 10 afferents further verifies the severe response attenuation among afferents from treated labyrinths. Second, the compromise of response capabilities among semicircular canal afferents, first observed at 1 month post-administration, persisted through 6 months post-administration, which provided evidence indicating the vestibular sensory epithelia do not exhibit capabilities for spontaneous recovery by 6 months. Third, despite the severe response attenuation spontaneous discharge remained robust at this post-administration time, with some afferents exhibiting rates exceeding 80 $spikes\cdot s^{-1}$ (e.g., **Figures 4B-iv,v,x**). This demonstrated an absence of any progressive compromise in spontaneous discharge through the 6 month post-administration interval.

Alterations in Spontaneous Discharge Associated with Intraperilymphatic Gentamicin

The principal finding from electrophysiologic recordings of vestibular afferents following intraperilymphatic administration of 1 μg gentamicin was the persistence of spontaneous discharge while modulation in response to head movement rotations was severely attenuated or lost. We tested the null hypothesis that spontaneous discharge characteristics of afferents recorded from gentamicin-treated preparations were similar to those of our laboratory's database of semicircular canal afferents recorded from untreated preparations. We also conducted parallel analyses of previously published spontaneous discharge data recorded from normal (untreated) semicircular canal and utricular afferents (Baird et al., 1988; Goldberg et al., 1990). These latter analyses provided an independent context for comparing distributions of spontaneous discharge characteristics derived from rotationally sensitive (semicircular canal) and rotationally insensitive (utricular) afferents, similar to the classifications of untreated semicircular canal (rotationally sensitive) and gentamicin-treated (rotationally insensitive) afferents.

The spontaneous discharge characteristics of afferents from gentamicin-treated preparations (green symbols) are shown in **Figure 5A**, against a backdrop of the characteristics obtained from our database of untreated semicircular canal afferents (black/gray symbols). The inset plot illustrates previously

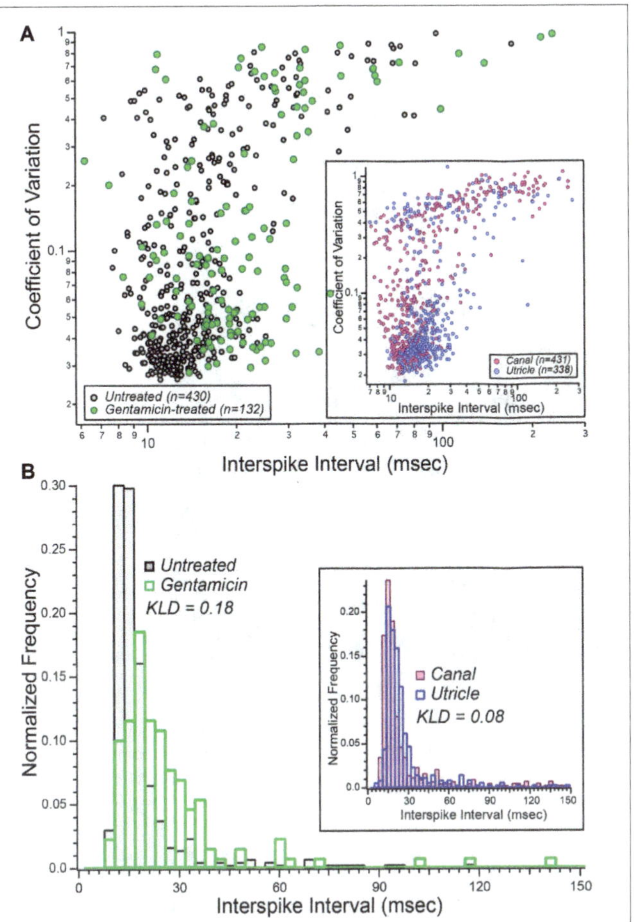

FIGURE 5 | Aggregate distributions of spontaneous discharge characteristics in vestibular afferents recorded after low-dose gentamicin administration. **(A)** Scatterplot illustrating the comparison of spontaneous discharge characteristics from gentamicin-treated specimens (green symbols) and the laboratory's database of 430 semicircular canal afferents from normal (untreated) specimens (black/gray symbols). These data illustrated that the mean spontaneous ISIs among afferents from gentamicin-treated preparations appeared to be greater (right-shifted in this scatter plot) than afferents recorded from untreated specimens. These data are interpreted in the context of published data from semicircular canal (Baird et al., 1988) and utricular (Goldberg et al., 1990) afferents, shown in the inset, representing a comparison of spontaneous discharge characteristics from canal and utricle afferents recorded from the same laboratory, and therefore under similar conditions. **(B)** Normalized histograms of mean ISIs from gentamicin-treated (green bars, $n = 132$) and untreated (black/gray bars, $n = 430$) preparations (i.e., mean ISI data from **A**). The Kullback–Leibler divergence between these two distributions was 0.18, and resampling analyses indicated the probability that this KLD could have been derived from random sampling of a single combined distribution was less than 10^{-6} (i.e., $p < 10^{-6}$). The inset histograms were derived from the published mean interspike interval (ISI) data of semicircular canal and utricular afferents (i.e., from inset in **A**). The KLD for these distributions was 0.08, reflecting the expected difference in mean intervals between canal and utricular afferents from the same preparations. See text for details.

published spontaneous discharge data of semicircular canal and utricular afferents (Baird et al., 1988; Goldberg et al., 1990), reconstructed as described in section "*Materials and Methods.*" The distribution of gentamicin-treated afferents appears to be right-shifted in the main plot, suggesting that the mean ISIs from this afferent group are, collectively, longer than untreated semicircular canal afferents. A similar impression is also given by the inset scatterplot, in which the cloud of utricular afferents appears to represent slightly greater mean ISIs. To compare the distributions of mean ISIs among untreated and gentamicin-treated populations (and between previously published semicircular canal and utricular afferents), histograms were prepared and are shown in **Figure 5B** (inset), in which the longer mean ISIs of gentamicin-treated afferents are visualized. The two distributions were compared by computing the KLD, after which a resampling strategy was implemented to test the hypothesis that the mean ISI distributions were derived from random sampling from a single underlying distribution. This probability was less than $1.0{\cdot}10^{-6}$, supporting rejection of the null hypothesis. Furthermore, this result indicated that the distribution of mean ISIs from our sample of gentamicin-treated preparations corresponded to longer mean intervals compared to those of untreated semicircular canal afferents.

The histograms within the inset of **Figure 5B** represent the distributions of ISIs for semicircular canal and utricular afferents previously reported (Baird et al., 1988; Goldberg et al., 1990). These data make an important contribution to the interpretation of the data reported herein in that they represent the expected differences in spontaneous discharge characteristics between semicircular canal and utricular afferents. The computed KLD between these distributions was 0.081, and resampling analyses supported the conclusion that the mean intervals for utricular afferents were longer than that of semicircular canal afferents ($p = 2{\cdot}10^{-6}$). The difference in mean interval distributions between semicircular canal and gentamicin-treated afferents (KLD = 0.18) was more than twice that expected between semicircular canal and utricular afferents from the same preparations. This finding supports the conclusion that the difference in mean ISI distributions of untreated and gentamicin-treated preparations is much greater than that expected from canal-utricle differences.

Spontaneous discharge coefficient of variation (CV) was also compared between untreated and gentamicin-treated distributions (KLD = 0.080), and between distributions of previously published data from semicircular canal and utricular afferents (KLD = 0.040). Through resampling analyses, we concluded that the CVs of gentamicin-treated afferents were greater than that of untreated afferents ($p = 2.6{\cdot}10^{-4}$). However, similar resampling analyses showed that the CVs of previously published data from semicircular canal and utricular afferents were similar ($p = 0.34$). This latter analysis further supports the conclusion that the difference in CV distributions between gentamicin-treated and untreated afferents cannot be explained by a mis-categorization of rotationally insensitive utricular afferents as a characteristic of a gentamicin-treated pathotype.

Morphologic Lesions Associated with Severe Functional Deficit

Intraperilymphatic administration of 1 μg gentamicin resulted in lesions of the vestibular epithelia characterized by afferent

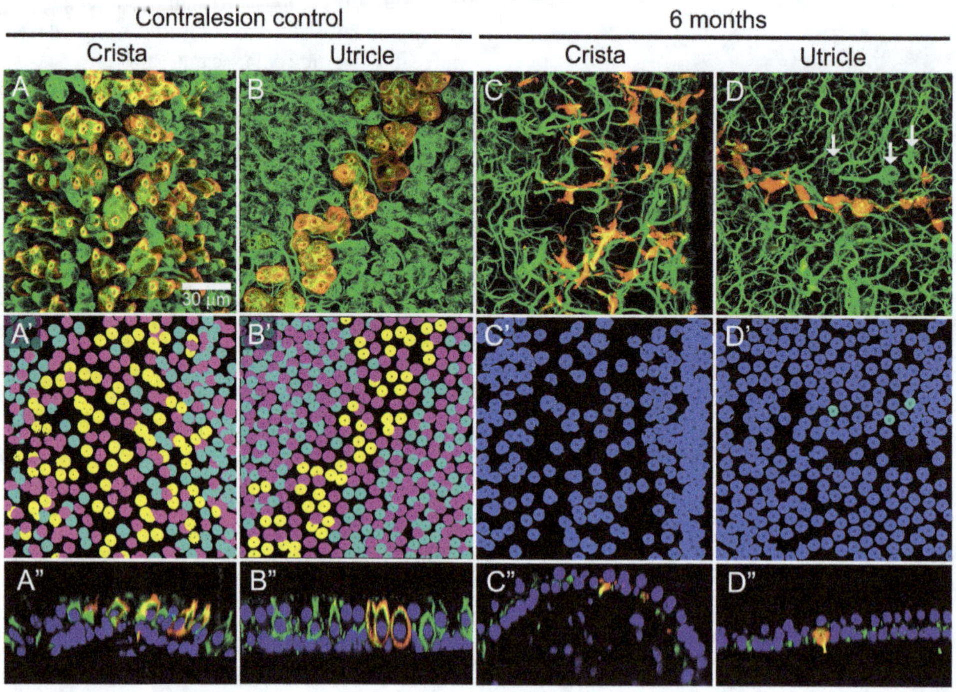

FIGURE 6 | Extensive calyx loss is seen in vestibular sensory epithelia exposed to 1 µg gentamicin. Horizontal semicircular canal cristae and utricles were immunolabeled with anti-CALB2 (red) and anti-TUBB3 (green) antibodies, and nuclei were labeled with a Nissl stain. **(A–D)** Confocal projections illustrating afferent calyces projecting to the cristae central-intermediate zones and utricle peristriola regions in contralesion control **(A,B)** and gentamicin-treated **(C,D)** specimens 6 months post-administration. Only three TUBB3+ calyces (arrows) can be seen in the micrograph of the treated utricle **(D)**. **(A′–D′)** Projections of hair cell nuclei of the neuroepithelial areas shown in **(A–D)**. Nuclei are colored in **(A′,B′)** to indicate type I_c (yellow), type I_d (cyan), and type II (magenta) hair cells. In the treated epithelia **(C′–D′)** most hair cell types were indistinguishable because of extensive calyx loss, and nuclei are colored to indicate uncharacterized (blue) and type I_d (cyan) hair cells. **(A″–D″)** Orthogonal optical sections illustrate diminished laminar organization of sensory and support cell nuclei (Nissl stain; blue) in gentamicin-treated specimens. Scale shown in **A** applies to all panels.

calyx retraction and modest hair cell loss. These pathotypes are illustrated in the maximum intensity projection micrographs of horizontal canal cristae (central zone) and utricles (peristriola) from contralesion control (**Figures 6A,B**) and gentamicin-treated (**Figures 6C,D**) specimens immunolabeled with anti-CALB2 (red) and anti-TUBB3 (green). In the contralesion control specimens (**Figures 6A,B,A″,B″**), anti-TUBB3 immunolabeling (TUBB3+) extends into the calyx neck as was found for the anti-CALB2 labeling (see also **Figure 1**). The CALB2+ calyx defined type I_c hair cells [i.e., those that received a CALB2+ calyx and associated with calyx-only afferents, (Li et al., 2008)], while the balance of type I hair cells associated with TUBB3+ calyces that were CALB2 negative represent type I_d [i.e., associated with dimorphic afferents (Li et al., 2008)]. This provided positive criteria to identify Nissl-stained hair cell nuclei belonging to types I_c, I_d, or II (i.e., hair cell nuclei not associated with a calyx) hair cells. Hair cell nuclei within the contralesion control confocal stacks that were identified in this way are shown in **Figures 6A′,B′** in yellow (type I_c), cyan (type I_d), or magenta (type II), providing a graphic illustration of hair cell density in the crista central zone and utricular peristriola.

The gentamicin-treated specimens exhibited sharp contrast to the contralesion control specimens as illustrated by the micrographs of horizontal crista and utricle specimens harvested 6 months after gentamicin administration (**Figures 6C,C′,C″,D,D′,D″**). Virtually all calyces (i.e., both CALB2+ and TUBB3+) are lost in the gentamicin-treated specimens, though CALB2+ and TUBB3+ parent axons remain within the neuroepithelia (**Figures 6C,D,C″,D″**). The absence of calyces and preservation of parent axons indicates a pathology that predominantly involved the calyx, which we refer to as *calyx retraction*. The extensive retraction was apparent for both CALB2+ and TUBB3+ calyces, indicating that CALB2+ calyx retraction is representative of all calyces at this post-administration time. **Figures 6C′,D′** illustrate the spatial density of hair cell nuclei, which was lower (i.e., more empty space) than that found in the contralesion control specimens (**Figures 6A′,B′**) and indicated partial hair cell loss. Because of extensive calyx loss and thinning of the epithelia, it was impossible to determine hair cell phenotype based on calyx innervation pattern or laminar organization of nuclei, except in the rare occurrence when partial calyces persisted (**Figure 6D′**, cyan nuclei). Therefore, the micrographs in **Figures 6C′,D′** illustrate all unsegregated hair cells.

The cristae from gentamicin-treated specimens were subject to histologic examination at 0.5, 1, 2, or 6 months post-administration times. At each interval, we found the effects of

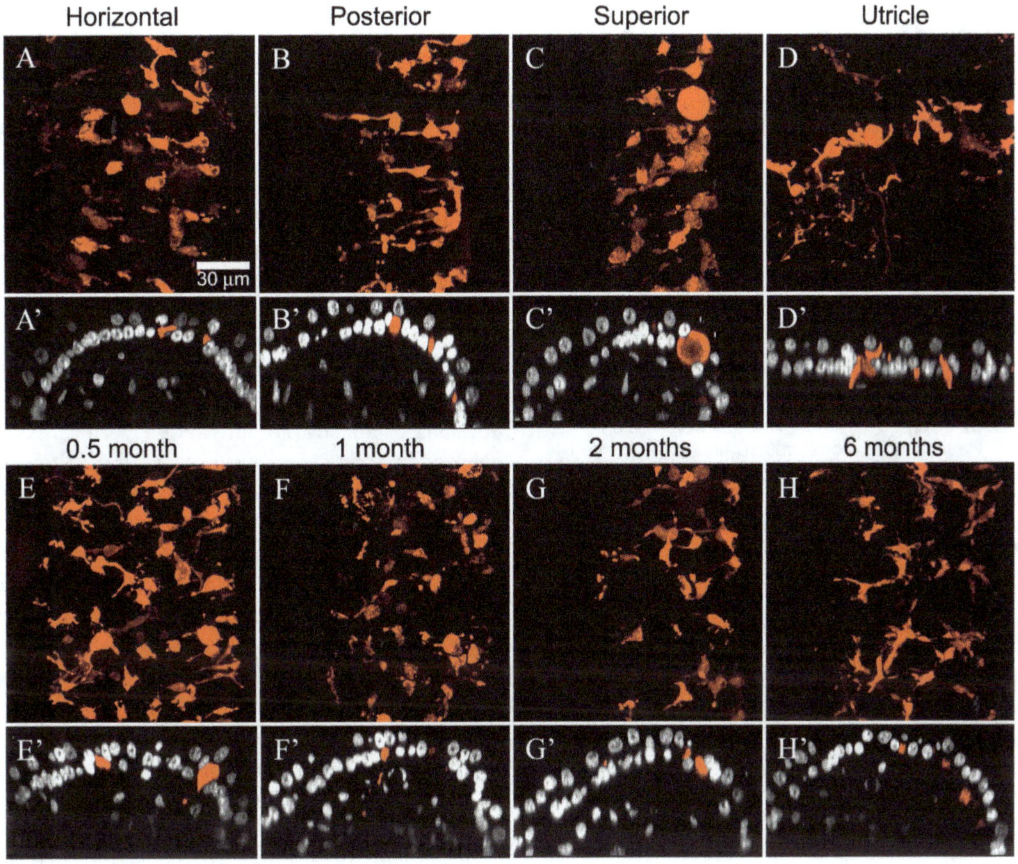

FIGURE 7 | Gentamicin induced damage is similar across vestibular endorgans and at all post-administration time periods. Damage as illustrated by CALB2 immunoreactivity (red) and Nissl stain (grayscale) for endorgans of a single animal 2 months after administration **(A–D)** and in horizontal cristae ampullaris 0.5, 1, 2, and 6 months after exposure **(E–H)** is shown. Maximum intensity projections of confocal image stacks taken from the central-intermediate zone of the cristae and the peristriola region of the utricle demonstrate extensive CALB2+ calyx loss in all endorgans **(A–D)** and at all time periods **(E–H)**. Orthogonal optical sections illustrate similar morphological characteristics in all endorgans **(A′–D′)** and at all time periods **(E′–H′)**. Scale shown in **A** applies to all micrographs.

1 µg gentamicin to be comparable across individual epithelia within a given labyrinth. This is illustrated in **Figures 7A–D** for one preparation analyzed 2 months following gentamicin treatment. These micrographs, representing maximum intensity projections of anti-CALB2 immunoreacted specimens, illustrate the retraction of all CALB2+ calyces in the cristae and utricle from a single labyrinth. Representative orthogonal sections are shown in **Figures 7A′–D′**. **Figures 7E–H** illustrate the time course of calyx retraction in horizontal cristae at the indicated post-administration times. Complete calyx retraction (CALB2+ and TUBB3+) was seen in 2 of 3 specimens examined at 0.5 and 1 month post-administration. Intact calyces were extremely rare at 2 and 6 months post-administration (shown for CALB2-immunoreacted specimens in **Figures 7G–H**). The morphologies of 0.5- and 1-month specimens were more variable; and while evidence of the lesion was observed in all specimens, some exhibited partially retracted calyces rather than complete retraction (see **Figure 3D**). At post-administration durations of 2–6 months, the majority of CALB2+ parent axons terminated as blunt endings within the sensory epithelia.

The Majority of Calyces Retracted While Most Hair Cells Survived Exposure to 1 µg Gentamicin

Calyces and Parent Axons

The quantifications of CALB2+ calyces, parent axons, and hair cells reflecting lesions to vestibular epithelia (**Figures 6, 7**) are illustrated in **Figures 8** and **9**, and summarized in **Tables 1** and **2**. The effects on CALB2+ calyces and parent axons are shown in **Figure 8**, depicting their densities at all post-administration times. We found only 36.9 ± 63.87% (n = 3; $p < 0.001$) and 38.80 ± 63.87% (n = 3; $p < 0.001$) of CALB2+ calyces remained 0.5 and 1 month after gentamicin exposure, respectively; however, nearly all CALB2+ calyces had retracted by 2 and 6 months post-administration ($p < 0.001$; **Figure 8**). No differences between cristae (i.e., horizontal, superior, or posterior) harvested at the same post-administration duration were found ($p > 0.05$). Although calyces were found in some samples, no complex calyces were observed in damaged specimens with the exception of two; a 0.5-month specimen that showed no signs of morphological damage or hair cell loss,

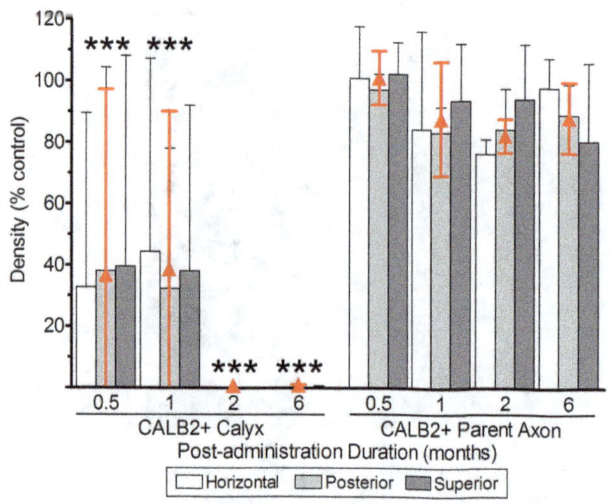

FIGURE 8 | CALB2+ afferent damage after 1 µg gentamicin administration. Normalized CALB2+ calyx and parent axon densities, expressed as percentages of contralesion controls, are shown for horizontal, posterior and superior cristae at the specified post-administration times (i.e., 0.5, 1, 2, and 6 months). ANOVAs indicated the absence of a main effect for crista type, and therefore the mean densities across all cristae are represented by the red triangles. All data are shown as mean ± SD. Triple asterisks (***) correspond to $p < 0.001$.

and a 1 month specimen that exhibited a more modest lesion than other comparably treated specimens with reduced hair cell density and malformations in calyx structure (i.e., calyces without necks and retracted calyces; **Figure 3D**). These specimens came from preparations made very early in our experience, and it is possible that they reflect incidences of incomplete gentamicin infusion.

Although most calyces within gentamicin-treated labyrinths retracted, the majority of CALB2+ parent axons remained at the sensory epithelium at all post-administration periods, supported by the finding that parent axon densities were not different from contralesion controls ($p > 0.05$; **Figure 8**). Damaged afferents (including CALB2+ dendrites and intermediate diameter TUBB3+ fibers without calyceal endings) remained at the sensory epithelia at least 6 months after gentamicin exposure (also represented in **Figure 6**). As illustrated in **Figure 8**, it was estimated that the fractions of CALB2+ parent axons (expressed as percent of contralesion control) present at the sensory epithelia were 100.0 ± 9.3 (0.5 months; $N = 3$), 87.2 ± 19.56 (1 month; $N = 3$), 83.0 ± 5.87 (2 months; $N = 3$) and 87.0 ± 12.19 (6 months; $N = 4$).

Hair Cells

The quantification of hair cell densities required a critical evaluation of lesioned epithelia to distinguish hair cell and support cell nuclei. Hair cell nuclei were identified predominantly by morphology and chromatin condensation as previously described. In general hair cell nuclei remained located more apical-ward in gentamicin-treated epithelia as found in untreated specimens, though this distinction became less clear in damaged specimens. In addition, hair cell nuclei often exhibited asymmetrical morphologies after gentamicin exposure. These variants were most pronounced in specimens with the heaviest damage as characterized by gross morphological changes and hair cell loss. For these specimens, a qualitative analysis of chromatin density became an important identifying criterion for hair cell nuclei.

The measures of hair cell densities following low-dose gentamicin administration portray a different picture than that of the afferents. This is illustrated in **Figure 9A**, showing densities of hair cell nuclei in the central zone of vertical and horizontal cristae at all post-administration durations, and in **Figure 9B** for the utricular striola at 6 months post-administration. The low-dose gentamicin exposure induced hair cell loss in vestibular epithelia at all post-administration periods. As shown for the calyx and parent axon counts, hair cell densities are expressed as percentages of contralesion controls (**Figure 9**) and counts per 100 μm^2 (**Table 2**). The central zones of horizontal, superior, and posterior cristae from treated specimens exhibited similar hair cell densities at all post-administration durations (**Table 2**), indicating that they exhibited comparable hair cell loss. We determined that over 60–80% of central zone hair cells survived following 1 µg gentamicin exposure (**Figure 9A**), where hair cell survival in pooled cristae (mean % of contralesion control, shown as red symbols, ±standard deviation) was 82.5 ± 14.01 at 0.5 months ($p < 0.01$), 73.7 ± 18.62 at 1 month ($p < 0.01$), 71.1 ± 2.68 at 2 months ($p < 0.001$) and 61.6 ± 9.55 at 6 months ($p < 0.001$). In addition, hair cell densities were measured in the utricular peristriola, as well as from lateral and medial extrastriola regions for 6 month specimens [the post-administration duration that exhibited the most damage (**Figure 9B**)]. Control specimen hair cell density (hair cell nuclei per 100 μm^2) of the peristriola region was estimated at 1.7 ± 0.15, and 2.5 ± 0.14 and 2.4 ± 0.12 for the lateral and medial extrastriola regions, respectively ($N = 4$). In comparison, hair cell densities of the gentamicin treated specimens were 1.1 ± 0.12 for the peristriola region, and 1.7 ± 0.51 and 1.5 ± 0.38 for the lateral and medial extrastriola regions ($N = 4$; $p < 0.001$). The relative densities computed from these absolute densities were similar to the central zone cristae at 6 months post-administration, which amounted to 64, 64, and 69% for the peristriola, medial extrastriola and lateral extrastriola (respectively).

It has been previously reported that the thickness of the sensory epithelium (lumenal surface to the basement membrane) decreases as a consequence of the morphologic alterations induced by gentamicin (Forge et al., 1998). Therefore, we evaluated whether such volumetric modifications alone could account for the quantitative changes in hair cell, calyx, or axon densities. For example, if gentamicin-induced decreases in epithelial volume resulted in a concomitant decrease in epithelial area without loss of its constituents, the analytical tendency would be to increase the density of components within these volumes. We evaluated the effects of any putative volumetric changes caused by gentamicin exposure by estimating support cell densities in the horizontal semicircular canal cristae central zones for normal and treated specimens. We posited that support cells would be minimally affected by low-dose

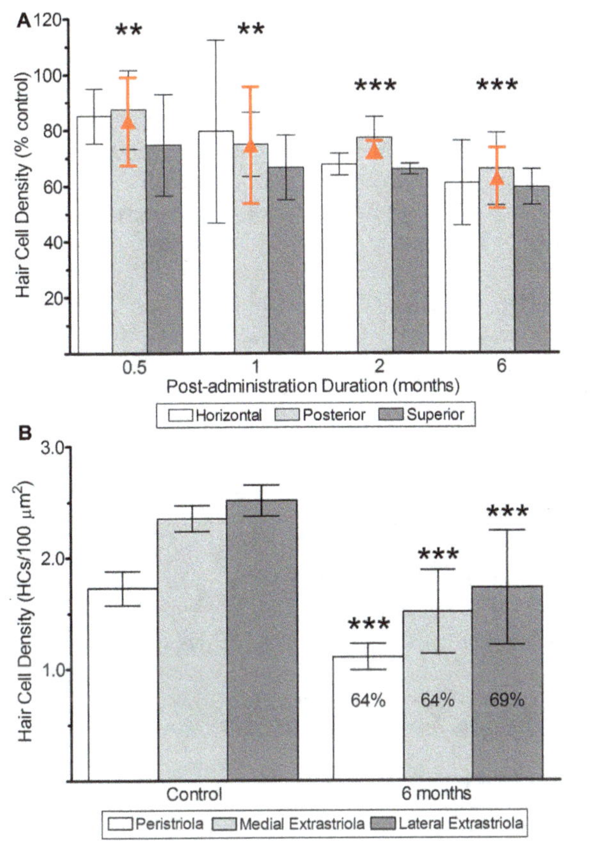

FIGURE 9 | Hair cell survival after 1 μg gentamicin administration. **(A)** Hair cell survival in cristae from labyrinths treated with 1 μg gentamicin. As noted above, two-factor ANOVA revealed the absence of a main effect of crista type, and therefore the mean densities (±*SD*) are represented by the red triangles (and error bars). **(B)** Hair cell survival in utricles determined 6 months after gentamicin administration. The mean hair cell survival at this post-administration time in the peristriola (64%), medial extrastriola (64%), and lateral extrastriola (69%) were similar. All data are shown as means (±*SD*). Double asterisks (**) correspond to $p < 0.01$; triple asterisks (***) correspond to $p < 0.001$.

gentamicin exposure, and that if gentamicin-induced volume changes did result in decreased epithelial areas we would find that untreated normal specimens would exhibit lower support cell densities than the gentamicin-treated specimens. We found that support cell densities (support cells/100 μm^2) were similar for the 0.5-month (2.1 ± 0.11; $N = 3$), 1-month (2.2 ± 0.01; $N = 2$), 2-month (2.1 ± 0.19; $N = 3$), 6-month (1.8 ± 0.18; $N = 3$), and normal (2.1 ± 0.19; $N = 3$) specimens. These data support the conclusion that the alterations in epithelia morphology concomitant with gentamicin treatment could not account for the quantitative changes in hair cell or CALB2+ afferent densities.

Previous assessments of the distribution of hair cell types (i.e., types I and II) indicated that type I hair cells represented approximately 60% of all hair cells within the central zones of chinchilla cristae (Desai et al., 2005a). The loss of all calyces and morphologic stereotypes precludes an evaluation of the remaining hair cell types in treated specimens. However, even if all lost hair cells were type I, the fact that the minimum mean fraction of surviving hair cells (i.e., at 6 months post-administration) was over 60% indicate that a notable number of type I hair cells survive the treatment that yields total loss of afferent calyces. Therefore, our hair cell density measures alone indicate that some type I hair cells remain viable - albeit functionally compromised - within the cristae central zones and utricular striolae in labyrinths exposed to 1 μg gentamicin, even when all calyces have retracted.

Viable, Morphologically Altered Hair Cells at 6 Months Post-administration

Anti-MYOVI and anti-CALB2 immunohistochemistry was used to visualize hair cell morphology and the association with intact and remnant CALB2+ calyces in contralesion-control and gentamicin-treated specimens. As shown for superior semicircular canal cristae in **Figure 10**, MYOVI immunoreactivity was robust in contralesion control hair cells that were tightly packed in the sensory epithelia (**Figures 10A,B**). Hair cells with type I (arrowhead; **Figure 10C**) and type II (arrow; **Figure 10C**) morphologies were easily recognizable in optical orthogonal sections of the untreated specimens. Most type II hair cells exhibited the stereotypical morphology being broad around the more apically located nuclei and narrow and cylindrical at their bases. Type I hair cells exhibited the prototypical "chalice" morphology with a thickened plate atop the thin apical neck. This is further illustrated in the reconstructions of two type I_c hair cells shown in **Figure 10D**, highlighted for comparison to hair cells from gentamicin-treated epithelia. In this reconstruction, the CALB2+ calyces (red) were made translucent for visualization of the encapsulated MYOVI+ hair cells.

The morphologic changes in hair cells resulting from low-dose gentamicin administration is shown in **Figures 10E–H**, representing the central zone of a superior crista 6 months post-administration. While plenty of viable hair cells are indicated by robust anti-MYOVI immunolabeling, they were less densely packed reflecting hair cell loss (**Figures 10E,F**). Hair cells exhibiting the stereotypical types I and II morphology were observed in few treated specimens (not shown); however, most hair cells lost distinguishing morphological characteristics as illustrated in the orthogonal optical section shown in **Figure 10G**. Some hair cells in damaged epithelia exhibited a "tear drop" morphology (arrowheads; **Figure 10G**) while others exhibited a "barrel" morphology (arrows; **Figure 10G**). The "tear drop" hair cells, although sharing similar morphological characteristics to type I hair cells, did not have the typical elongated neck of untreated type I hair cells. Some hair cells with 'tear drop" morphologies were contacted by a retracted CALB2+ partial calyx as illustrated by the reconstruction in **Figure 10H**. In addition, partial calyces were observed to encapsulate only the bases of such "tear-drop" hair cells, inferring that hair cells with such morphologies are remnant type I_c hair cells.

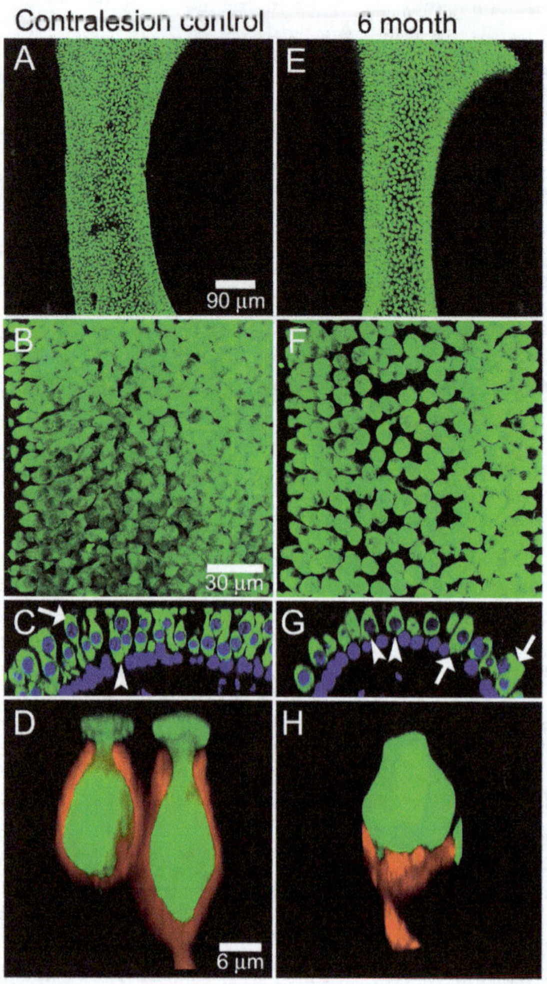

FIGURE 10 | Surviving hair cells following gentamicin exposure exhibit aberrant morphology. Contralesion control **(A–D)** and gentamicin-treated **(E–H)** superior semicircular canal cristae were immunolabeled with anti-MYOVI (green) and anti-CALB2 (red) antibodies, and were Nissl-stained (blue) 6 months after gentamicin administration. **(A,E)** Low magnification confocal projections illustrating the distribution of MyoVI+ hair cells. **(B,F)** Higher magnification confocal projections images of the central-intermediate zones illustrate reduced MYOVI+ hair cell densities in the lesioned epithelia. **(C,G)** Orthogonal optical sections of the untreated and treated specimens. Cells with morphologies characteristic of type I (arrowhead) and type II (arrow) hair cells can be seen in an optical orthogonal section of the undamaged specimen **(C)**. However, hair cells with aberrant morphologies resembling "tear drops" (arrowheads) and "barrels" (arrows) are observed in treated specimens **(G)**. **(D,H)** 3D volume reconstructions show two MYOVI+ type I hair cells enveloped by a CALB2+ complex calyx in a contralesion control specimen **(D)**, and a hair cell exhibiting "tear-drop" morphology is shown closely-apposed to a CALB2+ dendrite in a gentamicin-treated specimen **(H)**. The CALB2 signal in **(D)** was made translucent to enable visualization of MYOVI signal. Scale bars are the same for **(A,E)** (90 μm), **(B,C,F,G)** (30 μm), and **(D,H)** (6 μm).

Fine Dendritic Projections Persist in Gentamicin-Treated Epithelia

Although anti-TUBB3 immunohistochemistry revealed fine dendritic projections, it did not enable visualization of dendritic varicosities representing putative boutons of dimorphic afferent dendrites within the crista central zones or utricular striola (Fernandez et al., 1988, 1990). Therefore, retrograde labeling of TRITC-conjugated biocytin was used to visualize the fine dendritic branches and putative boutons innervating the central zones of superior and horizontal cristae and striolar region of the utricle. **Figures 11A,B** show TRITC-labeled fibers (represented in green) projecting to the horizontal canal crista and utricle 6 months after gentamicin treatment, illustrating patent fibers projecting to the central zone and striola of these epithelia. In addition, these fine dendritic branches have morphological features representative of *en passant* and terminal boutons, characterized by varicosities along the trajectories and at the terminations of thin dendritic branches (Fernandez et al., 1988, 1990). Extensive damage to this region is illustrated by the diminished hair cell densities observed in the maximum intensity projections of hair cell nuclei (**Figures 11C,D**). Three-dimensional reconstructions of representative labeled fibers further illustrate the varicosities on small diameter branches (arrows; **Figures 11E,F**) and show that large-intermediate diameter afferents with retracted calyces often were closely apposed to hair cell nuclei (**Figures 11G,H**). Some of these fibers exhibited a bowl-shaped "hemi-calyx" ending at the base of the closely apposed hair cell (**Figures 11G,G′**).

DISCUSSION

Through the present investigation we implemented a method for direct intraperilymphatic gentamicin administration to achieve three principal objectives. First, we sought to produce a limited lesion among hair cells of the vestibular epithelia, thereby unmasking potential effects on the dendrites of primary afferent neurons (i.e., to investigate dendritic lesions in cases of limited hair cell loss). Second, we believed the refined strategy would limit the dosing variability and, therefore, achieve greater consistency in the outcome parameters. Our third objective was to elucidate the effects of lesioning both potential targets (i.e., hair cells and afferents dendrites) on the discharge characteristics of afferent neurons. These results are summarized in the cartoon depicted in **Figure 12**, the discussion of which will include the limitations and impacts of the outcomes of this experimental approach.

Limitations of the Present Results

Limited Hair Cell Loss Unmasks Independent Calyx Retraction

The administration of 1 μg gentamicin to the perilymph resulted in the loss of hair cells that was determined by comparing counts within the cristae central zones and utricular striolae from treated and contralateral control labyrinths. The mean hair cell counts ranged between 82.5 and 61.6% of hair cells in the contralateral labyrinths (0.5 and 6 month specimens, respectively), corresponding to mean hair cell loss estimates between 17.5 and 38.4%. Since the fraction of type I hair cells found in the central zones and striolae of untreated epithelia are approximately 60% (Desai et al., 2005a,b), the measured

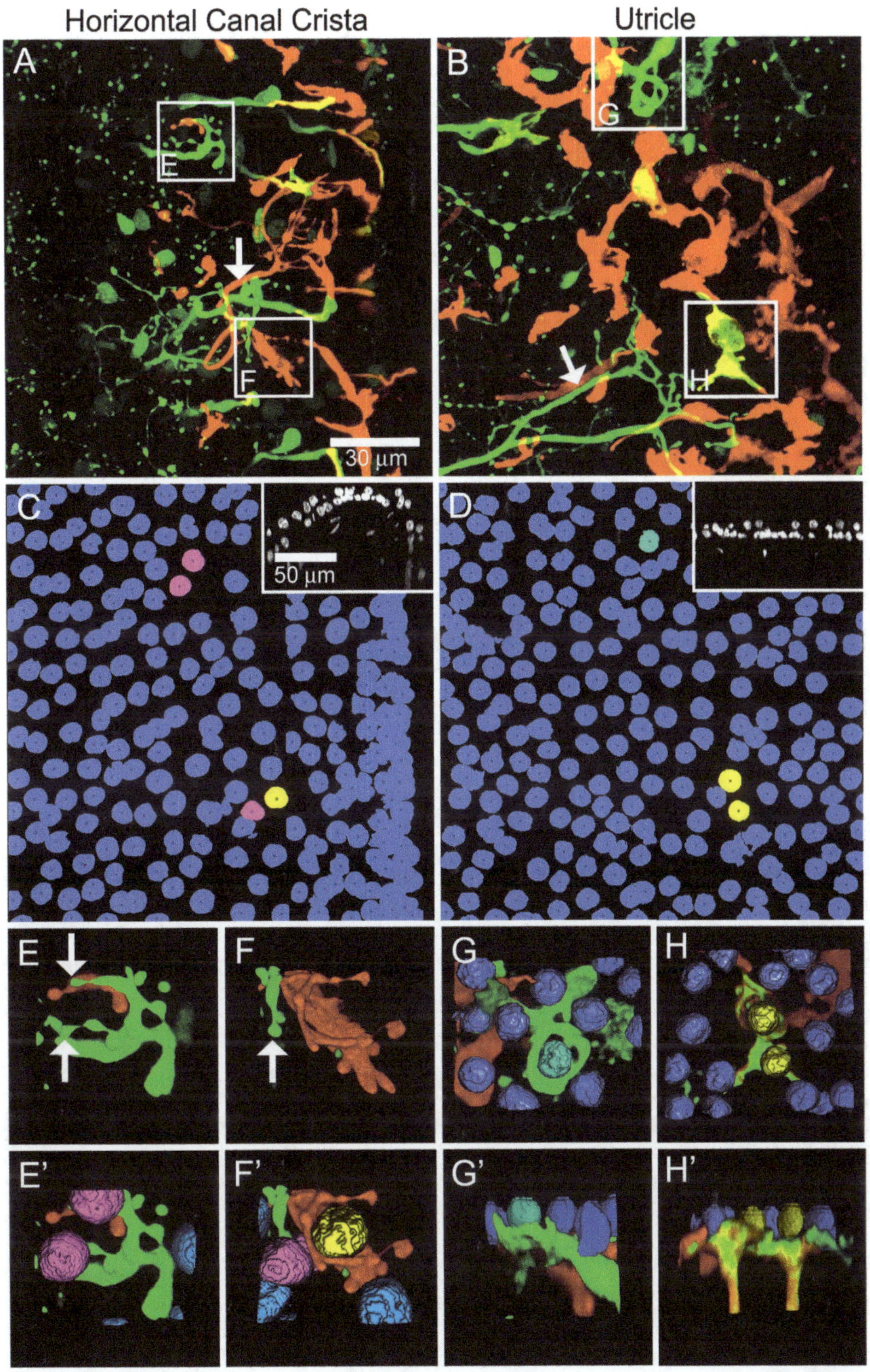

FIGURE 11 | Biocytin labeled fibers illustrate patent small diameter dendritic branches and endings exhibiting bouton-like morphology in lesioned vestibular epithelia. Shown are micrographs of the horizontal semicircular canal crista and utricle from a specimen whose superior vestibular nerve was retrogradely labeled with TRITC-biocytin (green) 6 months post-administration. The specimens were also labeled with anti-CALB2 antibody (red) and Nissl stain (blue; nuclei in insets are grayscale). **(A,B)** Maximum intensity projections from the central and intermediate zones of the crista **(A)** and peristriola region of the utricle **(B)** illustrate the presence of biocytin-labeled fibers (arrows) projecting to the neuroepithelial regions harboring CALB2+ fibers. These fibers, which in untreated specimens would exhibit dimorphic dendritic morphologies (i.e., CALB2-negative fibers within these crista zones), were also without calyces as expected (see **Figure 6**). However, they do *(Continued)*

FIGURE 11 | Continued
exhibit a number of putative boutons en passant, seen as varicosities along thin dendritic branches. **(C,D)** Maximum intensity projections of hair cell nuclei present in the confocal projections shown in **(A,B)**. Nuclei are colored to indicate representative hair cell nuclei closely apposed to a partially collapsed CALB2+ calyx (yellow in **C** and **D**), a partially collapsed biocytin-labeled calyx (cyan in **D**), and bouton-like endings (magenta in **C**). All other hair cell nuclei are shown in blue. Inset figures show representative orthogonal optical sections of stained nuclei (grayscale). **(E–H')**. Volume reconstructions of CALB2+ and biocytin-labeled dendrites illustrate the details of their projections in close proximity to hair cell nuclei. **(E,E')** A 3D volume rendering of the corresponding boxed area in **A** illustrates bouton type endings (arrows) in close apposition to hair cell nuclei (magenta; **E'**). **(F,F')** A 3D volume rendering of the corresponding boxed area in **A** shows a CALB2+ afferent wrapping around a hair cell nucleus (yellow) and a biocytin labeled neuron in close apposition to a hair cell nucleus (magenta). **(G,G')** 3D volume renderings of the corresponding boxed region in **B** exhibiting a large-intermediate diameter biocytin labeled fiber forming a bowl at the base of a hair cell nucleus (cyan). **(H,H')** 3D volume renderings of the corresponding boxed region in **B** show two CALB2+ fibers also labeled with TRITC-biocytin in close proximity to hair cells (nuclei shown in yellow). Note that CALB2 immunolabeling and TRITC-biocytin labeling closely overlap. Scale is the same for **(A–D)** (30 μm), and insets (72 μm). Scale is not shown for 3D volumes.

hair cell loss did not amount to the total number of type I hair cells. At the same time, virtually all calyces were lost in preparations investigated at 2 months post-administration and longer; **Figure 3** illustrates a case of extensive calyx loss even at 0.5 months. Some of the early calyx loss may be a downstream consequence of apoptosis (Forge and Li, 2000; Matsui et al., 2002, 2003, 2004; Cunningham et al., 2004; Ding et al., 2010; Zhang et al., 2012; Tao and Segil, 2015) among the most sensitive type I hair cells. However, the vast calyx loss found at the later post-administration times could not be wholly accounted for by loss of encapsulated hair cells. While the findings of the present study cannot exclude the possibility that calyx loss was induced by factors released by gentamicin-damaged (yet still viable) hair cells, these data also indicate a reasonable probability that gentamicin targeted the calyx directly. This component of the lesion did not involve loss of parent axons, which would have implied degeneration and perhaps apoptosis of Scarpa's ganglion neurons (**Figure 8**). Therefore, the restricted lesion involving retraction of the calyx can be characterized as *non-apoptotic*. Data from the present study indicates that this lesion component may exhibit greater sensitivity, and perhaps have a greater impact, than hair cell *loss* in terms of the gentamicin-induced vestibular dysfunction or hypofunction.

While data of the present investigation do not provide direct insight into the pathophysiologic mechanisms of the lesions induced by low-dose gentamicin, they do provide a foundation upon which to build future investigations of the most labile components of vestibular dysfunction. In view of broad evidence indicating the deleterious action of gentamicin on mitochondria (Dehne et al., 2002; Morales et al., 2010), and the large number of mitochondria within afferent calyces (Lysakowski and Goldberg, 1997, 2008), it would be far from surprising if afferent calyces were directly susceptible to direct gentamicin-induced damage. The density of mitochondria within calyces implies that considerable energy production is required for normal homeostasis of this structure, for example, to maintain the activity of the robust expression of Na^+/K^+ATPases within calyceal membranes (Cheng et al., 2006; Schuth et al., 2014). Gentamicin-induced mitochondrial compromise may lead to deteriorating function of the membrane ATPases and the inability to maintain membrane potential within the calyx, eventually leading to its morphologic collapse and retraction. Again, this does not necessarily lead to afferent apoptosis, as the accounting of CALB2+ parent axons indicated their numbers were similar to that found in untreated labyrinths (**Figure 8**).

The present investigation did not enable resolution of the hair cell phenotypes that were lost upon gentamicin administration. The afferent calyx is the only morphologic characteristic that unambiguously identifies a type I hair cell. Other characteristics, such as general chalice morphology or nuclear location within the epithelia, are less definitive. Since gentamicin exposure, even at the low doses used in the present study, leads to calyx retraction and distortion of the epithelia that precludes the use of other characteristics (even if less reliable), it was not possible to estimate the contribution of hair cell phenotype to their total loss. Furthermore, the temporal profile of the loss suggests that there may be differential sensitivities whereby the most sensitive (amounting to approximately 18% within the crista central zones) are lost by 2 weeks, and another less sensitive group (amounting to an additional approximately 17%) that is lost over the succeeding 5.5 months. The proclivity with which type I hair cells have been shown to take up and retain gentamicin (Lyford-Pike et al., 2007) suggests that they constitute the most sensitive fraction to gentamicin. However, this group cannot constitute the full complement of type I hair cells, and other type I hair cells are likely to be as insensitive as type II hair cells (evidenced in **Figure 10H**).

Intraperilymphatic Administration and Outcome Variability

The goal of direct administration of gentamicin to the perilymph was to limit the variability in outcome measures to that associated with gentamicin pharmacology within vestibular epithelia and subsequent detection methods, eliminating variability associated with dosing and the quantity reaching the labyrinth. In only one preparation (0.5 months post-administration) was there no evidence of hair cell loss or calyx retraction, which we attribute to a failure of gentamicin administration. During port placement in this preparation, the subarcuate fossa adjacent to the bony superior canal was violated, which likely provided a pathway for misdirecting the infusate away from the labyrinth leading to the administration failure. Every other preparation resulted in hair cell loss and calyx pathology, and in preparations investigated at 1 month post-administration and longer severe attenuation of stimulus-evoked afferent discharge modulation was found. This supports the conclusion that these results provide a perspective of the inherent pathophysiologic

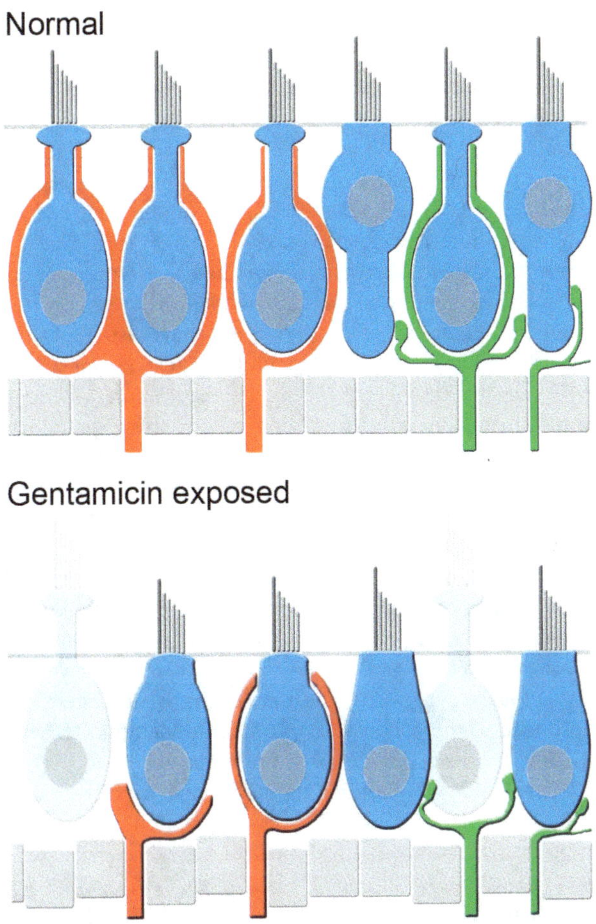

FIGURE 12 | Summary schematic of partial lesion induced by low-dose gentamicin in the cristae central zones and utricle striola. The *Normal* (untreated) panel **(top)** depicts the components of these neuroepithelial regions, including types I and II hair cells exhibiting stereotyped morphologies, CALB2+ afferents with simple and complex calyces (i.e., calyx-only, red), dimorphic afferents (green), spherical hair cell nuclei, and tightly packed support cell nuclei. Vestibular epithelia exposed to *Low-dose gentamicin* **(bottom)**, however, undergo several alterations that characterize the lesion. These include: (a) retraction of most calyces, including those of dimorphic afferents (right side of panel; **Figures 3**, **6**, **7**, **8**); (b) modest hair cell loss **(Figures 6, 9)**; (c) altered morphology of remaining hair cells, such that the stereotype morphologies of types I and II hair cells are not readily distinguished; these hair cells are viable as indicated by positive MYOVI immunolabeling **(Figure 10)**; (d) remaining non-CALB2+ afferents projecting to the crista central zones and utricular striola (i.e., afferents originally exhibiting dimorphic morphologies) retain fine dendritic branches and putative postsynaptic boutons **(Figure 11)**.

variability of gentamicin administration that is independent of dosing variability. This includes: (1) hair cell and calyx loss that ensues within 2 weeks post-administration, exhibits modest variability through 1 month post-administration, but is highly stable after that time; (2) though severe response attenuation can be apparent within 2 weeks, some weak residual responsiveness can remain through 2 months; and (3) severe response attenuation persists through 6 months post-administration.

CALB2+ Calyces as an Index of Central Zone and Striolar Calyces

We used the subpopulation of CALB2+ calyces as the marker with which to delineate defined regions of vestibular epithelia [i.e., cristae central zones and utricular striolae (Desai et al., 2005a,b)] for hair cell counts, and as indices of calyceal morphology. While this approach certainly served its purpose, it did not specifically address whether, in specimens examined a 0.5, 1, and 2 months post-administration, all central zone calyces exhibited pathology that paralleled CALB2+ calyces (i.e., CALB2− calyces). We do provide evidence that CALB2+ calyx pathology was representative of all central zone and striolar calyces at 6 months post-administration (**Figures 6C,D**), including those beyond the central zone and striolar boundaries. CALB2+ calyx pathology that was not representative of other calyces at shorter post-administration intervals would be indicative of a differential sensitivity to gentamicin, for which we are unaware of any evidence. **Figures 6C,D** demonstrate the absence of any such differential sensitivity at 6 months post-administration. As noted above, hair cell loss could not be distinguished by phenotype, including those designated type I_c (those encapsulated by CALB2+ calyces) and I_d hair cells (those encapsulated by CALB2− calyces) (Li et al., 2008), providing no insight into this level of gentamicin sensitivity. While we expect that all central zone and striolar calyces exhibit similar pathology as represented by CALB2+ calyces, this remains an issue to be confirmed in future experiments.

Response Attenuation with Intact Spontaneous Discharge

Hirvonen et al. (2005) first reported the remarkable finding of severely attenuated stimulus-evoked discharge modulation and preserved spontaneous discharge in chinchillas that underwent intratympanic gentamicin administration. They provided evidence for average hair cell loss of 57% across crista specimens evaluated (from serial cryostat sections), and without reference to crista zone distinctions. In the present study, we focused specifically upon the crista central zones and utricular striolae based upon prevailing evidence for these regions being the most sensitive to aminoglycoside-induced pathology (Wersall and Hawkins, 1962; Watanuki et al., 1972; Lii et al., 2004; Lyford-Pike et al., 2007; Lue et al., 2009). The principal focus was to investigate afferent dendritic pathology that could be not be accounted for by regional hair cell loss. Therefore, utilizing more focused histologic analyses with more modest hair cell loss (18–34%), we estimate that the effective gentamicin dose in the present study was less than that responsible for the lesions induced in the previous study that produced greater hair cell loss (Hirvonen et al., 2005). Despite a gentamicin dose leading to less hair cell loss, our physiologic findings, including severely attenuated responses to natural stimuli and spontaneous discharge that exhibited greater mean ISIs than found in untreated afferents, resembled those previously reported (Hirvonen et al., 2005).

In the present investigation evoked discharge modulation in vestibular afferent neurons was evaluated using stimulus characteristics for which robust responses were readily detected in untreated specimens (**Figures 2, 4**). The detection of stimulus-mediated responses was evaluated using stimulus–response coherence measures, which were determined from comparisons of frequency spectra contained in raw spike trains (Jarvis and Mitra, 2001) and the applied stimuli. Each coherence measure was accompanied by a probability measure corresponding to chance correlation. The untreated afferents included in the figures were selected for their low response sensitivities, which presented the greatest challenge for the coherence analyses in demonstrating representative coherence measures among semicircular canal afferents. These examples at the designated stimulus characteristics exhibited typically high coherence measures, and very low probabilities of chance coherence between stimulus and response (**Figures 2, 4**). Most coherence measures determined from the discharge of gentamicin-treated labyrinths were low by comparison, and the probabilities of chance correlation were typically high. Of course, it is always possible that increasing stimulus magnitude (e.g., by increasing stimulus frequency and/or peak velocity) would result in higher coherence between stimulus and response, as demonstrated by the superior canal afferent in **Figures 4A-vii,viii**. This reflects a threshold elevation due to the gentamicin treatment, which is not normally observed in mammalian afferents at comparable stimulus characteristics. Therefore, we interpret the low coherence measures among semicircular canal afferents from gentamicin-treated specimens, or the absence of stimulus–response coherence, as a severe attenuation in the capabilities for stimulus-evoked discharge modulation.

A limitation of the present study concerns our inability to apply linear acceleration stimuli in the electrophysiologic evaluation of untreated or treated afferents. Hirvonen et al. (2005) reported that 45 of 212 afferents recorded from gentamicin-treated afferents exhibited severely attenuated responses, demonstrating that, even under morphologic lesions induced in their preparations, responses were detected in 21% of recorded afferents. This indicates the likelihood that a small fraction of afferents that exhibited low response coherence to rotational stimuli projected from the utricle. This fraction may be estimated to be approximately 4%, representing the estimated combined probability of 21% response probability from Hirvonen et al. (2005) and the 20% probability of encountering a utricular afferent from our electrophysiologic approach (see **Figure 2A**). However, it is also important to note that Hirvonen et al. (2005) also reported severe response attenuation was a feature of both canal and utricular afferents, providing evidence that the gentamicin-induced dysfunction was induced in both epithelia (Hirvonen et al., 2005). Consequently, application of linear acceleration stimuli in our preparations would have yielded low response coherence measures in an additional small fraction of afferents, and likely would not have had additional impact on the resulting conclusions. Therefore, our findings were similar in that modest responses were detected in a small fraction of afferents (e.g., **Figure 4**), but the absence of stimulus-evoked discharge was the predominant finding among most afferents recorded in the present study.

The preservation of spontaneous discharge among afferents recorded in the present study, in addition to remnant and attenuated stimulus-evoked discharge modulation, indicated that synaptic transmission between hair cell and afferent neurons remained intact, to some degree, following administration of low-dose gentamicin. **Figure 10H** illustrates that the anatomical substrate for connectivity exists between viable hair cells and remnant parent axons even after calyces have retracted in putative calyx-only (CALB2+) afferents (Fernandez et al., 1988; Desmadryl and Dechesne, 1992). It is more plausible that spontaneous and remnant evoked discharge was driven by synaptic transmission between type II hair cells and remaining postsynaptic afferent boutons that were shown to exhibit intact morphology (**Figure 11**). Type II hair cells have also been shown to project onto parent axons through lateral extensions near the support cell layer (Pujol et al., 2014). This projection provides the anatomical substrate for type II hair cells to drive spontaneous discharge in CALB2+ calyx-only afferents even under conditions in which the calyces have retracted.

If synaptic transmission between hair cells and afferent dendrites was intact following administration of low-dose gentamicin, what could be the mechanism responsible for the severe attenuation or elimination of stimulus-evoked discharge? It is certainly most likely that this result stems from an effect to hair cells that does not lead to apoptotic events. It was previously suggested that this result is consistent with compromise to the hair cell transduction apparatus (Hirvonen et al., 2005), possibly resulting from stereocilia fusion (Duvall and Wersall, 1964; Takumida et al., 1989a) or disruption of stereocilia tip links (Takumida et al., 1989b). Gentamicin-induced transduction channel blockade is a reversible effect subject to washout (Jaramillo and Hudspeth, 1991; Nagata et al., 2005; Alharazneh et al., 2011), and is unlikely to persist at the long post-administration times investigated in the present and previous study (Hirvonen et al., 2005). Alternatively, the coexistence of spontaneous discharge preservation and evoked discharge compromise is also consistent with the condition found in some vestibular hair cells in mice lacking the gene coding for the protein otoferlin. Dulon and colleagues (Dulon et al., 2009; Vincent et al., 2014) reported that striolar type I hair cells did not exhibit depolarization-induced increases in membrane capacitance, a proxy for stimulus-induced transmitter exocytosis, while spontaneous discharge was intact in such preparations. In type II hair cells, while the relationship between membrane capacitance and local calcium concentration was found to be altered, they did not exhibit the same dependence upon otoferlin as striolar type I hair cells (Dulon et al., 2009). Otoferlin immunolabeling was diminished in apical turn mouse inner hair cells at day 10 following daily systemic administration of gentamicin (ShuNa et al., 2009), suggesting that otoferlin may be labile to gentamicin treatment (e.g., through diminished expression or induction of a post-translation modification). These data suggest that gentamicin may induce a condition in hair cells that compromises effective stimulus-induced neurotransmitter release, while spontaneous discharge remains intact. This is unlikely to be the complete story in view of the intact function of type II hair cells, but the similarities in physiologic outcomes between otoferlin-null and gentamicin-treated preparations are compelling.

The data of the present investigation demonstrate that stimulus-evoked discharge modulation is severely attenuated after administration of intraperilymphatic low-dose gentamicin, despite the presence of viable hair cells. We have shown that this gentamicin dose resulted in more modest hair cell loss than previously shown (Hirvonen et al., 2005), and while direct evidence is not offered in the present study we presume this occurred primarily through apoptotic mechanisms (Forge and Li, 2000; Matsui et al., 2002, 2003; Cunningham et al., 2004; Zhang et al., 2012). In specimens that reflected modest hair cell loss, other effects not directly related to hair cell apoptosis dominated the morphologic and physiologic aspects of the lesion, and included complete calyx retraction and drastic attenuation in the capabilities for stimulus-evoked discharge modulation. This supports the conclusion that non-apoptotic effects overwhelm the apoptotic effects in the vestibular dysfunction that resulted from modest gentamicin exposure [present study, (Hirvonen et al., 2005)].

Translational Impact on Clinical Applications of Intratympanic Gentamicin

Gentamicin-Induced Hypofunction

Intratympanic administration of gentamicin (ITG) has become a clinical treatment for conditions of intractable vertigo associated with Mèniére's syndrome (Carey, 2004; Cohen-Kerem et al., 2004; Casani et al., 2014; Marques et al., 2015; Rah et al., 2015; Syed et al., 2015; Espinosa-Sanchez and Lopez-Escamez, 2016; Junet et al., 2016) and as pretreatment in advance of vestibular schwannoma resection (Magnusson et al., 2007, 2009). The goals of ITG treatments are to induce vestibular hypofunction that would provide a reduction in the occurrence of vertigo and expedite intrinsic central compensatory mechanisms, while preserving cochlear function (e.g., Carey, 2004; Huon et al., 2012; Marques et al., 2015; Espinosa-Sanchez and Lopez-Escamez, 2016). Evidence in support of the efficacy of this strategy is provided by Magnusson et al. (2007, 2009), who report that patients requiring vestibular schwannoma resection exhibit a drastically reduced incidence of vertigo when they undergo "prehab" treatments of gentamicin-induced hypofunction and physical therapy regimens to promote central vestibular compensation. Ostensibly, the preoperative hypofunction and subsequent central compensation dampen the effects of the abrupt unilateral vestibular ablation resulting from tumor resection. In general, the efficacy of ITG treatments can be variable, which most likely is due to dosing variability resulting from individual patient factors leading to heterogeneity in the quantity of gentamicin that diffuses into the perilymph. Crane et al. (2009) identified factors in individual patients that improved outcomes in a second ITG treatment following an initial unsuccessful application. Hence, under these conditions it is difficult to interpret whether variability in treatment efficacy is due to dosing or intrinsic heterogeneity in the cellular response to gentamicin.

While the present investigation utilizing normal animal subjects cannot provide direct insight into the etiology of Mèniére's syndrome or other clinical conditions, it does provide important information regarding the pathophysiology of gentamicin-induced vestibular hypofunction. Direct intraperilymphatic administration eliminates potential dosing ambiguity associated with ITG, and while unlikely to be implemented as a clinical procedure it does provide insight into the outcomes that result under optimal administration conditions. Under the refined dosing conditions of the present investigation we found modest intrinsic variability within the first post-administration month across the limited number of subjects with respect to the morphologic (hair cell loss, calyx retraction) and physiologic (residual stimulus-evoked afferent discharge modulation) lesions. Hirvonen et al. (2005) reported similar findings, although the variability across subjects is difficult to assess in these data. In the present study, the induced lesion stabilized in the period between 2 and 6 months post-administration. Therefore, these findings provide insight into a temporal model for the development of hypofunction that may guide repeated treatment regimens.

A critical topic in ITG therapy for intractable Mèniére's syndrome concerns the relative level of induced hypofunction that optimizes the reduction in vertigo. Recent reviews of the clinical literature concerning ITG therapy are available (Casani et al., 2014; Rah et al., 2015; Syed et al., 2015; Espinosa-Sanchez and Lopez-Escamez, 2016) and summarize the findings associated with residual function and vertigo control. The contribution of the present investigation, as well as that of Hirvonen et al. (2005), is in providing important perspectives regarding the pathophysiology associated with the hypofunction. As noted above, we estimate that the direct intraperilymphatic dose used in the present study [approximately 130 μM, based upon 1 μg in a perilymph volume of 16 μl (Shinomori et al., 2001)] was lower than that achieved by ITG in chinchillas (Hirvonen et al., 2005). This conclusion was based upon the relative magnitude of hair cell loss, which was approximately half in the present study. Both studies demonstrated severe stimulus-evoked response attenuation in afferent neurons, representing a non-apoptotic effect that was independent of hair cell loss. If the goal of ITG therapy is to induce hypofunction (i.e., and not complete ablation), then the outcomes demonstrated herein and by Hirvonen et al. (2005) would seem to represent the maximum desirable functional reduction. That is, spontaneous discharge among vestibular afferents is a functional attribute that would provide residual input to central vestibular circuitry that is likely to be beneficial for compensatory mechanisms. The pathophysiologic substrates of smaller lesions resulting from lower gentamicin doses have yet to be comprehensively explored. However, preliminary studies from our laboratory showed that smaller intraperilymphatic quantities of gentamicin (e.g., 0.5 and 0.75 μg) resulted in greater function among semicircular canal afferents, though deficits were still apparent (Hoffman et al., 2013).

The present study provides insight into the dose required to achieve the maximum level of hypofunction consistent with optimizing central compensation. That is, abrupt elimination of afferent input associated with vestibular schwannoma resection appears to be suboptimal in promoting central compensation, supporting the "prehab" strategy (Magnusson et al., 2007, 2009). We have shown that 1 μg administered to the chinchilla labyrinth [estimated at 16 μl, the measured volume of the guinea pig labyrinth (Shinomori et al., 2001)] preserves vestibular afferent spontaneous discharge while inducing severe attenuation in stimulus-evoked activity modulation. If this represents the maximum level of desired hypofunction, then this gentamicin concentration, or 130 μM, represents an initial estimate of the dose that would achieve a corresponding level of hypofunction for ITG therapy in humans. The volume of the human perilymphatic space is approximately 10 times that of the chinchilla [158.3 μl (Buckingham and Valvassori, 2001)]. Therefore, these results suggest that the gentamicin quantity estimated to achieve maximally desired level of vestibular hypofunction would be 10 μg.

Post-treatment Recovery of Function

It stands to reason that a critical goal of intraperilymphatic gentamicin is to provide permanent vertigo relief, and quite apart from the cases of treatment failure there is evidence that vertigo symptoms may return after initial relief following ITG treatment for Mènière's syndrome. De Waele et al. (2002) reported cases of patients that exhibited a return of a positive caloric response after 12 months, following an initial post-ITG period during which no responses were measured. The presence of caloric responses 12 months after ITG therapy, during which vestibular hypofunction was documented, is not inconsistent with the results of the present investigation. These authors assumed that the gentamicin-induced loss of vestibular function was due to hair cell loss, and therefore reconciled the recovery of caloric responses was due to hair cell regeneration within the horizontal cristae (De Waele et al., 2002). However, it is also likely that the induced loss was due to non-apoptotic functional deficits (e.g., loss of stimulus-exocytosis coupling) as demonstrated in the present results. This potential recovery of the non-apoptotic component of the gentamicin-induced lesion was found only after the 6 months examination [when vestibular dysfunction persisted in all patients (De Waele et al., 2002)]. The longest post-administration interval examined in the present study was 6 months, which the results of De Waele et al. (2002) would suggest is insufficient to observe any modest recovery of the non-apoptotic lesion. It may be possible that the recovery of caloric responses could have reflected a direct thermal effect upon spontaneously discharging afferents (Peterka et al., 2004). However, the recovery was also accompanied by the absence of refixation saccades after head impulse testing, which would only result under conditions of functional hair cells and vestibulo-ocular reflex (De Waele et al., 2002). The absence of functional recovery following gentamicin-induced hypofunction at post-administration periods ≤6 months was also indicated the results by Hirvonen et al. (2005) and Bremer et al. (2014). The results of De Waele et al. (2002) are intriguing, and may be indicative of long-term recovery capabilities for non-apoptotic lesions.

Summary

While the use of small gentamicin doses unmasked a potentially critical effect on vestibular primary afferent dendrites, it also provides insight into other important aspects of vestibular pathophysiology. Certainly, establishment of precise ototoxicity protocols that render partial lesions to the vestibular epithelia are invaluable to the development of testing strategies for the early diagnosis of peripheral vestibular dysfunction. It also establishes a platform for the development of strategies for protection against ototoxicity resulting from systemic aminoglycoside therapy or chemotherapy. Furthermore, it must be recognized that the intratympanic administration (ITG) of gentamicin for the treatment of Mènière's disease is being conducted without an animal model exhibiting comparable level of pathology or dysfunction. That is, while partial dysfunction has been demonstrated in patients receiving ITG (Nguyen et al., 2009), a pathophysiologic model exhibiting similar hypofunction has not been produced. Such a model would be extremely valuable in providing a comprehensive pathophysiologic picture of the induced pathology.

AUTHOR CONTRIBUTIONS

DS and LH made substantial, direct, and intellectual contributions to the conception, execution, and analyses of the experimental work described, and approved it for publication.

REFERENCES

Alharazneh, A., Luk, L., Huth, M., Monfared, A., Steyger, P. S., Cheng, A. G., et al. (2011). Functional hair cell mechanotransducer channels are required for aminoglycoside ototoxicity. *PLOS ONE* 6:e22347. doi: 10.1371/journal.pone.0022347

Baird, R. A., Desmadryl, G., Fernandez, C., and Goldberg, J. M. (1988). The vestibular nerve of the chinchilla. II. Relation between afferent response properties and peripheral innervation patterns in the semicircular canals. *J. Neurophysiol.* 60, 182–203.

Bearzatto, B., Servais, L., Roussel, C., Gall, D., Baba-Aissa, F., Schurmans, S., et al. (2006). Targeted calretinin expression in granule cells of calretinin-null mice restores normal cerebellar functions. *FASEB J.* 20, 380–382. doi: 10.1096/fj.05-3785fje

Bignall, J. R., Crofton, J. W., and Thomas, J. A. (1951). Effect of streptomycin on vestibular function. *Br. Med. J.* 1, 554–559. doi: 10.1136/bmj.1.4706.554

Bremer, H. G., Versnel, H., Hendriksen, F. G., Topsakal, V., Grolman, W., and Klis, S. F. (2014). Does vestibular end-organ function recover after gentamicin-induced trauma in Guinea pigs? *Audiol. Neurootol.* 19, 135–150. doi: 10.1159/000357587

Buckingham, R. A., and Valvassori, G. E. (2001). Inner ear fluid volumes and the resolving power of magnetic resonance imaging: can it differentiate endolymphatic structures? *Ann.*

Otol. Rhinol. Laryngol. 110, 113–117. doi: 10.1177/000348940111000204

Burns, J. C., and Corwin, J. T. (2014). Responses to cell loss become restricted as the supporting cells in mammalian vestibular organs grow thick junctional actin bands that develop high stability. *J. Neurosci.* 34, 1998–2011. doi: 10.1523/JNEUROSCI.4355-13.2014

Carey, J. (2004). Intratympanic gentamicin for the treatment of Meniere's disease and other forms of peripheral vertigo. *Otolaryngol. Clin. North Am.* 37, 1075–1090. doi: 10.1016/j.otc.2004.06.002

Casani, A. P., Cerchiai, N., Navari, E., Dallan, I., Piaggi, P., and Sellari-Franceschini, S. (2014). Intratympanic gentamicin for Meniere's disease: short- and long-term follow-up of two regimens of treatment. *Otolaryngol. Head Neck Surg.* 150, 847–852. doi: 10.1177/0194599813520398

Chen, J. M., Kakigi, A., Hirakawa, H., Mount, R. J., and Harrison, R. V. (1999). Middle ear instillation of gentamicin and streptomycin in chinchillas: morphologic appraisal of selective ototoxicity. *J. Otolaryngol.* 28, 121–128.

Cheng, P. W., Liu, S. H., Young, Y. H., and Lin-Shiau, S. Y. (2006). D-Methionine attenuated cisplatin-induced vestibulotoxicity through altering ATPase activities and oxidative stress in guinea pigs. *Toxicol. Appl. Pharmacol.* 215, 228–236. doi: 10.1016/j.taap.2006.02.014

Cicchillitti, L., Penci, R., Di Michele, M., Filippetti, F., Rotilio, D., Donati, M. B., et al. (2008). Proteomic characterization of cytoskeletal and mitochondrial class III beta-tubulin. *Mol. Cancer Ther.* 7, 2070–2079. doi: 10.1158/1535-7163.MCT-07-2370

Cohen-Kerem, R., Kisilevsky, V., Einarson, T. R., Kozer, E., Koren, G., and Rutka, J. A. (2004). Intratympanic gentamicin for Meniere's disease: a meta-analysis. *Laryngoscope* 114, 2085–2091. doi: 10.1097/01.mlg.0000149439.43478.24

Crane, B. T., Minor, L. B., Della Santina, C. C., and Carey, J. P. (2009). Middle ear exploration in patients with Meniere's disease who have failed outpatient intratympanic gentamicin therapy. *Otol. Neurotol.* 30, 619–624. doi: 10.1097/MAO.0b013e3181a66d2b

Cunningham, L. L., Matsui, J. I., Warchol, M. E., and Rubel, E. W. (2004). Overexpression of Bcl-2 prevents neomycin-induced hair cell death and caspase-9 activation in the adult mouse utricle in vitro. *J. Neurobiol.* 60, 89–100. doi: 10.1002/neu.20006

Day, A. S., Lue, J. H., Yang, T. H., and Young, Y. H. (2007). Effect of intratympanic application of aminoglycosides on click-evoked myogenic potentials in Guinea pigs. *Ear Hear.* 28, 18–25. doi: 10.1097/01.aud.0000249765.76065.27

De Waele, C., Meguenni, R., Freyss, G., Zamith, F., Bellalimat, N., Vidal, P. P., et al. (2002). Intratympanic gentamicin injections for Meniere disease: vestibular hair cell impairment and regeneration. *Neurology* 59, 1442–1444. doi: 10.1212/WNL.59.9.1442

Dehne, N., Rauen, U., de Groot, H., and Lautermann, J. (2002). Involvement of the mitochondrial permeability transition in gentamicin ototoxicity. *Hear. Res.* 169, 47–55. doi: 10.1016/S0378-5955(02)00338-6

Desai, S. S., Ali, H., and Lysakowski, A. (2005a). Comparative morphology of rodent vestibular periphery. II. Cristae ampullares. *J. Neurophysiol.* 93, 267–280.

Desai, S. S., Zeh, C., and Lysakowski, A. (2005b). Comparative morphology of rodent vestibular periphery. I. Saccular and utricular maculae. *J. Neurophysiol.* 93, 251–266.

Desmadryl, G., and Dechesne, C. J. (1992). Calretinin immunoreactivity in chinchilla and guinea pig vestibular end organs characterizes the calyx unit subpopulation. *Exp. Brain Res.* 89, 105–108. doi: 10.1007/BF00229006

Dickman, J. D., and Lim, I. (2004). Posture, head stability, and orientation recovery during vestibular regeneration in pigeons. *J. Assoc. Res. Otolaryngol.* 5, 323–336. doi: 10.1007/s10162-004-4047-0

Ding, D., Jiang, H., and Salvi, R. J. (2010). Mechanisms of rapid sensory hair-cell death following co-administration of gentamicin and ethacrynic acid. *Hear. Res.* 259, 16–23. doi: 10.1016/j.heares.2009.08.008

Dulon, D., Safieddine, S., Jones, S. M., and Petit, C. (2009). Otoferlin is critical for a highly sensitive and linear calcium-dependent exocytosis at vestibular hair cell ribbon synapses. *J. Neurosci.* 29, 10474–10487. doi: 10.1523/JNEUROSCI.1009-09.2009

Duvall, A. J., and Wersall, J. (1964). Site of action of streptomycin upon inner ear sensory cells. *Acta Otolaryngol.* 57, 581–598. doi: 10.3109/00016486409137120

Espinosa-Sanchez, J. M., and Lopez-Escamez, J. A. (2016). Meniere's disease. *Handb. Clin. Neurol.* 137, 257–277. doi: 10.1016/B978-0-444-63437-5.00019-4

Fernandez, C., Baird, R. A., and Goldberg, J. M. (1988). The vestibular nerve of the chinchilla. I. Peripheral innervation patterns in the horizontal and superior semicircular canals. *J. Neurophysiol.* 60, 167–181.

Fernandez, C., Goldberg, J. M., and Baird, R. A. (1990). The vestibular nerve of the chinchilla. III. Peripheral innervation patterns in the utricular macula. *J. Neurophysiol.* 63, 767–780.

Flores-Otero, J., Xue, H. Z., and Davis, R. L. (2007). Reciprocal regulation of presynaptic and postsynaptic proteins in bipolar spiral ganglion neurons by neurotrophins. *J. Neurosci.* 27, 14023–14034. doi: 10.1523/JNEUROSCI.3219-07.2007

Forge, A., and Li, L. (2000). Apoptotic death of hair cells in mammalian vestibular sensory epithelia. *Hear. Res.* 139, 97–115. doi: 10.1016/S0378-5955(99)00177-X

Forge, A., Li, L., Corwin, J. T., and Nevill, G. (1993). Ultrastructural evidence for hair cell regeneration in the mammalian inner ear. *Science* 259, 1616–1619. doi: 10.1126/science.8456284

Forge, A., Li, L., and Nevill, G. (1998). Hair cell recovery in the vestibular sensory epithelia of mature guinea pigs. *J. Comp. Neurol.* 397, 69–88. doi: 10.1002/(SICI)1096-9861(19980720)397:1<69::AID-CNE6>3.0.CO;2-G

Goldberg, J. M., Desmadryl, G., Baird, R. A., and Fernandez, C. (1990). The vestibular nerve of the chinchilla. IV. Discharge properties of utricular afferents. *J. Neurophysiol.* 63, 781–790.

Halmagyi, G. M., Fattore, C. M., Curthoys, I. S., and Wade, S. (1994). Gentamicin vestibulotoxicity. *Otolaryngol. Head Neck Surg.* 111, 571–574. doi: 10.1177/019459989411100506

Haque, A., Zakir, M., and Dickman, J. D. (2009). Regeneration of vestibular horizontal semicircular canal afferents in pigeons. *J. Neurophysiol.* 102, 1274–1286. doi: 10.1152/jn.91000.2008

Harada, Y., Sera, K., Ohya, T., Tagashira, N., Suzuki, M., and Takumida, M. (1991). Effect of gentamicin on vestibular ganglion. *Acta Otolaryngol. Suppl.* 481, 135–138. doi: 10.3109/00016489109131365

Hasson, T., Gillespie, P. G., Garcia, J. A., MacDonald, R. B., Zhao, Y., Yee, A. G., et al. (1997). Unconventional myosins in inner-ear sensory epithelia. *J. Cell Biol.* 137, 1287–1307. doi: 10.1083/jcb.137.6.1287

Hilton, M., Chen, J., Kakigi, A., Hirakawa, H., Mount, R. J., and Harrison, R. V. (2002). Middle ear instillation of gentamicin and streptomycin in chinchillas: electrophysiological appraisal of selective ototoxicity. *Clin. Otolaryngol. Allied Sci.* 27, 529–535. doi: 10.1046/j.1365-2273.2002.00614.x

Hirvonen, T. P., Minor, L. B., Hullar, T. E., and Carey, J. P. (2005). Effects of intratympanic gentamicin on vestibular afferents and hair cells in the chinchilla. *J. Neurophysiol.* 93, 643–655. doi: 10.1152/jn.00160.2004

Hoffman, L. F., Choy, K. R., Sultemeier, D. R., and Lopez, I. A. (2013). Cellular correlates of coding deficits associated with partial lesions of the vestibular epithelia. *Abs. Assoc. Res. Otolaryngol.* 36, 192–193.

Hoffman, L. F., and Honrubia, V. (2002). Fiber diameter distributions in the chinchilla's ampullary nerves. *Hear. Res.* 172, 37–52. doi: 10.1016/S0378-5955(02)00390-8

Hong, S. H., Park, S. K., Cho, Y. S., Lee, H. S., Kim, K. R., Kim, M. G., et al. (2006). Gentamicin induced nitric oxide-related oxidative damages on vestibular afferents in the guinea pig. *Hear. Res.* 211, 46–53. doi: 10.1016/j.heares.2005.08.009

Hullar, T. E., and Minor, L. B. (1999). High-frequency dynamics of regularly discharging canal afferents provide a linear signal for angular vestibuloocular reflexes. *J. Neurophysiol.* 82, 2000–2005.

Huon, L. K., Fang, T. Y., and Wang, P. C. (2012). Outcomes of intratympanic gentamicin injection to treat Meniere's disease. *Otol. Neurotol.* 33, 706–714. doi: 10.1097/MAO.0b013e318259b3b1

Imamura, S., and Adams, J. C. (2003a). Changes in cytochemistry of sensory and nonsensory cells in gentamicin-treated cochleas. *J. Assoc. Res. Otolaryngol.* 4, 196–218. doi: 10.1007/s10162-002-2037-7

Imamura, S., and Adams, J. C. (2003b). Distribution of gentamicin in the guinea pig inner ear after local or systemic application. *J. Assoc. Res. Otolaryngol.* 4, 176–195. doi: 10.1007/s10162-002-2036-8

Jaramillo, F., and Hudspeth, A. J. (1991). Localization of the hair cell's transduction channels at the hair bundle's top by iontophoretic application of a channel blocker. *Neuron* 7, 409–420. doi: 10.1016/0896-6273(91)90293-9

Jarvis, M. R., and Mitra, P. P. (2001). Sampling properties of the spectrum and coherency of sequences of action potentials. *Neural Comput.* 13, 717–749. doi: 10.1162/089976601300014312

Junet, P., Karkas, A., Dumas, G., Quesada, J. L., and Schmerber, S. (2016). Vestibular results after intratympanic gentamicin therapy in disabling Meniere's disease. *Eur. Arch. Otorhinolaryngol.* 273, 3011–3018. doi: 10.1007/s00405-015-3889-x

Kawamoto, K., Izumikawa, M., Beyer, L. A., Atkin, G. M., and Raphael, Y. (2009). Spontaneous hair cell regeneration in the mouse utricle following gentamicin ototoxicity. *Hear. Res.* 247, 17–26. doi: 10.1016/j.heares.2008.08.010

King, E. B., Shepherd, R. K., Brown, D. J., and Fallon, J. B. (2017). Gentamicin applied to the oval window suppresses vestibular function in Guinea pigs. *J. Assoc. Res. Otolaryngol.* 18, 291–299. doi: 10.1007/s10162-016-0609-1

Li, A., Xue, J., and Peterson, E. H. (2008). Architecture of the mouse utricle: macular organization and hair bundle heights. *J. Neurophysiol.* 99, 718–733. doi: 10.1152/jn.00831.2007

Li, L., Nevill, G., and Forge, A. (1995). Two modes of hair cell loss from the vestibular sensory epithelia of the guinea pig inner ear. *J. Comp. Neurol.* 355, 405–417. doi: 10.1002/cne.903550307

Lii, M., Ding, D., Zheng, X. Y., and Salvi, R. (2004). Vestibular destruction by slow infusion of gentamicin into semicircular canals. *Acta Otolaryngol. Suppl.* 552, 35–41. doi: 10.1080/03655230410017102

Lindeman, H. H. (1969a). Regional differences in sensitivity of the vestibular sensory epithelia to ototoxic antibiotics. *Acta Otolaryngol.* 67, 177–189. doi: 10.3109/00016486909125441

Lindeman, H. H. (1969b). Studies on the morphology of the sensory regions of the vestibular apparatus with 45 figures. *Ergeb. Anat. Entwicklungsgesch.* 42, 1–113.

Lopez, I., Honrubia, V., Lee, S. C., Chung, W. H., Li, G., Beykirch, K., et al. (1999). The protective effect of brain-derived neurotrophic factor after gentamicin ototoxicity. *Am. J. Otol.* 20, 317–324.

Lue, J. H., Day, A. S., Cheng, P. W., and Young, Y. H. (2009). Vestibular evoked myogenic potentials are heavily dependent on type I hair cell activity of the saccular macula in guinea pigs. *Audiol. Neurootol.* 14, 59–66. doi: 10.1159/000156701

Lyford-Pike, S., Vogelheim, C., Chu, E., Della Santina, C. C., and Carey, J. P. (2007). Gentamicin is primarily localized in vestibular type I hair cells after intratympanic administration. *J. Assoc. Res. Otolaryngol.* 8, 497–508. doi: 10.1007/s10162-007-0093-8

Lysakowski, A., and Goldberg, J. M. (1997). A regional ultrastructural analysis of the cellular and synaptic architecture in the chinchilla cristae ampullares. *J. Comp. Neurol.* 389, 419–443. doi: 10.1002/(SICI)1096-9861(19971222)389:3<419::AID-CNE5>3.0.CO;2-3

Lysakowski, A., and Goldberg, J. M. (2008). Ultrastructural analysis of the cristae ampullares in the squirrel monkey (*Saimiri sciureus*). *J. Comp. Neurol.* 511, 47–64. doi: 10.1002/cne.21827

Mackay, D. J. C. (2003). *Information Theory, Inference, and Learning Algorithms.* Cambridge: Cambridge University Press.

Magnusson, M., Kahlon, B., Karlberg, M., Lindberg, S., and Siesjo, P. (2007). Preoperative vestibular ablation with gentamicin and vestibular 'prehab' enhance postoperative recovery after surgery for pontine angle tumours–first report. *Acta Otolaryngol.* 127, 1236–1240. doi: 10.1080/00016480701663433

Magnusson, M., Kahlon, B., Karlberg, M., Lindberg, S., Siesjo, P., and Tjernstrom, F. (2009). Vestibular "PREHAB". *Ann. N. Y. Acad. Sci.* 1164, 257–262. doi: 10.1111/j.1749-6632.2009.03778.x

Marques, P., Manrique-Huarte, R., and Perez-Fernandez, N. (2015). Single intratympanic gentamicin injection in Meniere's disease: VOR change and prognostic usefulness. *Laryngoscope* 125, 1915–1920. doi: 10.1002/lary.25156

Matsui, J. I., Gale, J. E., and Warchol, M. E. (2004). Critical signaling events during the aminoglycoside-induced death of sensory hair cells in vitro. *J. Neurobiol.* 61, 250–266. doi: 10.1002/neu.20054

Matsui, J. I., Haque, A., Huss, D., Messana, E. P., Alosi, J. A., Roberson, D. W., et al. (2003). Caspase inhibitors promote vestibular hair cell survival and function after aminoglycoside treatment in vivo. *J. Neurosci.* 23, 6111–6122.

Matsui, J. I., Ogilvie, J. M., and Warchol, M. E. (2002). Inhibition of caspases prevents ototoxic and ongoing hair cell death. *J. Neurosci.* 22, 1218–1227.

Minor, L. B. (1999). Intratympanic gentamicin for control of vertigo in Meniere's disease: vestibular signs that specify completion of therapy. *Am. J. Otol.* 20, 209–219.

Miyata, T., Maeda, T., and Lee, J. E. (1999). NeuroD is required for differentiation of the granule cells in the cerebellum and hippocampus. *Genes Dev.* 13, 1647–1652. doi: 10.1101/gad.13.13.1647

Morales, A. I., Detaille, D., Prieto, M., Puente, A., Briones, E., Arevalo, M., et al. (2010). Metformin prevents experimental gentamicin-induced nephropathy by a mitochondria-dependent pathway. *Kidney Int.* 77, 861–869. doi: 10.1038/ki.2010.11

Nagata, K., Duggan, A., Kumar, G., and Garcia-Anoveros, J. (2005). Nociceptor and hair cell transducer properties of TRPA1, a channel for pain and hearing. *J. Neurosci.* 25, 4052–4061. doi: 10.1523/JNEUROSCI.0013-05.2005

Nedzelski, J. M., Chiong, C. M., Fradet, G., Schessel, D. A., Bryce, G. E., and Pfleiderer, A. G. (1993). Intratympanic gentamicin instillation as treatment of unilateral Meniere's disease: update of an ongoing study. *Am. J. Otol.* 14, 278–282.

Nguyen, K. D., Minor, L. B., Della Santina, C. C., and Carey, J. P. (2009). Vestibular function and vertigo control after intratympanic gentamicin for Meniere's disease. *Audiol. Neurootol.* 14, 361–372. doi: 10.1159/000241893

Paulin, M. G., and Hoffman, L. F. (2001). Optimal firing rate estimation. *Neural Netw.* 14, 877–881. doi: 10.1016/S0893-6080(01)00058-2

Peterka, R. J., Gianna-Poulin, C. C., Zupan, L. H., and Merfeld, D. M. (2004). Origin of orientation-dependent asymmetries in vestibulo-ocular reflexes evoked by caloric stimulation. *J. Neurophysiol.* 92, 2333–2345. doi: 10.1152/jn.00174.2004

Popper, P., Lopez, I., Beizai, P., Li, G., Kim, J., Micevych, P. E., et al. (1999). Expression of BDNF and TrkB mRNAs in the crista neurosensory epithelium and vestibular ganglia following ototoxic damage. *Brain Res.* 846, 40–51. doi: 10.1016/S0006-8993(99)01941-1

Pujol, R., Pickett, S. B., Nguyen, T. B., and Stone, J. S. (2014). Large basolateral processes on type II hair cells are novel processing units in mammalian vestibular organs. *J. Comp. Neurol.* 522, 3141–3159. doi: 10.1002/cne.23625

Rah, Y. C., Han, J. J., Park, J., Choi, B. Y., and Koo, J. W. (2015). Management of intractable Meniere's disease after intratympanic injection of gentamicin. *Laryngoscope* 125, 972–978. doi: 10.1002/lary.25009

Robson, J. M., and Goulding, R. (1952). Streptomycin and dihydrostreptomycin. *Proc. R. Soc. Med.* 45, 777–778.

Roehm, P., Hoffer, M., and Balaban, C. D. (2007). Gentamicin uptake in the chinchilla inner ear. *Hear. Res.* 230, 43–52. doi: 10.1016/j.heares.2007.04.005

Schuknecht, H. F. (1956). Ablation therapy for the relief of Meniere's disease. *Laryngoscope* 66, 859–870. doi: 10.1288/00005537-195607000-00005

Schuknecht, H. F. (1957). Ablation therapy in the management of Meniere's disease. *Acta Otolaryngol. Suppl.* 132, 1–42.

Schuth, O., McLean, W. J., Eatock, R. A., and Pyott, S. J. (2014). Distribution of Na,K-ATPase alpha subunits in rat vestibular sensory epithelia. *J. Assoc. Res. Otolaryngol.* 15, 739–754. doi: 10.1007/s10162-014-0479-3

Shinomori, Y., Spack, D. S., Jones, D. D., and Kimura, R. S. (2001). Volumetric and dimensional analysis of the guinea pig inner ear. *Ann. Otol. Rhinol. Laryngol.* 110, 91–98. doi: 10.1177/000348940111000117

ShuNa, L., Zhong, R., and Ke, L. (2009). A pattern of otoferlin expression interrupted by gentamicin exposure in ribbon synapse of inner hair cell in C57BL/6J mice. *Acta Neurol. Belg.* 109, 221–225.

Stone, J. S., and Rubel, E. W. (2000). Temporal, spatial, and morphologic features of hair cell regeneration in the avian basilar papilla. *J. Comp. Neurol.* 417, 1–16. doi: 10.1002/(SICI)1096-9861(20000131)417:1<1::AID-CNE1>3.0.CO;2-E

Stone, J. S., Shang, J. L., and Tomarev, S. (2004). cProx1 immunoreactivity distinguishes progenitor cells and predicts hair cell fate during avian hair cell regeneration. *Dev. Dyn.* 230, 597–614. doi: 10.1002/dvdy.20087

Syed, M. I., Ilan, O., Nassar, J., and Rutka, J. A. (2015). Intratympanic therapy in Meniere's syndrome or disease: up to date evidence for clinical practice. *Clin. Otolaryngol.* 40, 682–690. doi: 10.1111/coa.12449

Takumida, M., Bagger-Sjoback, D., Harada, Y., Lim, D., and Wersall, J. (1989a). Sensory hair fusion and glycocalyx changes following gentamicin exposure in the guinea pig vestibular organs. *Acta Otolaryngol.* 107, 39–47.

Takumida, M., Bagger-Sjoback, D., Wersall, J., and Harada, Y. (1989b). The effect of gentamicin on the glycocalyx and the ciliary interconnections in vestibular sensory cells: a high resolution scanning electron microscopic investigation. *Hear. Res.* 37, 163–170.

Tao, L., and Segil, N. (2015). Early transcriptional response to aminoglycoside antibiotic suggests alternate pathways leading to apoptosis in sensory hair cells in the mouse inner ear. *Front. Cell. Neurosci.* 9:190. doi: 10.3389/fncel.2015.00190

Vincent, P. F., Bouleau, Y., Safieddine, S., Petit, C., and Dulon, D. (2014). Exocytotic machineries of vestibular type I and cochlear ribbon synapses display similar intrinsic otoferlin-dependent Ca^{2+} sensitivity but a different coupling to Ca^{2+} channels. *J. Neurosci.* 34, 10853–10869. doi: 10.1523/JNEUROSCI.0947-14.2014

Warchol, M. E. (2010a). Cellular mechanisms of aminoglycoside ototoxicity. *Curr. Opin. Otolaryngol. Head Neck Surg.* 18, 454–458. doi: 10.1097/MOO.0b013e32833e05ec

Warchol, M. E. (2010b). Sensory regeneration in the vertebrate inner ear: differences at the levels of cells and species. *Hear. Res.* 273, 72–79. doi: 10.1016/j.heares.2010.05.004

Warchol, M. E., Stone, J., Barton, M., Ku, J., Veile, R., Daudet, N., et al. (2017). ADAM10 and gamma-secretase regulate sensory regeneration in the avian vestibular organs. *Dev. Biol.* 428, 39–51. doi: 10.1016/j.ydbio.2017.05.014

Watanuki, K., Stupp, H. F., and Meyer zum Gottesberge, A. (1972). Toxic effects of gentamycin upon the peripheral vestibular sensory organs. *Laryngoscope* 82, 363–371. doi: 10.1288/00005537-197203000-00002

Weisleder, P., and Rubel, E. W. (1992). Hair cell regeneration in the avian vestibular epithelium. *Exp. Neurol.* 115, 2–6. doi: 10.1016/0014-4886(92)90211-8

Weisleder, P., and Rubel, E. W. (1993). Hair cell regeneration after streptomycin toxicity in the avian vestibular epithelium. *J. Comp. Neurol.* 331, 97–110. doi: 10.1002/cne.903310106

Wersall, J., and Hawkins, J. E. Jr. (1962). The vestibular sensory epithelia in the cat labyrinth and their reactions in chronic streptomycin intoxication. *Acta Otolaryngol.* 54, 1–23. doi: 10.3109/00016486209126917

Wersall, J., Lundquist, P. G., and Bjorkroth, B. (1969). Ototoxicity of gentamicin. *J. Infect. Dis.* 119, 410–416. doi: 10.1093/infdis/119.4-5.410

Zhang, D., Fan, Z., Han, Y., Bai, X., Liu, W., Lu, S., et al. (2012). Apoptosis-inducing factor is involved in gentamicin-induced vestibular hair cell death. *ORL J. Otorhinolaryngol. Relat. Spec.* 74, 1–5. doi: 10.1159/000333251

20

Non-Autonomous Cellular Responses to Ototoxic Drug-Induced Stress and Death

Shimon P. Francis and Lisa L. Cunningham *

National Institute on Deafness and Other Communication Disorders, National Institutes of Health, Bethesda, MD, United States

Edited by:
Michael E. Smith, Western Kentucky University, United States

Reviewed by:
Andy Groves, Baylor College of Medicine, United States
Gourav Roy Choudhury, Texas Biomedical Research Institute, United States

***Correspondence:**
Lisa L. Cunningham
lisa.cunningham@nih.gov

The first major recognition of drug-induced hearing loss can be traced back more than seven decades to the development of streptomycin as an antimicrobial agent. Since then at least 130 therapeutic drugs have been recognized as having ototoxic side-effects. Two important classes of ototoxic drugs are the aminoglycoside antibiotics and the platinum-based antineoplastic agents. These drugs save the lives of millions of people worldwide, but they also cause irreparable hearing loss. In the inner ear, sensory hair cells (HCs) and spiral ganglion neurons (SGNs) are important cellular targets of these drugs, and most mechanistic studies have focused on the cell-autonomous responses of these cell types in response to ototoxic stress. Despite several decades of studies on ototoxicity, important unanswered questions remain, including the cellular and molecular mechanisms that determine whether HCs and SGNs will live or die when confronted with ototoxic challenge. Emerging evidence indicates that other cell types in the inner ear can act as mediators of survival or death of sensory cells and SGNs. For example, glia-like supporting cells (SCs) can promote survival of both HCs and SGNs. Alternatively, SCs can act to promote HC death and inhibit neural fiber expansion. Similarly, tissue resident macrophages activate either pro-survival or pro-death signaling that can influence HC survival after exposure to ototoxic agents. Together these data indicate that autonomous responses that occur within a stressed HC or SGN are not the only (and possibly not the primary) determinants of whether the stressed cell ultimately lives or dies. Instead non-cell-autonomous responses are emerging as significant determinants of HC and SGN survival vs. death in the face of ototoxic stress. The goal of this review is to summarize the current evidence on non-cell-autonomous responses to ototoxic stress and to discuss ways in which this knowledge may advance the development of therapies to reduce hearing loss caused by these drugs.

Keywords: ototoxicity, cisplatin, aminoglycoside, macrophages, glial cells, non-autonomous

OTOTOXICITY

Ototoxicity refers to damage to the inner ear by toxic substances. Some of these substances are medications that are used to treat a variety of conditions. It is estimated that 130–200 therapeutic drugs are ototoxic (Lien et al., 1983; Seligmann et al., 1996; Lanvers-Kaminsky et al., 2017). These include antibiotic glycopeptides and macrolides, anti-malarials, loop diuretics, and non-steroidal anti-inflammatory drugs (NSAIDs). Hearing loss caused by some of these drugs is reversible. However, there are two important classes of ototoxic drugs that cause permanent hearing loss: the aminoglycoside antibiotics and the platinum-based antineoplastic agents. The aminoglycoside antibiotics are effective for the treatment of a wide range of bacterial infections, including *Mycobacterium tuberculosis, Pseudomonas, Escherichia coli, and Klebsiella* (Schacht et al., 2012; Krause et al., 2016). Administration of clinically relevant doses of aminoglycosides results primarily in damage to basal turn OHCs in the cochlea and both type I and type II vestibular HCs (Tsuji et al., 2000; Hinojosa et al., 2001). Damage in the cochlea progresses in a gradient from base to apex, and in the vestibular maculae in a gradient from the striolar to the extrastriolar region. Prolonged or high-dose treatment with aminoglycosides also results in changes in the stria vascularis, including thinning, shrinkage, and atrophy (Forge and Fradis, 1985; Forge et al., 1987). While many cell types in the inner ear internalize aminoglycosides, the HCs are particularly vulnerable to aminoglycoside-induced death. Aminoglycoside-induced HC death has been described as both apoptotic and necrotic (Nakagawa et al., 1998; Lenoir et al., 1999; Matsui et al., 2002, 2003; Cunningham et al., 2004; Jiang et al., 2005). The molecular and cellular mechanisms that result in HC death are not fully understood, but there are a number of signaling molecules that are associated with aminoglycoside ototoxicity. One of the earliest observed indicators of toxicity is the formation of reactive oxygen species (ROS) in HCs (Priuska and Schacht, 1995; Hirose et al., 1997; Sha and Schacht, 1999). Increased oxidative burden in HCs and spiral ganglion neurons (SGNs) has been linked to activation of the c-jun-N-terminal kinase (JNK) stress signaling pathway, which in-turn has been shown to be associated with activation of pro-apoptotic caspases -8, -9, and -3, and HC death (Hirose et al., 1999; Pirvola et al., 2000; Cunningham et al., 2002, 2004; Matsui et al., 2002, 2003, 2004; Ylikoski et al., 2002; Cheng et al., 2003; Wang et al., 2003; Lee et al., 2004; Mangiardi et al., 2004; Sugahara et al., 2006; Jeong et al., 2010).

The platinum-based antineoplastic agents, cisplatin, oxaliplatin, and carboplatin are among the most widely used anti-cancer drugs, and they are used to treat a variety of solid tumors in both pediatric and adult cancer patients. Cisplatin is the most commonly-used of these and is also the most ototoxic drug in clinical use (Muggia et al., 2015). As with aminoglycosides, cisplatin ototoxicity is associated with OHC loss in a basal to apical gradient, with the innermost row of OHCs being affected first (Schacht et al., 2012). Cisplatin-induced HC death is associated with oxidative stress, phosphorylation of STAT1, and activation of caspases -9 and -3 (Rybak et al., 2009; Schmitt et al., 2009). Reductions in both the endocochlear potential (EP) and compound action potential (CAP) are concomitant with OHC loss, indicating effects on the cells of the stria vascularis and SGNs (Schacht et al., 2012). *In vivo* studies indicate membrane blebbing and cytoplasmic vacuolization in strial marginal cells after cisplatin treatment, as well as shrinking and atrophy of intermediate cells, and demyelination, shrinkage, and apoptosis of SGNs (Cardinaal et al., 2000; Sluyter et al., 2003; van Ruijven et al., 2004; Ozkiris et al., 2013; Sun et al., 2016). Thus, unlike aminoglycosides, which primarily affect hair cells, cisplatin damages several cell types in the inner ear.

NON-AUTONOMOUS CELLULAR DISEASE PATHOLOGIES

Like most diseases, drug-induced hearing loss has been studied in terms of the cells that are killed, primarily the HCs and SGNs, and the molecular and cellular signals specific to those cells. Rudolph Virchow is commonly referred to as the father of pathology, and his 1858 treatise on the "cell state" helped to form the basis of how we view diseases and their etiologies. Central to his dogma is the idea of cell autonomy. Virchow's vision of the cells of an organism was comparable with citizens in a society, with each cell having autonomy from the larger body (Reynolds, 2007). Since then, many diseases have been considered to have cell-autonomous etiologies and outcomes, with the assumption that pathology is caused by damage to a specific class of autonomous cells. Biologists now recognize that cells are a community, and the behavior of one cell type can influence whether another cell type lives or dies after stress (Cleveland and Rothstein, 2001; Barbeito et al., 2004; Kemp et al., 2011; Popiel et al., 2012; May et al., 2013; Anttonen et al., 2016; Halievski et al., 2016; Macrez et al., 2016; Tognatta and Miller, 2016; Olson et al., 2017). Studies of CNS diseases have provided insights into non-autonomous cell death. Stress or injury in CNS neurons can induce phenotypic changes in both astrocytes and microglia (known as reactive astrocytosis or gliosis, respectively) that can either exacerbate or limit the extent of progressive neuronal cell death (Cleveland and Rothstein, 2001; Barbeito et al., 2004; Compston and Coles, 2008; Ilieva et al., 2009; Macrez et al., 2016; Kipp et al., 2017). Thus, glial cells are often mediators of whether a neuron under stress will live or die.

Examples of non-cell-autonomous pathologies are associated with many glial cell types of the CNS. Amyotrophic lateral sclerosis (ALS) is a neurodegenerative disease that results in progressive muscle deterioration and paralysis. This pathology is attributed to the death of motor neurons and activation of glial cells in the lumbar spinal cord (Cleveland and Rothstein, 2001; Rowland and Shneider, 2001; Barbeito et al., 2004; Vargas and Johnson, 2010). Several studies suggest that while the onset of ALS may begin in neurons, disease progression is due to reactive astrocytosis (Cleveland and Rothstein, 2001; Rowland and Shneider, 2001; Barbeito et al., 2004). These reactive astrocytes downregulate trophic machinery, such as glutamate transporters, and they induce the expression of pro-inflammatory cytokines (Cleveland and Rothstein, 2001; Rowland and Shneider, 2001; Barbeito et al., 2004). These changes result in deterioration of otherwise healthy motor neurons, initiating a positive feedback cascade and disease progression. Similarly, autism spectrum disorder (ASD) refers to a group of developmental disorders associated with abnormalities in language and social interaction. The etiology of ASD is still unknown, but there is an increasing body of research that suggests a link to defective microglia, abnormal synaptogenesis, inflammatory gliosis, and destruction of CNS connectivity by reactive microglia (Vargas et al., 2005; Bessis et al., 2007; Morgan et al., 2010; Suzuki et al., 2013). Finally, multiple sclerosis (MS) is a common autoimmune disease that is characterized by chronic inflammation and demyelination, resulting in motor, sensory, and cognitive defects (Compston and Coles, 2008; Domingues et al., 2016; Macrez et al., 2016; Kipp et al., 2017). MS arises from a nexus of non-cell-autonomous interactions between the adaptive (T and B cells) and innate (microglia) immune systems, along with astrocytes and oligodendrocytes (Kotter et al., 2006; Compston and Coles, 2008; Domingues et al., 2016; Duncan and Radcliff, 2016; Macrez et al., 2016; Tognatta and Miller, 2016; Kipp et al., 2017). Autoimmune responses of T and B cells result in activation of microglia and/or astrocytes, resulting in inflammation and possibly glutamate toxicity that converge on oligodendrocytes and ultimately neurons (Domingues et al., 2016; Duncan and Radcliff, 2016; Macrez et al., 2016; Tognatta and Miller, 2016). Thus, CNS diseases can be driven by non-autonomous cellular mechanisms in which non-neuronal cell types promote degeneration of neurons. Similarly, hearing loss is not simply a manifestation of autonomous HC and SGN dysfunction. Recent studies indicate that it is important to also consider the effects of ototoxic drugs on other cell types of the inner ear, including SCs and macrophages, and that these cells are critical determinants of recovery (or death) of sensory cells and neurons after ototoxic injury (Bichler et al., 1983; Sugawara et al., 2005; Ladrech et al., 2007; Lahne and Gale, 2008; Sato et al., 2010; May et al., 2013; Baker et al., 2015; Sun et al., 2015; Takada et al., 2015; Anttonen et al., 2016; Jadali and Kwan, 2016; Kim et al., 2016).

SUPPORTING CELL FUNCTIONS IN THE UNDAMAGED INNER EAR

Supporting cells of the inner ear are analogous to glial cells of the central nervous system, expressing glial markers, such as vimentin, glutamate-aspartate transporter (GLAST), and glial fibrillary acidic protein (GFAP) (Anniko et al., 1986; Furness and Lehre, 1997; Rio et al., 2002). Like glial cells, SCs also play important non-cell-autonomous roles by promoting either survival or death of HCs and/or SGNs in the inner ear during and after ototoxic challenge. Supporting cells are highly specialized and polarized accessory epithelial cells that support the functions and viability of sensory HCs and neurons by providing structural integrity, trophic factors, and potassium and glutamate recycling. The mammalian organ of Corti contains at least seven different SC types: Deiters' cells, pillar cells, Hensen's cells, inner phalangeal cells, inner border cells, Claudius' cells, and Boettcher cells in the basal turn. All of these supporting cell types are required for normal hearing function (Wan et al., 2013; Burns et al., 2015).

Supporting cells are integral to the maintenance of the integrity of the reticular lamina, ion recycling, and thus normal functioning of the inner ear. The inner ear consists of three fluid-filled compartments, each with different ionic compositions. Endolymph in the scala media is high in potassium and low in sodium, and it bathes the apical surfaces of the organ of Corti. Perilymph in the scala vestibuli and scala tympani is low in potassium and high in sodium, and it bathes the basolateral surfaces of HCs and SCs. The electrochemical gradient produced by the separation of these fluid compartments is essential for HC mechanotransduction and normal hearing (Wangemann, 2006). The reticular lamina provides an impermeable epithelial barrier between the endolymph and perilymph. This structure is formed by a network of special "very tight" junctions between HCs and their neighboring SCs (Anniko and Wroblewski, 1986). In the event of HC degeneration and death, SCs seal the resulting wound, maintaining the integrity of the reticular lamina (Forge, 1985; Cotanche and Dopyera, 1990; Li et al., 1995; Hordichok and Steyger, 2007; Anttonen et al., 2014). In addition to providing structural and trophic support to HCs, SCs also express neurotrophins and neurotrophin receptors that are required for the long-term survival of SGNs (Stankovic et al., 2004). Thus, supporting cells are specialized glia that promote the functions of both hair cells and SGNs and are required for hearing function.

SUPPORTING CELLS AND HAIR CELL DEATH

In the event of HC death and degeneration, a critical response of SCs is rapid expansion to fill the voids left by degenerating HCs in order to maintain the integrity of the reticular lamina (Forge, 1985; Cotanche and Dopyera, 1990; Li et al., 1995; Hordichok and Steyger, 2007; Anttonen et al., 2014). Ototoxic damage to HCs has the potential to disrupt the reticular lamina, reducing the EP, and potentially exacerbating the injury by exposing the lateral membranes of HCs and SCs to high levels of potassium in endolymph (Cody et al., 1980; Bohne and Rabbitt, 1983; Meiteles and Raphael, 1994). Supporting cells preserve the integrity of the reticular lamina by either extruding or engulfing dead HCs and forming an epithelial scar (Forge, 1985; Cotanche and Dopyera, 1990; Meiteles and Raphael, 1994; Li et al., 1995; Hordichok and Steyger, 2007; Bird et al., 2010; Anttonen et al., 2014; Monzack et al., 2015). The mode of HC clearance (extrusion vs. phagocytic engulfment) varies among species, and even between the auditory and vestibular systems within the same species (Dodson et al., 1982; Li et al., 1995; Nakagawa et al., 1997). Extrusion is the predominant mode for removal of dead hair cells in the chick auditory system and guinea pig vestibular system (Cotanche and Dopyera, 1990; Li et al., 1995; Mangiardi et al., 2004). HC extrusion is usually preceded by ballooning of the entire apical surface of the HC; this is followed by ejection of the entire HC with the stereocilia bundle generally still attached (Hirose et al., 2004; Mangiardi et al., 2004). In addition to dead HCs, it appears that even viable HCs may be extruded, since some extruded HCs maintain membrane integrity (Mangiardi et al., 2004). Scanning electron microscopic analysis of the vestibular organs of guinea pigs injected with aminoglycosides reveals that HC bodies are extruded from the sensory epithelium, and SCs rapidly expand apical processes that forms a scar and seals the reticular lamina (Li et al., 1995).

The second mode by which supporting cells remove dead hair cells and preserve the reticular lamina is sub-luminal phagocytosis, which is the dominant means of apoptotic HC clearance in the chick and most mammalian vestibular organs and the mammalian cochlea (Forge, 1985; Bird et al., 2010; Anttonen et al., 2014; Monzack et al., 2015). In this process, dead HCs are engulfed by neighboring SCs. In the chick and mouse utricle this HC removal process occurs as two distinct events, an initial excision of the stereocilia bundle and cuticular plate and a second phagocytic engulfment of the remainder of the HC body (Bird et al., 2010; Monzack et al., 2015). SCs initiate excision of the stereocilia bundle by extending a cable-like circumferential actin belt at the apical portion of the dying HC. Constriction of this actin belt results in the excision of the cuticular plate and hair bundle, which either remain attached to the epithelium or are ejected into the lumen. This process also results in the formation of an epithelial scar (Li et al., 1995; Bird et al., 2010; Monzack et al., 2015). The second phase is characterized by SC extension of an actin-based phagosome that engulfs the remaining HC soma (Bird et al., 2010; Monzack et al., 2015). The HC appears to be degraded within this phagosome. In the mammalian cochlea, the phalangeal processes of Deiters' cells expand below the cuticular plate, excising the stereocilia bundle and engulfing the bodies of dead HCs (Forge, 1985; Anttonen et al., 2014). Whether via extrusion or phagocytosis, SCs play critical roles in the removal of dead HCs, thus preserving the integrity of the reticular lamina and sensory epithelium.

NON-AUTONOMOUS CELLULAR RESPONSES TO OTOTOXIC DRUG-INDUCED HAIR CELL STRESS: RESPONSES OF SUPPORTING CELLS

Supporting cells play central roles in mediating HC survival and death after damage (**Figure 1**). Exposure to aminoglycosides results in SC-specific activation of ERK1/2 mitogen-activated protein kinase (MAPK) in neonatal rat cochlear explants (Lahne and Gale, 2008). ERK1/2 activation begins in SCs at the site of injury and spreads to adjacent SCs in the immediate region in a manner that depends on inter-cellular communication via gap junctions. Pharmacological inhibition of ERK1/2 signaling reduces aminoglycoside-induced HC death (Lahne and Gale, 2008). These data indicate that ERK1/2 is activated specifically in SCs in response to aminoglycoside ototoxicity, and that this activation promotes hair cell death. Thus, the factors that determine whether the aminoglycoside-exposed HC will live or die are not entirely autonomous to the hair cell. ERK-dependent signals from SCs can promote non-cell-autonomous HC death and thus determine the fate of HCs exposed to aminoglycosides.

The idea that SCs mediate the life vs. death fate of damaged HCs is further supported by *in vivo* data from the noise and aminoglycoside-damaged adult cochlea. Aminoglycoside ototoxicity results in activation of the c-Jun N-terminal protein kinase (JNK/c-Jun) pathway in hair cells, which is associated with ototoxic stress and cell death pathways (Pirvola et al., 2000; Ylikoski et al., 2002; Matsui et al., 2004; Sugahara et al., 2006; Francis et al., 2011, 2013; Anttonen et al., 2016). Inhibition of JNK signaling inhibits aminoglycoside-induced HC death both *in vitro* and *in vivo* (Pirvola et al., 2000; Ylikoski et al., 2002; Sugahara et al., 2006; Francis et al., 2013). Anttonen et al. (2016) observed an unexpected pattern of JNK activation in the organ of Corti of adult mice administered kanamycin (an aminoglycoside) and furosemide (a loop diuretic). Outer HC degeneration and apoptosis were accompanied by robust upregulation and phosphorylation of c-Jun (target of JNK activation) in cells that are not vulnerable to aminoglycoside-induced death, including IHCs and SCs, especially Deiters' cells. In contrast, OHCs were negative for both c-Jun expression and phosphorylation (JNK activation). OHCs are required for the damage-associated JNK activation in SCs, and blockade of JNK activation specifically in SCs resulted in partial protection against acoustic trauma. These data suggest that JNK activation in SCs may reflect damage signaling from HCs under stress. In addition, JNK activation in SCs may mediate OHC degeneration (Anttonen et al., 2016). Together these results indicate that stress signaling in SCs can promote HC death *in vivo*.

Non-cell-autonomous signaling from SCs may also influence HC death in response to cisplatin ototoxicity. The gap junction protein connexin 43 is expressed in SCs and not in HCs, yet it can function as a pro-apoptotic mediator of cisplatin-induced HC death (Kikuchi et al., 1995; Zhao and Santos-Sacchi, 1999; Zhao and Yu, 2006; Zhao et al., 2006; Yu and Zhao, 2009; Kim et al., 2016). Inhibition of gap junction signaling reduced cisplatin-induced hearing loss, as measured by auditory brainstem response (ABR), suggesting that SC signaling via gap junctions may promote cisplatin-induced hair cell death (Kim et al., 2016). Gap junctional intercellular communication may either promote cell survival or cell death, depending on the context of injury. Connexin hemi-channels can be conduits for ATP release, and it is reasonable to consider the possibility that SC intercellular communication can either enhance or inhibit the spread of an ototoxic insult (Lahne and Gale, 2008).

In addition to promoting HC death, SCs can also protect HCs undergoing ototoxic challenge. Induction of heat shock proteins (HSPs) is protective against both aminoglycoside- and cisplatin-induced HC death in adult mouse utricle explants (Cunningham and Brandon, 2006; Taleb et al., 2008, 2009; Francis et al., 2011; May et al., 2013). Following heat shock, inducible HSP70 is localized primarily in SCs, with little immunoreactivity detected in HCs, suggesting that SCs mediate the protective effect of HSP70 induction. Supporting-cell-specific expression of HSP70 by adenovirus (AdHSP70) is also protective against aminoglycoside-induced HC death, indicating that HSP70 expression in SCs is sufficient to protect HCs from aminoglycoside ototoxicity (May et al., 2013). SCs may confer their protective effect by secreting HSP70 into the extracellular environment (May et al., 2013). In support of this hypothesis, extracellular HSP70 is required for the protective effect of heat shock (May et al., 2013). These data indicate that non-cell-autonomous signaling from SCs can promote survival of HCs treated with aminoglycosides *in vitro*. Evidence for the protective effect of SC-derived HSP70 *in vivo* comes from a study in which cochleas of adult guinea pig were infected with AdHSP70,

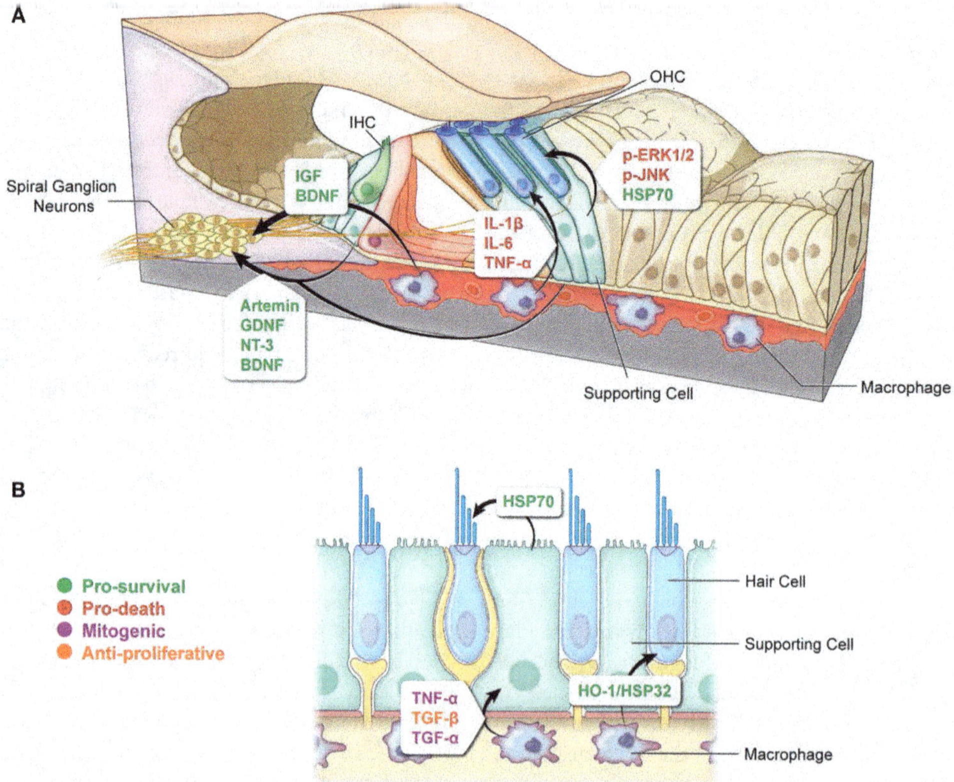

FIGURE 1 | Non-autonomous cellular signals influence survival of HCs and SGNs as well as SC proliferation after ototoxic insult. **(A)** In response to ototoxic stress in the cochlea, SCs can promote either survival (via induction of HSP70) (Takada et al., 2015) or death (via activation of ERK1/2 and JNK pathways) (Lahne and Gale, 2008; Anttonen et al., 2016) of HCs. Supporting cells can also support the survival of SGNs after ototoxic injury through the release of protective neurotrophins (Sugawara et al., 2007; Zilberstein et al., 2012; Bailey and Green, 2014). Similarly, macrophages can promote survival of SGNs by releasing cytoprotective neurotrophins (Kaur et al., 2015b), and they can also promote HC death after ototoxic injury by releasing pro-inflammatory cytokines (Sato et al., 2010; Sun et al., 2015). **(B)** Vestibular SCs and macrophages can promote HC survival during ototoxic stress through the release of HSP70 and HO-1/HSP32, respectively (May et al., 2013; Baker et al., 2015). Macrophages can promote SC proliferation in response to ototoxic stress through the release of mitogenic cytokines TNF-α and TGF-α, or they can suppress SC proliferation through release of TGF-β (Warchol, 1999). Arrows indicate which cell types are involved in each signaling event. Signaling molecules are indicated beside each arrow. Green, pro-survival signals; Red, pro-death signals; Purple, mitogenic signals; Orange, anti-proliferative signals.

resulting in robust HSP70 immunoreactivity in Deiters' cells and pillar cells, with no immunoreactivity observed in HCs (Takada et al., 2015). When the animals were treated with kanamycin and furosemide to kill HCs, over-expression of HSP70 in SCs reduced IHC death and improved ABR thresholds in ears receiving viral HSP70 infection relative to untreated ears. OHCs were not protected against aminoglycoside-induced death, even though the SCs adjacent to them were infected by Ad-HSP70. It is possible that the magnitude of the damage caused by the combination of kanamycin and furosemide results in OHC damage that overwhelms HSP70-mediated protection. Regardless, both *in vitro* and *in vivo* data indicate that HCs can be protected against ototoxic drug-induced death in a non-autonomous manner by HSP expression in supporting cells.

The above-described data indicate that induction of protective molecules in SCs can promote HC survival after ototoxic insult. Taken together with the data indicating that SCs can also promote HC death (Lahne and Gale, 2008; Anttonen et al., 2016), a model emerges in which non-cell-autonomous signals are critical determinants of whether a HC under stress will ultimately live or die.

SUPPORTING CELLS AND OTOTOXIC DRUG-INDUCED SPIRAL GANGLION NEURON DEATH: NON-AUTONOMOUS CELLULAR RESPONSES

In addition to HCs, ototoxic drugs also cause death of SGNs and degeneration of peripheral auditory fibers (PAFs). Animal models and analysis of human temporal bones suggest that SCs influence the survival of SGNs and maintenance or regrowth of degenerated PAFs after ototoxic insult. Aminoglycoside-induced loss of OHCs in cats had little effect on degeneration the of SGNs and PAFs; however, loss of IHCs and their "supporting structures" (SCs) was followed by rapid retrograde degeneration of SGNs (Leake and Hradek, 1988). Systemic aminoglycoside administration in chinchilla revealed that changes in SC morphology were accompanied by degeneration of outer spiral afferent dendrites (Ryan et al., 1980). Even in instances of aminoglycoside ototoxicity that result in near complete loss of both IHCs and OHCs, there was significantly more neuronal survival in areas where SCs remained intact (Sugawara et al., 2005). Studies of human temporal bones confirm that even in cases of severe HC loss, 5–10% of SGNs "resist retrograde degeneration" (Spoendlin, 1975). Schuknecht was one of the first to identify the correlation between surviving SCs and the presence of surviving PAFs (Schuknecht, 1953). Analysis of temporal bones from patients with a variety of inner ear pathologies including exposure to ototoxic drugs indicated that peripheral fibers were able to survive in the absence of IHCs and OHCs, but not in the absence of intact SCs (Johnsson, 1974; Otte et al., 1978; Johnsson et al., 1981; Suzuka and Schuknecht, 1988). The loss of these SCs was thought to lead to retrograde degeneration of PAF and SGNs, and the extent of SGN degeneration was directly correlated to the extent of SC loss (Suzuka and Schuknecht, 1988). Together these studies suggest that SCs (but not HCs) must be present in order for PAFs and SGNs to survive.

In contrast to the above studies suggesting that SGN survival requires SCs, there are also studies suggesting that intact differentiated SCs are not required for peripheral auditory fiber or SGN survival (Bichler et al., 1983; Leake and Hradek, 1988). These conflicting reports may be related to the identity of the cells that remain in the undifferentiated "flat" epithelium observed after severe ototoxicity. Are these cells de-differentiated SCs, or possibly cells from adjacent regions that have migrated to replace dead SCs (Kim and Raphael, 2007; Izumikawa et al., 2008; Oesterle and Campbell, 2009; Abbas and Rivolta, 2015)? Studies by Abbas and Rivolta (Abbas and Rivolta, 2015) suggest that the cells making up the flat epithelium are SCs. Although these cells have lost their characteristic morphologies, they continue to express SC markers, including OCP2 and acetylated αTubulin. Both IHCs and SCs provide SGNs with neurotrophic factors that are required for their survival (Ernfors et al., 1992; Farinas et al., 2001; Sobkowicz et al., 2002). NT-3 expression in SCs is required for the survival of SGNs in both the cochlea and vestibular organs (Sugawara et al., 2007). In the adult cochlea deafened by aminoglycosides, NT-3 is expressed primarily by surviving, differentiated SCs (Bailey and Green, 2014). Additional neurotrophins are also expressed in the organ of Corti after aminoglycoside-induced HC death, suggesting that even in the absence of HCs, neurotrophic factors produced by SCs are available to SGNs (Bailey and Green, 2014). Moreover, genetic studies have shown that SGNs can survive in the absence of IHCs through development and into maturity, and this survival is dependent on neurotrophins provided by SCs (Zilberstein et al., 2012). These data suggest that the cells constituting the flat epithelium retain a SC phenotype, and these de-differentiated SCs continue to provide neurotrophic support to remaining SGNs and PAFs. Thus, in the studies suggesting that SCs were not required for survival of SGNs and PAFs, there may have been de-differentiated SCs present that were providing trophic support after ototoxic insult. Overall the data are consistent with a model in which supporting cells release trophic factors that are required for proper innervation, SGN and PAF homeostasis under normal conditions and after ototoxic insult (**Figure 1**).

NON-AUTONOMOUS CELLULAR SIGNALING FROM MACROPHAGES IN THE UNDAMAGED AND LESIONED INNER EAR

The inner ear was long believed to be an immune-privileged organ, like the brain and retina, due to the presence of tight junctions within the stria vascularis that constitute the blood-labyrinth barrier (BLB) (Harris, 1983, 1984; Fujioka et al., 2014). Early studies of inflammation after ototoxic insult indicated that macrophages did not infiltrate the organ of Corti and were only identified in the endolymphatic sac, along with cellular debris (Wright and Meyerhoff, 1984). Systemic administration of a highly immunogenic protein, keyhole limpet hemocyanin (KLH), resulted in very little antibody production in perilymph (Harris, 1983). In contrast, when perilymph was directly injected with KLH, there was a significant increase in anti-KLH titers, indicating that there is a resident population of immune cells (later identified as macrophages) within the inner ear (Harris, 1983, 1984). Therefore, it was hypothesized that these resident macrophages are capable of mounting an immune response, but the BLB serves as a barrier that blocks: (a) immune cells, (b) antigens from the inner ear that may provoke a systemic immune response, and (c) antibodies from systemic circulation (Harris, 1983, 1984). However, recent studies suggest that the inner ear is not an immune-privileged compartment; instead it is permeable to hematopoietic stem cells, both after injury and under normal conditions (Lang et al., 2006; Okano et al., 2008; Sato et al., 2010).

Macrophages are myeloid cells of the innate immune system, first described by Elie Metchikoff in the late nineteenth century and recognized for being highly phagocytic (Davies et al., 2013; Varol et al., 2015). Resident macrophages are present in the majority of tissues in the body, where they are integral to the maintenance of homeostasis through phagocytosis and degradation of dead cells, cellular debris, and foreign materials (Davies et al., 2013; Varol et al., 2015). Resident macrophages are present in the undamaged mammalian inner ear, where they perform functions required for the maintenance of the extracellular environment and the BLB (Hirose et al., 2005; Shi, 2010; Zhang et al., 2012; O'Malley et al., 2016). Some of the first studies into the interplay between macrophages and HCs suggested that they may play a role in wound healing and regeneration of lost HCs. After tail amputation in salamander, macrophages are recruited to the tissues surrounding the neuromast most proximal to the site of injury, and macrophage recruitment precedes the onset of SC mitotic activity in these neuromasts (Jones and Corwin, 1993). When neuromast HCs were damaged by laser ablation, macrophage infiltration peaked shortly before the onset of SC proliferation, suggesting that these macrophages may function to influence HC regeneration through the secretion of growth factors and mitogenic cytokines (Corwin et al., 1991; Jones and Corwin, 1996;

Pei et al., 2016). Subsequent studies in chick utricle exposed to neomycin confirmed that cytokines secreted from activated macrophages influence the rate of SC proliferation (Warchol, 1999). These experiments suggest that macrophage activity is required for effective recovery of the sensory epithelium after injury, and macrophages have non-cell-autonomous effects on SC proliferation and regeneration of HCs after injury.

The undamaged chick auditory and vestibular organs contain a resident population of two distinct leukocyte-derived cells, identified as macrophages and "microglia-like" cells (MLCs), based on morphology and expression of the common leukocyte marker CD45 or monocyte marker CD68 (Bhave et al., 1998; Warchol, 1999). Macrophages (large round shape) are present immediately beneath the HC nuclear layer, whereas microglia-like cells are most often located in the SC layer. Numerous cells expressing macrophage markers (Bu-1, Cla, and 74.2) are also observed in regions outside of the sensory epithelium, such as the underlying stromal tissues (O'Halloran and Oesterle, 2004). After ototoxic injury, both macrophages and microglia-like cells are recruited to the sensory epithelium and luminal surface, suggesting that dying HCs attract them to sites of injury. In contrast, microglia-like cell numbers are increased in both damaged and undamaged regions (Bhave et al., 1998; Warchol, 1999). These data in conjunction with those on the release of mitogenic cytokines from macrophages (Warchol, 1999) suggest that macrophages/microglia-like cells are recruited to sites of ototoxic injury, where they may function to enhance the proliferation and/or differentiation of SCs after HC death in the avian inner ear.

Macrophages are also recruited to sites of ototoxic injury in the mammalian inner ear (Sato et al., 2010; Hirose and Sato, 2011; Sun et al., 2015). Potential roles for damage-recruited macrophages include phagocytosis of dead HCs and debris, and secretion of cytokines (Hirose et al., 2005; Sato et al., 2010; Kaur et al., 2015a,b; Sun et al., 2015). CD45+ macrophages were recruited to the tunnel of Corti as soon as the first week after systemic aminoglycoside administration in rats (Ladrech et al., 2007). The timing of macrophage infiltration coincided with the peak of HC death and ended when most of the OHCs and IHCs had been eliminated, suggesting that infiltration signals were mediated by HC death. This study provided no direct evidence for macrophage phagocytosis of apoptotic HCs or apoptotic bodies, but it suggested that macrophages may function in phagocytosis and/or wound repair. Transmission electron microscopic studies indicate that "microglia-like cells" are present in the rat organ of Corti after amikacin administration, and these cells contain endocytic vesicles filled with degenerated cellular material (Wang and Li, 2000). These data suggest that macrophages may assist SCs in the engulfment of dead HC debris after ototoxic insult. Further evidence for phagocytosis of dead HCs and HC debris by macrophages comes from studies using utricles from transgenic mice expressing the diphtheria toxin receptor (DTR) specifically in HCs (Kaur et al., 2015a). While these Pou4f3-huDTR mice are not a model of drug-induced ototoxicity, they do demonstrate some cellular changes that are similar to those that occur after ototoxic insult. CX3CR1-GFP (a leukocyte and/or macrophage-specific cell surface receptor that functions in macrophage recruitment) positive macrophages infiltrate the sensory epithelium in response to DT-mediated HC death. These macrophages appear to be recruited from the population of resident macrophages residing in the stromal tissues of the utricle (Kaur et al., 2015a). This increase in macrophage number is transient, suggesting that HC death was the driving force behind macrophage infiltration into the sensory epithelium. Macrophage processes were in frequent contact with potentially apoptotic HCs, and these macrophages were actively engulfing HC debris (Kaur et al., 2015a). Taken together these data indicate that a population of macrophages resides in the major compartments of the undamaged mammalian inner ear, and they are recruited to sites of ototoxic injury, where they may assist SCs in the phagocytosis of dead HCs and HC debris.

Macrophages may have functions beyond phagocytosis of HC corpses and debris after injury in the inner ear. Macrophage infiltration and signaling may mediate survival of HCs and SGNs after ototoxic insult. CX3CR1 KO mice show significantly more macrophage infiltration into the cochlea after aminoglycoside administration, compared to control and heterozygous mice (Sato et al., 2010). In addition, CX3CR1 KO mice are more susceptible to aminoglycoside-induced hearing loss and HC death. These studies indicate that CX3CR1 inhibits macrophage infiltration or cytokine secretion after ototoxic insult, and they suggest that macrophage infiltration can influence the extent of HC damage and hearing loss after ototoxic injury.

Further evidence for non-autonomous effects of macrophages on HC viability after ototoxic insult comes from examination of CX3CL1/CX3CR1 signaling during neomycin-induced HC death (Sun et al., 2015). CX3CL1 (fractalkine) is a chemokine located on the surface of neurons and endothelial cells, and it serves as a damage signal and ligand for CX3CR1 receptors on macrophages (Ransohoff et al., 2007). Systemic aminoglycoside administration in neonatal mice resulted in a significant increase in expression of the soluble form of CX3CL1 in HCs and induced migration and activation of macrophages or MLCs into the sensory epithelium. Exogenous application of CX3CL1 resulted in a significant increase in the number of MLCs in the sensory epithelium as well as increased pro-inflammatory cytokine secretion and increased HC death. Inhibition of MLC activation inhibited neomycin-induced IHC and OHC death and hearing loss, suggesting that cytokine production by activated MLCs exacerbates aminoglycoside-induced HC death (Sun et al., 2015). These data suggest that HCs communicate damage signals to macrophages through upregulation of soluble CX3CL1, and CX3CL1/CX3CR1 signaling is integral to macrophage recruitment after injury. In addition, macrophage recruitment and activation may exacerbate ototoxic lesions through inflammatory cytokine production (**Figure 1**).

Like SCs, macrophages also have the potential to promote survival of HCs after ototoxic injury. Treatment with an inducer of heme oxygenase 1 (HO-1, also called heat shock protein 32, HSP32) protected against cisplatin-induced hair cell death in utricle explants (Baker et al., 2015). HO-1 was induced only in resident macrophages with no induction in HCs or SCs. When macrophages were depleted from the explants, the protective effect of HSP32/HO-1 was abolished (Baker et al., 2015). These data indicate that HO-1 induction specifically in macrophages can protect hair cells against aminoglycoside-induced death. Thus, the protective effect of HO-1 induction against HC death is non-autonomous and is mediated by resident macrophages.

In addition to modulating the survival and death of HCs under stress, macrophages also modulate the survival of SGNs. Although it is not an ototoxic drug, diphtheria toxin injection in Pou4f3-huDTR/CX3CR1-GFP mice results in complete loss of OHCs and IHCs after 7 days, with no obvious effects on other cell types (Kaur et al., 2015b). Recruitment of resident macrophages was significantly increased in the cochlea after DT injection. Infiltrating macrophages were observed below the basilar membrane and in Rosenthal's canal in association with SGN cell bodies. CX3CR1 KO mice had fewer macrophages infiltrating into the sensory epithelium and after DT injection compared with WT DTR mice. Notably, the reduction in macrophages within Rosenthal's canal was accompanied by a significant decrease in SGN survival after DT injection in CX3CR1 null mice. SGN numbers were unaffected in CX3CR1 KO mice that did not receive DT, suggesting that macrophages are only required for SGN survival after HC death. This is in contrast to previous studies showing an increase in macrophage infiltration in the cochleas of CX3CR1 KO mice administered aminoglycosides, which indicates that CX3CR1 and fractalkine signaling is complex, and maybe dependent on the cytotoxic insult or possibly the inner ear organ being analyzed (Sato et al., 2010; Kaur et al., 2015a). These data suggest that like SCs, macrophages can have either pro-death or pro-survival effects on both HCs and SGNs after injury, and these effects are likely mediated through the induction of cytotoxic cytokines, or protective molecules, such as HSPs and neurotrophins (**Figure 1**).

CONCLUSION

Important non-cell-autonomous signals from surrounding cell types (SCs and macrophages) can increase or reduce the extent of ototoxic injury to both HCs and SGNs. Significant questions remain about these intercellular communication events. First, how do SCs and macrophages sense that HCs and SGNs are damaged? The damage signals that activate SCs and macrophages after ototoxic insult remain unclear; however, in other models of tissue damage and wound healing, transcription-independent signals are rapidly released from damaged cells, including calcium, ROS, and ATP (Lahne and Gale, 2008; Cordeiro and Jacinto, 2013). Second, how do SCs and macrophages differentiate between a "help me" signal and a "kill me" signal and thus decide whether to promote survival vs. death of damaged cells? Are these signals mediated by different molecules, or does the magnitude of the damage signal perhaps determine whether the SCs and macrophages act to promote death vs. survival? Finally, once a HC or SGN dies, what are the signals that mediate recognition of the dying cell for engulfment or extrusion (i.e., the "eat me" signal)? The importance of non-cell-autonomous signals in determining these life-or-death outcomes in the inner ear has only recently emerged, and it will be important to take these intercellular signaling events into account when developing therapies aimed at protecting hearing from the deleterious effects of ototoxic drugs.

AUTHOR CONTRIBUTIONS

SF and LC conceived of and together outlined this review. SF wrote the manuscript. LC critiqued the manuscript.

ACKNOWLEDGMENTS

We would like to thank Dr. Jonathan Bird, Dr. Elyssa Monzack, and Dr. Doris Wu for their insightful comments on this manuscript. We would also like to thank Erina He and Alan Hoofring for the figure illustration. This work was supported by the Division of Intramural Research at the National Institute on Deafness and Other Communication Disorders (project number 1ZIADC000079).

REFERENCES

Abbas, L., and Rivolta, M. N. (2015). Aminoglycoside ototoxicity and hair cell ablation in the adult gerbil: a simple model to study hair cell loss and regeneration. *Hear. Res.* 325, 12–26. doi: 10.1016/j.heares.2015.03.002

Anniko, M., Thornell, L. E., Gustavsson, H., and Virtanen, I. (1986). Intermediate filaments in the newborn inner ear of the mouse. *ORL J. Otorhinolaryngol. Relat. Spec.* 48, 98–106. doi: 10.1159/000275854

Anniko, M., and Wroblewski, R. (1986). Ionic environment of cochlear hair cells. *Hear. Res.* 22, 279–293. doi: 10.1016/0378-5955(86) 90104-8

Anttonen, T., Belevich, I., Kirjavainen, A., Laos, M., Brakebusch, C., Jokitalo, E., et al. (2014). How to bury the dead: elimination of apoptotic hair cells from the hearing organ of the mouse. *J. Assoc. Res. Otolaryngol.* 15, 975–992. doi: 10.1007/s10162-014-0480-x

Anttonen, T., Herranen, A., Virkkala, J., Kirjavainen, A., Elomaa, P., Laos, M., et al. (2016). c-Jun N-terminal phosphorylation: biomarker for cellular stress rather than cell death in the injured cochlea. *eNeuro* 3:ENEURO.0047-16.2016. doi: 10.1523/ENEURO.0047-16.2016

Bailey, E. M., and Green, S. H. (2014). Postnatal expression of neurotrophic factors accessible to spiral ganglion neurons in the auditory system of adult hearing and deafened rats. *J. Neurosci.* 34, 13110–13126. doi: 10.1523/JNEUROSCI.1014-14.2014

Baker, T. G., Roy, S., Brandon, C. S., Kramarenko, I. K., Francis, S. P., Taleb, M., et al. (2015). Heat shock protein-mediated protection against Cisplatin-induced hair cell death. *J. Assoc. Res. Otolaryngol.* 16, 67–80. doi: 10.1007/s10162-014-0491-7

Barbeito, L. H., Pehar, M., Cassina, P., Vargas, M. R., Peluffo, H., Viera, L., et al. (2004). A role for astrocytes in motor neuron loss in amyotrophic lateral sclerosis. *Brain Res. Brain Res. Rev.* 47, 263–274. doi: 10.1016/j.brainresrev.2004.05.003

Bessis, A., Bechade, C., Bernard, D., and Roumier, A. (2007). Microglial control of neuronal death and synaptic properties. *Glia* 55, 233–238. doi: 10.1002/glia.20459

Bhave, S. A., Oesterle, E. C., and Coltrera, M. D. (1998). Macrophage and microglia-like cells in the avian inner ear. *J. Comp. Neurol.* 398, 241–256.

Bichler, E., Spoendlin, H., and Rauchegger, H. (1983). Degeneration of cochlear neurons after amikacin intoxication in the rat.

Arch. Otorhinolaryngol. 237, 201–208. doi: 10.1007/BF00453725

Bird, J. E., Daudet, N., Warchol, M. E., and Gale, J. E. (2010). Supporting cells eliminate dying sensory hair cells to maintain epithelial integrity in the avian inner ear. *J. Neurosci.* 30, 12545–12556. doi: 10.1523/JNEUROSCI.3042-10.2010

Bohne, B. A., and Rabbitt, K. D. (1983). Holes in the reticular lamina after noise exposure: implication for continuing damage in the organ of Corti. *Hear. Res.* 11, 41–53. doi: 10.1016/0378-5955(83)90044-8

Burns, J. C., Kelly, M. C., Hoa, M., Morell, R. J., and Kelley, M. W. (2015). Single-cell RNA-Seq resolves cellular complexity in sensory organs from the neonatal inner ear. *Nat. Commun.* 6, 8557. doi: 10.1038/ncomms9557

Cardinaal, R. M., de Groot, J. C., Huizing, E. H., Veldman, J. E., and Smoorenburg, G. F. (2000). Dose-dependent effect of 8-day cisplatin administration upon the morphology of the albino guinea pig cochlea. *Hear. Res.* 144, 135–146. doi: 10.1016/S0378-5955(00)00059-9

Cheng, A. G., Cunningham, L. L., and Rubel, E. W. (2003). Hair cell death in the avian basilar papilla: characterization of the *in vitro* model and caspase activation. *J. Assoc. Res. Otolaryngol.* 4, 91–105. doi: 10.1007/s10162-002-3016-8

Cleveland, D. W., and Rothstein, J. D. (2001). From Charcot to Lou Gehrig: deciphering selective motor neuron death in ALS. *Nat. Rev. Neurosci.* 2, 806–819. doi: 10.1038/35097565

Cody, A. R., Robertson, D., Bredberg, G., and Johnston, B. M. (1980). Electrophysiological and morphological changes in the guinea pig cochlea following mechanical trauma to the organ of Corti. *Acta Otolaryngol.* 89, 440–452. doi: 10.3109/00016488009127160

Compston, A., and Coles, A. (2008). Multiple sclerosis. *Lancet* 372, 1502–1517. doi: 10.1016/S0140-6736(08)61620-7

Cordeiro, J. V., and Jacinto, A. (2013). The role of transcription-independent damage signals in the initiation of epithelial wound healing. *Nat. Rev. Mol. Cell Biol.* 14, 249–262. doi: 10.1038/nrm3541

Corwin, J. T., Jones, J. E., Katayama, A., Kelley, M. W., and Warchol, M. E. (1991). Hair cell regeneration: the identities of progenitor cells, potential triggers and instructive cues. *Ciba Found. Symp.* 160, 103–120.

Cotanche, D. A., and Dopyera, C. E. (1990). Hair cell and supporting cell response to acoustic trauma in the chick cochlea. *Hear. Res.* 46, 29–40. doi: 10.1016/0378-5955(90)90137-E

Cunningham, L. L., and Brandon, C. S. (2006). Heat shock inhibits both aminoglycoside- and cisplatin-induced sensory hair cell death. *J. Assoc. Res. Otolaryngol.* 7, 299–307. doi: 10.1007/s10162-006-0043-x

Cunningham, L. L., Cheng, A. G., and Rubel, E. W. (2002). Caspase activation in hair cells of the mouse utricle exposed to neomycin. *J. Neurosci.* 22, 8532–8540.

Cunningham, L. L., Matsui, J. I., Warchol, M. E., and Rubel, E. W. (2004). Overexpression of Bcl-2 prevents neomycin-induced hair cell death and caspase-9 activation in the adult mouse utricle *in vitro*. *J. Neurobiol.* 60, 89–100. doi: 10.1002/neu.20006

Davies, L. C., Jenkins, S. J., Allen, J. E., and Taylor, P. R. (2013). Tissue-resident macrophages. *Nat. Immunol.* 14, 986–995. doi: 10.1038/ni.2705

Dodson, H. C., Bannister, L. H., and Douek, E. E. (1982). The effects of combined gentamicin and white noise on the spiral organ of young guinea pigs. A structural study. *Acta Otolaryngol.* 94, 193–202. doi: 10.3109/00016488209128905

Domingues, H. S., Portugal, C. C., Socodato, R., and Relvas, J. B. (2016). Oligodendrocyte, astrocyte, and microglia crosstalk in myelin development, damage, and repair. *Front. Cell Dev. Biol* 4:71. doi: 10.3389/fcell.2016.00071

Duncan, I. D., and Radcliff, A. B. (2016). Inherited and acquired disorders of myelin: the underlying myelin pathology. *Exp. Neurol.* 283, 452–475. doi: 10.1016/j.expneurol.2016.04.002

Ernfors, P., Merlio, J. P., and Persson, H. (1992). Cells expressing mRNA for neurotrophins and their receptors during embryonic rat development. *Eur. J. Neurosci.* 4, 1140–1158. doi: 10.1111/j.1460-9568.1992.tb00141.x

Farinas, I., Jones, K. R., Tessarollo, L., Vigers, A. J., Huang, E., Kirstein, M., et al. (2001). Spatial shaping of cochlear innervation by temporally regulated neurotrophin expression. *J. Neurosci.* 21, 6170–6180.

Forge, A. (1985). Outer hair cell loss and supporting cell expansion following chronic gentamicin treatment. *Hear. Res.* 19, 171–182. doi: 10.1016/0378-5955(85)90121-2

Forge, A., and Fradis, M. (1985). Structural abnormalities in the stria vascularis following chronic gentamicin treatment. *Hear. Res.* 20, 233–244. doi: 10.1016/0378-5955(85)90028-0

Forge, A., Wright, A., and Davies, S. J. (1987). Analysis of structural changes in the stria vascularis following chronic gentamicin treatment. *Hear. Res.* 31, 253–265. doi: 10.1016/0378-5955(87)90195-X

Francis, S. P., Katz, J., Fanning, K. D., Harris, K. A., Nicholas, B. D., Lacy, M., et al. (2013). A novel role of cytosolic protein synthesis inhibition in aminoglycoside ototoxicity. *J. Neurosci.* 33, 3079–3093. doi: 10.1523/JNEUROSCI.3430-12.2013

Francis, S. P., Kramarenko, I. I., Brandon, C. S., Lee, F. S., Baker, T. G., and Cunningham, L. L. (2011). Celastrol inhibits aminoglycoside-induced ototoxicity via heat shock protein 32. *Cell Death Dis.* 2:e195. doi: 10.1038/cddis.2011.76

Fujioka, M., Okano, H., and Ogawa, K. (2014). Inflammatory and immune responses in the cochlea: potential therapeutic targets for sensorineural hearing loss. *Front. Pharmacol.* 5:287. doi: 10.3389/fphar.2014.00287

Furness, D. N., and Lehre, K. P. (1997). Immunocytochemical localization of a high-affinity glutamate-aspartate transporter, GLAST, in the rat and guinea-pig cochlea. *Eur. J. Neurosci.* 9, 1961–1969. doi: 10.1111/j.1460-9568.1997.tb00763.x

Halievski, K., Kemp, M. Q., Breedlove, S. M., Miller, K. E., and Jordan, C. L. (2016). Non-cell-autonomous regulation of retrograde motoneuronal axonal transport in an SBMA mouse model. *eNeuro* 3:ENEURO.0062-16.2016. doi: 10.1523/ENEURO.0062-16.2016

Harris, J. P. (1983). Immunology of the inner ear: response of the inner ear to antigen challenge. *Otolaryngol. Head Neck Surg.* 91, 18–32. doi: 10.1177/019459988309100105

Harris, J. P. (1984). Immunology of the inner ear: evidence of local antibody production. *Ann. Otol. Rhinol. Laryngol.* 93(2 Pt 1), 157–162.

Hinojosa, R., Nelson, E. G., Lerner, S. A., Redleaf, M. I., and Schramm, D. R. (2001). Aminoglycoside ototoxicity: a human temporal bone study. *Laryngoscope* 111, 1797–1805. doi: 10.1097/00005537-200110000-00025

Hirose, K., Discolo, C. M., Keasler, J. R., and Ransohoff, R. (2005). Mononuclear phagocytes migrate into the murine cochlea after acoustic trauma. *J. Comp. Neurol.* 489, 180–194. doi: 10.1002/cne.20619

Hirose, K., Hockenbery, D. M., and Rubel, E. W. (1997). Reactive oxygen species in chick hair cells after gentamicin exposure *in vitro*. *Hear. Res.* 104, 1–14. doi: 10.1016/S0378-5955(96)00169-4

Hirose, K., and Sato, E. (2011). Comparative analysis of combination kanamycin-furosemide versus kanamycin alone in the mouse cochlea. *Hear. Res.* 272, 108–116. doi: 10.1016/j.heares.2010.10.011

Hirose, K., Westrum, L. E., Cunningham, D. E., and Rubel, E. W. (2004). Electron microscopy of degenerative changes in the chick basilar papilla after gentamicin exposure. *J. Comp. Neurol.* 470, 164–180. doi: 10.1002/cne.11046

Hirose, K., Westrum, L. E., Stone, J. S., Zirpel, L., and Rubel, E. W. (1999). Dynamic studies of ototoxicity in mature avian auditory epithelium. *Ann. N.Y. Acad. Sci.* 884, 389–409. doi: 10.1111/j.1749-6632.1999.tb08657.x

Hordichok, A. J., and Steyger, P. S. (2007). Closure of supporting cell scar formations requires dynamic actin mechanisms. *Hear. Res.* 232, 1–19. doi: 10.1016/j.heares.2007.06.011

Ilieva, H., Polymenidou, M., and Cleveland, D. W. (2009). Non-cell autonomous toxicity in neurodegenerative disorders: ALS and beyond. *J. Cell Biol.* 187, 761–772. doi: 10.1083/jcb.200908164

Izumikawa, M., Batts, S. A., Miyazawa, T., Swiderski, D. L., and Raphael, Y. (2008). Response of the flat cochlear epithelium to forced expression of Atoh1. *Hear. Res.* 240, 52–56. doi: 10.1016/j.heares.2008.02.007

Jadali, A., and Kwan, K. Y. (2016). Activation of PI3K signaling prevents aminoglycoside-induced hair cell death in the murine cochlea. *Biol. Open* 5, 698–708. doi: 10.1242/bio.016758

Jeong, S. W., Kim, L. S., Hur, D., Bae, W. Y., Kim, J. R., and Lee, J. H. (2010). Gentamicin-induced spiral ganglion cell death: apoptosis mediated by ROS and the JNK signaling pathway. *Acta Otolaryngol.* 130, 670–678. doi: 10.3109/00016480903428200

Jiang, H., Sha, S. H., Forge, A., and Schacht, J. (2005). Caspase-independent pathways of hair cell death induced by kanamycin *in vivo*. *Cell Death Differ.* 13, 20–30. doi: 10.1038/sj.cdd.4401706

Johnsson, L. G. (1974). Sequence of degeneration of Corti's organ and its first-order neurons. *Ann. Otol. Rhinol. Laryngol.* 83, 294–303. doi: 10.1177/000348947408300303

Johnsson, L. G., Hawkins, J. E. Jr., Kingsley, T. C., Black, F. O., and Matz, G. J. (1981). Aminoglycoside-induced cochlear pathology in man. *Acta Otolaryngol. Suppl.* 383, 1–19.

Jones, J. E., and Corwin, J. T. (1993). Replacement of lateral line sensory organs during tail regeneration in salamanders: identification of progenitor cells and analysis of leukocyte activity. *J. Neurosci.* 13, 1022–1034.

Jones, J. E., and Corwin, J. T. (1996). Regeneration of sensory cells after laser ablation in the lateral line system: hair cell lineage and macrophage behavior revealed by time- lapse video microscopy. *J. Neurosci.* 16, 649–662.

Kaur, T., Hirose, K., Rubel, E. W., and Warchol, M. E. (2015a). Macrophage recruitment and epithelial repair following hair cell injury in the mouse utricle. *Front. Cell. Neurosci.* 9:150. doi: 10.3389/fncel.2015.00150

Kaur, T., Zamani, D., Tong, L., Rubel, E. W., Ohlemiller, K. K., Hirose, K., et al. (2015b). Fractalkine signaling regulates macrophage recruitment into the cochlea and promotes the survival of spiral ganglion neurons after selective hair cell lesion. *J. Neurosci.* 35, 15050–15061. doi: 10.1523/JNEUROSCI.2325-15.2015

Kemp, M. Q., Poort, J. L., Baqri, R. M., Lieberman, A. P., Breedlove, S. M., Miller, K. E., et al. (2011). Impaired motoneuronal retrograde transport in two models of SBMA implicates two sites of androgen action. *Hum. Mol. Genet.* 20, 4475–4490. doi: 10.1093/hmg/ddr380

Kikuchi, T., Kimura, R. S., Paul, D. L., and Adams, J. C. (1995). Gap junctions in the rat cochlea: immunohistochemical and ultrastructural analysis. *Anat. Embryol.* 191, 101–118. doi: 10.1007/BF00186783

Kim, Y. H., and Raphael, Y. (2007). Cell division and maintenance of epithelial integrity in the deafened auditory epithelium. *Cell Cycle* 6, 612–619. doi: 10.4161/cc.6.5.3929

Kim, Y. J., Kim, J., Kim, Y. S., Shin, B., Choo, O. S., Lee, J. J., et al. (2016). Connexin 43 acts as a proapoptotic modulator in cisplatin-induced auditory cell death. *Antioxid. Redox Signal.* 25, 623–636. doi: 10.1089/ars.2015.6412

Kipp, M., Nyamoya, S., Hochstrasser, T., and Amor, S. (2017). Multiple sclerosis animal models: a clinical and histopathological perspective. *Brain Pathol.* 27, 123–137. doi: 10.1111/bpa.12454

Kotter, M. R., Li, W. W., Zhao, C., and Franklin, R. J. (2006). Myelin impairs CNS remyelination by inhibiting oligodendrocyte precursor cell differentiation. *J. Neurosci.* 26, 328–332. doi: 10.1523/JNEUROSCI.2615-05.2006

Krause, K. M., Serio, A. W., Kane, T. R., and Connolly, L. E. (2016). Aminoglycosides: an overview. *Cold Spring Harb. Perspect. Med.* 6:a027029. doi: 10.1101/cshperspect.a027029

Ladrech, S., Wang, J., Simonneau, L., Puel, J. L., and Lenoir, M. (2007). Macrophage contribution to the response of the rat organ of Corti to amikacin. *J. Neurosci. Res.* 85, 1970–1979. doi: 10.1002/jnr.21335

Lahne, M., and Gale, J. E. (2008). Damage-induced activation of ERK1/2 in cochlear supporting cells is a hair cell death-promoting signal that depends on extracellular ATP and calcium. *J. Neurosci.* 28, 4918–4928. doi: 10.1523/JNEUROSCI.4914-07.2008

Lang, H., Ebihara, Y., Schmiedt, R. A., Minamiguchi, H., Zhou, D., Smythe, N., et al. (2006). Contribution of bone marrow hematopoietic stem cells to adult mouse inner ear: mesenchymal cells and fibrocytes. *J. Comp. Neurol.* 496, 187–201. doi: 10.1002/cne.20929

Lanvers-Kaminsky, C., Zehnhoff-Dinnesen, A. A., Parfitt, R., and Ciarimboli, G. (2017). Drug-induced ototoxicity: mechanisms, Pharmacogenetics, and protective strategies. *Clin. Pharmacol. Ther.* 101, 491–500. doi: 10.1002/cpt.603

Leake, P. A., and Hradek, G. T. (1988). Cochlear pathology of long term neomycin induced deafness in cats. *Hear. Res.* 33, 11–33. doi: 10.1016/0378-5955(88)90018-4

Lee, J. E., Nakagawa, T., Kim, T. S., Iguchi, F., Endo, T., Kita, T., et al. (2004). Signaling pathway for apoptosis of vestibular hair cells of mice due to aminoglycosides. *Acta Otolaryngol. Suppl.* 551, 69–74. doi: 10.1080/03655230310016799

Lenoir, M., Daudet, N., Humbert, G., Renard, N., Gallego, M., Pujol, R., et al. (1999). Morphological and molecular changes in the inner hair cell region of the rat cochlea after amikacin treatment. *J. Neurocytol.* 28, 925–937. doi: 10.1023/A:1007034508547

Li, L., Nevill, G., and Forge, A. (1995). Two modes of hair cell loss from the vestibular sensory epithelia of the guinea pig inner ear. *J. Comp. Neurol.* 355, 405–417. doi: 10.1002/cne.903550307

Lien, E. J., Lipsett, L. R., and Lien, L. L. (1983). Structure side-effect sorting of drugs. VI. Ototoxicities. *J. Clin. Hosp. Pharm.* 8, 15–33. doi: 10.1111/j.1365-2710.1983.tb00893.x

Macrez, R., Stys, P. K., Vivien, D., Lipton, S. A., and Docagne, F. (2016). Mechanisms of glutamate toxicity in multiple sclerosis: biomarker and therapeutic opportunities. *Lancet Neurol.* 15, 1089–1102. doi: 10.1016/S1474-4422(16)30165-X

Mangiardi, D. A., McLaughlin-Williamson, K., May, K. E., Messana, E. P., Mountain, D. C., and Cotanche, D. A. (2004). Progression of hair cell ejection and molecular markers of apoptosis in the avian cochlea following gentamicin treatment. *J. Comp. Neurol.* 475, 1–18. doi: 10.1002/cne.20129

Matsui, J. I., Gale, J. E., and Warchol, M. E. (2004). Critical signaling events during the aminoglycoside-induced death of sensory hair cells *in vitro*. *J. Neurobiol.* 61, 250–266. doi: 10.1002/neu.20054

Matsui, J. I., Haque, A., Huss, D., Messana, E. P., Alosi, J. A., Roberson, D. W., et al. (2003). Caspase inhibitors promote vestibular hair cell survival and function after aminoglycoside treatment *in vivo*. *J. Neurosci.* 23, 6111–6122.

Matsui, J. I., Ogilvie, J. M., and Warchol, M. E. (2002). Inhibition of caspases prevents ototoxic and ongoing hair cell death. *J. Neurosci.* 22, 1218–1227.

May, L. A., Kramarenko, I. I., Brandon, C. S., Voelkel-Johnson, C., Roy, S., Truong, K., et al. (2013). Inner ear supporting cells protect hair cells by secreting HSP70. *J. Clin. Invest.* 123, 3577–3587. doi: 10.1172/JCI68480

Meiteles, L. Z., and Raphael, Y. (1994). Scar formation in the vestibular sensory epithelium after aminoglycoside toxicity. *Hear. Res.* 79, 26–38. doi: 10.1016/0378-5955(94)90124-4

Monzack, E. L., May, L. A., Roy, S., Gale, J. E., and Cunningham, L. L. (2015). Live imaging the phagocytic activity of inner ear supporting cells in response to hair cell death. *Cell Death Differ.* 22, 1995–2005. doi: 10.1038/cdd.2015.48

Morgan, J. T., Chana, G., Pardo, C. A., Achim, C., Semendeferi, K., Buckwalter, J., et al. (2010). Microglial activation and increased microglial density observed in the dorsolateral prefrontal cortex in autism. *Biol. Psychiatry* 68, 368–376. doi: 10.1016/j.biopsych.2010.05.024

Muggia, F. M., Bonetti, A., Hoeschele, J. D., Rozencweig, M., and Howell, S. B. (2015). Platinum antitumor complexes: 50 years since barnett rosenberg's discovery. *J. Clin. Oncol.* 33, 4219–4226. doi: 10.1200/JCO.2015.60.7481

Nakagawa, T., Yamane, H., Shibata, S., Sunami, K., and Nakai, Y. (1997). Cell death caused by the acute effects of aminoglycoside and zinc in the ampullary cristae of guinea pigs. *Eur. Arch. Otorhinolaryngol.* 254, 153–157. doi: 10.1007/BF02471281

Nakagawa, T., Yamane, H., Takayama, M., Sunami, K., and Nakai, Y. (1998). Apoptosis of guinea pig cochlear hair cells following chronic aminoglycoside treatment. *Eur. Arch. Otorhinolaryngol.* 255, 127–131. doi: 10.1007/s004050050027

Oesterle, E. C., and Campbell, S. (2009). Supporting cell characteristics in long-deafened aged mouse ears. *J. Assoc. Res. Otolaryngol.* 10, 525–544. doi: 10.1007/s10162-009-0183-x

O'Halloran, E. K., and Oesterle, E. C. (2004). Characterization of leukocyte subtypes in chicken inner ear sensory epithelia. *J. Comp. Neurol.* 475, 340–360. doi: 10.1002/cne.20162

Okano, T., Nakagawa, T., Kita, T., Kada, S., Yoshimoto, M., Nakahata, T., et al. (2008). Bone marrow-derived cells expressing Iba1 are constitutively present as resident tissue macrophages in the mouse cochlea. *J. Neurosci. Res.* 86, 1758–1767. doi: 10.1002/jnr.21625

Olson, O. C., Kim, H., Quail, D. F., Foley, E. A., and Joyce, J. A. (2017). Tumor-associated macrophages suppress the cytotoxic activity of antimitotic agents. *Cell Rep.* 19, 101–113. doi: 10.1016/j.celrep.2017.03.038

O'Malley, J. T., Nadol, J. B. Jr., and McKenna, M. J. (2016). Anti CD163+, Iba1+, and CD68+ cells in the adult human inner ear: normal distribution of an unappreciated class of macrophages/microglia and implications for inflammatory otopathology in humans. *Otol. Neurotol.* 37, 99–108. doi: 10.1097/MAO.0000000000000879

Otte, J., Schuknecht, H. F., and Kerr, A. G. (1978). Ganglion cell populations in normal and pathological human cochleae. Implications for cochlear implantation. *Laryngoscope* 88(8 Pt 1), 1231–1246. doi: 10.1002/lary.25219

Ozkiris, M., Kapusuz, Z., Karacavus, S., and Saydam, L. (2013). The effects of lycopene on cisplatin-induced ototoxicity. *Eur. Arch. Otorhinolaryngol.* 270, 3027–3033. doi: 10.1007/s00405-013-2352-0

Pei, W., Tanaka, K., Huang, S. C., Xu, L., Liu, B., Sinclair, J., et al. (2016). Extracellular HSP60 triggers tissue regeneration and wound healing by regulating inflammation and cell proliferation. *Npj Regen. Med.* 1:16013. doi: 10.1038/npjregenmed.2016.13

Pirvola, U., Xing-Qun, L., Virkkala, J., Saarma, M., Murakata, C., Camoratto, A. M., et al. (2000). Rescue of hearing, auditory hair cells, and neurons by CEP-1347/KT7515, an inhibitor of c-Jun N-terminal kinase activation. *J. Neurosci.* 20, 43–50.

Popiel, H. A., Takeuchi, T., Fujita, H., Yamamoto, K., Ito, C., Yamane, H., et al. (2012). Hsp40 gene therapy exerts therapeutic effects on polyglutamine disease mice via a non-cell autonomous mechanism. *PLoS ONE* 7:e51069. doi: 10.1371/journal.pone.0051069

Priuska, E. M., and Schacht, J. (1995). Formation of free radicals by gentamicin and iron and evidence for an iron/gentamicin complex. *Biochem. Pharmacol.* 50, 1749–1752. doi: 10.1016/0006-2952(95)02160-4

Ransohoff, R. M., Liu, L., and Cardona, A. E. (2007). Chemokines and chemokine receptors: multipurpose players in neuroinflammation. *Int. Rev. Neurobiol.* 82, 187–204. doi: 10.1016/S0074-7742(07)82010-1

Reynolds, A. (2007). The theory of the cell state and the question of cell autonomy in nineteenth and early twentieth-century biology. *Sci. Context* 20, 71–95. doi: 10.1017/S0269889706001141

Rio, C., Dikkes, P., Liberman, M. C., and Corfas, G. (2002). Glial fibrillary acidic protein expression and promoter activity in the inner ear of developing and adult mice. *J. Comp. Neurol.* 442, 156–162. doi: 10.1002/cne.10085

Rowland, L. P., and Shneider, N. A. (2001). Amyotrophic lateral sclerosis. *N. Engl. J. Med.* 344, 1688–1700. doi: 10.1056/NEJM200105313442207

Ryan, A. F., Woolf, N. K., and Bone, R. C. (1980). Ultrastructural correlates of selective outer hair cell destruction following kanamycin intoxication in the chinchilla. *Hear. Res.* 3, 335–351. doi: 10.1016/0378-5955(80)90027-1

Rybak, L. P., Mukherjea, D., Jajoo, S., and Ramkumar, V. (2009). Cisplatin ototoxicity and protection: clinical and experimental studies. *Tohoku J. Exp. Med.* 219, 177–186. doi: 10.1620/tjem.219.177

Sato, E., Shick, H. E., Ransohoff, R. M., and Hirose, K. (2010). Expression of fractalkine receptor CX3CR1 on cochlear macrophages influences survival of hair cells following ototoxic injury. *J. Assoc. Res. Otolaryngol.* 11, 223–234. doi: 10.1007/s10162-009-0198-3

Schacht, J., Talaska, A. E., and Rybak, L. P. (2012). Cisplatin and aminoglycoside antibiotics: hearing loss and its prevention. *Anat. Rec.* 295, 1837–1850. doi: 10.1002/ar.22578

Schmitt, N. C., Rubel, E. W., and Nathanson, N. M. (2009). Cisplatin-induced hair cell death requires STAT1 and is attenuated by epigallocatechin gallate. *J. Neurosci.* 29, 3843–3851. doi: 10.1523/JNEUROSCI.5842-08.2009

Schuknecht, H. F. (1953). Lesions of the organ of Corti. *Trans. Am. Acad. Ophthalmol. Otolaryngol.* 57, 366–383.

Seligmann, H., Podoshin, L., Ben-David, J., Fradis, M., and Goldsher, M. (1996). Drug-induced tinnitus and other hearing disorders. *Drug Saf.* 14, 198–212. doi: 10.2165/00002018-199614030-00006

Sha, S. H., and Schacht, J. (1999). Stimulation of free radical formation by aminoglycoside antibiotics. *Hear. Res.* 128, 112–118. doi: 10.1016/S0378-5955(98)00200-7

Shi, X. (2010). Resident macrophages in the cochlear blood-labyrinth barrier and their renewal via migration of bone-marrow-derived cells. *Cell Tissue Res.* 342, 21–30. doi: 10.1007/s00441-010-1040-2

Sluyter, S., Klis, S. F., de Groot, J. C., and Smoorenburg, G. F. (2003). Alterations in the stria vascularis in relation to cisplatin ototoxicity and recovery. *Hear. Res.* 185, 49–56. doi: 10.1016/S0378-5955(03)00260-0

Sobkowicz, H. M., August, B. K., and Slapnick, S. M. (2002). Influence of neurotrophins on the synaptogenesis of inner hair cells in the deaf Bronx waltzer (bv) mouse organ of Corti in culture. *Int. J. Dev. Neurosci.* 20, 537–554. doi: 10.1016/S0736-5748(02)00084-9

Spoendlin, H. (1975). Retrograde degeneration of the cochlear nerve. *Acta Otolaryngol.* 79, 266–275. doi: 10.3109/00016487509124683

Stankovic, K., Rio, C., Xia, A., Sugawara, M., Adams, J. C., Liberman, M. C., et al. (2004). Survival of adult spiral ganglion neurons requires erbB receptor signaling in the inner ear. *J. Neurosci.* 24, 8651–8661. doi: 10.1523/JNEUROSCI.0733-04.2004

Sugahara, K., Rubel, E. W., and Cunningham, L. L. (2006). JNK signaling in neomycin-induced vestibular hair cell death. *Hear. Res.* 221, 128–135. doi: 10.1016/j.heares.2006.08.009

Sugawara, M., Corfas, G., and Liberman, M. C. (2005). Influence of supporting cells on neuronal degeneration after hair cell loss. *J. Assoc. Res. Otolaryngol.* 6, 136–147. doi: 10.1007/s10162-004-5050-1

Sugawara, M., Murtie, J. C., Stankovic, K. M., Liberman, M. C., and Corfas, G. (2007). Dynamic patterns of neurotrophin 3 expression in the postnatal mouse inner ear. *J. Comp. Neurol.* 501, 30–37. doi: 10.1002/cne.21227

Sun, C., Wang, X., Chen, D., Lin, X., Yu, D., and Wu, H. (2016). Dexamethasone loaded nanoparticles exert protective effects against Cisplatin-induced hearing loss by systemic administration. *Neurosci. Lett.* 619, 142–148. doi: 10.1016/j.neulet.2016.03.012

Sun, S., Yu, H., Yu, H., Honglin, M., Ni, W., Zhang, Y., et al. (2015). Inhibition of the activation and recruitment of microglia-like cells protects against neomycin-induced ototoxicity. *Mol. Neurobiol.* 51, 252–267. doi: 10.1007/s12035-014-8712-y

Suzuka, Y., and Schuknecht, H. F. (1988). Retrograde cochlear neuronal degeneration in human subjects. *Acta Otolaryngol. Suppl.* 450, 1–20. doi: 10.3109/00016488809098973

Suzuki, K., Sugihara, G., Ouchi, Y., Nakamura, K., Futatsubashi, M., Takebayashi, K., et al. (2013). Microglial activation in young adults with autism spectrum disorder. *JAMA Psychiatry* 70, 49–58. doi: 10.1001/jamapsychiatry.2013.272

Takada, Y., Takada, T., Lee, M. Y., Swiderski, D. L., Kabara, L. L., Dolan, D. F., et al. (2015). Ototoxicity-induced loss of hearing and inner hair cells is attenuated by HSP70 gene transfer. *Mol. Ther. Methods Clin. Dev.* 2:15019. doi: 10.1038/mtm.2015.19

Taleb, M. B., Brandon, C. S., Lee, F.-S., Harris, K. C., Dillmann, W. H., and Cunningham, L. L. (2009). Hsp70 inhibits aminoglycoside-induced hearing loss and cochlear hair cell death. *Cell Stress Chaperones.* 14, 427–437. doi: 10.1007/s12192-008-0097-2

Taleb, M., Brandon, C. S., Lee, F. S., Lomax, M. I., Dillmann, W. H., and Cunningham, L. L. (2008). Hsp70 inhibits aminoglycoside-induced hair cell death and is necessary for the protective effect of heat shock. *J. Assoc. Res. Otolaryngol.* 9, 277–289. doi: 10.1007/s10162-008-0122-2

Tognatta, R., and Miller, R. H. (2016). Contribution of the oligodendrocyte lineage to CNS repair and neurodegenerative pathologies. *Neuropharmacology* 110(Pt B), 539–547. doi: 10.1016/j.neuropharm.2016.04.026

Tsuji, K., Velazquez-Villasenor, L., Rauch, S. D., Glynn, R. J., Wall, C. III., and Merchant, S. N. (2000). Temporal bone studies of the human peripheral vestibular system. Aminoglycoside ototoxicity. *Ann. Otol. Rhinol. Laryngol. Suppl.* 181, 20–25. doi: 10.1177/00034894000109S504

van Ruijven, M. W., de Groot, J. C., and Smoorenburg, G. F. (2004). Time sequence of degeneration pattern in the guinea pig cochlea during cisplatin administration. A quantitative histological study. *Hear Res.* 197, 44–54. doi: 10.1016/j.heares.2004.07.014

Vargas, D. L., Nascimbene, C., Krishnan, C., Zimmerman, A. W., and Pardo, C. A. (2005). Neuroglial activation and neuroinflammation in the brain of patients with autism. *Ann. Neurol.* 57, 67–81. doi: 10.1002/ana.20315

Vargas, M. R., and Johnson, J. A. (2010). Astrogliosis in amyotrophic lateral sclerosis: role and therapeutic potential of astrocytes. *Neurotherapeutics* 7, 471–481. doi: 10.1016/j.nurt.2010.05.012

Varol, C., Mildner, A., and Jung, S. (2015). Macrophages: development and tissue specialization. *Annu. Rev. Immunol.* 33, 643–675. doi: 10.1146/annurev-immunol-032414-112220

Wan, G., Corfas, G., and Stone, J. S. (2013). Inner ear supporting cells: rethinking the silent majority. *Semin. Cell Dev. Biol.* 24, 448–459. doi: 10.1016/j.semcdb.2013.03.009

Wang, J., Van De Water, T. R., Bonny, C., de Ribaupierre, F., Puel, J. L., and Zine, A. (2003). A peptide inhibitor of c-Jun N-terminal kinase protects against both aminoglycoside and acoustic trauma-induced auditory hair cell death and hearing loss. *J. Neurosci.* 23, 8596–8607.

Wang, Z., and Li, H. (2000). Microglia-like cells in rat organ of Corti following aminoglycoside ototoxicity. *Neuroreport* 11, 1389–1393. doi: 10.1097/00001756-200005150-00008

Wangemann, P. (2006). Supporting sensory transduction: cochlear fluid homeostasis and the endocochlear potential. *J. Physiol.* 576(Pt 1), 11–21. doi: 10.1113/jphysiol.2006.112888

Warchol, M. E. (1999). Immune cytokines and dexamethasone influence sensory regeneration in the avian vestibular periphery. *J. Neurocytol.* 28, 889–900. doi: 10.1023/A:1007026306730

Wright, C. G., and Meyerhoff, W. L. (1984). Ototoxicity of otic drops applied to the middle ear in the chinchilla. *Am. J. Otolaryngol.* 5, 166–176. doi: 10.1016/S0196-0709(84)80008-3

Ylikoski, J., Xing-Qun, L., Virkkala, J., and Pirvola, U. (2002). Blockade of c-Jun N-terminal kinase pathway attenuates gentamicin-induced cochlear and vestibular hair cell death. *Hear. Res.* 163, 71–81. doi: 10.1016/S0378-5955(01)00380-X

Yu, N., and Zhao, H. B. (2009). Modulation of outer hair cell electromotility by cochlear supporting cells and gap junctions. *PLoS ONE* 4:e7923. doi: 10.1371/journal.pone.0007923

Zhang, W., Dai, M., Fridberger, A., Hassan, A., Degagne, J., Neng, L., et al. (2012). Perivascular-resident macrophage-like melanocytes in the inner ear are essential for the integrity of the intrastrial fluid-blood barrier. *Proc. Natl. Acad. Sci. U.S.A.* 109, 10388–10393. doi: 10.1073/pnas.1205210109

Zhao, H. B., Kikuchi, T., Ngezahayo, A., and White, T. W. (2006). Gap junctions and cochlear homeostasis. *J. Membr. Biol.* 209, 177–186. doi: 10.1007/s00232-005-0832-x

Zhao, H. B., and Santos-Sacchi, J. (1999). Auditory collusion and a coupled couple of outer hair cells. *Nature* 399, 359–362. doi: 10.1038/20686

Zhao, H. B., and Yu, N. (2006). Distinct and gradient distributions of connexin26 and connexin30 in the cochlear sensory epithelium of guinea pigs. *J. Comp. Neurol.* 499, 506–518. doi: 10.1002/cne.21113

Zilberstein, Y., Liberman, M. C., and Corfas, G. (2012). Inner hair cells are not required for survival of spiral ganglion neurons in the adult cochlea. *J. Neurosci.* 32, 405–410. doi: 10.1523/JNEUROSCI.4678-11.2012

Permissions

All chapters in this book were first published in CMO, by Frontiers; hereby published with permission under the Creative Commons Attribution License or equivalent. Every chapter published in this book has been scrutinized by our experts. Their significance has been extensively debated. The topics covered herein carry significant findings which will fuel the growth of the discipline. They may even be implemented as practical applications or may be referred to as a beginning point for another development.

The contributors of this book come from diverse backgrounds, making this book a truly international effort. This book will bring forth new frontiers with its revolutionizing research information and detailed analysis of the nascent developments around the world.

We would like to thank all the contributing authors for lending their expertise to make the book truly unique. They have played a crucial role in the development of this book. Without their invaluable contributions this book wouldn't have been possible. They have made vital efforts to compile up to date information on the varied aspects of this subject to make this book a valuable addition to the collection of many professionals and students.

This book was conceptualized with the vision of imparting up-to-date information and advanced data in this field. To ensure the same, a matchless editorial board was set up. Every individual on the board went through rigorous rounds of assessment to prove their worth. After which they invested a large part of their time researching and compiling the most relevant data for our readers.

The editorial board has been involved in producing this book since its inception. They have spent rigorous hours researching and exploring the diverse topics which have resulted in the successful publishing of this book. They have passed on their knowledge of decades through this book. To expedite this challenging task, the publisher supported the team at every step. A small team of assistant editors was also appointed to further simplify the editing procedure and attain best results for the readers.

Apart from the editorial board, the designing team has also invested a significant amount of their time in understanding the subject and creating the most relevant covers. They scrutinized every image to scout for the most suitable representation of the subject and create an appropriate cover for the book.

The publishing team has been an ardent support to the editorial, designing and production team. Their endless efforts to recruit the best for this project, has resulted in the accomplishment of this book. They are a veteran in the field of academics and their pool of knowledge is as vast as their experience in printing. Their expertise and guidance has proved useful at every step. Their uncompromising quality standards have made this book an exceptional effort. Their encouragement from time to time has been an inspiration for everyone.

The publisher and the editorial board hope that this book will prove to be a valuable piece of knowledge for researchers, students, practitioners and scholars across the globe.

List of Contributors

Jonathon W. Vargo, Steven N. Walker, Suhasini R. Gopal and Aditi R. Deshmukh
Department of Otolaryngology—Head and Neck Surgery, University Hospitals Cleveland Medical Center, Cleveland, OH, United States

Brian M. McDermott Jr.
Department of Otolaryngology—Head and Neck Surgery, University Hospitals Cleveland Medical Center, Cleveland, OH, United States
Department of Biology, Case Western Reserve University, Cleveland, OH, United States
Department of Neurosciences, Case Western Reserve University, Cleveland, OH, United States
Department of Genetics and Genome Sciences, Case Western Reserve University, Cleveland, OH, United States

Kumar N. Alagramam
Department of Otolaryngology—Head and Neck Surgery, University Hospitals Cleveland Medical Center, Cleveland, OH, United States
Department of Biology, Case Western Reserve University, Cleveland, OH, United States
Department of Genetics and Genome Sciences, Case Western Reserve University, Cleveland, OH, United States

Ruben Stepanyan
Department of Otolaryngology—Head and Neck Surgery, University Hospitals Cleveland Medical Center, Cleveland, OH, United States
Department of Neurosciences, Case Western Reserve University, Cleveland, OH, United States

Heather Wiedenhoft
College of Arts and Sciences, Washington State University, Vancouver, WA, United States

Lauren Hayashi
Knight Cancer Institute, Oregon Health & Science University, Portland, OR, United States

Allison B. Coffin
College of Arts and Sciences, Washington State University, Vancouver, WA, United States
Department of Integrative Physiology and Neuroscience, Washington State University, Vancouver, WA, United States

Anette E. Fransson, Marta Kisiel and Göran F. E. Laurell
Department of Surgical Science, Uppsala University, Uppsala, Sweden

Kristian Pirttilä and Curt Pettersson
Division of Analytical Pharmaceutical Chemistry, Department of Medical Chemistry, Uppsala University, Uppsala, Sweden

Pernilla Videhult Pierre
Division of Audiology, Department of Clinical Science, Intervention and Technology, Karolinska Institutet, Stockholm, Sweden

Meiyan Jiang and Farshid Taghizadeh
Oregon Hearing Research Center, Oregon Health & Science University, Portland, OR, United States

Peter S. Steyger
Oregon Hearing Research Center, Oregon Health & Science University, Portland, OR, United States
National Center for Rehabilitative Auditory Research, VA Portland Health Care System, Portland, OR, United States

Sandeep Sheth and Vickram Ramkumar
Department of Pharmacology, Southern Illinois University School of Medicine, Springfield, IL, United States

Debashree Mukherjea
Department of Surgery (Otolaryngology), Southern Illinois University School of Medicine, Springfield, IL, United States

Leonard P. Rybak
Department of Pharmacology, Southern Illinois University School of Medicine, Springfield, IL, United States
Department of Surgery (Otolaryngology), Southern Illinois University School of Medicine, Springfield, IL, United States

Mary E. O'Sullivan, Adela Perez, Randy Lin, Autefeh Sajjadi and Alan G. Cheng
Department of Otolaryngology–Head and Neck Surgery, Stanford University School of Medicine, Stanford, CA, United States

Anthony J. Ricci
Department of Otolaryngology-Head and Neck Surgery, Stanford University School of Medicine, Stanford, CA, United States
Department of Molecular and Cellular Physiology, Stanford University School of Medicine, Stanford, CA, United States

Bharath Ramaswamy
Fischell Department of Bioengineering, University of Maryland, College Park, MD, United States
Pfizer Inc., New York, NY, United States

Soumen Roy
Sensory Cell Biology, National Institute on Deafness and Other Communication Disorders (NIDCD), National Institutes of Health (NIH), Bethesda, MD, United States

Andrea B. Apolo
Genitourinary Malignancies Branch, Center for Cancer Research, National Cancer Institute, National Institutes of Health (NIH), Bethesda, MD, United States

Benjamin Shapiro
Fischell Department of Bioengineering, University of Maryland, College Park, MD, United States
Institute for Systems Research, University of Maryland, College Park, MD, United States
Otomagnetics, Rockville, MD, United States

Didier A. Depireux
Institute for Systems Research, University of Maryland, College Park, MD, United States
Otomagnetics, Rockville, MD, United States
Department of Otorhinolaryngology/Head and Neck Surgery, University of Maryland School of Medicine, Baltimore, MD, United States

Volker Noack, Rahul Jalota and Arwa Kurabi
Department of Surgery and Otolaryngology, School of Medicine, University of California, San Diego, La Jolla, CA, United States

Allen F. Ryan and Kwang Pak
Department of Surgery and Otolaryngology, School of Medicine, University of California, San Diego, La Jolla, CA, United States
VA San Diego Healthcare System, San Diego, CA, United States

Chao-Hui Yang
Kresge Hearing Research Institute, Department of Otolaryngology, University of Michigan, Ann Arbor, MI, United States
Department of Otolaryngology, Kaohsiung Chang Gung Memorial Hospital, Chang Gung University College of Medicine, Kaohsiung, Taiwan

Zhiqi Liu, Deanna Dong and Su-Hua Sha
Department of Pathology and Laboratory Medicine, Medical University of South Carolina, Charleston, SC, United States

Jochen Schacht
Kresge Hearing Research Institute, Department of Otolaryngology, University of Michigan, Ann Arbor, MI, United States

Dev Arya
Department of Chemistry, Clemson University, Clemson, SC, United States

Azadeh Jadali
Department of Cell Biology and Neuroscience, Rutgers University, Piscataway, NJ, USA
Stem Cell Research Center and Keck Center for Collaborative Neuroscience, Rutgers University, Piscataway, NJ, USA
3D Biotek, Bridgewater, NJ, USA

Yu-Lan M. Ying
Department of Otolaryngology—Head and Neck Surgery, Rutgers New Jersey Medical School, Newark, NJ, USA

Kelvin Y. Kwan
Department of Cell Biology and Neuroscience, Rutgers University, Piscataway, NJ, USA
Stem Cell Research Center and Keck Center for Collaborative Neuroscience, Rutgers University, Piscataway, NJ, USA

Paromita Majumder and Paulette A. Moore
UCL Ear Institute, University College London, London, UK

Guy P. Richardson
Sussex Neuroscience, School of Life Sciences, University of Sussex, Falmer, UK

Jonathan E. Gale
UCL Ear Institute, University College London, London, UK
Department of Cell and Developmental Biology, University College London, London, UK

Mark A. Crumling and R. Keith Duncan
Department of Otolaryngology-Head & Neck Surgery, Kresge Hearing Research Institute, University of Michigan, Ann Arbor, MI, United States

Kelly A. King
Audiology Unit, Otolaryngology Branch, National Institute on Deafness and Other Communication Disorders, National Institutes of Health, Bethesda, MD, United States

Nerissa K. Kirkwood, Molly O'Reilly, Emma J. Kenyon and Guy P. Richardson
Sussex Neuroscience, School of Life Sciences, University of Sussex, Brighton, United Kingdom

Rosemary Huckvale, Simon E. Ward and Marco Derudas
Sussex Drug Discovery Centre, School of Life Sciences, University of Sussex, Brighton, United Kingdom

Sietse M. van Netten
Institute of Artificial Intelligence and Cognitive Engineering, University of Groningen, Groningen, Netherlands

Megan B. Wood and Jian Zuo
Department of Developmental Neurobiology, St. Jude Children's Research Hospital, Memphis, TN, USA

Meiyan Jiang and Takatoshi Karasawa
Oregon Hearing Research Center, Oregon Health & Science University, Portland, OR, United States

Peter S. Steyger
Oregon Hearing Research Center, Oregon Health & Science University, Portland, OR, United States
National Center for Rehabilitative Auditory Research, Portland VA Medical Center (VHA), Portland, OR, United States

Shin Hye Kim
Department of Otorhinolaryngology-Head and Neck Surgery, Korea University Medical Center, Korea University College of Medicine, Seoul, South Korea

Gaon Jung
Department of Otorhinolaryngology-Head and Neck Surgery, Seoul National University Bundang Hospital, Seoul National University College of Medicine, Seongnam, South Korea

Sangjae Kim
GemVax & Kael Co., Ltd, Seongnam, South Korea

Ja-Won Koo
Sensory Organ Research Institute, Seoul National University Medical Research Center, Seoul, South Korea

Martin Mwangi, Sung-Hee Kil, David Phak, David J. Lim and Sung K. Moon
Department of Head and Neck Surgery, David Geffen School of Medicine, University of California, Los Angeles, Los Angeles, CA, United States

Hun Yi Park
Department of Otolaryngology, Ajou University School of Medicine, Suwon, South Korea

Raekil Park
Gwangju Institute of Science and Technology, Gwangju, South Korea

Brian D. Nicholas, Shimon Francis, Elizabeth L. Wagner, Sibo Zhang and Jung-Bum Shin
Department of Neuroscience, University of Virginia, Charlottesville, VA, United States

David R. Sultemeier
Department of Head and Neck Surgery, David Geffen School of Medicine, University of California, Los Angeles, Los Angeles, CA, United States

Larry F. Hoffman
Department of Head and Neck Surgery, David Geffen School of Medicine, University of California, Los Angeles, Los Angeles, CA, United States
Brain Research Institute, David Geffen School of Medicine, University of California, Los Angeles, Los Angeles, CA, United States

Shimon P. Francis and Lisa L. Cunningham
National Institute on Deafness and Other Communication Disorders, National Institutes of Health, Bethesda, MD, United States

Index

N

O

P

R

S

T

U

Z

www.ingramcontent.com/pod-product-compliance
Lightning Source LLC
LaVergne TN
LVHW080928210926
848485LV00004B/756
* 9 7 8 1 6 3 9 8 9 4 0 1 7 *